Ethnomedicinal Practices and Application of Traditional Medicinal Plants in Contemporary Indian Society

Critical Plant Studies

Series Editor

Douglas Vakoch

This series calls us to re-examine in fundamental ways our understanding of and engagement with plants, drawing on diverse disciplinary perspectives. The series encourages work grounded in the humanities and social sciences that provides innovative reformulations of the scope and practice of critical plant studies. Books in this series include both monographs and edited volumes that target academic audiences. To introduce critical plant studies to readers not familiar with this field, the series publishes work that is relevant to those engaged in critical plant studies, while also being of interest to scholars from the author's primary discipline. Among the books of special interest for the series are those that examine plants with reference to particular countries or regions of the world, or with respect to specific cultural, philosophical, religious, or literary traditions. Contemporary and historical works are equally appropriate. We especially welcome books that bridge academia and activism.

Recent Titles in the Series

Ethnomedicinal Practices and Application of Traditional Medicinal Plants in Contemporary Indian Society, edited by Arun Makal & Gour Gopal Satpati

Shaped by Vegetal Matters: Phyto-Influence on Humans, Other Animals, and Place, by Elizabeth Oriel

Cartographies of Postcolonial Vegetal Politics: Deleuze, Guattari and Mathema of Vegetality,

by Abhisek Ghosal

Critical Plant Studies in Taiwan, edited by Iping Liang

Human-Plant Entanglement and Vegetal Agency in the Poetry of Thomas Hardy and Sylvia Plath, by Dilek Bulut Sarıkaya

Ethnomedicinal Practices and Application of Traditional Medicinal Plants in Contemporary Indian Society

Edited by Arun Makal and Gour Gopal Satpati

BLOOMSBURY ACADEMIC
NEW YORK • LONDON • OXFORD • NEW DELHI • SYDNEY

BLOOMSBURY ACADEMIC
Bloomsbury Publishing Inc, 1359 Broadway, New York, NY 10018, USA
Bloomsbury Publishing Plc, 50 Bedford Square, London, WC1B 3DP, UK
Bloomsbury Publishing Ireland, 29 Earlsfort Terrace, Dublin 2, D02 AY28, Ireland

First published in the United States of America 2026

Cover design:
©DrAfter123/Getty Images

Library of Congress Cataloging-in-Publication Data

Names: Makal, Arun editor | Satpati, Gour Gopal editor
Title: Ethnomedicinal practices and application of traditional medicinal plants in contemporary Indian society / edited by Arun Makal & Gour Gopal Satpati.
Description: New York, NY : Bloomsbury Academic, 2026. | Series: Critical Plant Studies | Includes bibliographical references and index. | Summary: "This book provides an opportunity for students, academicians, and researchers in India and around the World to develop their concept on application of indigenous medicinal plants and traditional medical practices of various ethnic groups across India. Comprised of twenty-four chapters written by a diverse group of scholars and researchers, Ethnomedicinal Practices and Application of Traditional Medicinal Plants in Contemporary Indian Society explores various current issues and perspectives of ethnomedicinal knowledge and practices of different sections of people of contemporary India"-- Provided by publisher.
Identifiers: LCCN 2025034172 (print) | LCCN 2025034173 (ebook) | ISBN 9781666982077 hb | ISBN 9798216254591 pdf | ISBN 9781978771727 epub
Subjects: LCSH: Traditional medicine--India | Ethnobotany--India | Materia medica, Vegetable--India | Medicinal plants--India
Classification: LCC GR880 .E825 2026 (print) | LCC GR880 (ebook)
LC record available at https://lccn.loc.gov/2025034172
LC ebook record available at https://lccn.loc.gov/2025034173

ISBN: HB: 978-1-6669-8207-7
ePDF: 979-8-2162-5459-1
eBook: 978-1-9787-7172-7

Series: Critical Plant Studies

Typeset by Deanta Global Publishing Services, Chennai, India

Contents

Figures viii
Tables x
Foreword xii
Acknowledgments xiv

Introduction 1

Part I Ethnomedicine, Environment, and Sustainable Development

1 Recent Advances in Ethnobotany: Strategies to Rejuvenate Our Green Planet by Sustainable Development 23
2 Ethnomedicinal Knowledge among the Tribal Communities to Sustain the Economy and Socio-Environmental Infrastructure 39
3 Ethnomedicine: A Vital Component for Sustainable Development 53

Part II Ethnobotanical Knowledge and Medicinal Plants

4 Ethnomedicinal and Indigenous Knowledge of Some Locally Available Important Medicinal Plants 77
5 Plausible Ethnobotanical Perception of Indigenous Mangrove Flora of the Indian Sundarbans 85
6 Mangroves of Indian Sundarbans: A Treasure Trove of Medicinal Properties and Ethnomedicinal Significance 101
7 Possible Application and Ethnomedicinal Use of Aquatic and Semiaquatic Plants 127

Part III Medicinal Plants

8 Use of Ethnomedicines as an Elixir of Life: Phytochemical Analysis of Traditional Medicinal Plants in India 149
9 An Exploration into the Phytochemical Enrichment of *Lawsonia inermis* L. and Its Medicinal Implications 167

10 Antimicrobial Activity of Some Ethnomedicinal Plants of India and Their Potential Application in Modern Medicine 183
11 Utilization of Ethnomedicinal Plants for Their Potential Antimicrobial Activity 213
12 Bioactive Compounds from Ethnomedicinal Plants with Antimicrobial Properties 241
13 Nutraceutical, Phytochemical, and Pharmacological Value of Lactuca: A Review 267

Part IV Indigenous Communities

14 Indigenous Medicines and Rituals: The Traditional Indian Medicine System 319
15 Indigenous Healing, Social Beliefs, and Practices among the Onges of Little Andaman of Andaman Archipelagos 333
16 Perception of Health and Traditional Health-Seeking Behavior among the Tai Ahom, Tai Khamte, and Tai Phake Communities of Northeastern Part of India 345
17 Indigenous Knowledge Systems of the Great Andamanese Community Residing in Port Blair and Strait Island of Andaman Archipelagos 365

Part V Indian Knowledge System and Ethnomedicinal Values

18 Concept of Ayurveda, Siddha, and Unani in Indian Traditional Knowledge System and Ethnomedicinal Values 381
19 Ethnomedicinal Practices and Traditional Healthcare Systems of the Nicobarese Tribe of Nicobar Archipelagos 389
20 Elements and Wellness Application of Botany and Medicinal Plants in Ancient India: A Systematic Review 401

Part VI Current Healthcare Sector and Benefits of Medicinal Plants

21 Benefits and Contributions of Medicinal Plants to Health Sector 423
22 Presence of Trans-α-bergamotene from Young Leaves of *Aegle marmelos* (L.) Correa: An Insight to the Future Therapeutic Potential of a Plant Used in Traditional Healing Practices 453

23 Ethnomedicinal Practices and Effect of Socioeconomic Factors on Health among the Rabhas of Garo Basti in Alipurduar of West Bengal, India 463
24 Indigenous Knowledge and Healthcare Practices among the Limbu Community of Darjeeling Hills: Insights from the Covid-19 Pandemic 481

Index 493
About the Editors 502
About the Contributors 503

Figures

1.1	Different fields of ethnobotanical research	28
1.2	Schematic representation showing how planet and ethnobotanist remain in an interwoven way essential for the sustainable development goals	29
1.3	Flowchart representing the ways by which ethnobotany can help in solving various problems and achieving sustainable development	30
1.4	Schematic representation showing different aspects of ethnobotany and how it helps in conserving nature	30
3.1	Perception of ethnomedicine in daily life	59
3.2	Sustainability of current harvesting practices	60
3.3	Integration of ethnomedicine and modern medicine	60
3.4	Role of the community in environmental practices	61
3.5	Variety of medicinal plants used in Aadi Nippani	62
4.1	Photographs of important medicinal plants. A. *Justicia spicigera*, B. *Moringa oleifera*, C. *Glinus oppositifolius*, D. *Typhonium trilobatum*, E. *Anisomeles indica*, F. *Rauvolfia*	80
4.2	Some important medicinal plants. A. *Ficus pumila*, B. *Hygrophila auriculata*, C. *Hyptis suaveolens*, D. *Cassia alata*	82
5.1	Bioactive Compounds Found in Members of Avicenniaceae	90
5.2	Compounds contributing to the antioxidant potential of *Avicennia* sp.	94
5.3	Antimicrobial potentialities of Avicenniaceae members	94
5.4	Antibacterial effect of *Avicennia marina* proven against four renowned bacterial strains	95
5.5	Anti-inflammatory properties of Avicenniaceae members	95
5.6	Anticancer property of *Avicennia marina* against five important cancer cell lines	96
5.7	Wound-healing mechanism of *Avicennia* sp.	96
6.1	Ethnomedicinal plants of Indian Sundarbans	104
7.1	Midnapore Sadar block of the district Paschim Medinipur of West Bengal, India	130
7.2	Aquatic medicinal plants of the Midnapore Sadar block	135
7.3	Semiaquatic medicinal plants of the Midnapore Sadar block	136
9.1	Lawsone Biosynthesis Pathway found in the Plant Metabolic Network (PMN) Database	170
9.2	Mechanism of action of elicitors	172
9.3	A pictorial presentation of elicitor classification	172

10.1 a. Ocimum tenuiflorum plant, b. Chemical structure of Eugenol, c. Chemical structure of Linalool 187
10.2 a. Allium sativum bulb, b. Chemical structure of Allicin 189
10.3 a. Curcuma longa rhizome, b. Chemical structure of Curcumin 191
10.4 a. Chemical structure of Turmerones 191
10.5 a. Zingiber officinale rhizome, b. Chemical structure of Gingerol 194
10.6 a. Azadirachta indica plant, b. Chemical structure of Nimbin 196
10.7 a–b. Aloe vera plant, c. Inflorescence of Aloe vera, d. *Phyllanthus emblica*, e–f. Lantana camara 199
11.1 Names of bioactive compounds and their family 226
11.2 Extraction methods of bioactive compounds 228
12.1 Ethnomedicinal plant parts contribution (%) 243
14.1 The three humors or tridosha of the human body 324
16.1 Distributions of Tai people residing in Assam and Arunachal Pradesh 348
19.1 Map of the Nicobar district in Andaman and Nicobar Islands 392
20.1 Ayurvedic medicinal plants able to fight with a number of diseases 417
21.1 Lignan compounds of *Phyllanthus amarus* and anti-inflammatory function of nirtetralin 430
21.2 Bioactivities of catechin 432
22.1 Structure of bergamotene 457
22.2 GCMS result of analysis of young leaf showing probable presence of Trans-α-Bergamotene 459
23.1 Map of the district Alipurduar showing the village Garo Basti in the Rajabhat Khawa region 465
23.2 Ojha, a Rabha Medicine Man, providing knowledge about the medicinal plant use 476
24.1 Primary Health Centre (PHC), Lamagaon 486
24.2 Pillar of Pradhan Mantri Gram Sadak Yojana (PMGSY) 487
24.3 A local medicinal plant named Titepati 488
24.4 Mostly used medicinal plant locally called as Tulsi 488
24.5 Phedangba, a Limbu priest, mostly relies on herbal medicines than modern alternatives 489
24.6 A local medicinal flower used by the Limbu community called Chuwa-Ko-Phool 489
24.7 A well-known medicinal plant used by the Limbu community, locally called Makiba 490

Tables

1.1	New Drugs and Compounds Obtained from Various Medicinal Plants by Ethnopharmacological Research	33
2.1	Various Medicinal Plants Utilized by Indigenous Communities of North East India	41
3.1	Traditional Medicinal Plants and their Uses	62
5.1	Therapeutic Uses of Several Mangrove Specimens of the Indian Sundarbans	87
5.2	Phytoconstituents Revealed Upon Metabolic Profiling of *Avicennia* sp.	92
6.1	Ethnomedicinal Plants of Indian Sundarbans	105
7.1	Aquatic Medicinal Plants Used by the Local People of Midnapore Sadar Block	133
7.2	Semiaquatic Medicinal Plants Used by the Local People of Midnapore Sadar Block	134
8.1	Qualitative Study of Different Phytochemicals of Twenty Different Plant Samples	155
8.2	List of Studied Plant Taxa along with the Major Phytochemicals and Their Medicinal Uses	156
8.3	Ethnomedicinally Used Plants along with the Parts Used in Treatment of Human Diseases	158
9.1	Medicinal Properties of *L. inermis* L. Respecting Nature of Phytochemicals	169
9.2	Main Phytochemicals and Their Associative Pathways	170
9.3	Elicitors of Shikimic Acid and Naphthoquinones in Plants	176
10.1	Antimicrobial Activity of Tulsi	187
10.2	Antibacterial Activity of Compounds and Secondary Metabolites of Garlic	190
10.3	Antibacterial Activity of Compounds and Secondary Metabolites of Turmeric	192
10.4	Antimicrobial Activities of Ginger	195
10.5	Antimicrobial Activity of Neem	198
10.6	Antimicrobial Activity of Some Other Ethnomedicinal Plants	200
11.1	Name of the Tribes and Parts of Plants They Use for Particular Microbial Disease	216
11.2	Name of the Ethnomedicinal Plants with Their Family and Their Parts Used Against Bacteria	221
12.1	Comprehensive Overview of Medicinal Plants, Plant Parts, and Biological Activities of Key Phytochemicals	245
13.1	Terpenoids Isolated from Members of the Genus *Lactuca*	274

13.2 Phenolic Compounds and Flavonoids Isolated from Members of the Genus *Lactuca* 287
13.3 Lignans and Coumarins Isolated from Members of the Genus *Lactuca* 299
14.1 List of Some Common Healing Techniques and Rituals in Traditional Medicine 322
14.2 Some Common Medicinal Plants and Their Use in Traditional Medicine 326
15.1 Endemic Plants Used by the Onges of Little Andaman for Indigenous Healing and Social Practices 339
16.1 Medicinal Plants Used by the Tai People 353
17.1 Knowledge Systems and Different Endemic Plants Used by the Great Andamanese 368
18.1 Plant-Based Substances or Plants Used in the Indian Ayurvedic System 383
18.2 Plant-Based Remedies in Siddha 385
18.3 Common Plants Used in the Unani System 386
20.1 Common Medicinal Plants Used in Ancient India 406
22.1 Molecular Characters of Trans-α-Bergamotene 457
23.1 List of Medicinal Plants Used by the Rabhas of the Village Garo Basti, Rajabhat Khawa, Alipurduar 474

Foreword

Ethnomedicine is the study of traditional medicinal practices and knowledge of different ethnic groups, particularly those of indigenous peoples. The indigenous people, by tradition, have identified various plants and animals with medicinal properties and have used them for curing several ailments. The history of ethnomedicine dates back thousands of years with evidence of plants and animals being used for medicine in the Middle Paleolithic Period. Paleolithic people started their life in the forest. Living close to the forest, they had acquired unique knowledge about the ambient biodiversity by nature, trial or error and experimentation, and used a variety of plants to meet their essential requirements like food, fuel, fiber, and also medicine. The ethnic groups or tribes in China, India, Romania, and Africa have practiced ethnomedicine for many generations. According to the World Health Organization, around 88 percent of people still depend on traditional medicines and herbs for their primary health care requirements. India is a country that reports a vast history of the knowledge and practice of traditional medicine. Ayurveda is a well-known form of traditional medicine with its roots extending to the time of the Indus Valley Civilization. One of the pillars of Ayurveda is resources used by ethnic communities that use different parts of a plant comprising stems, roots, leaves, seeds, bark, and fruits for healing. Other healing procedures like Yoga and Naturopathy, Unani, Siddha, and Homeopathy have also become traditional ways of healing. With around 645 indigenous tribes that inhabit India, the majority of its traditional knowledge is passed on through generations without any formal documentation. Therefore, the documentation and research on ethnomedicinal practices in India is important for preserving traditional knowledge, developing herbal drugs, conserving local and wild plants and animals, as well as protecting intellectual property.

Ethnomedicinal Practices and Application of Traditional Medicinal Plants in Contemporary Indian Society, edited by Arun Makal and Gour Gopal Satpati, has selected some of the significant studies that are prepared recently in the field of ethnomedicine in India. The twenty-four chapters included in the volume have focused on ethnomedicinal practices of different regions of India. The contributing chapters deal with a wide range of topics focusing on ethnomedicine, environment and sustainable development; ethnobotanical knowledge; phytochemical analysis and antimicrobial activities of medicinal plants; concept of health, illness, beliefs, and practices of indigenous communities; Indian knowledge system and ethnomedicinal values as well as important issues related to current healthcare sector and benefits of medicinal plants. Most of the authors in this volume have written their own recent investigation in the field of ethnobiology, ethnobotany, ethnomedicine, and traditional knowledge with special reference to India. Thus, this edited book volume is very significant in the broad academic field of ethnomedicine. It contributed a complete overview of the folk therapeutic practices by the different communities (Onges, Tai, Andamanese, Nicobarese, Rabhas, and Limbu) of contemporary Indian society. Besides, it presented diverse applications of traditional medicinal herbs and plants by different sections of people of contemporary India for the treatment of disease and healthcare. This volume is timely and important because it shows the existing cultural events, knowledge, and interpretation regarding health, diseases, and illness among the different communities of India. Therefore, this volume is unique for its rich contents from various expert academicians, researchers, and scholars of different regions of India who presented their diverse viewpoints, experiences, and extensive exploration on the significant themes of ethnobotany, ethnomedicinal practices, traditional knowledge, concept of health beliefs, and values. This volume will help researchers and scholars from various disciplines of social-cultural anthropology, medical anthropology, medical sociology, ethnobiology, cultural geography, cultural ecology, tribal studies, public health, liberal studies, sustainability, and development. It can prepare undergraduate and graduate students to become creative thinkers and communicators in the broad field of ethnomedicine. It will also help other general readers to develop their concept on the application of indigenous medicinal plants and traditional medical practices of various ethnic groups across India. This volume will be useful for the scholars and students of anthropology, ethnobiology, and ethnobotany not only for the knowledge and information but also for planning future research. The editors are credited for this scholarly effort.

Dr. Yadvinder Singh
Assistant Professor of Botany
School of Basic Sciences
Central University of Punjab, India

Acknowledgments

First of all, we wrote together a project proposal, "Ethno-Medicinal Knowledge and Practices after Covid-19 among the Tribal People of Bankura District of West Bengal, India," in October 2023. Apart from this, we also wrote another article, "Traditional Knowledge of Medicinal Plants among the Tribal People of Bankura District of West Bengal, India." That was the beginning of our work with ethnomedicinal knowledge, practice, and usage of various traditional medicinal plants in different regions of our country India. Then we both discussed if an edited volume could be written and published with these keywords. As usual, we prepared a proposal and sent it to various young scholars, researchers, teachers, and professors. We got a good response from them and divided their abstracts into various themes and started writing the contents accordingly. So we are very grateful to each and every contributor of this edited book volume for their responses and for writing the chapters according to the theme.

Then, after arranging the contents, we discussed the publishing. In that case, one of our friends and colleagues named Dr. Abhradip Banerjee, Assistant Professor, Department of Anthropology, Government General Degree College, Singur, Hooghly, India, gave us knowledge about Lexington Books, an imprint of Bloomsbury Publishing Inc., New York, United States. He also provided the contact as well as email address of Ms. Courtney Morales, Senior Acquisitions Editor at Bloomsbury Academic. On that account, our heartfelt thanks to Dr. Banerjee for his valuable suggestions and help. Accordingly, we emailed Ms. Courtney, and she gave us a very quick response as well as publishing agreement, guides, and forms. Therefore, we would like to extend our utmost gratitude to Ms. Courtney for her prompt response, positive feedback, valuable suggestions, and insightful comments.

Furthermore, we must thank Nicolette Amstutz, Director of Editorial, Bloomsbury Publishing Inc., and other authorities associated with Lexington Books for offering us the wonderful opportunity to collaborate with their publishing house and bring this edited book volume into reality. We would like to extend our utmost gratitude to them for their invaluable support.

We also must acknowledge Dr. Yadvinder Singh, Assistant Professor of Botany, Central University of Punjab, India, for writing the foreword of this edited book volume despite his busy schedule.

Last of all, we are highly obliged to all our family members, college staff, and all the people who have directly and indirectly helped to complete this edited book volume. Hope this volume will help the researchers and scholars from various disciplines of social-cultural anthropology, medical anthropology, medical sociology, ethnobiology, cultural geography, cultural ecology, tribal studies, public health, liberal studies, sustainability, and development. It will help to prepare the undergraduate and graduate students to become creative thinkers and communicators in the broad field of ethnomedicine. It will also help other general readers to develop their concept on the application of indigenous medicinal plants and traditional medical practices of various ethnic groups across India.

Arun Makal
Gour Gopal Satpati

Introduction

Arun Makal and Gour Gopal Satpati

Ethnomedicine is an interdisciplinary field that combines the study of natural pharmaceuticals with ethnobotany and medical anthropology. It is the study of traditional medicine of ethnic communities, their knowledge and practices that are transmitted orally over centuries and evolved over millennia of human existence. Specifically, ethnomedicine studies traditional healing practices and cultural beliefs about health and illness as practiced by various ethnic groups. Therefore, ethnomedicine is the study of traditional medical practices that use plants and animals to treat diseases and is often practiced by indigenous peoples or those with limited access to Western medicine (Helman 1984; Maheshwari, Painuli, and Dwivdi 1997; Erickson 2007; Chattopadhyay 2009, 2010). This ethnomedicine was practiced by many ancient civilizations including Indian Ayurveda, Chinese Traditional Medicine, Indian Yoga, Muti of Africa, and Unani medicine of Mughal India, and so on. Indian Ayurveda is a traditional medical practice that depends on the balance between the body and soul. Conversely, Chinese Traditional Medicine uses herbs, acupuncture, *tai-chi*, and *ai-gong* to treat and prevent diseases. Moreover, Indian Yoga is a mainstream medical practice in the Indus-Sarasvati civilization in Northern India that was used to maintain health and long life. In addition, the Muthi is a traditional medicine practice in Southern Africa as far north as Lake Tanganyika. African traditional medicine uses various natural products derived from trees and plants. Here the botanical medicine prescribed by herbal healers or *inyanga* is generally known as *muthi*. The same term *muthi* can apply to other traditional medical formulations including those that are zoological or mineral in composition. Besides, the Unani system of medicine was developed in India during the Mughal period. It is a traditional system of healing and health maintenance observed in South Asia. The origins of Unani medicine are found in the doctrines of the ancient Greek physicians. As a field, it was later developed and refined through systematic experiments by the Arabs. Furthermore, the Native Hawaiians use the nut, sap, and leaves of the candlenut tree for food, medicine, and other purposes. The nut is used as a laxative, the sap is used to speed up healing, and the leaves and flowers are used to make leis. Other examples of ethnomedicine practices include Traditional Korean Medicine, Celtic Medicine, Japanese Kampo Medicine, and Haitian Folk Medicine.

Thus, ethnomedicine is a cultural heritage all over the world, including India. However, presently, this ethnomedicine is threatened by a number of factors, including the exploitation of natural resources, dependency on chemical resources, and limited knowledge. These factors have opened a corridor for future insecurity of natural resources and ultimately the loss of human lives. In such contexts, ethnomedicine is an alternative for future generations because it is a practice which contains sustainable use of natural resources. It is a knowledge of people which uses nature in balance for the welfare of society by treating their diseases and illnesses with the help of herbs and medicinal animals. It is the cultural heritage of rural and tribal people in which they heal and cure disease by using some zoo-botanical products and practicing magico-religious rituals (Vaidya and Devasagayam 2007; Roy Burman 1982; Banik and Nema 2014). Besides, due to limitation of medicinal knowledge to only few persons of the society, status of local culture not universal, absence of written form, treatment, and healing of only small-scale diseases, its future is supposed to be in danger. Therefore, in India, coexistence of both complementary and alternative medicine system is very much demanding in present scenario. Thus, we can not only preserve our traditional healing system and culture for future generations but will also struggle with alarming diseases and future challenges. Consequently, the documentation of ethnomedicinal knowledge and practices, as well as record of application of traditional medicinal plants, will help in preservation of cultural legacy and sustainable development of the contemporary Indian society.

Ethnomedicinal Research and Its Importance

Ethnomedicine is a traditional knowledge that is thought to disappear in the near future, so for that reason, it should be preserved. Ethnomedicinal research deals with medicines derived from plants, animals, and minerals and used in the treatment of various diseases and ailments based on indigenous pharmacopoeia, folklore, and herbal attractions. This research is involved with distinctive knowledge about plant wealth and search of new resources for the preparation of herbal medicines, edible plants for consumption, and other aspects of plants, as well as understanding healing practices for different diseases. Thus, ethnomedicinal practices are important because they can help identify new sources of antivirals and other drugs. It has been used as a starting point for drug discovery, particularly through reverse pharmacological methods. Ethnomedicinal investigation can be used for anthropological or ethnobotanical research and in the field of drug discovery. For example, researchers have used ethnomedicine to identify new sources of antivirals. Some modern drugs, such as aspirin, have been discovered by following leads from folk uses. Accordingly, ethnomedicinal research is the study of traditional medicine practices and knowledge of plants and animals and is important for several reasons like drug discovery, public health, understanding cultural context, preserving knowledge and health of indigenous communities.

Drug discovery in ethnomedicinal research is the process of using traditional knowledge and natural resources to identify new drugs. It involves a multidisciplinary approach that combines botanical, biological, phytochemical, and molecular techniques. Thus, ethnomedicinal research has led to the discovery of new drugs and compounds that can be used in pharmaceuticals, supplements, and cosmetics. Conversely, ethnomedicinal research can help identify ways to incorporate traditional medical practices into public health efforts. Moreover, ethnomedicinal research can help understand the cultural context and perception of traditional medicines. Besides, ethnomedicinal research can help preserve traditional knowledge that is often passed down orally. All over again, ethnomedicinal research can help improve the health of indigenous communities who may have limited access to modern healthcare.

Therefore, ethnomedicinal research is interdisciplinary, drawing on methods from ethnobotany and medical anthropology. It is involved with (a) documenting or recording traditional knowledge about medicinal plants and their uses; (b) using quantitative value indices to analyze data on the relative importance of plants; (c) conducting chemical and pharmacological studies to determine the safety and efficacy of ethnomedicines. Consequently, ethnomedicinal research is the study of unique knowledge about plant wealth and search of new resources for the preparation of herbal medicines, edible plants for consumption, and other aspects of plants (Chandra, Nautiyal, and Nautiyal 2013; Purohit 2004). This ethnomedicinal research is also important in the context of India where 20 percent of plant species are reported for medicinal values. Besides, 98.55 percent of the sixty-nine animal species are used by traditional healers in India for medicinal purposes or as food products (Kala, Farooquee, and Dhar 2004; Malik et al. 2015). Accordingly, ethnomedicinal research in India can help (a) to preserve traditional healers' knowledge, (b) to promote collaboration to preserve ethnomedicinal practices, (c) to support the development of herbal drug formulations, and (d) to conserve and sustainably utilize threatened and endangered species.

Ethnomedicine as a Synonym for Traditional Medicine

The word "ethnomedicine" is sometimes used as a synonym for traditional medicine, which is concerned with the study of old-fashioned medical practices, beliefs, and knowledge based on cultural perspectives. The traditional medicine, also known as indigenous medicine or folk medicine, comprises medical aspects of traditional knowledge that developed over generations within the folk beliefs of various societies, including indigenous peoples, before the era of modern medicine. Indigenous medicine or folk medicine is relevant to today's world because many people in developing countries depend on traditional medicine and medicinal plants. This traditional or folk medicine also includes health beliefs, disease classifications, and cultural values. Some examples of traditional medical systems that are considered ethnomedicine include Indian Ayurveda, Chinese medicine, Arabic Unani, medicines of Egypt, Africa, America, and the Mediterranean.

Ethnomedicine and Medicinal Plants

Ethnomedicine is the study of traditional medicine practices that use plants and animals for health and healing and the cultural interpretation of health and disease. However, the plants are the significant part of ethnomedicine. Plants are used to treat a variety of illnesses including jaundice, diabetes, dysentery, typhoid, and so on. Various plants and their parts like herbs, roots, leaves, fruits, and flowers are used in ethnomedicine or traditional medicine. With this intention, the plants are a vital source of both curative and preventive medical therapy preparations for human beings, which are also used for the extraction of important bioactive compounds (Lambert, Srivastava, and Vietmeyer 1997; Thirumalai et al. 2009; Rasool 2012). On the other hand, ethnomedicine may be defined broadly as the use of plants by humans as medicines, but these uses could be called to be more precise as ethnobotanic medicine, and it is estimated that around 200,000 plant species are known all over the world for the treatment of a variety of diseases (Jain 1991; Fransworth 1994; Chandel, Shukla, and Sharma 1996).

In the context of ethnomedicine, phytochemical studies of plants are vital because plants can produce a large number of bioactive compounds such as alkaloids, flavonoids, coumarins, anthraquinones, steroids, tannins, and vitamins that may complement the needs of the human body by acting as natural antioxidants (Das et al. 2014; Altemimi et al. 2017). Besides, the phytochemical studies of plants are significant for a number of reasons including identifying biological activity, understanding health risks, developing therapeutic drugs, commercial applications, documenting traditional knowledge, and conservation. Accordingly, the phytochemical analysis is a way to identify the unique biological activity of medicinal plants by analyzing the chemicals they contain or phytochemicals. For example, terpenoids are phytochemicals that can have antiviral, antibacterial, and anti-inflammatory properties. On the other hand, phytochemical analysis can help determine the health risks associated with the medicinal plants. In addition, the phytochemical screening can help identify bioactive constituents that may be useful in developing therapeutic drugs. Besides, phytochemicals have commercial applications in drugs, cosmetics, flavors, fragrances, fuels, preservatives, and enzymes. Moreover, the phytochemical studies can help document traditional knowledge and practices of medicinal plants. This is important because traditional knowledge is at risk of being lost, especially among younger generations. Last of all, the phytochemical studies can help identify the most valuable plants and develop conservation initiatives.

Medicinal plants are also an important source of compounds with therapeutic potential and still represent a significant pool for the discovery of new drugs. The medicinal properties of plants are mainly due to the presence of active primary metabolites. Yet again, medicinal plants are rich in a wide variety of chemical compounds which have been found in vitro to have antimicrobial activities. Thus, in the consideration of ethnomedicine, the antimicrobial activity of plants is imperative because it can help identify new compounds for therapeutic use to treat infectious diseases. Accordingly, studying the antimicrobial activity of plants is significant because it can help identify new antimicrobial agents and develop safer alternatives to chemical preservatives.

Presently, the rise of drug-resistant pathogens is a global health threat. Studying medicinal plants can help identify new compounds to treat these pathogens. Plants contain secondary metabolites like alkaloids, phenols, and terpenoids that play a role in their survival and adaptation to the environment. These compounds can be used to develop new antibiotics. Further, many plants used in ethnomedicine have been shown to be effective against disease-causing microorganisms. Some plants that have antimicrobial activity may reduce the side effects of synthetic drugs. Also, the traditional medicinal plants are often less expensive than other treatments.

Therefore, plants are a good source of new medicines and many plants used in ethnomedicine have shown promising antimicrobial activity against disease-causing microorganisms. Conversely, the chemical preservatives as well as chemical residues in food and feed chains can have negative impacts on human health and the environment. Plant extracts can be used to preserve food and control food poisoning diseases. Besides, the antimicrobial compounds from medicinal plants may inhibit the growth of bacteria, fungi, viruses, and protozoa by different mechanisms than those of presently used antimicrobials and may have significant clinical value in the treatment of resistant microbial strains (Cowan 1999; Lewis and Ausubel 2006; Shankar et al. 2010).

Cultural Beliefs, Health, Illness, and Indigenous Healers

Ethnomedicine is a field that studies cultural interpretation, beliefs, and notions related to illness and health by the ethnic or indigenous communities around the world over centuries. Moreover, it also involves understanding the healing practices for different diseases (Krippner and Staples, 2003). Consequently, ethnomedicine is a society's cultural knowledge about the management of health and treatments for illness, sickness, and disease. This includes the culturally appropriate process for seeking health care and the culturally defined signs and symptoms of illness that raise a health concern. Ethnomedical systems are frequently closely related to belief systems and religious practices. Healing can include rituals and natural treatments drawn from the local environment. Therefore, ethnomedicine studies how different cultures in various environments interpret health, illness, and disease, and the practices used to treat them. Cultural beliefs are central to ethnomedicine and are often closely linked to religious practices. Some examples of ethnomedicinal beliefs and practices include bioenergy, natural remedies, social behavior, and incantations.

Ethnomedical systems lack the division between mind and body. Many ethnomedical systems support a belief in a singular body force or bioenergy as the source of human health, including the traditional systems of Chinese medicine and Ayurvedic medicine of India. On the other hand, many ethnomedicinal systems focus strongly on preventative measures and the use of natural remedies or elements such as herbs, food, and spices, as well as exercise and massage components to heal. In addition, some ethnomedicinal systems associate disease with the social behavior of the affected person. However, some ethnomedicinal systems use incantations that are endowed with magical potency (Micozzi 2002; Rothstein and Rajapaksa 2003).

Ethnomedicinal systems have healers who are knowledgeable about how to heal and inflict harm. The healing specialists or indigenous healers in an ethnomedical system are experienced individuals who undergo training or apprenticeship. Indigenous healers or the practitioners of traditional medicines follow their traditions, observations, and beliefs but are unaware of the modern system of treatment. However, their proof of concept is based on the end result of using such therapy for generations. The main theme of their treatment is to provide relief to the sufferer and then find the real cause of the suffering with the belief of healing from within. Those traditional practitioners or indigenous healers do have a great knowledge about herbalism and ethnobotany as well as about human nature, which may not be based on modern anatomy, physiology, biochemistry, and genetics.

Some examples of indigenous healers are midwives, doulas, herbalists, bonesetters, surgeons, and shamans whose ethnomedicine existed in cultural traditions around the world prior to biomedicine. Anthropologists and ethnobotanists frequently note that indigenous healers possess knowledge of both how to heal and how to inflict harm by physical and sometimes metaphysical means. Consequently, ethnomedicine does not only emphasize traditional medicine but instead permits cross-cultural comparison of medical systems. Some forms of healing depend on spiritual knowledge as a form of medicine. Some indigenous healers in shamanism intentionally enter into the spirit world to treat diseases with the culture's shaman acting as a representative. The goal may be to eliminate the illness or to identify its source. Similarly, faith healing depends on a shared understanding of belief and local customs with spirituality permeating the healing process. Exorcizing individuals of possession by negative spirits is a common form of faith healing that occurs within Christian, Islamic, Buddhist, and shamanic frameworks. In many cases, cultures that utilize biomedicine also utilize some forms of faith healing.

Ethnomedicine, Environment, and Sustainable Development

Ethnomedicinal and ethnobotanical knowledge arises from a complex interaction between human beings and their neighboring environment, which is again governed by various factors like local classification systems, communication through language, human cognition, cultural history, beliefs and religion, social networks, and access to information (Pieroni and Quave 2005; Maffi 2005; Bandiera and Rasul 2006; Ellen 2009; Leonti and Casu 2013). Thus, ethnomedicine is a practice that uses knowledge of natural plants and animals to promote wellness for people, animals, plants, soil, water, and the environment. The relationship between ethnomedicine and the environment is complex and includes both the impact of ethnomedicine on the environment and the impact of the environment on ethnomedicine. In these contexts, ethnomedicine can contribute to ecological degradation, but it can also help to conserve and preserve the environment. So promoting ethnomedicine can help to protect biodiversity and environmental conservation by establishing traditional medicine preserves. Conversely, environment can impact ethnomedicine through ecological degradation and destruction. Deforestation can threaten the natural resources used in ethnomedicine and put many species at risk of extinction. For example, the tribal people in India generally live in forest areas where they become familiar with a variety of plant and animal species, which they sustainably use for their food and medicinal purposes. But presently, deforestation and displacement to other places very much affect their culture and economy. Besides, the loss of medicinal plants and animal species very much affects their ethnomedicinal practices like cure of general diseases, fever, gynecological problems, and so on (Roy Burman 1982; Chakraborty, Kosariya, and Chakravarty 2015).

Some other considerations related to ethnomedicine and the environment include traditional knowledge, replacement of ingredients, and endangered species. Ethnomedicinal research can help record the traditional knowledge of indigenous people about ethnomedicines. This knowledge can be important for future use and conservation. Alternatively, when replacing ingredients in remedies, it's important to be cautious. Different species may not have the same effectiveness, and it is important to ensure the sustainability of the substitute species. Then again, some medicinal species are endangered. For example, in Brazil, fifty-four medicinal species are listed as endangered and thirty-three of them are commercialized.

Therefore, ethnomedicine or traditional medicine is a sustainable way to use natural resources and can help environmental conservation. In other words, ethnomedicine is a traditional knowledge system that uses natural resources in a sustainable way to treat illnesses and diseases. It can help sustainable development by preserving natural resources, recording indigenous knowledge, developing new medicines, and supporting local communities and the economy. Accordingly, ethnomedicine can help to preserve natural resources by teaching people to use them in a balanced way. Ethnomedicinal research can help to record the knowledge of indigenous people about their traditional medicines. Ethnomedicine can help to discover new medicines by providing a basis for research. Ethnobotanical knowledge can contribute to sustainable development goals like ending poverty, improving health, and combating climate change. In such a way, indigenous people and local communities have traditional knowledge and practices that can help with environmental management and sustainable development. So, ethnomedicinal research in a sustainable way will be a good option for future generations as it is a practice involved with justifiable use of natural resources, which is very important for life on the earth.

Ethnomedicinal Values and Indian Knowledge System

Ethnomedicinal values are the traditional knowledge of plants and animals used for healing and are a key part of the Indian knowledge system. India's traditional medicine systems such as Ayurveda, Siddha, Unani, and Homeopathy are based on ethnomedicinal values. These systems have been used for centuries to treat a variety of illnesses. In addition, India's knowledge of ethnomedicinal plants has been used to develop herbal medicines with few side effects. The World Health Organization (WHO) recognizes the benefits of drugs made from natural products. For example, in the sub-Himalayan region of West Bengal, home gardens are a traditional source of ethnomedicinal plants. These home gardens are a vital part of the livelihood of the local ethnic communities.

As well, the ethnomedicinal values are found mentioned even in the ancient Vedas and other scriptures. The Indian Ayurvedic teachings traditionally suggest that every disease has several reasons and psychological factors like fear, anger, grief, greed, pride, and jealousy. So from the perspective of Ayurveda, all diseases, whether mental or physical, are caused by the imbalance of the *doshas*. Endogenous causes of the disease include internal variations of the *doshas*, and exogenous causes refer to injuries caused by factors from outside. Terminologically, the *dosha* is a Sanskrit word that refers to three types of substances that are believed to be present in a person's body. It is a central term in Ayurveda, which is the Indian science of medicine, herbalism, and more. In Ayurveda, *dosha* is a dynamic principle that determines a person's health and personality. It is based on the ratio of the five elements of nature: air, earth, space, water, and fire. The three main *doshas* are *Vata*, *Pitta*, and *Kapha*. Indian Ayurveda believes that an imbalance in *dosha* can lead to disease and poor health. However, there is little evidence to support the belief in personal *doshas*. Thus, *dosha* is a key concept in Ayurvedic assessments for disease management and prevention. A state of health called *swasthya*, which means "established in the self," is when a person's *doshas* and *prakriti* are balanced.

Moreover, in the context of the Indian knowledge system, the traditional or indigenous healers play a key role in passing down ethnomedicinal knowledge orally. However, presently this knowledge is at risk of being lost due to environmental degradation, social and economic change, and limited knowledge sharing. The traditional healers in India are recognized by their communities as competent to provide healthcare using a variety of methods, including herbal medicines, cultural practices, religious practices, and folk knowledge. In the case of herbal medicines, the traditional healers use medicinal formulas made from animal, vegetable, and mineral substances. Conversely, in the matter of cultural and religious practices, the healers consider the social, cultural, and religious backgrounds of their community, as well as their beliefs about health and disease. In addition, regarding folk knowledge, the healers may use indigenous knowledge about medicinal plants and their uses. Some examples of traditional healers in India are *bhopas* or *bhagats* and headmen. The *bhopas* or *bhagats* are traditional healers in Maharashtra who use rituals, prayers, and herbal medicines to treat physical and spiritual illnesses. Equally, the headmen are well-versed in the identification and uses of medicinal herbs in their surrounding forests. They treat skin diseases, digestive illnesses, and fevers. The Quality Council of India has a system for evaluating and certifying traditional healers.

Ethnomedicinal Practices in India

As an ancient civilization, present-day India has inherited a rich culture of traditional systems of medicine. So, India has a rich history of traditional systems of medicine based upon six systems, out of which Ayurveda is the most ancient, most widely accepted, practiced, and flourished indigenous system of medicine. This Ayurvedic concept appeared and developed between 2500 and 500 BC in India. The literal meaning of Ayurveda is science of life because ancient Indian system of health care focused on views of man and his illness (Subhose, Srinivas, and Narayana 2005; Patwardhan et al. 2005). Besides Ayurveda, the other allied systems of medicine in India are Yoga and Naturopathy, Unani, Siddha, and Homeopathy, which are collectively known as AYUSH. These six Indian systems of medicine are prevalent and practiced in India and some of the neighboring Asian countries with very few exceptions in some of the developed countries. In addition, these systems are based on definite medical philosophies and represent a way of healthy living with established concepts on prevention of diseases and promotion of health. But the individual treatment systems show region-wise variations. For example, the state of Uttar Pradesh has more Unani doctors whereas Maharashtra has more Ayurvedic doctors (Sen Gupta 2008; Sharma, Singh, and Sharma 2022).

Therefore by tradition, about 65 percent of the population in India relies mostly on the traditional medicines for their health care needs. Besides, there are more than 1.5 million traditional medical practitioners in the country who use natural products including medicinal plants and animals to prevent disease, maintain health, and cure diseases (Singh et al. 2017). In India, 20 percent of plant species are reported for medicinal values. So, India has a large number of medicinal plants with over 8,000 species in the Himalayas alone. These plants are used in traditional medicine for a variety of purposes including treating common diseases like respiratory problems, aches, pains, and wounds. Also, the plant-based medicines are at the root of modern health care and are now being increasingly recognized for their economic potentials in India.

Accordingly, the traditional knowledge including ethnomedicinal practices is a vital part of the lives of indigenous and local communities in India, especially for food and health. India is inhabited by about 645 indigenous tribes having rich knowledge of wild flora and fauna to manage or cure diseases with other incredible uses. So, the tribal people living in different parts of India are one of the significant participants of traditional medicinal knowledge. They have their own medicinal knowledge and remedial systems which are non-codified and passed orally from one generation to another. For example, in Jharkhand state, the *hodopathy* system of healing is widely practiced and relies on vegetation growing in jungles and wild bushes. Apart from these, it is estimated that tribal and ethnic communities in India use approximately 8,000 plant species with 25,000 effective plant-based preparations for healthcare (Sreedevi et al. 2013; Sen and Chakraborty 2015).

Thus, India has a rich tradition of ethnomedicinal practices with traditional healers using around 2,500 plant species for medicinal purposes (Jain 1991; Chandel, Shukla, and Sharma 1996). But now the medicinal plants have considerable global impact in recent years. As a result, due to various human activities such as deforestation, rapid industrialization, urbanization, and other developmental activities, there is a fast decline of both natural vegetation and traditional practices in India (Bhattacharjee 2001). On the other hand, the use of traditional plant and animal-based medicine is also declining due to the availability of synthetic drugs and other factors like lack of research, lack of standardization, lack of documentation, exploitation of the environment, increased demand for medicinal plants, changing lifestyles, and lack of affordability. Consequently, ethnomedicinal studies are very much important in India for many reasons, including preserving traditional knowledge, developing new drugs, understanding traditional healthcare, as well as understanding the relationship between humans and nature by supporting local communities.

Ethnomedicine: Benefits and Contributions

Ethnomedicine is presently valuable for the development of healthcare and conservation programs in different parts of the world. The documentation of ethnomedicinal studies helps to preserve knowledge before traditional folklores are lost forever. The World Health Organization estimates that 80 percent of the world's population depends on traditional systems of medicine. These traditional systems of medicine are mainly based on the use of plants and animals, of which medicinal plants form an important part of the world's economy, as many modern medicines are derived from these plants. Presently, the trade of medicinal plant and animals is growing rapidly, and rural communities depend largely on herbal resources for curing diseases. This culture continues today in the form of folk medicine in different parts of the world and has led to the development of traditional systems of medicine.

Besides, the systematic and scientific research on the traditional systems of medicine has also provided many valuable drugs in Western medicine. In addition, the traditional medicines from plants and animals are often cost-effective, safe, and nontoxic. Ethnomedicinal plants can be used to develop pharmaceuticals, supplements, and cosmetics. Also, ethnomedicinal research can help to explore the economy, society, culture, and livelihood of indigenous people. Therefore, considering the value of medicinal plant and animal documentation for further preservation is very significant before they disappear from nature. Consequently, the valuable plant and animal information from various regions of India needs to be systematically recognized and documented for generations to come apart from conserving these precious plant and animal resources of high economic utility.

Objectives of the Volume

The objective of this book volume is to provide an opportunity to the academicians, students, scholars, and researchers in various parts of India and across the world to gain insight into the cultural significance of healing practices and how they have contributed to the preservation of biodiversity. It also highlights the benefits of traditional medicinal plants and animals as well as ethnomedicinal values of various indigenous communities across India in the context of the current healthcare system. The present volume is designed to document the use of ethnomedicinal plants and animals in various regions of India. It considers finding information on the use of plants and animals. It also tries to understand the socioeconomic status of the people and their potential use and practice of traditional medicine and knowledge.

This volume may assist researchers and scholars from various disciplines of social-cultural anthropology, medical anthropology, medical sociology, ethnobiology, cultural geography, cultural ecology, tribal studies, public health, liberal studies, sustainability, and development. It can prepare undergraduate and graduate students to become creative thinkers and communicators in the broad field of ethnomedicine. It may help the general readers to develop their concept on application of indigenous medicinal plants and traditional medical practices of various ethnic groups across India.

Organization of the Volume

This edited book volume is a collection of twenty-four chapters which are organized into six parts. Part I is about ethnomedicine, environment, and sustainable development. This part comprises three chapters namely Chapter 1, Chapter 2, and Chapter 3. Chapter 1, "Recent Advances in Ethnobotany: Strategies to Rejuvenate Our Green Planet by Sustainable Development," written by Sandip More, Sutibra Narayan Mondal, and Dola Boral, shows that ethnobotany is the study of the interrelationship between human and plants and has played a valuable role in the conservation of biodiversity and sustainable development, especially when related to knowledge and practices on the use in agriculture and pharmaceutical industries. This chapter explains the interrelationships between the current ecological crisis and the changes occurring in the practice of ethnomedicine. It also reflects the vital role of ethnobotanical studies from various parts of the world to preserve biodiversity in the greater interest of people and the planet. Next, Chapter 2, "Ethnomedicinal Knowledge among the Tribal Communities to Sustain the Economy and Socio-Environmental Infrastructure," written by Barsha Majumder, describes that health depends on a plethora of socio-physical and cultural attributes and is a state of equilibrium among mental, social, and physical well-being, which is intricately connected to the environment. This chapter is concerned with the development of indigenous knowledge about herbal plants for sustainable human health to mitigate several aspects of environmental stresses on human lifestyle occurring in recent decades that will lead to an increase in interest in clinical and nonclinical use of plants related to physical and mental health of human beings. Then, Chapter 3, titled "Ethnomedicine: A Vital Component for Sustainable Development," written by Aishwarya B. Patil, illustrates that ethnomedicine is rooted in the traditional medical practices of indigenous cultures and plays a crucial role in promoting sustainable healthcare systems and environmental stewardship. This chapter explores the intersection of ethnomedicine, the environment, and sustainable development, highlighting how diverse ethnomedical practices contribute to ecological balance. It also addresses challenges in integrating ethnomedicine into modern systems, including issues of intellectual property rights, cultural appropriation, and standardization. Additionally, this chapter advocates for recognizing and integrating ethnomedicine as a vital component of sustainable development. By incorporating traditional medical knowledge, modern sustainability efforts can achieve a more holistic approach to health and environmental well-being, fostering a resilient and sustainable future for all.

Part II of this volume addresses ethnobotanical knowledge and traditional medicinal plants. This part includes four chapters namely Chapter 4, Chapter 5, Chapter 6, and Chapter 7. Chapter 4, entitled "Ethnomedicinal and Indigenous Knowledge of Some Locally Available Important Medicinal Plants," written by Mimosa Ghosh, Sunipa Sen, and Gour Gopal Satpati, discourses that ethnomedicine may be defined broadly as the use of plants by humans as medicine, but these uses could be called, more accurately, ethnobotanical medicine. It is estimated that around 200,000 plant species are known all over the world. This chapter reports on the virtues of five ethnomedicinal plants, such as one from the Acanthaceae family, one from the Moringaceae family, one from the Molluginaceae family, one from the Araceae family, and one from the Poaceae family. Thereafter, Chapter 5, titled "Plausible Ethnobotanical Perception of Indigenous Mangrove Flora of the Indian Sundarbans," written by Renia Mullick, Debleena Roy, Suchita Sinha, and Dipu Samanta, brings forth the Sundarbans is the largest contiguous deltaic mangrove ecosystem in the world, spanning through West Bengal and Bangladesh. The people living in this area have developed unique ways of livelihood due to the challenges they face. They profoundly rely on plants for daily needs and traditional medicine, which has been passed down orally through generations. This chapter focuses on documenting knowledge regarding the medicinal properties of the Sundarbans mangrove flora. It also draws attention to the sustainable utilization of the mangrove resources, advocating long-term conservation planning. Subsequently, Chapter 6, entitled "Mangroves of Indian Sundarbans: A Treasure Trove of Medicinal Properties and Ethnomedicinal Significance," written by Sreemanti Banerjee, Chirabrata Sarkar, and Suparna Sardar, reveals that mangroves represent highly productive ecosystems, offering a multitude of benefits. The Sundarbans, the largest single block of tidal halophytic mangrove forest in the world, is home to 334 plant species from 245 genera and 75 families, as well as 165 algae and 13 orchid species, as per the latest records of UNESCO. The residents of Sundarbans have been using the remedial and healing effects of the native flora since the initial settlement. This chapter aims to provide a comprehensive account of the medicinal properties and ethnomedicinal relevance of Indian Sundarban mangroves, as well as the conservation and utilization of these species as sources of bioactive agents. Afterward, Chapter 7, titled "Possible Application and Ethnomedicinal Use of Aquatic and Semiaquatic Plants," written by Kankana De and Arun Makal, brings forth that aquatic and semiaquatic medicinal plants play a vital role in humans' lives. They have biological, pharmacological, and commercial uses. This chapter aims to explore the current evidence on the ethnomedicinal and pharmacological uses of aquatic and semiaquatic medicinal plants belonging to various families like Acanthaceae, Amaranthaceae, Ceratophyllaceae, Fabaceae, Hydrocharitaceae, Lythraceae, Marsileaceae, Nymphaeaceae, Onagraceae, Plantaginaceae, Pontederiaceae, Scrophulariaceae, and Zingiberaceae of some lakes and wetland areas of the district Paschim Medinipur of the Indian state of West Bengal.

Part III describes phytochemical analysis and antimicrobial activities of various medicinal plants in many regions of India. This part contains six chapters namely Chapter 8, Chapter 9, Chapter 10, Chapter 11, Chapter 12, and Chapter 13. Chapter 8, "Use of Ethnomedicines as an Elixir of Life: Phytochemical Analysis of Traditional Medicinal Plants in India," written by Sutibra Narayan Mondal, Souhardya Ray, Dola Boral, and Sandip More, clarifies that plants have been used since time immemorial for the treatment of various diseases and even today the knowledge of medicinal plants is commonly used in developing countries like India. Traditional medical science like Homeopathy, Ayurveda, Unani uses the knowledge of ethnomedicinal plants for the ailments of human diseases. Plants contain a plethora of various bioactive compounds in them which serve as the base for the treatment of diseases. This particular chapter highlights the holistic knowledge about bioactive compounds found in the ethnomedicinal plants that have been harvested for the treatment of diseases mostly in the underdeveloped regions in India. Then, Chapter 9, "An Exploration into the Phytochemical Enrichment of Lawsonia inermis L. and Its Medicinal Implications," written by Debapriya Das, Debleena Roy, and Dipu Samanta highlights that secondary metabolites are the intermediates of metabolism, which are not entirely essential for growth, but play an important role in interaction with other organisms, helping the specific organism adapt to environmental constraints. *Lawsonia inermis* L. (Henna) has long been established as a commercially significant plant, being the sole source of dye, *mehendi*. This chapter has tried to analyze the secondary metabolite pool of the plant, *Lawsonia inermis*, L. the prevalent pathways present, the phytochemicals which can make the plant medicinally important, and ways by which the secondary metabolite content of the plant can be increased, which can aid the industrial sector immensely. Afterward, Chapter 10, titled "Antimicrobial Activity of Some Ethnomedicinal Plants of India and Their Potential Application in Modern Medicine," written by Camellia Nandi, depicts that ethnomedicine can be defined as a field involving cultural beliefs, and interpretations related to different ailments and health by the ethnic communities around the globe. It involves the use of traditional knowledge and healing practices for different diseases. Plants have been used since the beginning of civilization for their medicinal properties. This specific chapter reviews the antimicrobial activities of some ethnomedicinal plants of India and their potential application in modern medicine. Then, Chapter 11, entitled "Utilization of Ethnomedicinal Plants for Their Potential Antimicrobial Activity," written by Jit Sarkar, brings forth that infectious diseases cause major threats to human health in both developing and developed countries. The growing number of drug-resistant diseases necessitates the rapid identification and isolation of novel bioactive compounds from medicinal plants utilizing standardized modern analytical technologies. In this context, this chapter makes an attempt to provide a brief overview on utilization of ethnomedicinal plants for their potential antimicrobial activity. Subsequently, Chapter 12, titled "Bioactive Compounds from Ethnomedicinal Plants with Antimicrobial Properties," written by Atreyi Ghosh and Tanzila Alvi, signifies that ethnomedicinal plants have for a long time been necessary to traditional methods of healing across various cultures, celebrated for their wide exhibit of remedial properties. Because of the rise in antimicrobial resistance, ethnomedical plants, which are crucial for conventional healing, are being investigated in increasing numbers for their antibacterial characteristics. Based on this, this specific chapter encompasses the possibility of combining pharmacological research with ethnomedical knowledge, novel antimicrobial treatments can be created, safeguarding traditional information and advancing global health initiatives against antibiotic resistance and infectious illnesses. Next, the last chapter of this part, Chapter 13, titled "Nutraceutical, Phytochemical, and Pharmacological Value of Lactuca: A Review," written by Saroj Kumar Pradhan, Raspinder Kaur, Pooja Mawal, Jyoti Rani, and Rohita Singla, highlights that the *Lactuca* species are used in the traditional medicine system for the treatment of asthma, pain, insomnia, inflammation, intestinal, urinary tract infections, and various other health problems. This chapter reviews the nutraceutical value, phytochemistry, and associated bioactivity, which can be used for the future pharmacological applications of the *Lactuca* species.

Part IV discusses the indigenous communities and their concept of health, illness, beliefs, and practices based on empirical studies. This part covers four chapters, namely Chapter 14, Chapter 15, Chapter 16, and Chapter 17. Chapter 14, "Indigenous Medicines and Rituals: The Traditional Indian Medicine System," written by Shruti Chattaraj, articulates that indigenous medicine, also called traditional medicine or folk medicine, has a long history. Different indigenous medicine systems include traditional Chinese medicine, traditional European medicine, traditional African medicine, traditional Korean medicine, and traditional Indian medicine system. India has a long history of medicine; the oldest and most widely used medicine system is Ayurveda in traditional Indian medicine. In this chapter, an overview of Ayurveda's diagnosis method, various techniques, therapies, drugs, and rituals used for the treatment of individuals is discussed to provide a preliminary idea and understanding of indigenous medicine system and various rituals of Indian Ayurveda. Then, Chapter 15, titled "Indigenous Healing, Social Beliefs, and Practices among the Onges of Little Andaman of Andaman Archipelagos" written by Satyaki Paul and Sabatini Chatterjee, depicts that Onges are wanderlust tribal people of the Andaman and Nicobar archipelagos considering their identifying and naming of all islands in their language from north to south, as documented by ethnographers in the past. The Onges call their home *Guabolambe* or the Little Andaman, which was exclusive to them until the 1960s. They call themselves *En-iregale* or the perfect person to demarcate their prowess of knowing the unknown facets of the Andaman and Nicobar archipelagos. Due to their closeness to nature, their social beliefs and practices have harmony with the natural and supernatural context, which predominates their lives. This particular chapter seeks to identify and document the indigenous healing, social beliefs, and practices of the Onges of the Little Andaman of Andaman Archipelagos, considering their contemporary shift toward becoming a welfare-dependent community. Following this, Chapter 16, "Perception of Health and Traditional Health Seeking Behavior among the Tai Ahom, Tai Khamte, and Tai Phake Communities of Northeastern Part of India," written by Yikham Gogoi and Satyaki Paul, exemplifies that the Ahom, Khamte, and Phake are three significant communities among the total six groups of Tai peoples residing in the northeastern part of India. These Buddhist communities have significantly developed traditional knowledge systems regarding the flora endemic to their region and their uses in ethnomedicinal practices for mundane maladies. This knowledge of endemic flora is usually transferred from one generation to another through oral traditions, which have protected the Tai people since time immemorial. This chapter tries to document the ethnomedicinal and spiritual practices of the Tai people, as well as their benefits and the social change in health-seeking behavior that took place due to the advent of global influences. Subsequently, the last chapter of this part, Chapter 17, "Indigenous Knowledge Systems of the Great Andamanese Community Residing in Port Blair and Strait Island of Andaman Archipelagos," written by Sabatini Chatterjee, Satyaki Paul, and Jurol, describes that the Great Andamanese were the most dominant tribal group when the penal settlement was established in Andaman and Nicobar archipelagos for the second time in March 1858. In those times, there were ten distinctive groups spread from north to south of the Great Andaman archipelagos. They are further classified into creek (*adajig*) dwellers, coast (*ar-yauto*) dwellers, and forest (*erem-taga*) dwellers. The *Aka-Bea-Da*, residents of South Andaman, were in close contact with the colonial administrators, which led to their evanescing in 1901, becoming the first group to evanesce due to the white man's burden causing excessive encroachments in cultural patterns and mundane lives. At present, only two subgroups of Great Andamanese have survived, that is, *Aka-Cari* (Sare) and *Aka-Jeru*, who are mainly residing in Strait Island (after shifting from Bluff Island in 1969) and Port Blair of the Andaman archipelagos. Their entire indigenous knowledge system of *buamoh* making (only sounding board/musical instrument among Andaman and Nicobar tribes), canoe making, cane basket making, and using clay at calendrical festivals is evanescing slowly due to global influences and their over-admixture with mainstream people. This particular chapter tries to document all the social components of indigenous knowledge systems that were once present among the Great Andamanese tribe by revisiting all past ethnographic and anthropological studies done amid them.

Part V deliberates about the Indian knowledge system and ethnomedicinal values. This part includes three different chapters, namely Chapter 18, Chapter 19, and Chapter 20. Chapter 18, entitled "Concept of Ayurveda, Siddha, and Unani in Indian Traditional Knowledge System and Ethnomedicinal Values," written Gour Gopal Satpati, portrays the traditional knowledge about the three main pillars, namely, Ayurveda, Siddha, and Unani, of recognized Indian traditional medicines. This chapter tries to outline the historical background, research, and development related to ancient herbal medicines, as well as the overall idea about the three recognized systems, that is, Ayurveda, Siddha, and Unani in Indian perspective. After that, Chapter 19, namely "Ethnomedicinal Practices and Traditional Healthcare Systems of the Nicobarese Tribe of Nicobar Archipelagos," written by Satyaki Paul, Anstice Justin, and Sabatini Chatterjee, shows that the Nicobarese tribe is one of the most dominant tribes of the Andaman and Nicobar archipelagos considering its sheer size in comparison to other neighboring tribal groups. From the seventeenth century onwards, global influences have affected the Nicobarese people since time immemorial. However they have strong sociocultural ties among each other, although they have accepted several cultural traits from non-autochthons, making their sociocultural practices and beliefs more diverse and robust. The ethnomedicinal practices and traditional healthcare systems play a crucial part in the Nicobarese community, which is usually transmitted orally from one generation to another. This specific chapter essentially seeks to delve into the ethnomedicinal practices and traditional healthcare systems intertwined in the mundane lives of Nicobarese people, considering the prevalent availability of modern medicinal practices at the turn of the twenty-first century. Subsequently, Chapter 20, "Elements and Wellness Application of Botany and Medicinal Plants in Ancient India: A Systematic Review," written by Arun Makal, enlightens that the beginning of the relationship between humans and plants can be traced back to prehistoric times. Similarly, medical botany, or the study of medicinal plants and their traditional uses, has been a part of Indian culture for thousands of years. The earliest evidence of plants being used for medicine in India can be found in the Rig Veda. Post-Vedic literature also shows that botany developed as an independent science that served as the basis for medicine, agriculture, and arboriculture. Keeping all these understandings in mind, this chapter has tried to examine the elements and wellness application of botany and medicinal plants in ancient India by extensive review and reflections from the available secondary evidences.

Lastly, Part VI describes the situation of the current health care sector and benefits of medicinal plants among the various sections of people of contemporary Indian society. This last part comprises four chapters, namely Chapter 21, Chapter 22, Chapter 23, and Chapter 24. Chapter 21, titled "Benefits and Contributions of Medicinal Plants to Health Sector," written by Piyasa Ghosh, Shinjini Dey, and Srijita Ghosh, demonstrates that plants have been a source of support and sustenance for humans throughout their shared history in nature. The bioactive compounds present in medicinal plants exhibit significant potential for the development of new drugs as they possess antimicrobial, anti-inflammatory, anticancer, neuroprotective, and immunomodulatory properties. Additionally, plant-based medicines possess advantages over synthetic drugs in their synergistic effects on specific target sites with reduced risk of side effects and ready availability in nature. Thus, the growing demand for medicinal plants and their derivatives is compelling the global health industry to adopt herbal medicines to combat serious illnesses. Subsequently, Chapter 22 entitled "Presence of Trans-α-bergamotene from Young Leaves of Aegle marmelos (L.) Correa: An Insight to the Future Therapeutic Potential of a Plant Used in Traditional Healing Practices," written by Mitu De and Santi Ranjan Dey, presents that *Aegle marmelos* (L.) Correa has been used in Indian traditional medicinal practices. Different parts of this plant have been used in different ethnobotanical systems of traditional healing. The plant, commonly called *bael*, is native to India. *Aegle marmelos* (L.) Correa has been mentioned in Ayurvedic texts and Charaka Samhita. Recent research by different groups is now identifying various bioactive chemicals with potential medicinal properties. Common plant chemicals called bergamotenes are usually present in essential oils that are derived from various plant components such as flowers, fruits, leaves, and bark. Bergamotes, a type of bicyclic sesquiterpene, are found in plants, insects, and fungi, with trans-α-bergamotene as the most abundant compound. This chemical, trans-α-bergamotene, has been described for the first time in this book chapter from young *Aegle marmelos* (L.) Correa leaves using GC-MS analysis. Afterward, Chapter 23 entitled "Ethnomedicinal Practices and Effect of Socioeconomic Factors on Health among the Rabhas of Garo Basti in Alipurduar of West Bengal, India," written by Nabanita Goswamy and Somenath Bhattacharjee, shows that the Rabhas are one of the indigenous ethnic tribes residing in the forest fringe village of Garo Basti, Raja Bhat Khaoa of Alipurduar, West Bengal, considering themselves a part of the Bodo family. They apply and consume different parts of medicinal plants and local remedies on a regular basis. Furthermore, a number of socioeconomic factors like education, occupation, and marital status affect their health status and health care system. In this context, this particular chapter has tried to explore different ethnomedicinal practices and effect of various socioeconomic factors on the health of the Rabha community of the village Garo Basti in Alipurduar. Then, the last chapter of this last part is Chapter 24, entitled "Indigenous Knowledge and Healthcare Practices among the Limbu Community of Darjeeling Hills: Insights from the Covid-19 Pandemic," written by Niten Chhetri and Somenath Bhattacharjee, describes that the district Darjeeling of the Indian state of West Bengal, renowned for its rich biodiversity, is the ancestral land of the indigenous Limbu community. Their deep-rooted connections to nature and spiritual practices are intricately woven into their history and cultural development, particularly their relationship with the Khangchendzonga mountain range. This particular chapter has investigated the Limbu community's indigenous healthcare beliefs and practices amid the Covid-19 pandemic. The prime objective of this chapter is to understand ethnomedicinal practices, perspectives on Covid-19 vaccination, factors influencing traditional medicinal preferences, and its long-term implications during the pandemic. Further, this research has explored the role of traditional healers in providing healthcare services during the pandemic and their perceptions of Covid-19. The study has focused on the Limbu community's traditional healthcare practices, the perception of illness and healthcare, quarantine rituals, and medicinal plant use during and before Covid-19. This chapter has provided an emic perspective on the rituals of the Limbus, offering insights into their cultural significance and scientific value through a qualitative approach. Also, this chapter has incorporated both primary and secondary data sources. It has underscored the enduring relevance of traditional knowledge in times of crisis and called for further exploration and preservation of these practices.

References

Altemimi, A., N. Lakhssassi, A. Baharlouei, D. G. Watson, and D. A. Lightfoot. "Phytochemicals: Extraction, Isolation, and Identification of Bioactive Compounds from Plant Extracts." *Plants* 6, no. 42 (2017): 1–23.

Bandiera, O., and I. Rasul. "Social Networks and Technology Adoption in Northern Mozambique." *The Economic Journal* 116, no. 514 (2006): 869–902.

Banik, A., and S. Nema. "Ethnomedical Practices and Indigenous Household Remedies Used by the Tribals and Rurals of the Bastar Region (Chhattisgarh)." *The Indian Forester* 140, no. 2 (2014): 192–200.

Bhattacharjee, S. K. *Hand Book of Medicinal Plants*. Jaipur: Pointer Publishers, 2001.

Chandel, K. P. S., G. Shukla, and N. Sharma. *Biodiversity in Medicinal and Aromatic Plants in India*. Conservation and Utilization, New Delhi: Indian Council of Agricultural Research, National Bureau of Plant Genetic Resources, Pusa Campus, 1996.

Chattopadhyay, D. "Ethnomedicinal Phytophores in Disease Management." *International Journal of Pharmaceutical and Bio-Medical Science* 3, no. 11 (2009): 1–25.

Chattopadhyay, D. *Ethnomedicine: A Source of Complementary Therapeutics-A Review*. Trivandrum: Research Signpost, 2010.

Chakraborty, A., S. S. Kosariya, and M. Chakravarty. "A Review of Ethnomedicinal Practices for Gynaecological Disorders among the Various Tribes of Chhattisgarh." *IOSR Journal of Environmental Science, Toxicology and Food Technology* 1, no. 2 (2015): 55–62.

Chandra, K., B. Nautiyal, and M. C.Nautiyal. "Ethno-botanical Resources as Supplementary Foods and Less Known Wild Edible Fruits in District Rudraprayag, Uttarakhand, India." *Journal of Human Ecology* 42 (2013): 259–71.

Cowan, M. M. "Plant Products as Antimicrobial Agents." *Clinical Microbiology Reviews* 12, no. 4 (1999): 564–82.

Das, A., D. Chaudhuri, N. B. Ghate, A. Chatterjee, and N. Mandal. "Phytochemical Analysis, Antioxidant and Anticancer Potential of Leaf Extracts from Edible Greater Yam, Dioscorea Alata L., from North-East India." *International Journal of Phytopharmacology* 5, no. 2 (2014): 109–19.

Ellen, R. F. "Classification." In *The Routledge Encyclopedia of Social and Cultural Anthropology*, edited by A. Barnard and J. Spencer, 129–33. London: Routledge, 2009.

Erickson, P. I. *Ethnomedicine*. Long Grove, Illinois: Waveland Press, 2007.

Helman, C. G. *Culture, Health and Illness*. Florida: CRC Press, 1984.

Fransworth, N. R. "Ethnopharmacology and Drug Development." *Ciba Foundation Symposium* 185 (1994): 42–51.

Jain, S. K. *Dictionary of Indian Folk Medicines and Ethnobotany*. New Delhi: Deep Publications, 1991.

Kala, C. P., N. A. Farooquee, and U. Dhar. "Prioritization of Medicinal Plants on the Basis of Available Knowledge, Existing Practices and Use Value Status in Uttaranchal, India." *Biodiversity & Conservation* 13 (2004): 453–69.

Krippner R., and J. Staples "Suspected Allergy to Artemether-Lumefantrine Treatment of Malaria." *Journal of Travel Medicine* 10, no. 5 (2003): 303–5.

Lambert, J., J. Srivastava, and N. Vietmeyer. *Medicinal Plants: Rescuing a Global Heritage.* Washington, DC: World Bank, 1997.

Leonti, M., and L. Casu. "Traditional Medicines and Globalization: Current and Future Perspectives in Ethnopharmacology." *Frontiers in Pharmacology* 4 (2013): 1–13.

Lewis, K., and F. M. Ausubel. "Prospects for Plant-Derived Antibacterials." *Nature Biotechnology* 24 (2006): 1504–7.

Maffi, L. "Linguistic, Cultural, and Biological Diversity." *Annual Review of Anthropology* 34 (2005): 599–617.

Maheshwari, J. K., R. M. Painuli, and R. P. Dwivdi. "Notes on Ethnobotany of the Oraon and Korwa Tribes of Madhya Pradesh." In *Contribution to Indian Ethnobotany*, edited by S. K. Jain, 67–82. Jodhpur: Scientific Publishers, 1997.

Malik, Z. A., J. A. Bhat, R. Ballabha, R. W. Bussmann, and A. B. Bhatt. "Ethnomedicinal Plants Traditionally Used in Health Care Practices by Inhabitants of Western Himalaya." *Journal of Ethnopharmacology* 172 (2015): 133–44.

Micozzi, M. S. "Culture, Anthropology, and the Return of 'Complementary Medicine.'" *Medical Anthropology Quarterly* 16, no. 4 (2002): 398–403.

Patwardhan, B., D. Warude, P. Pushpangadan, and N. Bhatt. "Ayurveda and Traditional Chinese Medicine: A Comparative Overview." *Evidence-Based Complementary and Alternative Medicine* 2, no. 4 (2005): 465–73.

Pieroni, A., and C. Quave. "Traditional Pharmacopoeias and Medicines among Albanians and Italians in Southern Italy: A Comparison." *Journal of Ethnopharmacology* 101 (2005): 258–70.

Purohit, A. N. "Overview of State Policies, Plans and Interventions to Promote the Medicinal Plant Sector in Uttaranchal." *Searching Synergy, KIT Bulletin 359, Royal Tropical Institute: Amsterdam, The Netherlands* (2004): 21–9.

Rasool, H. B. "Medicinal Plants. Importance and Uses." *Pharmaceutica Analytica Acta* 3, no. 10 (2012): e139.

Rothstein, W. G., and S. Rajapaksa. "Health Beliefs of College Student Born in the United States, China, and India." *Journal of American College Health* 51, no. 5 (2003): 189–94.

Roy Burman, B. K. *Report of Committee on Forest and Tibals in India.* TD Division, Ministry of Home Affairs, Govt. of India, 1982.

Sen Gupta, A. "Medical Tourism in India: Winners and Losers." *Indian Journal of Medical Ethics* 5, no. 1 (2008): 4–5.

Sen, S., and R. Chakraborty. "Toward the Integration and Advancement of Herbal Medicine: A Focus on Traditional Indian Medicine." *Botanics: Targets and Therapy* 5 (2015): 33–44.

Shankar, S. R., R. Rangarajan, D. V. L. Sarada, and C. S. Kumar. "Evaluation of Antibacterial Activity and Phytochemical Screening of Wrightia Tinctoria L." *Pharmacognosy Journal* 2, no. 14 (2010): 19–22.

Sharma, P. K., A. Singh, and N. K. Sharma. "A Socio-Ecological Critique on India's Local Health Traditions amidst Rising Incidence of Global Pandemics." *Journal of Herbal Medicine* 34 (2022): 100578.

Singh, A., M. C. Nautiyal, R. M.Kunwar, and R. W. Bussmann. "Ethnomedicinal Plants Used by Local Inhabitants of Jakholi Block, Rudraprayag District, Western Himalaya, India." *Journal of Ethnobiology and Ethnomedicine* 13, no. 49 (2017): 1–29.
Sreedevi, P., T. P. Ijinu, S. Anzar, A. J. Bincy, V. George, and P. Pushpangadan. "Ethnobiology, Ethnobotany, Ethnomedicine and Traditional Knowledge with Special Reference to India." *Annals of Phytomedicine* 2, no. 2 (2013): 4–12.
Subhose, V., P. Srinivas, and A. Narayana. "Basic Principles of Pharmaceutical Science in Ayurvĕda." *Bulletin of the Indian Institute of History of Medicine* 35, no. 2 (2005): 83–92.
Thirumalai, T., E. Kelumalai, B. Senthilkumar, and E. David. "Ethnobotanical Study of Medicinal Plants Used by the Local People in Vellore District, Tamilnadu. India." *Ethnobotanical Leaflets,* 13 (2009): 1302–11.
Vaidya, A. D., and T. P. Devasagayam. "Current Status of Herbal Drugs in India: An Overview." *Journal of Clinical Biochemistry and Nutrition* 41, no. 1 (2007): 1–11.

Part I

Ethnomedicine, Environment, and Sustainable Development

1

Recent Advances in Ethnobotany

Strategies to Rejuvenate Our Green Planet by Sustainable Development

Sandip More*, Sutibra Narayan Mondal, and Dola Boral

PG Department of Botany, Murshidabad University, Murshidabad, West Bengal, India

*Corresponding Author's Email: smbot@msduniv.ac.in

Introduction

Plants have been extensively utilized by people for an assortment of things, such as food, medicine, shelter, decoration, building materials, and clothing (Balick 1996). The uses of plants as the source of medicines have been known since time immemorial. US botanist J. W. Harshberger in 1895 coined the term "ethnobotany." Ethnobotany deals with the interrelationship between plants and humans. Plants as the source of medicine and other cultures have been interwoven with humans since prehistoric times. Traditional ethnobotanical knowledge, which has been transmitted orally and vertically from generation to generation but is not extensively documented by indigenous people, comprises the methods by which indigenous and local communities use plants for an array of purposes (Garnatje, Peñuelas, and Vallès 2017). Ethnobotanical studies can interpret how each section of society interacts with their local environment. Knowledge about using plants for the treatment of various diseases depends upon the local environment and types of plants available in that region. Ethnobotany forms the science of the survival of human society since ancient times (Prance 2007). Ethnobotany helps to understand the interrelationship between humans and environment from traditional times to the present day. Ethnobotanical knowledge helps in preserving biodiversity and can help to achieve sustainable development (Pei, Alan, and Wang 2020). Ethnobotany helps in preserving the environment with the help of local communities and assists in achieving the biocultural conservation system, where local cultures are involved in association with the plants for their beneficial uses (Gaoue et al. 2017). Ethnobotanists can serve as a bridge between the two ends of the plant-human relationship and science because their field works at this crossroads (Alexiades 2003). Indigenous healers use the knowledge of ethnobotany to treat various human ailments. This knowledge has been used for collecting medicinal plants and helping in the treatment of diseases and also in biodiversity conservation. Proper documentation of the medicinal plants has been carried out by surveying and interviewing local communities and traditional healers by the ethnobotanist (Saha, Sundriyal, and Sundriyal 2014). Ethnobotanical knowledge has been preserved through generations orally and some of the usages of medicinal plants have been documented in various ancient literatures. Ancient literature like Ayurveda, Unani, Siddha, and Amchi provides the documented knowledge about different medicinal plants used in various parts of the world since time immemorial (Pushpangadan et al. 2018). Indian *Materia Medica* is a wealth of knowledge about the different plants used in traditional medicines that have been utilized for treating human problems since ancient times (Basu et al. 2023). The Indian traditional system of medicine like Ayurveda is years old and talks about the utilization of medicinal plants in the treatment of diseases in a holistic approach (Junaid et al. 2017). Ethnobotanical knowledge helps to understand nature and the important plants surrounding society and how plants and humans interact with them. This also helps in sustainable development of the environment.

Sustainable development means utilizing the natural resources in such a way that there is no overexploitation and still the needs of society can be fulfilled. Sustainable development encompasses a wider area that combines development and environment effectively, so that future generations can utilize natural resources (Parris and Kates 2003). Modern city development runs at such a fast pace that development hampers the natural environment. This rapid pace in urbanization, resulting from suburbanization, de-urbanization, and re-urbanization, leads to a loss of biodiversity (Van den Berg, Drewett, and Klaassen 2013). For the conservation of nature, certain steps, such as sustainable development, need to be taken for the betterment of the future. Ethnobotanical knowledge provides the link for the conservation of nature and helps in sustainable development. Indigenous people and local communities, with their knowledge about the environment, help in achieving sustainable development through their traditional knowledge (Kimerling 2002). Plants play an important role in the daily life of people, and human society is interwoven in many aspects (Zhao et al. 2020). Indigenous knowledge system is a complex and complete knowledge system which upholds a cultural belief unique to the particular locality and culture (Bates et al. 2009). Indigenous knowledge systems help in sustaining nature. Through their actions and flexibility to the environment, each ethnic group's cultural traits appear in the interaction between biodiversity in particular and natural resources in general (Sultana, Muhammad, and Zakaria 2018). Loss of biodiversity and urbanization leads to the destruction of natural resources, which is a major concern. Thus, the concept of sustainable development has emerged in recent years for the conservation of nature.

For the conservation of nature, the United Nations General Assembly in its seventieth meeting on September 25, 2015, formulated a resolution about the concept of sustainable development (Assembly 2015). The goals set by the United Nations for sustainable development are seventeen sets of goals which are aimed at various angles like ending poverty, protecting the planet, and ensuring prosperity for all. The idea about the sustainable development goals can be achieved with help from the government, private sector, and also from the traditional or indigenous people (Nyasimi and Peake 2015). The role of the indigenous people in contributing to the environment for sustainable development is immense. Their tradition, beliefs, culture, practices, and active participation in environmental knowledge can help to achieve the sustainable development goals (United Nations 1992). By the year 2030, the achievement of sustainable development can be predominantly achieved by the active participation of ethnobotanist groups with their vast knowledge about plants, culture, and society. The concept of ethnobotanical convergence has emerged which can also help in the concept of achieving sustainable development. "Ethnobotanical convergence" means that the independent knowledge about the traditional systems has converged by various confluence and influence in today's world and can be helped in achieving sustainable development (Hawkins and Teixidor-Toneu 2017). Thus, the traditional ethnobotanical knowledge (TEK) is used as an urgent basis for achieving sustainable development. TEK and the indigenous people can play an important role by providing information about the commonly used plants in that community. TEK can be incorporated into sustainable development and also in conserving biodiversity (Kumar et al. 2021). So, ethnobotanical knowledge paves a way in attaining the concept of sustainable development.

Biodiversity is the sum total of all the living organisms present on earth. Biodiversity is a broad sense which encompasses genetic, species, and ecosystem diversity. Conserving biodiversity is more of a moral issue because we are a part of this biodiversity. The knowledge of the ethnic groups, ethnolinguistic people, and their culture can be used and documented for the purpose of conservation of biodiversity (Basu 2009). There are approximately 50,000 to 80,000 plants from the angiosperms which are currently used as medicinal and aromatic plants (Leaman 2006). With the advent of civilization, there is a shrinking and loss of diversity of the medicinal and aromatic plants (MAP). With the commercialization of the medicinal plants, there is overexploitation and bioprospecting for medicinal plants (Kala 2000). This results in the loss of biodiversity of MAP. Almost 15,000 species of the medicinal plants are facing a problem of habitat destruction due to overexploitation. They are facing a threat of extinction due to continued harvesting and improper bioprospecting (Chen et al. 2016). The MAP can thus be conserved with the knowledge of the traditional people. Proper documentation can be done by conducting a proper survey about the different MAPs used among different traditions, and various concepts like sacred groves and medicinal plant gardens can be used for the biodiversity conservation of MAP (Kala 2010). With the concept of conserving MAP with the knowledge of ethnobotany, there arises the concept of knowledge of urban ethnobotany. The urban ethnobotanical knowledge, along with the cross-cultural heritages and pluralisms, helps in knowing the medicinally important plants growing in the urban areas which are useful in treatment of various human morbidities. So, urban ethnobotanical knowledge helps in assessing the medicinally important plants and also in their conservation of them (Dutta, Nandy, and Dey 2022).

Ethnobotanical knowledge, combined with modern scientific methods, helps in conserving plant diversity and in attaining sustainable development. Sustainable development can be achieved with the help of ethnobotanists and other ethnic communities. The concept of ethnobotany not only helps in conserving and protecting biodiversity but also aids in new drug development and the practice of sustainable agriculture. With concepts like ethnopharmacology and the knowledge of traditional medicines, new drugs have been developed and marketed (Bussmann 2002). With the advent of modern ethnopharmacological knowledge, it can be used to tap information about the medicinal plants used in Ayurveda and Siddha. Thus, the new drug delivery systems and new semi-synthetic drugs can be traced from traditional knowledge, aided by new ethnopharmacological research (Mukherjee and Wahile 2006). Traditional people used plants as the chief source for the cure of various ailments; the properties of the medicinal plants which help in curing various diseases are the presence of secondary metabolites in them. The ethnomedicinally important plants contain various secondary metabolites like alkaloids, tannins, phenolics, flavonoids, and glycosides, which help in combating various ailments (Mandal et al. 2023). These properties of the medicinal plants have been tapped since ancient times by local communities for using them as a cure to many diseases. With the advent of ethnobotany and its branch ethnopharmacology, the formulation of new drugs can be achieved by tracing the beneficial secondary metabolites present in the plants. Ethnobotanical knowledge helps to analyze the intrinsic knowledge about the medicinal plants that are used in drug discovery (Mehrotra and Mehrotra 2005).

The practice of sustainable agriculture is also contributed to by the knowledge of ethnobotany. With proper agricultural practices adapted from the traditional people, modern technologies can lead to greater improvement in agricultural practices. Thus, ethnobotanical knowledge helps in providing a proper idea about the practice of sustainable agriculture besides providing aid to the conservation of nature. Ethnobotanical research comprises various fields in an integrated manner, like the use of knowledge of anthropology, ecology, phytogeography, palynology, medicinal chemistry, and botany. These fields together develop the discipline of ethnobotany. Ethnobotany links the past and present knowledge in a comprehensive way. Ethnobotanical research provides ideas for the conservation of biodiversity and sustainable development. Both the conservation of biodiversity and sustainable development go hand in hand due to the knowledge of the traditional people and the combining of modern concepts in the field of ethnobotany (Pandey and Tripathi 2017). So, the ethnobotanical knowledge forms the base with traditional and modern science, which helps in the proper conservation of nature and natural resources.

Objectives

The study of ethnobotany helps to bridge the gap between traditional knowledge and modern concepts. It explores more about the traditional local communities and how their knowledge can impact the conservation of nature and natural resources. It also helps to document the various plant species used in various literatures which were used by the traditional people since ancient times. Ethnobotanical study also helps to conserve biodiversity and achieve sustainable development. Sustainable development goals can be achieved with the knowledge of ethnobotany and it helps in management of nature and natural resources. Ethnobotany forms the intersection between local and indigenous people and modern societies. The objective also implies the study of the various new compounds discovered from the plants which are essential for new drug discovery in the pharmaceutical industry. Drug discovery owes much of its credit to ethnobotanical knowledge, which has a great impact on it. Ethnobotanical study can help to assess the environmental impact due to certain anthropogenic causes. The result of modernization and how globalization affects the environment can be analyzed by various studies involved in ethnobotany. It can serve various ways for saving nature and ensuring sustainable utilization of natural resources.

Methodology

For the study about the role of ethnobotany in achieving sustainable development, various literatures and articles were studied for the proper presentation of the information in a concerted manner from the dispersed ideas. Reports from the various international organizations like WWF, UN, and IUCN were studied for preparation of the report on sustainable development and how it can be achieved by ethnobotanical research. This study explores the different ways identified from various literatures how ancient people used plants for their cure of diseases and the concept of ethnobotany. The concept provides a compact idea of how the traditional knowledge can be used nowadays for the proper management of the environment. The overexploitation of the environmental resources forms a threat to human society. The threat can be removed by sustainable development and proper use of the natural resources, which can be achieved with the help of ethnobotanical research.

Human survival on any part of the earth depends upon conservation of biodiversity resources. All types of biodiversity are overexploited. Deforestation is growing worldwide due to the overconsumption lifestyle of people. The high rate of deforestation poses a serious threat to human survival. The key to sustainable development in any forested region of the world lies in (a) empowering indigenous communities to coexist with biological diversity; (b) protecting biological wealth; (c) preventing the erosion of people's knowledge systems related to biological protection and conservation; (d) ensuring sustainable use of eco-health; (e) promoting a wider application of community knowledge, practices, and innovation related to biodiversity with their approval and participation; (f) ensuring equitable sharing of benefits arising from the utilization of indigenous knowledge systems, innovation, and practices. These basic concepts of sustainable development have been approved by the International Convention on Biological Diversity.

Different literatures were analyzed for the study of the new drug discovery, and the ancient people used certain plants for their treatment, which serves a purpose and certain chemical compounds can be identified, which is documented with the references that are used for the new drug discovery. These methods, based upon the literature study, have helped in documenting the various medicinal plants in this study.

Results

The results interpreted can be shown by the various schematic representations, flowcharts, and the tabulated formats which show how ethnobotanical knowledge is used for sustainable development. Figure 1.1 shows different fields in ethnobotany. The schematic diagram represents the interaction of the people, planet, and the plants which are working in an intersecting manner for sustainable development. This study searched various literatures to understand the role of ethnobotanical knowledge in the realization of sustainable development goals (Snyder 2019).

After a comprehensive study, seven goals related to ethnobotanical knowledge are identified which are SDG 1 (no poverty), SDG 2 (zero hunger), SDG 3 (good health and well-being), SDG 12 (responsible consumption and production), SDG 13 (climate

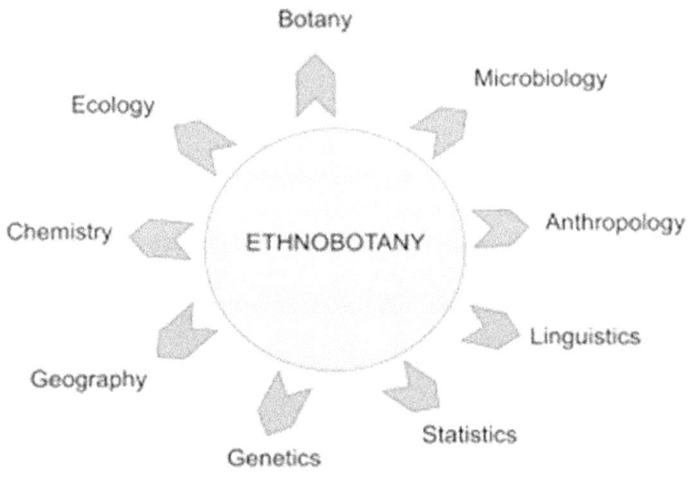

Figure 1.1. Different fields of ethnobotanical research. Source: Modified after Gaikwad et al. 2010.

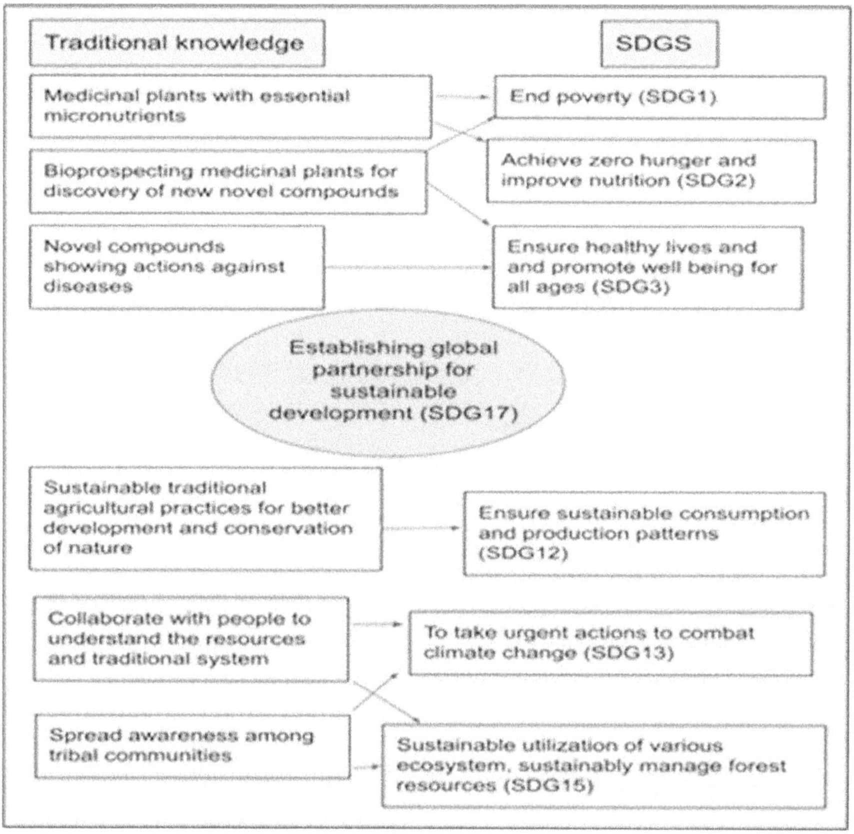

Figure 1.2. Schematic representation showing how planet and ethnobotanist remain in an interwoven way essential for the sustainable development goals. Source: Modified after Kumar et al. 2019.

action), SDG 15 (life and land), and SDG 17 (partnerships for the goals). The seven goals and their interrelationship are schematically present in Figure 1.2. Furthermore, various terms relating to sustainable development goals such as "traditional knowledge," ethnobotanical knowledge, traditional agricultural knowledge, food security, abiotic stress, climate change, end hunger, food security, medicinal plants, sustainable agriculture, climate resilience, and ethnobotanical knowledge, as well as various combinations of key terms, were searched from various database (Snyder 2019 and Kugley et al. 2017). Figure 1.3 shows the flowchart of how ethnomedicines and sustainable development are useful. Conversely, Figure 1.4 shows how ethnobotany is useful in conserving nature.

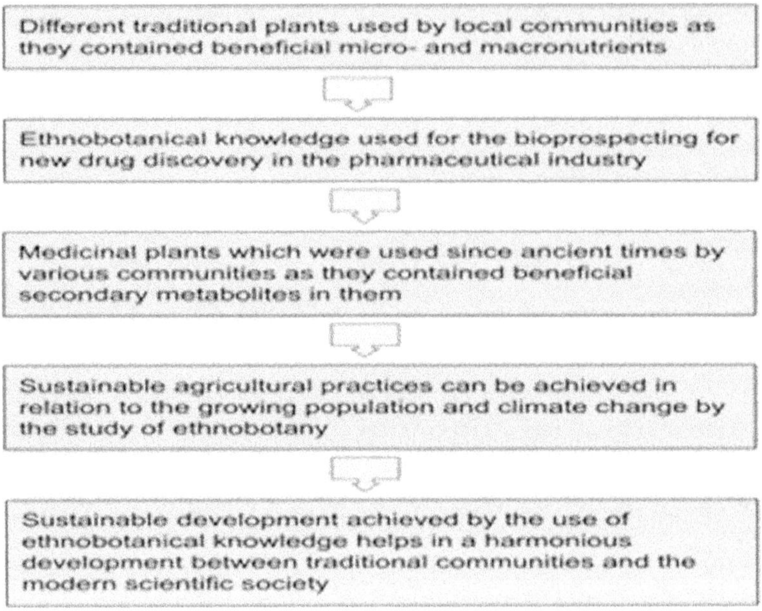

Figure 1.3. Flowchart representing the ways by which ethnobotany can help in solving various problems and achieving sustainable development. Source: Author.

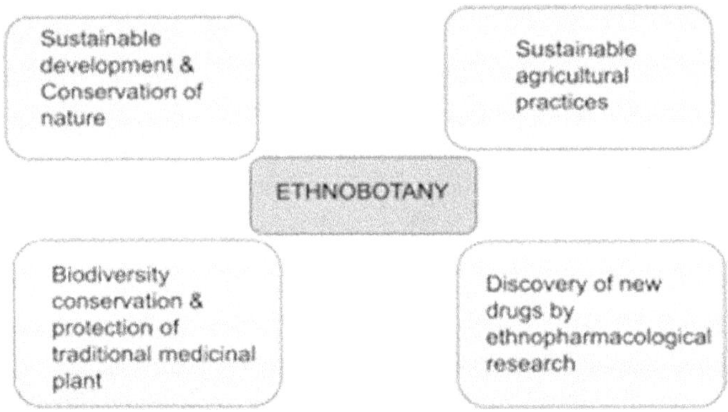

Figure 1.4. Schematic representation showing different aspects of ethnobotany and how it helps in conserving nature. Source: Author.

Discussions

In this chapter, it is seen how ethnobotany is useful in conserving nature and natural resources and helps in achieving sustainable development. Figure 1.1 shows the different branches of science and how, in an interdisciplinary way, the field of ethnobotany works.

Conversely, Figure 1.2 shows a schematic representation of the planet, people—mostly ethnobotanists and traditional healers—and the plants, which form an interactive Venn diagram. It shows that these three components are important and are interwoven and it is the responsibility of the people and the ethnobotanists to protect the environment through their proper knowledge of the plants and environment. Next, Figure 1.3 shows different positive roles of ethnobotany and its importance in many aspects. Ethnobotany helps in documenting the traditional knowledge and thus helps with the proper management of natural resources and achieving sustainable development. Knowledge about the medicinal plants is essential as it helps in documenting the traditional medicinal and aromatic plants used by various local communities. To prevent the overexploitation of these medicinal plants and to prevent the erosion of the knowledge from traditional people, ethnobotany has played an important role in documenting these plants. Thus, after proper documentation, this knowledge can be preserved, and it also helps in attaining the sustainable utilization of medicinal plants.

According to estimates by the World Health Organization (WHO), more than 80 percent of people worldwide depend upon traditional medicines. The demand for herbal medicine is growing daily, and the revitalized herbal industry has become a big business in today's global marketplace. India and China are two nations controlling the supply of herbal medicines in the global market. The scope and opportunities available for promotion of the herbal industry in the context of sustainable development and conservation of biodiversity are unlimited and bright. Proper knowledge of ethnobotany helps in new drug development, and there the role of ethnopharmacological knowledge comes, which serves as an important field in modern drug discovery in modern medical science.

Table 1.1 shows the different compounds identified from various medicinal plants by studying various literatures. Sixty different plants have been studied from various literatures, and the discovered plant compounds have been documented, which can be beneficial in modern drug discovery. These identified compounds form the base for new drug discovery, and the proper isolation of these compounds can help in combating various diseases. So, we can consider the importance of ethnobotany, the link between modern scientific society and traditional communities, which tries to harmonize them together. These aspects of ethnobotany are useful as they help in conserving nature and also help in preventing the loss of biodiversity. Preventing overexploitation and overuse of certain medicinal and aromatic plants thus causes their loss of diversity and helps in using them in a sustainable way. So, traditional ethnobotanical knowledge (TEK) and the local communities help in conserving the diversity of medicinal and aromatic plants (MAP) and also in sustainable development, which points out the main focus of present ever-changing environmental conditions.

Conclusion and Future Prospect

To sum up, new developments in ethnobotany highlight its enormous potential to revitalize our world by incorporating indigenous ecological knowledge with contemporary environmental policies and promoting sustainable development practices. Thus, this chapter shows the different aspects of ethnobotanical research. Ethnobotany is an integrative approach and comprises the various disciplines in an intermixed way. Different fields like botany, anthropology, palynology, and environmental sciences have played an important role in the development of ethnobotany. Ethnobotanical research provides valuable insights into how different plant species are used. It upholds significance not only from the ecological perspective but also from the social and cultural point of view. Ethnobotany deals with traditional medicinal knowledge and modern medicines. It forms a link between the two and helps to link a bridge between them. It is revealed from the various reviews that the knowledge of the traditional and local communities has paved a path for further documentation of important medicinal plants. This repository forms a valid document which has been utilized by modern scientists for new drug discovery.

Ethnopharmacological research helps to identify various compounds in the used plants for new and semi-synthetic drug discovery. Also, the ethnobotanical research shows how the ethnobotanist, planet, and the plants are related in an interdisciplinary way, those who work for the proper and sustainable development of the planet. For the proper conservation of nature and natural resources and the protection of the cause of the extinction of biodiversity, ethnobotany plays an important role. The knowledge of the traditional people also helps in the documentation of the various medicinal and aromatic plants used by the various communities in the treatment of various diseases. This documentation of the MAP, along with the traditional ethnobotanical knowledge (TEK), can help in conserving the various medicinal plants. Thus, it helps in conserving the biodiversity of the medicinal plants and prevents them from overexploitation and overuse. So, this study helps in the conservation of medicinal plants in various ways, like sacred gardens and medicinal plant gardens, which help in the protection and conservation of the essential medicinal plants.

The role of ethnobotanical knowledge is useful for the new drugs because herbal drugs are much more cost-effective, greener, and less toxic than the synthetic compounds used. The role of ethnobotany is useful in various aspects, as it helps in achieving sustainable development with the help of the local community, along with the TEK and the scientific community. With the continued effort of the ethnobotanist, it helps to document traditional knowledge, which helps in preventing biopiracy and also in preventing the erosion of the knowledge from society. Thus, encouraging an ethical and participatory approach to ethnobotanical research and implementation enhances indigenous communities' position as nature stewards while also honoring their intellectual legacy. By accepting these realizations, we open the door to a more resilient and greener world that blends in with its rich cultural and ecological legacy, ultimately ensuring a sustainable future for everybody. So, ethnobotanical research is interdisciplinary research which helps in many aspects to conserve nature and achieve sustainable development. Thus, preventing biodiversity loss and protecting the environment forms the key role of ethnobotanical research for a greener society and a clean environment, for the rejuvenation of mother earth.

Table 1.1. New Drugs and Compounds Obtained from Various Medicinal Plants by Ethnopharmacological Research

Sl. No.	Drug/Chemical	Plant Name	Action
1.	Acetyldigoxin	*Digitalis lanata*	Acts as cardiotonic
2.	Adoniside	*Adonis vernalis*	Acts as cardiotonic
3.	Aescin	*Aesculus hippocastanum*	Anti-inflammatory properties
4.	Aesculetin	*Frazinus rhychophylla*	Anti-dysentery
5.	Agrimophol	*Agrimonia supatoria*	Anthelminthic
6.	Ajmalicine	*Rauvolfia serpentina*	Circulatory disorder treatment
7.	Allyl isothiocyanate	*Brassica nigra*	Rubefacient
8.	Andrographolide	*Andrographis paniculata*	Hepatoprotective and dysentery protection
9.	Anisodine	*Anisodus tanguticus*	Anticholinergic
10.	Asiaticoside	*Centella asiatica*	Vulnerary in function
11.	Bromelain	*Ananas comosus*	Anti-inflammatory activity
12.	Caffeine	*Camellia sinensis*	Nervous system stimulant
13.	Codeine	*Papaver somniferum*	Analgesic, treatment of gout
14.	Colchicine	*Colchicum autumnale*	Antitumor, Antigout
15.	Convallatoxin	*Convallaria majalis*	Cardiotonic
16.	Cynarin	*Cynara scolymus*	Choleretic
17.	Danthron	*Cassia* spp.	Laxative
18.	Deserpidine	*Rauvolfia canescens*	Antihypertensive, Tranquilizer
19.	Digitoxin	*Digitalis purpurea*	Cardiotonic
20.	Emetine	*Cephaelis ipecacuanha*	Amoebicidal
21.	Ephedrine	*Ephedra sinica*	Sympathomimetic
22.	Etoposide	*Podophyllum peltatum*	Antitumor agent
23.	Gitalin	*Digitalis purpurea*	Cardiotonic
24.	Glaucarubin	*Glycyrrhiza glabra*	Amoebicide

(*Continued*)

Table 1.1 (Continued)

Sl. No.	Drug/Chemical	Plant Name	Action
25.	Gossypol	*Gossypium* spp.	Contraceptives for male
26.	Hemsleyadin	*Hemsleya amabilis*	Antibacterial dysentery
27.	Hyoscyamine	*Hyoscyamus niger*	Anticholinergic
28.	Irinotecan	*Camptotheca acuminata*	Anticancer, antitumor agent
29.	Kaibic acud	*Digenea simplex*	Ascaricide
30.	Kawain	*Piper methysticum*	Tranquilizer
31.	Kheltin	*Ammi visage*	Bronchodilator
32.	Lanatosides A, B, C	*Digitalis lanata*	Cardiotonic
33.	Lapachol	*Tabebuia species*	Anticancer, antitumor
34.	a-Lobeline	*Lobelia inflata*	Smoking deterrant, respiratory stimulant
35.	Monocrotaline	*Crotalaria sessiliflora*	Topical antitumor agent
36.	Morphine	*Papaver somniferum*	Analgesic
37.	Neoandrographolide	*Andrographis paniculata*	Treatment of dysentery
38.	Noscapine	*Papaver somniferum*	Antitussive
39.	Ouabain	*Strophanthus gratus*	Cardiotonic
40.	Papain	*Carica papaya*	Proteolytic, mucolytic
41.	Phyllodulcin	*Hydrangea macrophylla*	Sweetener
42.	Physostigmine	*Physostigma venenosum*	Cholinesterase inhibitor
43.	Picrotoxin	*Anamirta cocculus*	Analeptic
44.	Pilocarpine	*Pilocarpus jaborandi*	Parasympathomimetic
45.	Podophyllotoxin	*Podophyllum peltatum*	Antitumor, anticancer agent
46.	Protoveratrines A, B	*Veratrum album*	Antihypertensives
47.	Quinine	*Ephedra sinica*	Sympathomimetic
48.	Rescinnamine	*Rauvolfia serpentina*	Antihypertensive, tranquilizer
49.	Reserpine	*Rauvolfia serpentina*	Antihypertensive, tranquilizer

(Continued)

Table 1.1 (Continued)

Sl. No.	Drug/Chemical	Plant Name	Action
50.	Rhomitoxin	*Rhododendron molle*	Antihypertensive, tranquilizer
51.	Rorifone	*Rorippa indica*	Antitussive property
52.	Rotenone	*Lonchocarpus nicou*	Piscicide, Insecticidal property
53.	Rotundine	*Stephania sinica*	Analagesic, sedative, tranquilizer effect
54.	Salicin	*Salix alba*	Analgesic effect
55.	Santonin	*Artemisia maritma*	Ascaricide
56.	Scillarin A	*Urginea maritima*	Cardiotonic in function
57.	Scopolamine	*Datura* spp.	Sedative
58.	Sennosides A, B	*Cassia* spp.	Used as laxatives
59.	Silymarin	*Silybum marianum*	Act as antihepatotoxic drug
60.	Tetrahydropalmatine	*Corydalis ambigus*	Used as analgesic, sedatives

References

Alexiades, M. N. "Ethnobotany in the Third Millennium: Expectations and Unresolved Issues." *Delpinoa* 45, no. 1 (2003): 15–28.

Assembly, U. G. *Transforming Our World: The 2030 Agenda for Sustainable Development.* United Nations, 2015.

Balick, M. J. "Transforming Ethnobotany for the New Millennium." *Annals of the Missouri Botanical Garden* 83, no. 1 (1996): 58–66.

Basu, R. "Biodiversity and Ethnobotany of Sacred Groves in Bankura District, West Bengal." *The Indian Forester* 135, no. 6 (2009): 765–78.

Basu, R., S. Dasgupta, S. N. Babu, and A. Noor. "Medicinal Plants in the Indian Traditional Medicine and Current Practices." In *Bioprospecting of Tropical Medicinal Plants*, edited by K. Arunachalam, X. Yang, and S. Puthanpura Sasidharan, 253–86. Cham: Springer, 2023.

Bates, P., M. Chiba, S. Kube, and D. Nakashima. *Learning and Knowing in Indigenous Societies Today*, 95–105. Paris: UNESCO, 2009.

Bussmann, R. W. "Ethnobotany and Biodiversity Conservation." In *Modern Trends in Applied Terrestrial Ecology*, edited by R. S. Ambasht, and N. K. Ambasht, 343–60. Boston: Springer, 2002.

Chen, S. L., H. Yu, H. M. Luo, Q. Wu, C. F. Li, and A. Steinmetz. "Conservation and Sustainable Use of Medicinal Plants: Problems, Progress, and Prospects." *Chinese Medicine* 11, no. 37 (2016): 1–10.

Dutta, T., S. Nandy, and A. Dey. "Urban Ethnobotany of Kolkata, India: A Case Study of Sustainability, Conservation and Pluricultural Use of Medicinal Plants in Traditional Herbal Shops." *Environment, Development and Sustainability* 24, no. 1 (2022): 1207–40.

Farnsworth, N. R., O. Akerele, and A. S. Bingel. "Medicinal Plants in Therapy." *Journal of Ethnopharmacology* 19, no. 3 (1987): 336.

Gaikwad, J., K. Wilson, J. Kohen, S. Vemulpad, J. Jamie, and S. Ranganathan. "Combining Ethnobotany and Informatics to Discover Knowledge from Data." In *Ethnomedicinal Plants: Revitalization of Traditional Knowledge of Herbs*, edited by M. K. Rai, D. Acharya, J. L. Rios, 444–57. New Hampshire: Science Publishers, 2010.

Gaoue, O. G., M. A. Coe, M. Bond, G. Hart, B. C. Seyler, and H. McMillen. "Theories and Major Hypotheses in Ethnobotany." *Economic Botany* 71 (2017): 269–87.

Garnatje, T., J. Peñuelas, and J. Vallès. "Reaffirming Ethnobotanical Convergence." *Trends Plant Science* 22 (2017): 640–1.

Hawkins, J., and I. Teixidor-Toneu. "Defining Ethnobotanical Convergence." *Trends in Plant Science* 22, no. 8 (2017): 639–40.

Junaid, A., Anusooya, D., Tamilselvi, A., Suriani, I., and Rosliza, A. "The Concept of Ayurveda in Medical Science, an Indian Traditional Medicine: A Review." *International Journal of Public Health and Clinical Sciences* 4 (2017): 15–23.

Kala, C. P. "Ethnobotanical and Ecological Approaches for Conservation of Medicinal and Aromatic Plants." *Acta Horticulturae* 860 (2010): 19–26.

Kala, C. P. "Status and Conservation of Rare and Endangered Medicinal Plant in the Indian Trans-Himalaya." *Biological Conservation* 93 (2000): 371–9.

Kimerling, J. "Rio+ 10: Indigenous Peoples, Transnational Corporations and Sustainable Development in Amazonia." *Columbia Journal of Environmental Law* 27 (2002): 523.

Kugley, S., A. Wade, J. Thomas, Q. Mahood, A. K. Jørgensen, K. Hammerstrøm, and N. Sathe. "Searching for Studies: A Guide to Information Retrieval for Campbell Systematic Reviews." *Campbell Systematic Reviews* 13 (2017): 1–73.

Kumar, A., S. Kumar, Komal, N. Ramchiary, and P. Singh. "Role of Traditional Ethnobotanical Knowledge and Indigenous Communities in Achieving Sustainable Development Goals." *Sustainability* 13, no. 6 (2021): 3062.

Leaman, D. J. Medicinal *Plant Conservation, Newsletter of the Medicinal Plant Specialist Group of the IUCN Species Survival Commission*. IUCN-The World Conservation Union, 2006.

Mandal, A., S. More, M. Biswas, S. N. Mondal, S. Ray, and S. Ghosh. "Study on Secondary Metabolites of Some Ethnomedicinally Important Plants of Murshidabad District, West Bengal, India." *The Journal of Plant Science Research* 39, no. 2 (2023): 31–8.

Mehrotra, S., and B. N. Mehrotra. "Role of Traditional and Folk Lore Herbals in the Development of New Drugs." *Ethnobotany* 17 (2005): 104–11.

Mukherjee, P. K., and A. Wahile. "Integrated Approaches towards Drug Development from Ayurveda and Other Indian System of Medicines." *Journal of Ethnopharmacology* 103, no. 1 (2006): 25–35.

Nyasimi, M., and L. Peake. *Review of Targets for the* Sustainable Development Goals: *The Science Perspective*. Paris: International Council of Science and International Social Science Council, 2015.

Pandey, A. K., and Y. C. Tripathi. "Ethnobotany and Its Relevance in Contemporary Research." *Journal of Medicinal Plants Studies* 5, no. 3 (2017): 123–9.

Parris, T. M., and R. W. Kates. "Characterizing and Measuring Sustainable Development." *Annual Review of Environment and Resources* 28, no. 1 (2003): 559–86.
Pei, S., H. Alan, and Y. Wang. "Vital Roles for Ethnobotany in Conservation and Sustainable Development." *Plant Diversity* 42, no. 6 (2020): 399–400.
Prance, G. T. "Ethnobotany, the Science of Survival: A Declaration from Kaua'i." *Economic Botany* 61, no. 1 (2007): 1–2.
Pushpangadan, P., V. George, T. Ijinu, and M. A. Chithra. "Ethnomedicine, Health Food and Nutraceuticals-Traditional Wisdom of Maternal and Child Health in India." *Edelweiss Applied Science and Technology* 2, no. 1 (2018): 113–17.
Saha, D., M. Sundriyal, and R. C. Sundriyal. "Diversity of Food Composition and Nutritive Analysis of Edible Wild Plants in a Multi-ethnic Tribal Land, Northeast India: An Important Facet for Food Supply." *Indian Journal of Traditional Knowledge* 13, no. 4 (2014): 698–705.
Snyder, H. "Literature Review as a Research Methodology: An Overview and Guidelines." *Journal of Business Research*, 104 (2019): 333–9.
Sultana, R., N. Muhammad, and A. K. M. Zakaria. "Role of Indigenous Knowledge in Sustainable Development." *International Journal of Development Research* 8, no. 2 (2018): 18902–6.
United Nations. *Documentation, Reference, and Terminology Section.* Environment and Development, Vol. 2. New York: UN, 1992.
Van den Berg, L., R. Drewett, and L. H. Klaassen. *A Study of Growth and Decline: Urban Europe*. Elsevier: Pergamon Press, 2013.
Zhao, Y., Z. Yang, B. Lang, M. S. W. Meng, D. Xue, L. Gao, and L. Yang. "Skincare Plants of the Naxi of NW Yunnan, China." *Plant Diversity* 42, no. 6 (2020): 473–8.

2

Ethnomedicinal Knowledge among the Tribal Communities to Sustain the Economy and Socio-Environmental Infrastructure

Barsha Majumder*

Department of Botany, Netaji Nagar College for Women, Kolkata, West Bengal, India

*Corresponding Author's Email: barshamjmdr@gmail.com

Introduction

The study of interrelationships among nature, humans, and society has profound applications in various fields, namely, biodiversity conservation, food security, and human health, and has recently become significantly acknowledged. Human well-being and civilization depend on the adequate utilization and proper management of the resources around them, which leads to the prevention of biodiversity loss (Alves and Rosa 2007). Recently, the harmonious lifestyle of the indigenous people and tribal communities who are used to living in and around forest ecosystem is hampered due to immoderate utilization of plants and disrupted interrelationships between animals and plants with human beings that led to the destabilization of these precious traditional culture, lifestyle, and knowledge system (Schultes 1992; Pushpangadan 2005). An awareness of biodiversity and the unending utilization of medicinal plants, especially by indigenous people, support ecotourism, ecological progress, and sustainable development which helps to maintain ecological steadiness in nature and escalates the living standards of local inhabitants (Jarić et al. 2024). In Rio Earth Summit (1992), agenda 21, it was mentioned that sustainable development is a prerequisite for the management of environment for indigenous people and associated local communities because of their traditional ethnobotanical knowledge (TEK). To meet the sustainable development goals (SDGs), a balance between ecosystem resistance toward adverse conditions and social equity is essential that should be governed by civil society, governments, and different business firms (Sachs et al. 2019; Silvestre and Tîrca 2019; Kumar et al. 2021a).

A comprehensive interaction between humans and their surrounding ecosystem nourishes ethnobotanical knowledge through their cultural history, communication skills, religion and beliefs, regional classification system, and social network (Maffi 2005; Pieroni 2005; Bandiera and Rasul 2006; Ellen 2009). In recent times, decline in TEK has gained alarming global importance, resulting in altered eating habits, imbalanced lifestyles of human beings, and their relationship with the surrounding ecosystem, which has also disrupted local medical practices, health, and well-being. Plants have been used by people for several reasons, namely, medicine, food, building construction, shelter, textiles, ornamentation, and decoration, especially by indigenous people and regional communities because of their traditional ethnobotanical knowledge, which is scarcely documented and transferred mostly orally from generation to generation (Garnatje, Peñuelas, and Vallès 2017; Jarić et al. 2024). Sharma et al. (2009) documented in their findings that leaves are most commonly used as a prime ingredient of herbal ointments in comparison to other parts of the plants, which is in accordance with the study of Ignacimuthu, Ayyanar, and Sankarasivaraman (2006) where medicinal utilization of leaves was reported for the treatment of a plethora of serious health illnesses.

Objectives and Methods

Both scientific and systematic inspections of ethnomedicinal plants have provided key compositions of several important drugs in the Western medicine system (Thakur et al. 2014). According to WHO, around 80 percent of the world's population depends on an ethnomedicinal system, and herbal plants constitute a prerequisite part of the world's economy due to the emergence of most ingredients of modern medicines from these medicinal plants (Kumar et al. 2021). Kunwar and Bussmann 2008 reported that the study of ethnobotany has profound significance in different parts of the world with respect to conservation of this traditional knowledge before folktales are lost forever. This present study intends to highlight the recent state of ethnomedicines and ethnobotanical research as a result of environmental changes and incorporates the value of ethnomedicine in both rural and urban areas as a basic healthcare system and how to conserve traditional ethnobotanical knowledge that would assist in comprehending the manufacturing of modern-day medicines for acute disease management. Besides, this study is concerned with the development of indigenous knowledge about herbal plants for sustainable human health to mitigate several aspects of environmental stresses on human lifestyle occurring in recent decades that will lead to an increase in interest in clinical and nonclinical use of plants related to physical and mental health of human beings. Additionally, with the upsurge of ethnomedicinal research, the efficiency of herbal plants needs to be standardized and validated in the laboratory by understanding the mode of action of their principal bioactive ingredients which have become the most significant resources for pharmaceutical industries.

Medicinal Plants and Indigenous Communities

About 16,000 species of higher groups of plants are present in India, of which around 7,500 plant species are utilized for health treatment as a part of ethnomedicine by several indigenous communities (Arora 1987). It has been noted that North East India, principally comprised of Nagaland, Arunachal Pradesh, Meghalaya, Tripura, Assam, Manipur, Sikkim, and Mizoram, is the native land for plenty of ethnic groups, namely, Khasi, Naga, Mishing, Abor, Apatani, and Rabha, which are characterized by various sociocultural traditions and utilize approximately 1,963 plants for ethnomedicinal purposes to heal several diseases (Kala 2005; Sajem and Gosai 2006; Bhuyan 2015). Likewise, in Uttarakhand, well-known for its diverse forest types, which cover around 12.18 percent of the Indian Himalaya, and ethnic communities, namely, Tharu, Bhotia, Garhwali, and Jaunsari, people utilize the resources of natural forests for their primary health treatment and disease management (Uniyal 2003; Kala, Farooquee, and Dhar 2004). In the present study, a few common medicinal plants that are very useful for different indigenous communities of North East India are represented in Table 2.1.

Table 2.1. Various Medicinal Plants Utilized by Indigenous Communities of North East India

Medicinal Plants	Parts Used	Utilization For	Communities	Sources
Argemone mexicana L. (Family: Papaveraceae)	Leaves	Malaria, Jaundice, and Leprosy	Bodo-Kachari	Basumatary, Teron, and Saikia 2014
Calotropis gigantea L (Family: Apocynaceae)	Leaves	Swelling of liver and Dog Bite	Bodo-Kachari and Apatani	Kala 2005; Basumatary, Teron, and Saikia 2014
Oroxylum indicum (L) vent (Family: Bignoniaceae)	Stem, bark	Diarrhea and Dysentery	Chutia	Borah, Borah, and Nath 2012
	Flower, Seed	To cure burns	Nepali, Lepcha, and Bhutia	Idrisi, Badola, and Singh 2010
Amomum aromaticum Roxb. (Family: Zingiberaceae)	Fruits	To cure cough, fever, pox and in case of abortion	Bodo-Kachari and Apatani	Kala 2005; Basumatary, Teron, and Saikia 2014
Centella asiatica L. (Family: Apiaceae)	Whole Plant	Leprosy, Tuberculosis, and Asthma	Lushai	Sajem and Gosai 2006
Curcuma longa L. (Family: Zingiberaceae)	Rhizome	To counteract dyspepsia	Lushai	Sajem and Gosai 2010
		Used as an antiseptic in wounds and cuts for blood clotting	Adi-Miniyong	Baruah et al. 2013

(*Continued*)

Table 2.1 (Continued)

Medicinal Plants	Parts Used	Utilization For	Communities	Sources
Terminalia chebula Retz. (Family: Combretaceae)	Fruit, Bark	Indigestion, Fever, and Diarrhea	Nepali, Lepcha, and Bhutia	Idrisi, Badola, and Singh 2010
	Seed	Asthma	Chutia	Borah, Borah, and Nath 2012
Paederia foetida (L) (Family: Rubiaceae)	Stem	Diarrhea, Gastritis, Stomach Disorder	Apatani	Kala 2005
	Leaves	Skin Diseases	Adi-Miniyong	Baruah et al. 2013
Clerodendrum Viscosum vent (Family: Lamiaceae)	Leaves	Asthma, Diabetes, and High Blood Pressure	Jaintia	Sajem and Gosai 2006
Houttuynia cordata Thunb (Family: Saururaceae)	Leaves	Bodyache	Santal and Goreswar	Das et al. 2006
	Root, Leaves	Treatment for Amoebic Dysentery	Tribes of Meghalaya	Lahoo and Hemalatha 2011
Murraya Koenigii (L) Spreng (Family: Rutaceae)	Leaves	Stomach problem	Apatani	Kala 2005
		High fever	Bodo-Kachari	Basumatary, Teron, and Saikia 2014

Source: Author.

Rationalization of Ethnobotany

Rationalization of ethnobotanical study relies on the potentiality of traditional knowledge systems to integrate both scientific and local information regarding the use of plants as medicine to achieve the goal of biocultural conservation, which focuses mostly on in-depth research of pharmacological implications of medicinal herbs used by indigenous people and local communities (Prance 2007; Gaoue et al. 2017). The degree of global warming is rapidly elevating, even in high-altitude areas, resulting in irreparable adversities with respect to alterations in types and growth of vegetation, species, and their habitats (Liu and Chen 2000; McCarty 2001). Different plant species, especially the indigenous plants, reflect their responses to climatic change by reducing species diversity or by transposing their habitats (Parmesan and Yohe 2003; Krajick 2004). The modulations in the structure, posture, habitats, and species diversity of native medicinal plants are threatened by environmental changes, leading to severe impact on surrounding communities (Shrestha et al. 1999; Cavaliere 2009).

The interconnection between human well-being and the environment may be seen with respect to sustained good health of local communities that are mainly based on sustainable use and management of social resources, climate regulation, and natural ecosystems (McMichael and Beaglehole 2000). Additionally, the changes in ecosystems and their influence on indigenous people and local communities have a direct effect on traditional knowledge of native medicinal plants (Pirker et al. 2012). Ethnomedicine, which is often termed traditional medicine (TM), is principally used to refer to Indian Ayurvedic medicine, several types of indigenous medicine, Unani medicine, as well as traditional Chinese medicine (Alves and Rosa 2007). It is well-known that ethnomedicine plays a pivotal role in the health care of the large population of low- and middle-income countries (LMIC) in addition to indigenous people. These traditional medicines have been widely utilized as efficient health treatments in different cultures for a long time. Moreover, ethnomedicine was the only prime trusted means of various disease management systems to people in every aspect of life, namely, socioeconomic, health, well-being, culture, and communication, and has existed before the conventional medicine system (Wanzala, Wekesa, and Minyoso 2023; WHO 2023a).

In 1978, the World Health Organization (WHO), in association with the United Nations Children's Fund (UNICEF), acknowledged ethnomedicine as a vital constituent to be used by states and governments of the twentieth century to attain a disease-free health system for different populations by 2000, especially in underdeveloped countries (Wanzala and Minyoso 2024). Plethora of ethnopharmaceutical systems developed by local indigenous communities, namely, Unani medicine, traditional Chinese medicine, ancient Greek medicine, Ayurveda, ancient Iranian medicine, herbal medicine, Siddha medicine, Persian traditional medicine, American traditional herbal medicine, Georgian folk medicine, integrative medicine, Japanese Kampo medicine, ancient Egyptian medicine, Celtic traditional medicine, Arabic indigenous medicine, Islamic medicine, traditional African medicine, acupuncture, anthroposophic medicine, traditional Korean medicine, quackery medical practices, magical medical practices, and homeopathy have been employed by governments, international communities, and states to fulfill the target set by WHO/UNICEF in 1978 (Heinrich 2010; Wanzala et al. 2012; Wanzala and Walingo 2019; Wanzala and Minyoso 2024).

Although ethnomedicine has very few limitations because of its ineffectiveness for some deadly ailments, such as cancer, kidney disease, and pancreatitis, these are major warnings to this indigenous knowledge. Mainly, ethnomedicines are employed in common cough, cold, fever, jaundice, joint pain, and gastric problems. In rural areas, most people rely on agriculture for their existence and are characterized by different traditional ethnobotanical knowledge of curing ailments by using forest resources (Uniyal 2003). Conversely, lack of documentation regarding ethnomedicine practice by healers leads to the neglect of ethnomedicine in the present generation (Chakraborty, Roy, and Mandal 2016). The utilization of these traditional resources plays a predominant role in the sustenance of local communities and maintains a steady income for many tribal households (Schippmann, Leaman, and Cunningham 2002).

It has been found that the current market for herbal medicine is estimated at forty billion and expected to elevate by around 16 percent in the next four to five years, but the collection of many herbal drugs failed to attain the required amount of market, which resulted in the addition of adulterants in the Ayurvedic drugs to maintain profit level (Semwal et al. 2019). The traditional knowledge about the conservation of herbal plants and their usefulness has developed awareness regarding environmental conservation (Cameron 2008). However, in recent days, the practice of ethnomedicine has been significantly reduced even in the same places where the concept of using native plants as herbal medicines emerged and was nurtured by generation after generation of tribal and local communities. This reduction is caused by the preferences of people toward allopathic medicines over ethnomedicines, despite the fact of possible side effects of the former that will eventually lead to the loss of precious and traditional knowledge about the medicinal plants used in both rural areas and developing countries for disease management (Harsha et al. 2002).

Environmental Change and Human Health

Environmental changes can impact human health in many ways, including climate change, air pollution, and exposure to chemicals. Climate change can increase the risk of extreme heat waves, heavy storms, and flooding. This climate change can increase the amount of ground-level ozone, which can damage lung tissue and aggravate asthma. Again, the rising temperatures can lead to more heat-related deaths and illnesses. Besides, this climate change can change the spread of diseases carried by ticks and mosquitoes. Thus, every year environmental changes disrupt ecosystem balance, resulting in biodiversity loss, thousands of deaths worldwide, and are responsible for the origin of multiple categories of human diseases (Haines et al. 2006; Confalonieri et al. 2007). Such loss of biodiversity leads to less resilient habitat for medicinal plants and will not be capable of supplying required health care to people during their need. Biodiversity loss in terms of disappearance of medicinal plant species due to environmental changes also has deleterious effects on the supply of raw material in pharmaceutical industries, leads to spreading of ailments, and threatens human lives significantly (Chivian 2002). The alterations in biodiversity and forest resources have been widely documented, but very few studies have paid attention to their severe impact on human well-being (Di Napoli et al. 2022).

It has been observed that ethnomedicinal plants are very susceptible to current environmental crises, namely, alteration in vegetation types, savannahs, and growth of forest that have adverse effects on the cost of herbal medicine (Anyinam 1995). Moreover, in current days, forest degradation due to environmental factors and climate change, especially in the Brazilian Amazon, has impacted the availability of various medicinal plants, which eventually resulted in reduction in the production of potent pharmaceutical drugs and severely affected the healthcare options for different Brazilian ethnic communities as well as for urban people (Shanley and Luz 2003). In our country, environmental change, primarily driven by climate change, significantly affects human health through increased heat stress, altered vector-borne disease patterns (like malaria, dengue), air pollution, waterborne infections, and disturbances to food security, particularly affecting vulnerable populations due to existing poor sanitation and malnutrition conditions; these impacts can lead to increased morbidity and mortality, especially from respiratory and cardiovascular diseases. These types of environmental changes in India are significantly impacting the practice of ethnomedicine, primarily due to the dwindling availability of medicinal plants caused by deforestation, climate change, and unsustainable harvesting practices, which are crucial to traditional healing systems like Ayurveda, leading to concerns about the preservation of this knowledge and access to vital remedies for indigenous communities.

Ethnomedicine and Tribal Health

Long time ago, during the origin of life on earth, man-made ecosystems were developed to satisfy different types of requirements along with socioeconomic needs of which fitness of the body, healthcare, and disease management became prerequisites for their survival (Tripathi and Panigrahi 2017). Since prehistoric times, our early ancestors utilized the natural world for gathering food, hunting, shelter, and for disease curative purposes by identifying various plants and their useful parts (Alves and Rosa 2012; Rekka, Murugesh, and Prabakaran 2013). In India, other than Allopathy, various ancient medical systems of healing exist, namely, Siddha, Unani, Ayurveda, Homeopathy, and Naturopathy, along with the treatment of disease with ethnomedicinal plants by tribal communities, of which Ayurveda is known as the oldest system of disease management, having emerged first during the Vedic period (Magner 2005; Tripathi 2019). In India, more than 70 percent of people believe in herbal treatment of ailments where around 15,000 plant species have been identified as ethnomedicine and utilized by both tribal and herbal medical practitioners (Vaidya and Devasagayam 2007; Dhamija, Parashar, and Singh 2011). Tribal communities prefer to settle near forest ecosystems where they can evaluate the medicinal properties of the native plants and utilize them for their disease management purposes (Tripathi 2017).

Several indigenous tribes and communities of India have their own beliefs related to illness, health, and medicine. They often possess deep knowledge about medicinal plants and practices passed down through generations, which are studied under the field of ethnomedicine. The "tribal healers" or "ethno-physicians" are individuals within a community who hold expertise in traditional medicine and diagnose and treat ailments using local remedies. Thus, ethnomedicine refers to the study of traditional healing practices and beliefs related to health and illness within a specific ethnic or tribal community, often relying on locally available plants, animals, and minerals to treat various ailments, essentially encompassing the indigenous medical knowledge of a particular group of people; while "tribal health" specifically focuses on the overall health status and medical needs of indigenous or tribal communities, often including access to healthcare, disease patterns, and the role of traditional medicine within their culture. Various factors like geographic isolation, limited access to modern healthcare, poverty, and cultural barriers can significantly impact the health of tribal communities. Sharma et al. (2014) reported that the use of tribal medicine and their traditional formulations have always been associated with the social life of indigenous communities and found to be intensely useful in handling adverse situations caused by different diseases and gynecological problems. Reliance of tribal communities on medicinal plants elevated due to scarcity of other healthcare systems present in their households; as a result, the rural population included traditional ethnomedicinal knowledge in their decision-making procedures for a greater level of disease management (Kumar et al. 2021). Additionally, evaluation of toxicity of these ethnomedicinal products should be checked prior to their use by indigenous people and the transmission of knowledge to others (Zhou et al. 2013).

In present times, deforestation, rapid changes in urbanization, and displacement of people to different places modulate cultural settings, loss of medicinal plants, and reduction in traditional knowledge in local communities, especially surrounding Himalayan regions, that eventually lead to a disorganized way of knowledge transmission to the new generation and disturb the ethnomedicinal practices (Roy Burman 1982; Bhattarai, Chaudhary, and Taylor 2006). This state of eradication of traditional ethnomedicinal knowledge of a particular region can be mitigated by proper documentation by herbal practitioners, and the influence of tribal medicine in disease management should be highly recognized at both national and regional levels. Rokaya et al. (2014) proposed that the new generation should get detailed education regarding ethnomedicinal practices that will provide a significant effect on the sustainability of traditional knowledge about medicinal plants. Additionally, there is an intense need to develop a database where crucial information will be stored regarding the collection, habitats, identifying characters, along with the usage of medicinal plants for future research and to manufacture potent herbal medicines as it is adversely decreasing because of the influence of modern pharmaceutical medicines (Singh et al. 2017; Tripathi 2019).

Ethnobotany, Ethnomedicine, and Sustainable Development

Ethnobotany plays a critical role in drug discovery, conservation, and sustainable development. By valuing traditional knowledge and integrating it with modern practices, we can enhance health outcomes, preserve biodiversity, and empower communities. In other words, ethnobotany is known as the science of existence, and it can conserve biodiversity in terms of sustenance of local and indigenous knowledge of medicinal plants, where different ethnic communities have acquired innovative practices to maintain their plant diversity and resources. Throughout the world, different types of documentation regarding collection and employment of herbal plants for multiple disease management, which are provided by traditional healers and indigenous healthcare practitioners, have become one of the promising topics of ethnobotany. Several ethnobotanical researches have been published, of which few are documented in the present study to justify the influence of ethnobotanical study in conservation of ethnomedicinal practices and sustainable development. Study of Xiong et al. (2020) exhibited in their article that in eastern Yunnan, about 121 plant species were used formerly for disease management by the Buyi community of Luoping County, but many of them have not been listed in any literature, leading to disappearance of ethnomedicinal knowledge of the Buyi community. The authors suggested a few schemes to regain and restore this knowledge using the aforementioned plants in severe ailments.

Similarly, another ethnobotanical study of Zhejiang Province, China, documented the use of about 129 plant species comprising 75 families and 113 genera for treating almost thirty-one types of diseases (Liu et al. 2020). They also reported that in recent days, the use of these medicinal plants declined significantly along with the reduction in transmission of traditional knowledge regarding the ethnomedicinal properties of native plants in Qingtian, and they also provide protective measures to stabilize the rich store of that ethnic knowledge that will escalate the interest of indigenous communities to preserve native medicinal plants. In East Asia, a traditional medicinal plant—*Cistanche deserticola* is utilized as a tonic in different medicine systems, namely, Mongolian Medicine, Traditional Chinese Medicine (TCM), Tibetan Medicine, and so on, where about ninety-six plant species of the *Cistanche* community have been documented as an important resource in ethnomedicine of Mongolia and can be very useful for formulating different techniques for plant biodiversity preservation (Mandakh et al. 2020).

In addition to the ethnobotanical research articles that documented the way out to conserve medicinal plant biodiversity for sustainable development, different herbal markets also play a predominant role in the usage of medicinal plants along with the distribution of related knowledge. In Kahramanmaras, Turkey, about sixty-two plants are traded, and almost 50 percent of plant species are globally threatened due to overutilization of these species owing to increased demand in the market (Palabas Uzun and Koca 2020). Kathambi, Mutie, and Rono (2020) reported an ethnobotanical research study performed in Kenya where around 214 plant species, composed of seventy-three families, having medicinal properties have been documented with the hope that this documentation will enhance the value of indigenous plant resources among people, help in proper sustenance and conservation of herbal plants, along with the restoration of traditional knowledge about ethnomedicine among local inhabitants.

Conclusion and Recommendation

Traditional ethnobotanical knowledge should be conserved for future generations as the use of ethnomedicine involves sustainable utilization of natural resources by human beings and can be used as a remedy to overexploitation of natural resources for the existence of lives. In the present decades, significant alteration in environmental conditions dramatically influenced vegetation growth of a specific geographical region, resulting in biodiversity loss. Hence, with a view to keep our planet green, we need to follow traditional ethnic culture, especially by using medicinal plants for major health care purposes, which provide routes for sustainable development by restricted and balanced utilization of natural resources.

In order to achieve the goal of sustainable development, it is a prerequisite to document the traditional knowledge in the form of universal databases regarding the sustainable use of medicinal plants, conservation of biodiversity, ethnic cultures along with general properties and identifying characters of folk medicines that have progressed over the centuries. This digitization process could be utilized by modern scientists after further study in the field of pharmacology to inspect the key components of ethnomedicines and medicinal plants which are responsible for curing several ailments of indigenous and local tribal communities, so that it will help to develop side effects-free modern medicine for safer human consumption.

References

Alves, R. R. N., and I. L. Rosa. *Animals in Traditional Folk Medicine: Implications for Conservation.* Berlin Heidelberg: Springer, 2012.

Alves, R. R. N., and I. M. L. Rosa. "Biodiversity, Traditional Medicine and Public Health: Where Do They Meet?" *Journal of Ethnobiology and Ethnomedicine* 3, no. 14 (2007): 1–9.

Anyinam, C. "Ecology and Ethnomedicine: Exploring Links between Current Environmental Crisis and Indigenous Medical Practices." *Social Science & Medicine* 40, no. 3 (1995): 321–9.

Arora, R. K. "Ethnobotany and Its Role in the Conservation and Use of the Genetic Resources in India." *Ethnobotany* 9 (1987): 6–15.

Bandiera, O., and I. Rasul. "Social Networks and Technology Adoption in Northern Mozambique." *The Economic Journal* 116, no. 514 (2006): 869–902.

Baruah, S., S. K. Borthakur, P. Gogoi, and M. Ahmed. "Ethnomedicinal Plants Used by Adi-Miniyong Tribe of Arunachal Pradesh, Eastern Himalaya." *Indian Journal of Natural Products and Resources* 4, no. 3 (2013): 278–82.

Basumatary, N., R. Teron, and M. Saikia. "Ethnomedicinal Practices of the Bodo-Kachari Tribe of Karbi Anglong District of Assam." *International Journal of Life Sciences Biotechnology and Pharma Research* 3, no. 1 (2014): 161–7.

Bhattarai, S., R. P. Chaudhary, and R. S. L. Taylor. "Ethnomedicinal Plants Used by the People of Manang District, Central Nepal." *Journal of Ethnobiology and Ethnomedicine* 2 (2006): 41.

Bhuyan, M. "Comparative Study of Ethnomedicine among the Tribes of North East India." *International Research Journal of Social Sciences* 4, no. 2 (2015): 27–32.

Borah, S. M., L. Borah, and S. C. Nath. "Ethnomedicinal Plants from Disoi Valley Reserve Forest of Jorhat District, Assam." *Plant Sciences Feed* 2, no. 4 (2012): 59–63.

Cameron, M. M. "Modern Desires, Knowledge Control, and Physician Resistance: Regulating Ayurvedic Medicine in Nepal." *Asian Medicine* 4, no. 1 (2008): 86–112.

Cavaliere, C. "The Effects of Climate Change on Medicinal and Aromatic Plants." *Herbalgram* 81 (2009): 44–57.

Chakraborty, A., S. S. Kosariya, and M. Chakravarty. "A Review of Ethnomedicinal Practices for Gynaecological Disorders among the Various Tribes of Chhattisgarh." *IOSR- Journal of Environmental Science, Toxicology and Food Technology* 1, no. 2 (2016): 55–62.

Chakraborty, R., S. Roy, and V. Mandal. "Assessment of Traditional Knowledge of the Antidiabetic Plants of Darjeeling and Sikkim Himalayas in the Context of Recent Phytochemical and Pharmacological Advances." *Journal of Integrative Medicine* 14 (2016): 336–58.

Chivian, E. *Biodiversity: Its Importance to Human Health Center for Health and the Global Environment*. Harvard Medical School, 2002.

Confalonieri, U., B. Menne, R. Akhtar, K. L. Ebi, M. Hauengue, R. S. Kovats, B. Revich, A. Woodward, M. L. Parry, O. F. Canziani, J. P. Palutikof, P. J. V. Linden, and C. E. Hanson. *Human Health. Climate Change: Impacts, Adaptation and Vulnerability*. Contribution of Working Group II to the Fourth Assessment Report of the Intergovernmental Panel on Climate Change. Cambridge University Press, Cambridge, 2007.

Das, N. J., S. P. Saikia, S. Sarkar, and K. Devi. "Medicinal Plants of North-Kamrup District of Assam Used in Primary Healthcare System." *Indian Journal of Traditional Knowledge* 5, no. 4 (2006): 489–93.

Dhamija, H. K., B. Parashar, and J. Singh. "Anti-depression Potential of Herbal Drugs: An Overview." *Journal of Chemical and Pharmaceutical Research* 3, no. 5 (2011): 725–35.

Di Napoli, C., A. McGushin, M. Romanello, S. Ayeb-Karlsson, W. Cai, J. Chambers, S. Dasgupta, L. E. Escobar, I. Kelman, T. Kjellstrom, D. Kniveton, Y. Liu, Z. Liu, R. Lowe, J. Martinez-Urtaza, C. McMichael, M. Moradi-Lakeh, K. A. Murray, M. Rabbaniha, J. C. Semenza, L. Shi, M. Tabatabaei, J. A. Trinanes, B. N. Vu, C. Brimicombe, and E. J. Robinson. "Tracking the Impacts of Climate Change on Human Health via Indicators: Lessons from the Lancet Countdown." *BMC Public Health* 22 (2022): 663.

Ellen, R. F. *Classification*. Routledge Encyclopedia of Social and Cultural Anthropology. London: Routledge, 2009.

Gaoue, O. G., M. A. Coe, M. Bond, G. Hart, B. C. Seyler, and H. McMillen. "Theories and Major Hypotheses in Ethnobotany." *Economic Botany* 71 (2017): 269–87.

Garnatje, T., J. Peñuelas, and J. Vallès. "Reaffirming 'Ethnobotanical Convergence.'" *Trends in Plant Science* 22 (2017): 640–1.

Haines, A., R. S. Kovats, D. Campbell-Lendrum, and C. Corvalan. "Climate Change and Human Health: Impacts, Vulnerability and Public Health." *Public Health* 120, no. 7 (2006): 585–96.

Harsha, V. H., S. S. Hebbar, G. R. Hegde, and V. Shripathi. "Ethnomedical Knowledge of Plants Used by Kunabi Tribe of Karnataka in India." *Fitoterapia* 73 (2002): 281–7.

Heinrich, M. "Ethnopharmacology in the 21st Century – Grand Challenges." *Frontiers in Pharmacology* 1 (2010): 8.

Idrisi, M. S., H. K. Badola, and R. Singh. "Indigenous Knowledge and Medicinal Use of Plants by Local Communities in Ranjit Valley, South Sikkim, India." *NeBOI* 1, no. 2 (2010): 34–5.

Ignacimuthu, S., M. Ayyanar, and K. Sankarasivaraman. "Ethnobotanical Investigations among Tribes in Madurai District of Tamil Nadu (India)." *Journal of Ethnobiology and Ethnomedicine* 2 (2006): 25.

Jarić, S., O. Kostić, Z. Miletić, M. Marković, D. Sekulić, M. Mitrović, and P. Pavlović. "Ethnobotanical and Ethnomedicinal Research into Medicinal Plants in the Mt Stara Planina Region (South-Eastern Serbia, Western Balkans)." *Journal of Ethnobiology and Ethnomedicine* 20 (2024): 7.

Kala, C. P. "Ethnomedicinal Botany of the Apatani in the Eastern Himalayan Region of India." *Journal of Ethnobiology and Ethnomedicine* 1 (2005): 11.

Kala, C. P., N. A. Farooquee, and U. Dhar. "Prioritization of Medicinal Plants on the Basis of Available Knowledge, Existing Practices and Use Value Status in Uttaranchal, India." *Biodiversity and Conservation* 13 (2004): 453–69.

Kathambi, V., F. M. Mutie, and P. C. Rono. "Traditional Knowledge, Use and Conservation of Plants by the Communities of Tharaka-Nithi County, Kenya." *Plant Diversity* 42 (2020): 479–87.

Krajick, K. "All Downhill from Here?" *Science* 303, no. 5664 (2004): 1600–2.

Kumar, A., S. Kumar, Komal, N. Ramchiary, and P. Singh. "Role of Traditional Ethnobotanical Knowledge and Indigenous Communities in Achieving Sustainable Development Goals." *Sustainability* 13, no. 6 (2021a): 1–14.

Kumar, M., S. Rawat, B. Nagar, A. Kumar, N. A. Pala, J. A. Bhat, R. W. Bussmann, M. Cabral-Pinto, and R. Kunwar. "Implementation of the Use of Ethnomedicinal Plants for Curing Diseases in the Indian Himalayas and Its Role in Sustainability of Livelihoods and Socioeconomic Development." *International Journal of Environmental Research and Public Health* 18, no. 4 (2021b): 1509.

Kunwar, R. M., and R. W. Bussmann. "Ethnobotany in the Nepal Himalaya." *Journal of Ethnobiology and Ethnomedicine* 4, no. 24 (2008): 1–8.

Lahoo, D., and S. Hemalatha. "Ethnomedicinal Plants Used for Diarrhea by Tribals of Meghalaya." *Pharmacognosy Reviews* 5, no. 10 (2011): 147–54.

Liu, X., and B. Chen. "Climatic Warming in the Tibetan Plateau during Recent Decades." *International Journal of Climatology* 20, no. 14 (2000): 1729–42.

Liu, Y., R. Hu, S. Shen, Z. Zhang, J. Zhang, X. Song, and S. Qiang. "Plant Diversity on Herbal Tea and its Traditional Knowledge in Qingtian County, Zhejiang Province, China." *Plant Diversity* 42 (2020): 464–72.

Maffi, L. "Linguistic, Cultural, and Biological Diversity." *Annual Review of Anthropology* 34 (2005): 599–617.

Magner, L. N. *A History of Medicine*. Florida: Taylor and Francis group, 2005.

Mandakh, U., M. Battseren, D. Ganbat, T. Ayanga, Z. Adiya, A. Borjigidai, and L. Chunlin. "Folk Nomenclature of Plants in *Cistanche deserticola* – Associated Community in South Gobi, Mongolia." *Plant Diversity* 42, no. 6 (2020): 434–42.

McCarty, J. P. "Ecological Consequences of Recent Climate Change." *Conservation Biology* 15, no. 2 (2001): 320–31.

McMichael, A. J., and R. Beaglehole. "The Changing Global Context of Public Health." *Lancet* 356 (2000): 495–9.

Palabas Uzun, S., and C. Koca. "Ethnobotanical Survey of Medicinal Plants Traded in Herbal Markets of Kahramanmaras." *Plant Diversity*, 42 (2020): 443–54.

Parmesan, C., and G. Yohe. "A Globally Coherent Fingerprint of Climate Change Impacts across Natural Systems." *Nature* 421, no. 6918 (2003): 37–42.

Pieroni, A., and C. Quave. "Traditional Pharmacopoeias and Medicines among Albanians and Italians in Southern Italy: A Comparison." *Journal of Ethnopharmacology* 101 (2005): 258–70.

Pirker, H., R. Haselmair, E. Kuhn, C. Schunko, and C. R. Vogl. "Transformation of Traditional Knowledge of Medicinal Plants: The Case of Tyroleans (Austria) Who Migrated to Australia, Brazil and Peru." *Journal of Ethnobiology and Ethnomedicine* 8 (2012): 2–26.

Prance, G. T. "Ethnobotany, the Science of Survival: A Declaration from Kaua'I." *Economic Botany* 61, no. 1 (2007): 1–2.

Pushpangadan, P. "The Concept of Golden Triangle." *Herbal Tech. Industry* 1, no. 5 (2005): 12–15.

Rekka, R., S. Murugesh, and R. Prabakaran. "Plants Used by Malayali Tribes in Ethnogynaecological Disorders in Yercaud Hill, Southern Eastern Ghats, Salem District, Tamil Nadu." *Science Research Reporter* 3 (2013): 190–2.

Rokaya, M. B., Y. Uprety, R. C. Poudel, B. Timsina, Z. Münzbergová, H. Asselin, A. Tiwari, S. S. Shrestha, and S. R. Sigdel. "Traditional Uses of Medicinal Plants in Gastrointestinal Disorders in Nepal." *Journal of Ethnopharmacology* 158 (2014): 221–9.

Roy Burman, B. K. *Report of Committee on Forest and Tibals in India*. Ministry of Home Affairs, Govt. of India, 1982.

Sachs, J. D., G. Schmidt-Traub, M. Mazzucato, D. Messner, N. Nakicenovic, and J. Rockström. "Six Transformations to Achieve the Sustainable Development Goals." *Nature Sustainability* 2, no. 9 (2019): 805–14.

Sajem, A. L., and K. Gosai. "Ethnobotanical Investigations among the Lushai Tribes in North Cachar Hills District of Assam, Northeast India." *Indian Journal of Traditional Knowledge* 9, no. 1 (2010): 108–13.

Sajem, A. L., and K. Gosai. "Traditional Use of Medicinal Plants by the Jaintia Tribes in North Cachar Hills District of Assam, Northeast India." *Journal of Ethnobiology and Ethnomedicine* 2 (2006): 33.

Schippmann, U., D. J. Leaman, and A. B. Cunningham. *Impact of Cultivation and Gathering of Medicinal Plants on Biodiversity: Global Trends and Issues*. Biodiversity and the Ecosystem Approach in Agriculture, Forestry and Fisheries; Food and Agriculture Organization (FAO): Rome, Italy, 2002.

Schultes, R. E. "Ethnobotany and Technology in the Northwest Amazon: A Partnership." In *Sustainable Harvest and Marketing of Rain Forest Products*, edited by M. Plotkin and L. Famolare. Washington, DC: Island Press, 1992.

Semwal, D. K., A. Chauhan, A. Kumar, S. Aswal, R. B. Semwal, and A. Kumar. "Status of Indian Medicinal Plants in the International Union for Conservation of Nature and the Future of Ayurvedic Drugs: Shouldn't Think about Ayurvedic Fundamentals?" *Journal of Integrative Medicine* 17 (2019): 238–43.

Shanley, P., and L. Luz. "The Impacts of Forest Degradation on Medicinal Plant Use and Implications for Health Care in Eastern Amazonia." *BioScience* 53, no. 6 (2003): 573–84.

Sharma, C. M., S. Gairola, S. K. Ghildiyal, and S. Suyal. "Forest Resource Use Patterns in Relation to Socioeconomic Status." *Mountain Research and Development* 29 (2009): 308–19.

Sharma, J., S. Gairola, Y. P. Sharma, and R. Gaur. "Ethnomedicinal Plants Used to Treat Skin Diseases by Tharu Community of District Udham Singh Nagar, Uttarakhand, India." *Journal of Ethnopharmacology* 158 (2014): 140–206.

Shrestha, A. B., C. P. Wake, P. A. Mayewski, and J. E. Dibb. "Maximum Temperature Trends in the Himalaya and Its Vicinity: An Analysis Based on Temperature Records from Nepal for the Period 1971–94." *Journal of Climate* 12, no. 9 (1999): 2775–86.

Silvestre, B. S., and D. M. Tîrcˇa. "Innovations for Sustainable Development: Moving toward a Sustainable Future." *Journal of Cleaner Production* 208 (2019): 325–32.

Singh, A., M. C. Nautiyal, R. M. Kunwar, and R. W. Bussmann. "Ethnomedicinal Plants used by Local Inhabitants of Jakholi Block, Rudraprayag District, Western Himalaya, India." *Journal of Ethnobiology and Ethnomedicine* 13 (2017): 1–29.

Thakur, K. S., M. Kumar, R. Bawa, and O. B. Mohammed. "Ethnobotanical Study of Herbaceous Flora along an Altitudinal Gradient in Bharmour Forest Division, District Chamba of Himachal Pradesh, India." *Evidence Based Complementary and Alternative Medicine* 42 (2014): 1–7.

Tripathi, S. *Birhor and Their Culture: An Ethnographic Account of Particularly Vulnerable Tribal Group of Chhattisgarh*. JalJangal- Jameen Aur Janjatiyan, Allahabad, 2017.

Tripathi, S. "Ethnomedicine and Future Challenges." *Global Journal of Archaeology and Anthropology* 10, no. 5 (2019): 87–90.

Tripathi, S., and N. Panigrahi. "Changing Sacred Status of Village Pond in the Context of People-Pond-Spirit Complex: An Empirical Study." *The Oriental Anthropologist* 17, no. 1 (2017): 149–61.

Uniyal, B. "Utilization of Medicinal Plants by the Rural Women of Kullu Himachal." *Indian Journal of Traditional Knowledge* 2 (2003): 366–70.

United Nations. "Report of the United Nations Conference on Environment and Development (Rio de Janeiro, 3–14 June 1992), Vol 1: Resolutions adopted by the Conference" (1992): 1–5.

Vaidya, A. D., and T. P. Devasagayam. "Current Status of Herbal Drugs in India: An Overview." *Journal of Clinical Biochemistry and Nutrition* 41, no. 1 (2007): 1–11.

Wanzala, W., and S. I. Minyoso. "Ethnomedicines in the 21st Century: Challenges and Opportunities in the Contemporary World." *Journal of Medicinal Herbs and Ethnomedicine* 10 (2024): 12–36.

Wanzala, W., and K. M. Walingo. "Ethnomedicines and Health Management in Kenya: Which Way Forward?" *Journal of Complementary Medicine and Alternative Healthcare* 10, no. 3 (2019): 555788.

Wanzala, W., W. Takken, R. W. Mukabana, A. O. Pala, and A. Hassanali. "Ethnoknowledge of Bukusu Community on Livestock Tick Prevention and Control in Bungoma District, Western Kenya." *Journal of Ethnopharmacology* 140, no. 2 (2012): 298–324.

Wanzala, W., L. K. Wekesa, and S. I. Minyoso. "Some of the Commonly Used Bukusu Proverbs and Their Literal Meanings in the Society." *Journal of Natural and Ayurvedic Medicine* 7, no. 4 (2023): 000421.

World Health Organization (WHO). *Global Partners Commit to Advance Evidence-based Traditional, Complementary and Integrative Medicine*. World Health Organization. The First WHO Traditional Medicine Global Summit held in in Gandhinagar, Gujarat, India, 2023a.

World Health Organization (WHO)/United Nations Children's Fund (UNICEF). *Declaration of Alma-Ata*. International Conference on Primary Health Care, Almaty, Kazakh Soviet Socialist Republic, Soviet Union, 1978.

Xiong, Y., X. Sui, S. Ahmedet, Z. Wang, and C. Long. "Ethnobotany and Diversity of Medicinal Plants Used by the Buyi in Eastern Yunnan, China." *Plant Diversity* 42 (2020): 401–14.

Zhou, J., M. Ouedraogo, F. Qu, and P. Duez. "Potential Genotoxicity of Traditional Chinese Medicinal Plants and Phytochemicals: An Overview." *Phytotherapy Research* 27 (2013): 1745–55.

3

Ethnomedicine

A Vital Component for Sustainable Development

Aishwarya B. Patil*

MIT Art Design and Technology University, Rajbaugh, Pune, Maharashtra, India

*Corresponding Author's Email: pruthasmi@gmail.com

Introduction

Ethnomedicine, based on traditional medical practices deeply rooted in indigenous cultural systems, holds significant potential for fostering sustainable healthcare and environmental preservation. This branch of medicine encompasses a range of healing methods that draw on local knowledge and natural resources, promoting biodiversity and ecological sustainability. Indigenous practices often rely on medicinal plants and traditional healing, forming an essential part of healthcare in various communities. By aligning with the principles of ecological conservation, ethnomedicine plays a pivotal role in the sustainability discourse, integrating cultural practices with environmental stewardship. Thus, at its core, ethnomedicine is founded on an intimate understanding of local ecosystems. Indigenous communities possess detailed knowledge of their surrounding environments, which has been developed and refined over generations. For example, the knowledge systems within Ayurveda in India and traditional Chinese medicine exemplify holistic approaches to health that emphasize balance and preventive care. These systems rely on medicinal plants and organic compounds for treatment, fostering sustainable resource use and minimizing environmental degradation. The sustainable harvesting techniques often practiced in these traditions help maintain biodiversity, which is crucial for the availability of resources in the long term (Singh 2016; Zhang, Sun, and Wang 2015).

Ethnomedicine's role in sustainable development extends beyond healthcare, as it supports resource management and conservation efforts. For example, many indigenous practices involve selective harvesting techniques that protect plant species and allow for natural regeneration. This symbiotic relationship with the environment has led to sustainable resource use models, whereby communities use only what is necessary, fostering an ecological balance. Empirical studies have demonstrated that such practices contribute to the preservation of medicinal plant species, which is beneficial not only to the communities themselves but also to broader biodiversity conservation goals (WHO 2013). Despite these contributions, integrating ethnomedicine with modern healthcare and conservation systems presents challenges. Issues surrounding intellectual property rights and cultural appropriation often arise when traditional knowledge is commercialized. Indigenous communities, for example, may find their traditional medicinal practices used without proper acknowledgment or compensation. To address these concerns, legal protections and ethical guidelines must be established to ensure that indigenous knowledge is preserved and used responsibly. Intellectual property laws, as well as frameworks that ensure equitable benefit-sharing, are essential to prevent exploitation and ensure that indigenous communities benefit from the use of their knowledge (Correa 2001).

Standardization is another challenge in incorporating ethnomedicine into mainstream healthcare. Variability in traditional practices and a lack of standardized dosages can complicate efforts to apply ethnomedicine universally. This variability may limit its acceptance within modern medical frameworks, where consistency is highly valued. However, research collaborations that respect and preserve the cultural context of these practices could bridge this gap, allowing for the integration of ethnomedicine into contemporary healthcare in a way that is culturally sensitive and scientifically valid (Sharma, Singh, and Patwardhan 2020). The integration of ethnomedicine into sustainable development efforts holds promise for a more inclusive and holistic approach to healthcare and environmental conservation. As awareness grows around the need for sustainable practices, ethnomedicine offers a model of healthcare that emphasizes harmony with nature and community well-being. Recognizing the value of traditional medical knowledge can support resilient and sustainable healthcare systems that cater to diverse cultural needs and promote environmental sustainability. Through collaboration and respectful engagement with indigenous knowledge, modern sustainability efforts can become more robust, helping to build a sustainable future for all.

Conceptual Framework

Ethnomedicine, which is fundamentally tied to the social and cultural practices of indigenous societies, provides important insights into sustainable healthcare methods that both respect and preserve biodiversity. The World Health Organization (WHO), in its Traditional Medicine Strategy for 2014–23, highlights the significance of traditional medicine, noting its potential to complement modern healthcare by providing accessible, culturally relevant care (WHO 2013). Ethnomedicine typically emphasizes sustainable resource use, particularly through medicinal plants, aligning with ecological balance and minimal environmental impact (Sharma, Singh and

Patwardhan 2020). This review examines literature on the relationship between ethnomedicine and environmental conservation, focusing on how these practices can contribute to sustainable development.

Traditional medical systems, such as Ayurveda in India and traditional Chinese medicine (TCM), demonstrate sustainable healthcare models that incorporate principles of environmental conservation. Ayurveda, for example, promotes preventive health and balance, relying on plant-based treatments sustained by eco-friendly harvesting and local biodiversity. Similarly, TCM's reliance on natural elements offers a culturally informed approach that prioritizes ecological considerations (Singh 2016; Zhang, Sun, and Wang 2015). Research on these practices reveals how indigenous knowledge of local ecosystems enables sustainable management of resources, helping to conserve medicinal plants for future use (Correa 2001).

On the other hand, ethnomedicine significantly contributes to biodiversity conservation by using a broad spectrum of plant species for medicinal purposes. Indigenous knowledge systems are deeply embedded in local ecosystems, leading to unique, resource-preserving practices, such as selective harvesting and rotation of collection sites, which reduce overexploitation and encourage natural species regeneration. Studies on ethnomedicine's impact on biodiversity highlight how traditional knowledge fosters the sustainable management of natural resources (Bodeker and Ong 2005). These practices are essential for preserving biodiversity in areas where plant species face risks of extinction due to industrialization and habitat degradation.

Despite the valuable sustainability models presented by ethnomedicine, integrating this into the modern healthcare and conservation frameworks poses challenges. A primary issue is intellectual property rights, as Correa (2001) explains that the commercialization of traditional knowledge often leads to cultural appropriation, where indigenous groups may not receive appropriate recognition or compensation for their contributions. Additionally, Western medicine's emphasis on standardization presents difficulties for the personalized, adaptable nature of ethnomedicine. Standardization efforts, if not carefully managed, could diminish ethnomedicine's effectiveness or cause cultural erosion by disregarding traditional practices (Sharma, Singh, and Patwardhan 2020).

The literature stresses the importance of strong legal and ethical frameworks to safeguard indigenous knowledge and support fair benefit-sharing. Intellectual property laws that uphold indigenous rights are critical to preventing the exploitation of traditional knowledge. Moreover, ethical guidelines are needed to ensure cultural respect while enabling scientific research. Collaborative efforts among policymakers, researchers, and indigenous communities can establish frameworks that respect both traditional practices and the rights of those who hold them (Posey 1990). These ethical approaches to ethnomedicine promote shared knowledge, protect cultural heritage, and support sustainable development.

Thus, ethnomedicine has gained recognition as a crucial component of sustainable development, especially regarding health, well-being, sustainable consumption, and environmental conservation. Traditional medicine aligns with several United Nations Sustainable Development Goals (SDGs), including SDG 3 (Good Health and

Well-being) and SDG 15 (Life on Land). Integrating ethnomedical practices within sustainability frameworks enables modern systems to adopt a holistic approach to health and environmental conservation, fostering community resilience. The emphasis on sustainable resource use, local healthcare autonomy, and conservation underscores ethnomedicine's potential as a significant asset in addressing global environmental and health challenges (IUCN 2018).

This particular ethnobotanical study conducted in Aadi Nippani, Karnataka, has unveiled a wealth of traditional medicinal knowledge that aligns with sustainable environmental practices. This research aimed to document the diverse medicinal plants used in local ethnomedical practices, assess sustainable resource management by indigenous communities, and explore the integration of traditional knowledge into sustainable development frameworks.

Methodology

A sample of fifty participants was engaged in the study, comprising traditional healers, community elders, women, local farmers, and younger community members. Data collection methods included semi-structured interviews, focus group discussions, participant observation, and case studies, all of which provided comprehensive insights into traditional knowledge and sustainable practices within the community. A total of fifty participants were engaged in this ethnobotanical study of the Aadi Nippani, representing a cross-section of the community. These participants were selected based on their involvement in traditional medicine, local agriculture, and environmental practices, ensuring a diverse range of perspectives. Here is the breakdown of the study sample:

A. Gender Distribution

(i) Thirty women (60 percent): Women played a central role in the study, as they are the primary custodians of medicinal plant knowledge and the practice of ethnomedicine in the community. Many of the women participants were involved in domestic healing practices, such as using plants like *Tulsi*, *Ashwagandha*, and *Neem* for treating family ailments.

(ii) Twenty men (40 percent): Men in the community were predominantly involved in farming, with many also serving as herbalists or healers specializing in certain ailments. Some men were also part of the younger generation who are learning traditional practices from elders.

B. Age Distribution

(i) Ten participants (20 percent) aged sixty and above: These individuals, often community elders or traditional healers, have the most in-depth knowledge of medicinal plants and the sustainable methods of harvesting them. Their practices have been passed down through generations, often orally.

(ii) Twenty participants (40 percent) aged 30–59: These middle-aged participants represent the active workforce of the community. Many of them are farmers who also engage in the cultivation of medicinal plants like *Amla* and *Turmeric* and practice herbal healing.

(iii) Fifteen participants (30 percent) aged 18–29: This younger demographic represents a more modernized segment of the community. While they may not possess as much traditional knowledge, they are learning from elders and adapting these practices to modern life, particularly in home gardening and sustainable agriculture.

(iv) Five participants (10 percent) under the age of eighteen: These younger participants, though still in school, were involved through their families in cultivating medicinal plants and assisting in the harvesting process. Their involvement signifies the generational transfer of knowledge.

C. Occupation and Role in the Community

(i) Fifteen traditional healers (30 percent): This group included individuals who practice ethnomedicine and are considered local experts in treating common ailments using plant-based remedies. They are often consulted by community members for their expertise.

(ii) Twenty farmers (40 percent): Many participants in this group were directly involved in agricultural activities. They grow not only food crops but also medicinal plants. They played a crucial role in the study by discussing their agricultural practices, including sustainable methods for cultivating and harvesting medicinal plants.

(iii) Ten women (20 percent) involved in household healthcare: This group of participants is responsible for providing daily healthcare solutions within the family, using plants grown at home. Many women also contribute to passing down medicinal knowledge to younger generations.

(iv) Five youth (10 percent): These participants were mostly involved in the study through educational outreach and discussions about the future of traditional medicine in Aadi Nippani. They represent a future generation that is balancing modern education with traditional practices.

D. Educational Background

(i) Fifteen participants (30 percent) had completed high school or higher education, often being part of the younger demographic.

(ii) Twenty participants (40 percent) had minimal formal education, particularly the older generation, who learned about medicinal plants and healing through familial transmission rather than schooling.
(iii) Fifteen participants (30 percent) were still in school and represented a future generation of potential guardians of ethnomedicinal knowledge.

The diversity of this sample, in terms of gender, age, occupation, and education, ensured that the study captured a well-rounded view of how traditional medicinal knowledge is passed down, applied, and conserved in Aadi Nippani. Furthermore, it highlighted the importance of engaging both the older and younger generations to ensure the sustainability of ethnomedicinal practices.

Ethnomedicine and Sustainability in Context

Ethnomedicine and sustainability are intertwined as traditional knowledge often emphasizes the sustainable use of natural resources for healthcare and well-being. This includes understanding the importance of local ecosystems and the potential for both conservation and exploitation of medicinal plants. Accordingly, ethnomedical practices are deeply rooted in the environment, with many traditional healers relying on plants, animals, and other natural resources for medicinal purposes. Traditional knowledge often includes practices for sustainable harvesting and utilization of resources, ensuring that they are available for future generations. On the other hand, ethnomedical practitioners often possess a deep understanding of local ecosystems and the interconnectedness of plants, animals, and the environment, which is crucial for sustainable resource management. The preservation of ethnomedical knowledge is essential for maintaining biodiversity and promoting sustainable resource management. This ethnomedicine can provide economic opportunities for local communities through the sustainable use of medicinal plants and other resources. It can also play a crucial role in promoting health and well-being, particularly in areas with limited access to modern healthcare, while also fostering sustainable practices. By understanding the traditional knowledge of local communities, we can better protect biodiversity and promote sustainable ecosystems.

In this context, Figure 3.1 shows the perception of ethnomedicine in daily life among the communities of Aadi Nippani. This figure also states that 76 percent of participants use ethnomedicine regularly for treating common ailments like fevers, colds, and digestive issues. On the other hand, only 16 percent felt ethnomedicine was important but used it only for minor ailments, preferring modern medicine for more serious health concerns. Again, only 8 percent considered ethnomedicine outdated, favoring the use of modern medical services exclusively (see Figure 3.1). Besides, this study also explores that 84 percent of the participants emphasized the importance of conserving medicinal plants, viewing them as crucial for community health, culture,

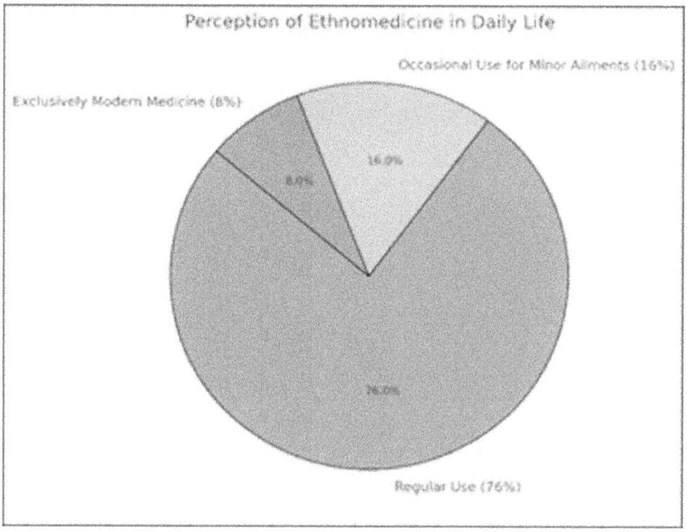

Figure 3.1. Perception of ethnomedicine in daily life. Source: Author.

and biodiversity. On the other hand, about 12 percent recognized the importance but felt that conservation should be managed by external bodies like NGOs or the government. In addition, only 4 percent felt that conservation was not a priority for the community, focusing instead on immediate health needs.

Figure 3.2 presents the sustainability of current harvesting practices. This figure states that about 68 percent of the participants believed that sustainable harvesting practices, such as selective picking, rotational harvesting, and seasonal collection, were being actively practiced within the community. Conversely, about 24 percent acknowledged that some overharvesting occurred, particularly for popular plants like neem, turmeric, and amla, but hoped that awareness would lead to better practices. Again, about 8 percent did not engage with or fully understand sustainable harvesting methods (see Figure 3.2). Moreover, Figure 3.3 exhibits the integration of ethnomedicine and modern medicine. By this figure we can see that about 90 percent of participants supported the idea of integrating ethnomedicine with modern medicine. They felt this approach would offer a more comprehensive healthcare system, combining the preventive and accessible nature of ethnomedicine with the advanced capabilities of modern healthcare. Besides, about 8 percent were uncertain about integration, preferring to rely on one system over the other. Further, only 2 percent felt that traditional practices should be phased out in favor of modern medical treatments (see Figure 3.3). Furthermore,Figure 3.4 displays the role of the community in environmental practices. By this figure, we can see that about 72 percent of participants believed that the community should play an active role in sustainable practices such as educating younger generations, conserving

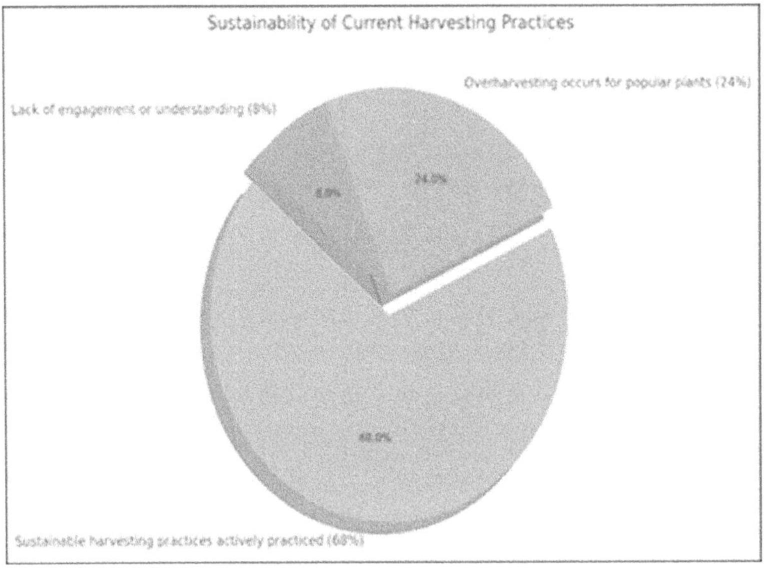

Figure 3.2. Sustainability of current harvesting practices. Source: Author.

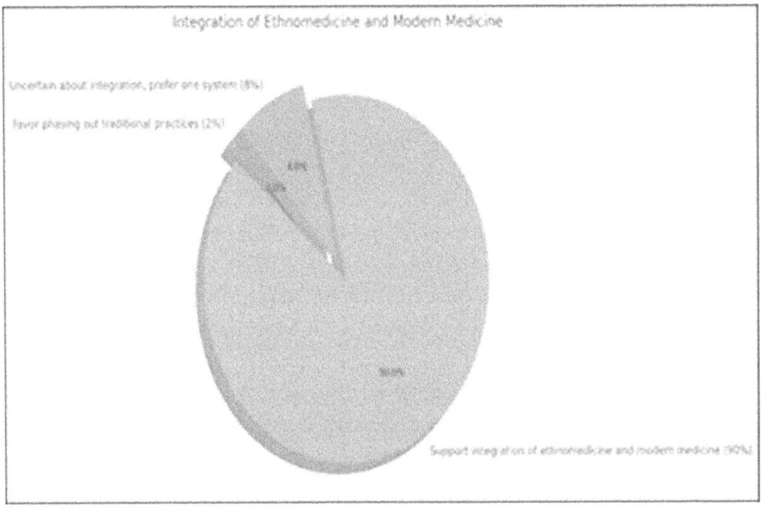

Figure 3.3. Integration of ethnomedicine and modern medicine. Source: Author.

medicinal plants, and creating protected areas for rare species. Conversely, about 20 percent thought that responsibility for conservation should lie with external organizations or government bodies, while 8 percent felt that their current efforts were sufficient.

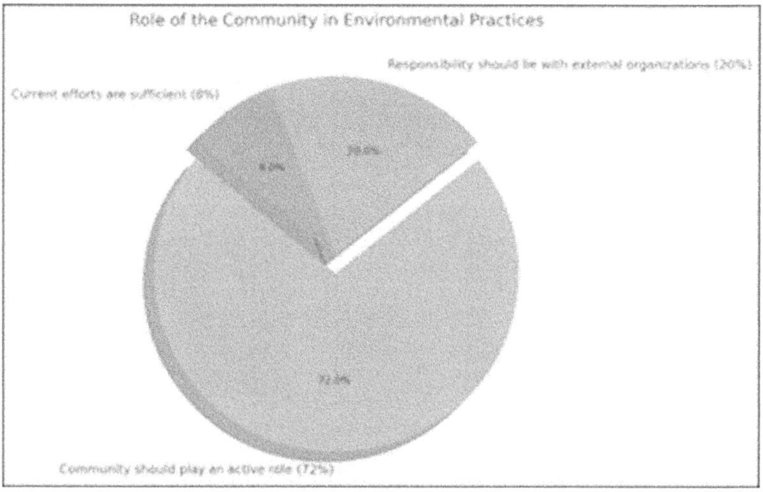

Figure 3.4. Role of the community in environmental practices. Source: Author.

Identified Medicinal Plants

The study identified a variety of medicinal plants used in Aadi Nippani, many of which were harvested sustainably through selective picking and rotational harvesting practices. Here are some of the key plants and their uses:

i. Neem (*Azadirachta indica*): Widely used for its antibacterial properties, neem leaves are employed to treat skin infections and as an antiseptic in wound cleaning (see Figure 3.5).
ii. Tulsi (*Ocimum tenuiflorum*): Known as holy basil, tulsi is used to treat colds, fevers, and respiratory ailments. Many households grow tulsi in home gardens, making it readily accessible.
iii. Ashwagandha (*Withania somnifera*): Known for its rejuvenating properties, ashwagandha roots are used to alleviate stress, anxiety, and inflammation. Local healers demonstrated how they carefully harvested roots only from mature plants to ensure sustainable growth.
iv. Turmeric (*Curcuma longa*): Used extensively for its anti-inflammatory properties, turmeric is grown locally and used in poultices to treat wounds, insect bites, and skin conditions.
v. Amla (*Phyllanthus emblica*): This fruit, rich in vitamin C, is used to boost immunity, enhance digestion, and promote skin health. Seasonal harvest and careful collection ensure no overharvesting.
vi. Giloy (*Tinospora cordifolia*): An adaptogen, giloy is used to boost immunity and treat fever, especially during seasonal changes. Harvesting is done with great care to protect the plant's vines and leaves.

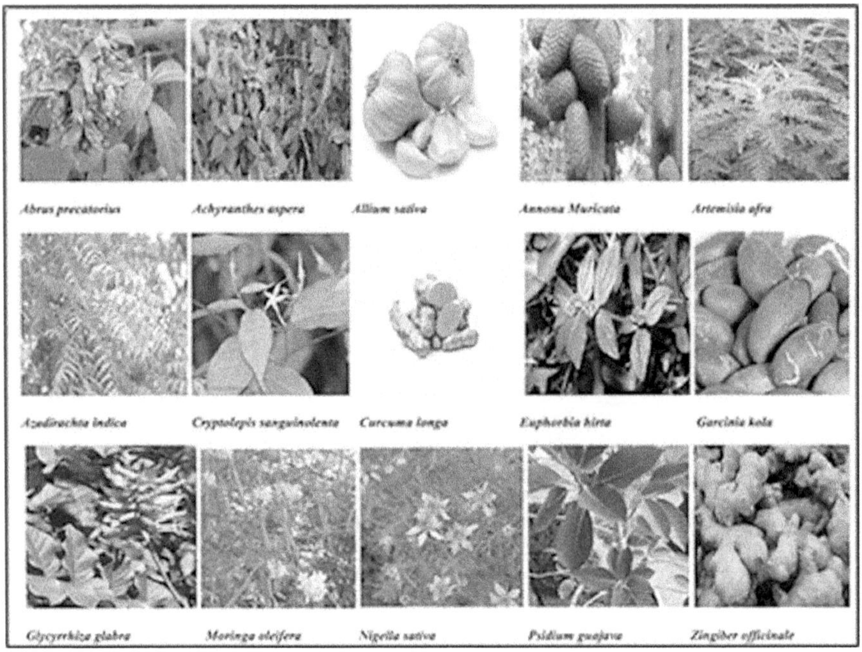

Figure 3.5. Variety of medicinal plants used in Aadi Nippani. Source: Author.

Table 3.1. Traditional Medicinal Plants and Their Uses

Medicinal Plants	Primary Uses
Neem (*Azadirachta indica*)	Antibacterial, wound cleaning
Tulsi (*Ocimum tenuiflorum*)	Respiratory ailments, colds, fevers
Ashwagandha (*Withania somnifera*)	Stress, anxiety, inflammation
Turmeric (*Curcuma longa*)	Anti-inflammatory, skin conditions
Amla (*Phyllanthus emblica*)	Immunity, digestion, skin health
Giloy (*Tinospora cordifolia*)	Immunity, fever management
Nagarmotha (*Cyperus rotundus*)	Digestive, anti-inflammatory
Kalmegh (*Andrographis paniculata*)	Fevers, liver health, immunity
Betel Leaf (*Piper betle*)	Antiseptic, anti-inflammatory
Baheda (*Terminalia bellirica*)	Digestive health, rejuvenation
Safed Musli (*Chlorophytum borivilianum*)	Vitality, immunity
Guggul (*Commiphora wightii*)	Arthritis, inflammation

In the Aadi Nippani region, several unique medicinal plants were documented, each with specific uses in traditional healthcare and locally adapted harvesting practices (see Table 3.1). Here are some notable examples:

(a) Nagarmotha (*Cyperus rotundus*): Commonly known as nutgrass, this plant is valued for its digestive and anti-inflammatory properties. Traditional healers in Aadi Nippani use it to treat gastrointestinal issues, and its roots are carefully harvested to prevent plant depletion.

(b) Kalmegh (*Andrographis paniculata*): Known for its bitter taste and powerful healing properties, kalmegh is used to manage fevers, liver ailments, and respiratory conditions. Healers selectively harvest its leaves to sustain its population, as it is highly regarded for immune support.

(c) Betel Leaf (*Piper betle*): Locally grown and culturally significant, betel leaves are used for their antiseptic and anti-inflammatory benefits. In Aadi Nippani, the leaves are used to treat wounds and alleviate headaches through topical applications. Harvesting is done rotationally to ensure consistent plant growth.

(d) Baheda (*Terminalia bellirica*): This tree is one of the "three fruits" in the Ayurvedic formula Triphala, used for digestive health and as a rejuvenating tonic. Healers in Aadi Nippani harvest its fruits seasonally, allowing natural regeneration.

(e) Safed Musli (*Chlorophytum borivilianum*): Valued for its adaptogenic properties, safed musli is a rare herb known for boosting vitality and immunity. Due to its increasing commercial demand, community members practice limited harvesting to ensure the plant's survival in its natural habitat.

(f) Guggul (*Commiphora wightii*): Traditionally used to treat arthritis and inflammation, guggul resin is collected with care to avoid overharvesting. The community observes strict harvesting limits to protect this endangered species.

Traditional Healers and Practices: Some Cases

Some case studies present the indigenous knowledge of Aadi Nippani healers and highlight sustainable harvesting and healthcare practices. Case 1 was taken from the local healer Rukmini Amma (pseudo names have been used). Rukmini Amma, a healer specializing in women's health, uses a combination of Ashoka bark (*Saraca asoca*) and Neem to treat menstrual disorders and skin issues. She demonstrated how she only collects bark from mature trees, applying techniques that avoid harm to the plants. Her knowledge of herb preparation using natural oils and turmeric enhances efficacy while preserving the natural resource.

On the other hand, case 2 was taken from the traditional healer Basavaraj (pseudo names have been used). Basavaraj, another well-respected healer, specializes in treating respiratory conditions. He combines Tulsi, Ginger, and Black Pepper in formulations for coughs and colds. Basavaraj has been teaching younger members of his family to grow these plants locally, encouraging sustainable farming practices that avoid overdependence on wild sources.

Next, case 3 was taken from the local herbalist Lakshmi Bai (pseudo names have been used). Lakshmi Bai, a community herbalist, uses amla and giloy to boost immunity and address fevers, particularly during the monsoon season. She emphasized sustainable harvesting by instructing villagers to collect only what they need, thus avoiding the depletion of these critical plants. Her approach reflects the community's collective effort toward ecological preservation.

Environmental Conservation Practices

Ethnomedicine often incorporates environmental conservation practices, including sustainable harvesting techniques, knowledge of plant ecology, and the preservation of traditional knowledge to protect biodiversity and ecosystems. The traditional healers and communities often have specific rules and practices for harvesting medicinal plants, ensuring that only a sustainable amount is taken, leaving enough for regeneration and reproduction. In this case, practices like avoiding uprooting entire plants, especially lone individuals, and covering exposed roots are common to promote plant survival. Again, some cultures have restrictions on excessive debarking, recognizing the importance of the bark for the tree's health. In addition, the harvesting of primary roots is often prohibited to ensure the plant's survival. Moreover, traditional knowledge often includes a deep understanding of plant growth cycles, seasons, and the specific habitats where medicinal plants thrive. Thus, ethnomedical practices can play a role in identifying and protecting endangered or rare medicinal plants, as their use is often tied to cultural and medicinal importance. Accordingly, by promoting the sustainable use of medicinal plants, ethnomedicine contributes to the overall conservation of biodiversity.

The present study found that community members of Aadi Nippani practice unique conservation strategies to protect medicinal plants like rotational harvesting, seasonal collection, and protected zones. In the case of rotational harvesting, the local healers use periodic harvesting resources, moving from one area to another to avoid overharvesting any single area. This allows plants time to regenerate naturally. This rotational harvesting aims to ensure the long-term sustainability of medicinal plant populations by preventing overharvesting and allowing for natural regeneration. On the other hand, in case of seasonal collection, plants are collected according to seasonal cycles to ensure optimal potency and sustainability. For example, Neem leaves are primarily gathered during the monsoon season, ensuring regrowth and minimal impact on the plant's health. It is because the concentration of medicinal compounds (phytochemicals) in plants varies throughout the year, influencing their therapeutic efficacy. Besides, the Ayurvedic and other traditional systems of medicine emphasize the importance of collecting plants during specific seasons for optimal results. Lastly, in the case of protected zones, certain forest patches have been designated as no-harvest zones, particularly areas with rare medicinal plants. These zones reflect a community-led approach to environmental stewardship, where plants are allowed to thrive undisturbed.

Impact on Sustainable Development Goals (SDGs)

Ethnomedicine, with its focus on traditional knowledge and practices, can significantly contribute to achieving the sustainable development goals (SDGs), particularly in areas like health, well-being, and sustainable livelihoods, by promoting access to affordable healthcare, preserving biodiversity, and empowering local communities. In the case of SDG 3 (Good Health and Well-being), ethnomedicine can offer accessible and affordable healthcare options, especially in underserved areas, by utilizing locally available resources and traditional healing practices. Traditional knowledge can be used to prevent and manage diseases, including communicable and noncommunicable ones, through the use of medicinal plants and other natural remedies. Integrating traditional medicine into healthcare systems can contribute to achieving universal health coverage, ensuring that everyone has access to quality healthcare services.

On the other hand, in case of SDG 12 (Responsible Consumption and Production), ethnomedicine promotes the sustainable use of natural resources, ensuring the long-term availability of medicinal plants and other resources for future generations. Traditional practices often involve minimal waste and pollution, contributing to environmental sustainability. Moreover, in case of SDG 15 (Life on Land), ethnomedicine can play a crucial role in biodiversity conservation by promoting the sustainable use of medicinal plants and other natural resources. Traditional knowledge can help in preventing deforestation and promoting sustainable land management practices. Also, in case of SDG 17 (Partnerships for the Goals), ethnomedicine can empower local communities by recognizing and valuing their traditional knowledge and practices. Ethnomedicine facilitates the sharing of traditional knowledge with the wider world, contributing to a more holistic understanding of health and well-being.

Keeping all these understandings in mind, the practices in Aadi Nippani align well with several sustainable development goals like SDG 3 and SDG 15. In Aadi Nippani, ethnomedicine enhances community health by providing accessible healthcare solutions, reducing dependence on external medical systems, and fostering local resilience following SDG 3. Conversely, the conservation practices among indigenous communities promote biodiversity and sustainable land use, directly supporting ecosystem integrity and habitat protection following SDG 15.

Policy Implication and Recommendation

The findings underscore the importance of protecting and promoting ethnomedicine practices, for both their healthcare value and their ecological benefits. The following policy recommendations arise from the study:

(i) Intellectual Property Rights for Indigenous Knowledge: Ensuring that healers and community knowledge bearers receive recognition and benefits from any commercial use of traditional medicinal knowledge. This would require legal frameworks that protect indigenous intellectual property.

(ii) Incorporation of Ethnomedicine into Local Healthcare: Establishing support for local healthcare systems that include traditional healers in Aadi Nippani, creating a complementary system alongside modern medicine.

(iii) Training Programs for Sustainable Harvesting: Government or NGO-led workshops could teach sustainable harvesting techniques, ensuring long-term availability of medicinal plants and avoiding overexploitation.

(iv) Community-Led Conservation Initiatives: Establishing formal conservation areas within community forests managed by local councils and guided by traditional practices, to protect biodiversity and medicinal plant species.

Holistic Approach for Ecological Balance

Ethnomedicine, deeply rooted in indigenous knowledge and cultural practices, is intricately connected to environmental stewardship and sustainable development. Drawing from local biodiversity and generations of ecological knowledge, ethnomedicine represents a comprehensive approach to healthcare that is attuned to ecological balance. This chapter explores how ethnomedical practices contribute to sustainability and environmental conservation, focusing on case studies from India, including Ayurvedic practices and other region-specific indigenous traditions, which serve as exemplary models of environmental and healthcare integration.

(a) **Ethnomedicine and Ecological Balance:** Ethnomedicine, particularly in India, is fundamentally tied to environmental sustainability, emphasizing the use of local plant species and natural resources. Unlike industrial medicine, which relies on synthesized compounds, traditional Indian medicine uses whole plants and natural extracts, resulting in minimal environmental disturbance (Ravishankar and Shukla 2007). Indigenous communities employ sustainable practices to manage natural resources, such as selective harvesting and seasonal gathering, allowing for the continued regeneration of plant species. A study on the ethnobotanical practices of the indigenous Baiga and Gond tribes in Madhya Pradesh highlighted the depth of local knowledge in harvesting and conserving medicinal plants, ensuring both efficacy and resource renewal (Pandey and Tripathi 2017).

(b) **Indigenous Knowledge and Sustainable Resource Management:** Indian indigenous communities possess rich ecological insights that guide their resource management practices. This traditional knowledge, developed through centuries of coexistence with nature, extends beyond plant use to include climate, soil, and species interdependence. For instance, the Raikas in Rajasthan, known for their medicinal knowledge, manage local resources by rotating collection sites and timing harvests to avoid disrupting plant cycles, thus preserving biodiversity (Choudhary and Singh 2018). Indian ethnomedicine prioritizes natural regeneration, ensuring long-term availability of resources. These practices demonstrate a sustainable model of healthcare that aligns with modern environmental objectives by fostering resilience within the ecosystem.

(c) **Indian Case Studies in Ethnomedicine and Sustainable Development:** Ayurveda in India is one of the oldest examples of ethnomedicine, illustrating a deeply ecological approach to health that emphasizes balance within the individual and the environment. Ayurveda relies on a diverse range of medicinal plants like neem, ashwagandha, and tulsi, which are sustainably harvested and cultivated in regions throughout India. Studies reveal that Ayurvedic practices encourage conservation by promoting sustainable agriculture and the ethical harvesting of medicinal plants (Patwardhan et al. 2005). The benefits extend beyond healthcare to include ecosystem preservation, as these practices minimize soil depletion, support biodiversity, and reduce the carbon footprint through local sourcing. Similarly, the Bhils and Bhilalas in Madhya Pradesh incorporate plant-based remedies in ways that align with sustainable principles. These communities adhere to strict seasonal guidelines for harvesting, which reduces the pressure on vulnerable species and fosters natural regeneration. Their use of the Amaltas (*Cassia fistula*) and Satawar (*Asparagus racemosus*) plant species demonstrates a sustainable approach that limits resource depletion. In the case of traditional Chinese medicine (TCM) in East Asia, which has some practices mirrored in Northeastern Indian regions, local agroforestry systems incorporate medicinal plant cultivation alongside staple crops. This method improves biodiversity while protecting the ecosystem and supporting sustainable livelihoods, showing that integrating traditional practices with modern agricultural models can be mutually beneficial (Ravishankar and Shukla 2007).

(d) **Ethnomedicine's Role in Biodiversity Conservation:** Ethnomedicine in India is a crucial factor in biodiversity conservation, helping protect diverse plant species from overharvesting or habitat loss. Ethnomedical practices often include in situ conservation methods that align with the cultural beliefs of many indigenous groups, ensuring plants are harvested sustainably. Research into the practices of the Konda Reddis in Andhra Pradesh, for example, found that indigenous healers implement selective harvesting and enforce community-wide rules to preserve rare medicinal species (Sinha and Biswal 2015). Such community-led efforts contribute not only to biodiversity but also to ecological resilience, allowing plants and other species to coexist in balanced ecosystems. The conservation focus in Indian ethnomedicine is especially relevant in light of rapid biodiversity loss due to urbanization, climate change, and deforestation. By valuing a wide range of plant species for their medicinal properties, ethnomedicine fosters a holistic view of nature that aligns with modern conservation goals. Additionally, ethnomedical practices align with the Indian government's biodiversity preservation initiatives, as they encourage traditional ecological knowledge and support sustainable use of biodiversity resources (Pandey 2009).

(e) **Challenges in Integrating Ethnomedicine into Modern Systems:** Integrating Indian ethnomedicine into mainstream healthcare systems presents several challenges. Intellectual property rights (IPR) are a significant concern, as traditional knowledge is frequently commercialized without compensation for indigenous communities. Legal scholars such as Correa (2001) argue for intellectual property protections that respect indigenous ownership and prevent cultural appropriation. Additionally, the drive to standardize ethnomedical practices can threaten cultural practices, as traditional Indian medicine is highly individualized and context-dependent. Governmental organizations such as the National Biodiversity Authority (NBA) have recognized the importance of protecting indigenous knowledge from exploitation, advocating for frameworks that ensure benefit-sharing and the protection of community rights (Sharma, Singh, and Patwardhan 2020).

(f) **Ethnomedicine's Alignment with Sustainable Development Goals:** Ethnomedicine in India supports several Sustainable Development Goals (SDGs), notably SDG 3 (Good Health and Well-being) and SDG 15 (Life on Land). Traditional medicine aligns with SDG targets by offering accessible healthcare that emphasizes prevention, which reduces strain on resources and infrastructure. Furthermore, ethnomedicine encourages biodiversity and ecosystem health, reinforcing SDG 15 through practices that prevent deforestation and habitat loss (Bodeker and Ong 2005). Indian case studies in sustainable development illustrate that adopting holistic healthcare models that incorporate ethnomedicine contributes significantly to the conservation and sustainable use of terrestrial ecosystems, ensuring long-term environmental and social benefits.

Ethnomedicine and Sustainability: Action-oriented Approach

Ethnomedicine, environmental conservation, and sustainable development are interconnected, as traditional knowledge of medicinal plants can promote sustainable resource management and contribute to both environmental protection and human well-being. In addition, environmental conservation and sustainability are two related but distinct concepts that aim to protect the natural world and our relationship with it. Environmental conservation is the practice of preserving the natural habitat, while sustainability is the practice of improving the environment for human health. Thus, to develop effective policies supporting ethnomedicine, environmental conservation, and sustainable development, a collaborative, action-oriented anthropological approach is essential. Here are policy suggestions informed by real-life examples of Indian initiatives, with future plans to foster sustainable practices in ethnomedicine.

I. Policy for Protection and Recognition of Indigenous Knowledge

(a) Policy Suggestion: Create and enforce legal protections for indigenous knowledge and intellectual property rights. This includes recognizing and compensating communities for their contributions to ethnomedicine, ensuring they benefit from the commercial use of their traditional knowledge.

(b) Real-Life Example: The Biological Diversity Act of 2002 in India protects biodiversity and acknowledges the traditional knowledge of indigenous communities. It mandates benefit-sharing when traditional knowledge is commercialized, aligning with global norms on intellectual property rights for indigenous knowledge.

(c) Future Plan: As an action anthropologist, advocate for enhanced community involvement in biodiversity councils and intellectual property boards. Establish local Intellectual Property Resource Centers to assist indigenous communities in documenting and protecting their knowledge.

II. Policy on Sustainable Cultivation and Conservation of Medicinal Plants

(a) Policy Suggestion: Develop programs that support the sustainable cultivation of medicinal plants while conserving wild species. This includes financial incentives for cultivating medicinal plants, promoting agroforestry, and creating protected medicinal plant conservation zones.

(b) Real-Life Example: National Medicinal Plants Board (NMPB) under India's Ministry of AYUSH works to promote the cultivation of medicinal plants by providing subsidies to farmers. It also sets up conservation areas and implements awareness programs on sustainable harvesting practices.

(c) Future Plan: Action anthropologists can facilitate workshops with indigenous communities, botanists, and policymakers to co-create guidelines for medicinal plant conservation. Additionally, implement community-driven conservation zones where indigenous groups receive training in sustainable cultivation practices, enhancing both biodiversity and local economies.

III. Policy on Integrating Ethnomedicine into Primary Healthcare

(a) Policy Suggestion: Incorporate ethnomedicine into primary healthcare by establishing guidelines for safe and effective integration with modern medicine. This policy should allow ethnomedicine practitioners to work in collaboration with medical professionals in rural healthcare settings.

(b) Real-Life Example: The National Rural Health Mission (NRHM) and Ministry of AYUSH have integrated traditional health practices in public health systems, particularly in underserved areas. Programs such as "AYUSH Wellness Clinics" promote Ayurvedic, Unani, Siddha, and Homeopathy (AYUSH) systems, providing patients with alternative healthcare options alongside allopathic treatments.

(c) Future Plan: Develop ethnomedicine accreditation programs, empowering indigenous healers to be certified as primary healthcare providers within rural clinics. Action anthropologists can also support capacity-building for these healers, establishing an accessible and culturally relevant healthcare system that can reduce healthcare costs and improve health outcomes.

IV. Policy on Sustainable Development Education and Community Involvement

(a) Policy Suggestion: Include ethnomedicine and biodiversity conservation in educational curricula at local and national levels, focusing on sustainable development principles. Engage indigenous youth through educational programs that honor their heritage while equipping them with modern sustainability practices.

(b) Real-Life Example: The Ekta Parishad's Jeevan Vidya Program works with local communities in central India to promote sustainable practices and educate youth on environmental conservation. The program combines traditional knowledge with modern ecological insights to help communities manage resources sustainably.

(c) Future Plan: Action anthropologists could collaborate with indigenous elders, educational institutions, and environmental NGOs to develop school curricula that emphasize ethnomedicine, ecological knowledge, and sustainable practices. Organize cultural exchange programs for students to learn directly from indigenous practitioners, fostering cross-generational knowledge transfer and building community pride.

V. Policy on Community-Led Resource Management and Biodiversity Conservation

(a) Policy Suggestion: Designate indigenous communities as primary stakeholders in managing local biodiversity and implementing sustainable resource practices. Establish participatory resource management councils where community members make decisions on the use and conservation of medicinal resources.

(b) Real-Life Example: The Joint Forest Management (JFM) initiative in India engages local communities in forest conservation, allowing them a share in forest produce and decision-making powers in forest resource management.

(c) Future Plan: Expand JFM-like models to medicinal plant conservation by creating Community Medicinal Plant Reserves where communities control sustainable harvesting and conservation efforts. Encourage indigenous women and youth to play leading roles in these councils, recognizing their central role in traditional medicine. This model, with community empowerment at its core, would safeguard biodiversity and enhance the livelihoods of local communities.

1. **VI. Policy on Research and Development with Equitable Benefit-Sharing**

(a) Policy Suggestion: Form partnerships between government research institutions, universities, and indigenous communities for research on ethnomedicine that includes equitable benefit-sharing agreements. This would protect indigenous knowledge rights and ensure fair compensation.
(b) Real-Life Example: India's Traditional Knowledge Digital Library (TKDL) has digitized traditional medicinal knowledge to protect it from misappropriation by ensuring only licensed users, such as patent examiners, can access it. This allows India to challenge any biopiracy claims on traditional knowledge.
(c) Future Plan: Establish community-led digital knowledge repositories for ethnomedicine that operate with consent-based sharing models. Action anthropologists can work with indigenous communities to document and control access to this knowledge, ensuring that research collaborations bring tangible benefits back to the communities.

2. **VII. Policy on Cultural Heritage and Sustainable Tourism**

(a) Policy Suggestion: Encourage sustainable tourism that respects and promotes indigenous ethnomedical practices while ensuring local communities benefit economically. This policy could support community-owned ecotourism and health tourism initiatives, creating new income streams linked to ethnomedicine.
(b) Real-Life Example: The Pochampally Village in Telangana, known for its weaving heritage, combines tourism with cultural heritage, enabling visitors to experience local crafts and purchase products directly from artisans, benefiting the community economically.
(c) Future Plan: Develop similar ethnomedicine-focused ecotourism programs where visitors learn about traditional healing and conservation methods. Action anthropologists can facilitate respectful cultural exchanges by setting up guidelines for tourists, educating them about the significance of these practices, and ensuring tourism benefits are reinvested in the local communities for sustainable development.

Conclusion

In conclusion, the study conducted in Aadi Nippani, Karnataka, underscores the deep connection between indigenous knowledge systems, sustainable healthcare practices, and environmental conservation. The unique ethnomedicine practices in the region, particularly the use of medicinal plants like Nagarmotha, Kalmegh, Betel Leaf, Baheda, Safed Musli, and Guggul, demonstrate a remarkable understanding of the local ecosystem. This knowledge is not only integral to the health and well-being of the community but also plays a vital role in maintaining ecological balance and conserving biodiversity. On the other hand, the sustainable harvesting practices observed in Aadi Nippani, such as selective collection, rotational harvesting, and seasonal plant use, reflect a conscious effort to protect medicinal plant populations from overexploitation. This tradition of responsible resource management, passed down through generations, ensures that valuable medicinal plants remain available for future use while promoting ecological sustainability.

The case studies of traditional healers like Rukmini Amma, Basavaraj, and Lakshmi Bai (pseudo names have been used) further emphasize the importance of preserving and promoting indigenous healthcare systems. Their role as custodians of traditional knowledge highlights the need for greater recognition and support of ethnomedicine within the broader context of modern healthcare and environmental conservation. These healers not only act as practitioners but also as stewards of the environment, blending health practices with the principles of sustainability. Ultimately, the Aadi Nippani example serves as a powerful model for integrating ethnomedicine into contemporary sustainability frameworks. By valuing and preserving the traditional practices of indigenous communities, we can foster a more holistic approach to health and environmental well-being. This study not only contributes to the body of knowledge on sustainable development but also calls for the integration of indigenous wisdom into global discussions on biodiversity conservation and sustainable healthcare.

References

Bodeker, G., and C. K. Ong. *WHO Global Atlas of Traditional, Complementary and Alternative Medicine*. World Health Organization, 2005.

Choudhary, K., and M. Singh. "Ethnobotanical Practices among the Raika Community in Rajasthan, India." *International Journal of Ecology and Environmental Sciences* 44, no. 3 (2018): 295–303.

Correa, C. M. *Traditional Knowledge and Intellectual Property: Issues and Options Surrounding the Protection of Traditional Knowledge*. Geneva: Quaker United Nations Office, 2001.

International Union for Conservation of Nature. IUCN 70 Years: Annual Report 2018. IUCN, 2018.

Pandey, D. N. "Ethnomedicine and Biodiversity Conservation: A Synthesis of Socio-Ecological Perspectives." *Indian Journal of Traditional Knowledge* 8, no. 1 (2009): 132–39.

Pandey, A. K., and Y. C. Tripathi. "Medicinal Plants in Indian Ethnobotany." *Ethnobotany Research and Applications* 4, no. 11 (2017): 352–62..

Patwardhan, B. D., Warude, P. Pushpangadan, and N. Bhatt. "Ayurveda and Traditional Chinese Medicine: A Comparative Overview." *Evidence-Based Complementary and Alternative Medicine* 2, no. 4 (2005): 465–73.

Posey, Darrell A. *The 'Balance Sheet' and the 'Sacred Balance': Valuing the Knowledge of Indigenous and Traditional Peoples*. Oxford: Oxford Centre for the Environment, Ethics and Society, Mansfield College, 1990.

Ravishankar, B., and V. J. Shukla. "Indian Systems of Medicine: A Brief Profile." *African Journal of Traditional, Complementary and Alternative Medicines* 4, no. 3 (2007): 319–37.

Sharma, A., R. Singh, and B. Patwardhan. "Ethnomedicine and Sustainable Development in India." *Indian Journal of Traditional Knowledge* 19, no. 1 (2020a): 177–82.

Sharma, R., S. Singh, and B. Patwardhan. "Ethnopharmacology and Integration of Ethnomedicine into Global Healthcare." *Journal of Ethnopharmacology* 258 (2020b): 112726.

Singh, R. H. "Ayurveda in India: Past and Present." *Journal of Alternative and Complementary Medicine* 22, no. 6 (2016): 411–16.

Sinha, B., and U. C. Biswal. "Ethnomedicine among the Konda Reddi Tribes of Andhra Pradesh." *Journal of Medicinal Plants Studies* 3, no. 6 (2015): 1–11.

World Health Organization (WHO). *Traditional Medicine Strategy 2014–2023*. WHO, 2013.

Zhang, A., H. Sun, and X. Wang. "Ethnopharmacology, Traditional Chinese Medicine, and the Transformation to Modern Research." *Journal of Ethnopharmacology* 166 (2015): 5–15.

Part II

Ethnobotanical Knowledge and Medicinal Plants

4

Ethnomedicinal and Indigenous Knowledge of Some Locally Available Important Medicinal Plants

Mimosa Ghosh,[1] Sunipa Sen,[2] and Gour Gopal Satpati[2*]

[1]Department of Botany, Vidyasagar University, Midnapore, West Bengal, India

[2]Department of Botany, Bangabasi Evening College, Kolkata, West Bengal, India

*Corresponding Author's Email: gour_satpati@yahoo.co.in[2]

Introduction

Individuals from various cultures have historically relied on plants to meet essential needs such as food, shelter, warmth, and medicine, leading to a rich understanding of plant uses.[1] As they moved from place to place, this knowledge was shared with nearby tribes, allies, and adversaries, gradually growing richer in the process. Consequently, the wisdom regarding plants has circulated globally since ancient times, often accompanied by the plants themselves as they spread (Pandey and Tripathi 2017). The emphasis of ethnobotany is on the ways plants have been utilized, handled, and viewed within human communities, encompassing their use for food, medicinal purposes, divination, cosmetic applications, dyeing processes, textiles, construction, tools, currency, clothing, rituals, social interactions, and music. The connection between humans and plants has always held significant value. Plants are vital to every facet of our existence, and life cannot be sustained without them (Pandey and Tripathi 2017).

The use of scientific understanding regarding bioresources for the benefit of humanity requires information on socioeconomic factors, environmental impacts, and biodiversity conservation. Ethical considerations necessitate the maintenance of the knowledge base, the development of skills among indigenous communities, and equitable distribution of benefits gained from the commercial utilization of traditional knowledge (Mbuni et al. 2020). A contemporary scientific perspective on ethnobotany requires accurate information, statistical backing for data, and either quantitative or semi-quantitative analysis of field observations (Jain 2004).

Approximately 80 percent of the people in developing countries rely heavily on traditional medicine for health care needs, a majority of which involve the use of plant extracts or their active principles. South Africans regularly use traditional plant medicine; one of the criticisms of herbal medicine is the lack of standardization and quality control profiles. This misclassification of species and the mistaken substitutions present a real danger in the preparation and administration of herbal medicine. Medicinal plants have started to be considered an essential source in treating and preventing various kinds of disease (Satpati 2020; Manzoor et al. 2023). Each plants considered to have several important ingredients that can be used in the medical field and can be involved in the development of different kinds of drugs. Many developing countries, or even developed countries, are using herbal medicine to maintain human well-being, improve personal health conditions, and treat certain types of diseases, such as coughs, asthma, fever, bronchitis, and other diseases (Mbuni et al. 2020). This chapter highlights the locally available medicinal plants from our surroundings and their usefulness as traditional medicines.

Objectives and Methods

The present study gathered knowledge about medicinal plants which are observed in our surroundings and easily available. Then this study surveyed our surroundings and asked questions about the uses of medicinal plants nowadays. It tries to identify the medicinal plants and their traditional uses. It also tries to explore the symptoms related to many types of diseases. It attempts to raise awareness of medicinal plants as well as to find medicine from herbs for various diseases.

Medicinal Plants and Their Uses

Many locally available plants of India possess medicinal properties and are used traditionally and increasingly in modern medicine for treating various ailments. Some locally available well-known medicinal plants are *Justicia spicigera* (Acanthaceae), *Moringa oleifera* (Moringaceae), *Glinus oppositifolius* (Molluginaceae), *Typhonium trilobatum* (Araceae), *Anisomeles indica* (Lamiaceae), *Rauvolfia serpentina* (Apocynaceae), *Ecbolium linneanum* (Acanthaceae), *Azadirachta indica* (Meliaceae), *Ficus pumila* (Moraceae), *Hygrophila auriculata* (Acanthaceae), *Hyptis suaveolens* (Lamiaceae), and *Senna alata* (Fabaceae). The common or local names, plant parts used, and medicinal uses of these plants are given here:

1. ***Justicia spicigera* Schltdl.:** The family of this plant is Acanthaceae. Many common names are used for this plant like Mexican Honeysuckle, Firecracker Bush, and Lal basak. Mostly, leaves, roots, and barks of this plant are used for therapeutic purposes. Leaf decoction is used to treat rheumatism, asthma,

diarrhea, dysentery, piles, and pox; juice with honey is taken to treat chronic bronchitis, cough and cold, diabetes, and dysentery. On the other hand, the root bark decoction with a paste of black pepper is given to cattle for safe discharge of the placenta after delivery. Next, the bark is useful in acidity, indigestion, and heart disease.

2. ***Moringa oleifera* Lam.:** The family of this plant is Moringaceae. Some common names are used for this plant like drumstick tree, Sajina/sajne, and horseradish tree. Various parts of this plant are used for remedial purposes like roots, leaves, flowers, and fruits. Roots are used as an abortifacient, cardiac and circulatory tonic, and juice useful for asthma, nervous debility, epilepsy, gout, rheumatism, historia, and to treat enlarged liver and spleen. Conversely, the leaf extract is used for scurvy and catarrhal affection; cooked leaves are beneficial in influenza and control blood pressure and blood sugar. Next, the flowers of this plant are used to be stomachic, aphrodisiac, antilithic, and antiasthmatic. Then, fruits are used to treat diseases of liver and spleen, joint pain, tetanus and paralysis, and as anthelmintics.
3. ***Glinus oppositifolius* (L.) Aug DC.:** The family of this plant is Molluginaceae. A number of common names are used for this plant like Gima/Jima, Hill Mollugo. Whole plant is used for healing purposes. Whole plant used as stomachic, aperient, antiseptic, and is used to treat earache, itch, skin infection, ophthalmia, vomiting due to acidity; juice of fermented leaves is used as eye drops in eye disease. It is also used as a blood purifier, improves lactation, general weakness, and diabetes.
4. ***Typhonium trilobatum* (L.) Schott.:** The family of this plant is Araceae. Various local names are used by the people for this plant like Kharkol, Ghatkol, Bengal Arum. Essentially, the tuber and root of this plant are used for curative purposes. The tuber is used as a stimulant, used in hemorrhoids, windy colic, boils, eruption, and as an antidote to snake bite, paste applied as a poultice on scirrhous tumors. On the other hand, the roots are used in cases of venomous bites. Next, the aerial part of this plant is used mainly as an antidote to snake bite. It is also used as a traditional vegetable in Bengal.
5. ***Anisomeles indica* (L.) Kuntze:** The family of this plant is Lamiaceae. Many common names are used for this plant like Indian Catmint, Gopati, and Chodhara. The whole plant is used for therapeutic purposes. This plant is used as carminative, astringent, and tonic, and for problems of the uterus.
6. ***Rauvolfia serpentina* (L.) Benth. ex Kurz:** The family of this plant is Apocynaceae. Some common names of this plant are Sarpagandha, Indian Snakeroot. Largely, the roots and leaves of this plant are used for therapeutic purposes. The roots of this plant are used to treat high blood pressure, rheumatism, epilepsy, eczema, and snake bite. On the other hand, the leaves are used in removal of opacities of the cornea; paste and decoction of black pepper are used to treat pneumonia.
7. ***Ecbolium linneanum* Kurz.:** The family of this plant is Acanthaceae. A number of local names are used by the people for this plant like Blue Fox Tail and Green

Shrimp Plant. The whole plant, roots, and leaves are applied for medicinal purposes. The whole plant is used to treat dysuria and gout. Conversely, the leaf decoctions are used for stricture, jaundice, and rheumatism. Also, the roots are used in menorrhagia, crushed with water and taken to treat jaundice (Figure 4.1).

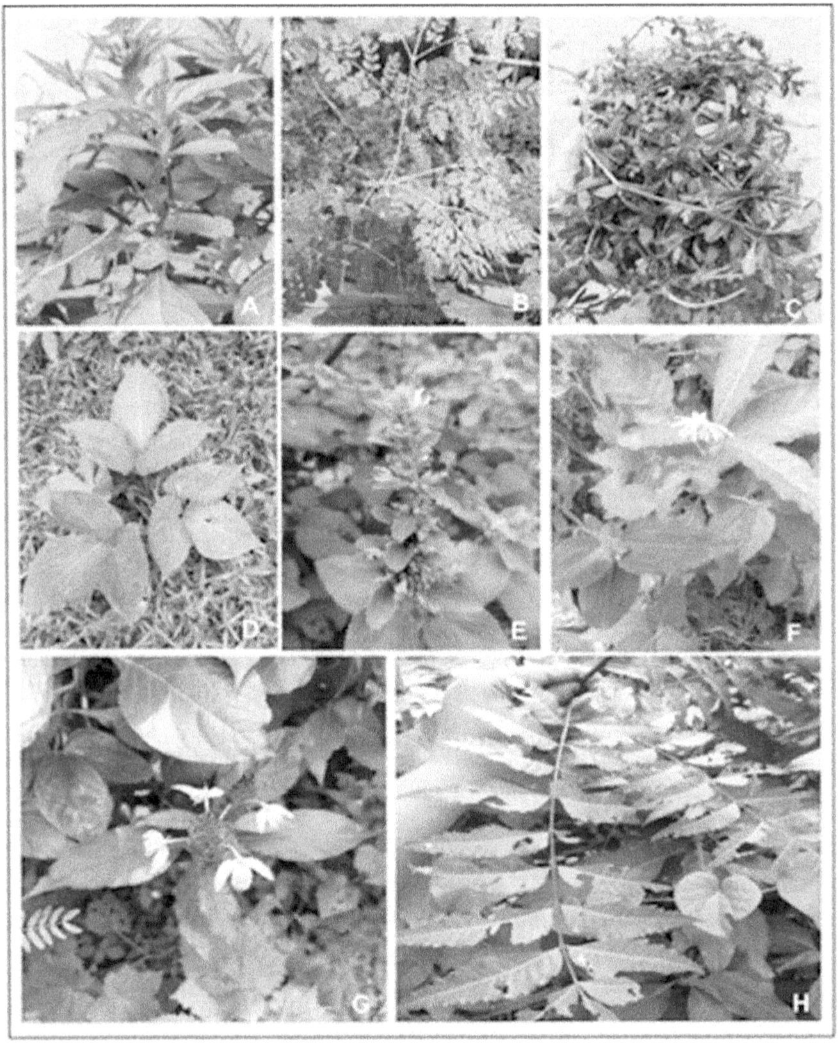

Figure 4.1. Photographs of important medicinal plants. A. *Justicia spicigera*, B. *Moringa oleifera*, C. *Glinus oppositifolius*, D. *Typhonium trilobatum*, E. *Anisomeles indica*, F. Rauvolfia. Source: Author.

8. ***Azadirachta indica* A. Juss.:** The family of this plant is Meliaceae. Various names are used by the local people for this plant like neem, Indian lilac, and margosa tree. Many parts of this plant are used for remedial purposes like bark, leaves, young branches, unripe fruit, stem, and neem seed oil. The barks of this plant are used in vomiting, burning sensation near the heart, fatigue, fever, thirst, cough, intermittency, ulcer, and inflammation. On the other hand, leaves are used to treat ophthalmia, leprosy, jaundice, consumed as preventive medicine for pox, paste applied to cure skin diseases, decoction is used for washing septic wounds, and leaf extract is used as a febrifuge, blood purifier, and to treat diabetes. Also, the young branches of this plant are used to cure cough, asthma, piles, and tumors. Again, the unripe fruit of this plant is used in urinary discharge, skin disease, piles, and toothache. Besides, the neem seed oil is applied to skin disease, ulcer, rheumatism, ringworm, and contraceptive use. Moreover, the stem and bark decoction is used by women after the menstruation period as a contraceptive.
9. ***Ficus pumila* L.:** The family of this plant is Moraceae. The common names of this plant are creeping fig and climbing fig. The medicinally usable parts of this plant are bark, fruits, and leaves. The bark is used as an antidote in snake bites. Also, fruit juice is used as an emetic and anthelmintic, mixed with turmeric and butter, and used to treat asthma; infusion is used in ulcer and skin disease. Besides, the leaves and fruits are used to treat bleeding, swelling, and hemorrhoids. The leaves and fruits are also used to treat intestinal disorder. Moreover, the leaves are used to treat skin infection, injury, and tuberculosis. In addition, the traditional East Asian medicine *Ficus pumila* (creeping fig) has been used for various ailments, including fever, diabetes, high blood pressure, joint pain, and as a tonic, with its leaves and fruits used in beverages and decoctions. Sometimes the leaves of this plant are used in beverages to treat diabetes and high blood pressure. A decoction of fruits, stems, and leaves is used to treat joint pain due to arthritis, rheumatism, and sprains. Fruits are said to promote lactation for mothers and cure impotency.
10. ***Hygrophila auriculata* (Schumach.) Heine:** The family of this plant is Acanthaceae. Various common names are used for this plant like Kulekhara, Talimkhana, Marsh Barbel, and Gokul Kanto. Many parts of this plant are used for therapeutic purposes like the whole plant, leaves, stem, and roots. The entire plant is used to treat swelling, anemia, sleeplessness, stones in kidney, and to stop bleeding. Besides, warm juice of leaves of this plant is used to treat anemia, and a decoction with long pepper is given to treat dropsy. Moreover, the root paste with country liquor is used to treat body pain. Also, the stem decoction with black pepper is given to women to treat constitutional disorders.
11. ***Hyptis suaveolens* (L.) Poit.:** The family of this plant is Lamiaceae. The common names of this plant are Wild Spikenard and Bush tea. The whole plant, as well as many other parts of this plant, like roots, flowering shoot, and leaves, is applied for medicinal purposes. The whole plant is used as carminative, sudorific,

lactagogue, stomachic, and stimulant; infusion is used as an anecephalic for uterine infection. On the other hand, the root decoction is used as an appetizer. The root is also chewed with betel nuts to treat stomach problems. Besides, the flowering shoot is used as antirheumatic, antisoporific, antispasmodic, applied to rheumatism and paralysis. Further, the juice obtained from the leaves is used as colic.

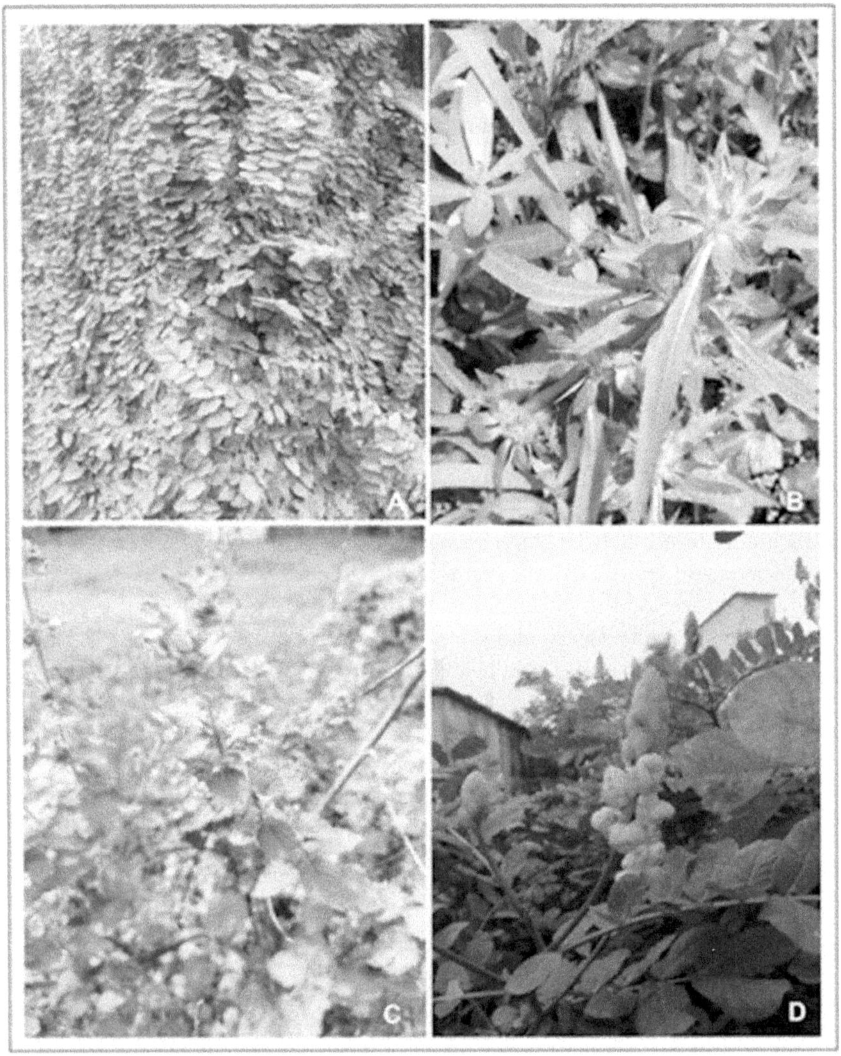

Figure 4.2. Some important medicinal plants. A. *Ficus pumila*, B. *Hygrophila auriculata*, C. *Hyptis suaveolens*, D. *Cassia alata*. Source: Author.

12. ***Cassia alata* L. [*Senna alata* (L.) Roxb.]:** The family of this plant is Fabaceae (Caesalpinioideae). The local names of this plant are Candle bush, ringworm plant, ringworm bush, Dadmari, Dadmardan. The medicinally usable parts of this plant are leaves, flowers, and bark. The leaves paste is applied to various types of skin diseases such as ringworm and itch; it is also used to treat cough, asthma, and leprosy. On the other hand, flower infusions are used to treat urinary infections as a diuretic. Moreover, the bark is used to treat hernia, syphilis, diabetes, and intestinal parasites (Figure 4.2).

Conclusion

Ethnobotany is the organized examination of how plants and humans are interconnected. Research in ethnobotany focuses on the relationships between plants and humans, as well as how indigenous communities manage plant diversity and utilize plants traditionally. For centuries, India has been the most ethnically diverse country in the world. Ethnobotany promotes an understanding of the connection between cultural diversity and biodiversity. Various tribal communities across India utilize plant species for food, animal feed, fibers, construction, and medicinal purposes. This study correlates with present-day utilization of local medicinal plants among the indigenous people, which has tremendous importance in research in terms of sustainable development.

Note

1 Acknowledgments: Authors are thankful to the Department of Botany, Bangabasi Evening College for working facilities. Conflict of interest: Authors declare that there is no conflict of interest.

References

Jain S. K. "Credibility of Traditional Knowledge Criterion of Multilocational and Multiethnic Use." *Indian J Traditional Knowledge* 3 (2004): 137–53.

Manzoor, M., M. Ahmad, M. Zafar, S. W. Gillani, H. Shaheen, A. Pieroni, A. A. Al-Ghamdi, M. S. Elshikh, S. Saqib, T. Makhkamov, and K. Khaydarov. The Local Medicinal Plant Knowledge in Kashmir Western Himalaya: A Way to Foster Ecological Transition Via Community-centred Health Seeking Strategies. *Journal of Ethnobiology and Ethnomedicine* 20, no. 19 (2023).

Mbuni, Y. M., S. Wang, B. N. Mwangi, N. J. Mbari, P. M. Musili, N. O. Walter, G. Hu, Y. Zhou, and Q.Wang. "Medicinal Plants and Their Traditional Uses in Local Communities around Cherangani Hills, Western Kenya." *Plants (Basel)* 9, no. 3 (2020): 331.

Pandey, A. K., and Y. C. Tripathi. "Ethnobotany and Its Relevance in Contemporary Research." *Journal of Medicinal Plants Studies* 5, no. 3 (2017): 123–9.

Satpati, G. G. "A Preliminary Report on Plant Based Immunity Against SARS-CoV-2 (COVID-19) in Pandemic 2020." *Research Journal of Biotechnology* 15, no. 10 (2020): 174–6.

5

Plausible Ethnobotanical Perception of Indigenous Mangrove Flora of the Indian Sundarbans

Renia Mullick,[1] Suchita Sinha,[1] Debleena Roy,[1] and Dipu Samanta[2*]

[1] PG Department of Botany, Lady Brabourne College, Kolkata, West Bengal, India

[2] Department of Botany, Dr. Kanailal Bhattacharyya College, Howrah, West Bengal, India

*Corresponding Author's Email: dipusamanta2010@gmail.com[2]

Introduction

Since ancient civilization, the medicinal plants of India have served as the rudiment of traditional medical practices involving Ayurveda (Dhakar et al. 2023).[1] The Indian subcontinent has discrete zones constituting unique flora of medicinal origin that are being used traditionally as therapeutics (Banerjee et al. 2014). Indigenous knowledge is increasingly recognized by prominent international conservation organizations, underscoring the significance of traditional methods of ecosystem management as a burgeoning area of research (Kassam et al. 2010). The Sundarbans mangrove forest, one of the largest forests in the world (140,000 ha), lies on the deltaic confluence of the Ganga, Brahmaputra, and Meghna River systems on the Bay of Bengal (Mullick, Sinha, and Roy 2024). This site is intersected by a complex network of tidal waterways, mudflats, and small islands bearing salt-tolerant mangrove species, and presents an excellent example of ongoing ecological processes. Its exceptional biodiversity is expressed in a wide range of flora and fauna consisting of 334 plant species belonging to 245 genera and 75 families, 165 algae, and 13 orchid species (Labadi 2014). The Sundarbans are quite infamous not only due to the challenging circumstances the locals face almost on a daily basis but more owing to the invaluable repository of ethnobotanically significant medicinal flora this ecosystem possesses (Chowdhury, Sanyal, and Maiti 2014). The traditional healthcare practices in the Indian Sundarbans are aligned in accordance with the local communities, influencing both the medical and cultural sectors. Furthermore, this extensive knowledge is transmitted through generations as part of the folk traditions within the community of the Sundarbans (Chowdhury, Sanyal, and Maiti 2014).

The island communities located in the Sundarbans face a multitude of challenges that disrupt their everyday activities, including transportation, access to markets, healthcare, electricity, education, and general awareness. As a repercussion to these day-to-day lifestyle struggles, the locals here have started adopting unique coping strategies (Rodriguez et al. 2012). One such strategy acknowledges the medicinal benefits of mangrove plants around them that they can utilize to cure both common and chronic health issues (Mondal et al. 2012). For example, the leaves and stem of *Acanthus illicifolius* is used in curing fever, colds, malaria, bronchitis, asthma, and skin conditions. On the other hand, *Avicennia alba* is effective against leprosy, smallpox, and ulcers. *Bruguiera gymnorrhiza*, then again, can treat diarrhea, dysentery, diabetes, and infertility (Table 5.1).

Thus, mangrove plants have been used for a long time in traditional medicine to treat a variety of ailments, including skin issues, stomach problems, and infectious diseases. Numerous medicines derived from mangroves (ashes or bark infusions) can be applied for skin disorders. Besides, these mangrove plants are rich in nutrients and secondary metabolites, including flavonoids, alkaloids, saponins, tannins, steroids, triterpenes, and glycosides. Also, mangrove plants are less toxic to humans and environmentally friendly. In addition, these mangrove plants have inhibitory activity against human, animal, and plant pathogens. Beyond their medicinal roles, these plants are deeply embedded in the community's cultural practices, rituals, and economic activities. They contribute to livelihoods through crafts, construction, and sustenance (Mondal and Das 2023).

Objectives and Methods

From the above understandings, it is revealed that the extensive usage of the mangrove medicinal plants emphasizes the interrelationship of humans with nature, highlighting the former's dependency on natural resources for therapeutic purposes (Smith-Hall, Larsen, and Pouliot 2012). This traditional knowledge, along with scientific support for the therapeutic potentials of these mangrove plants, opens up valuable opportunities for merging traditional medicine with modern healthcare practices (Mondal et al. 2012; Biswas et al. 2022). The focus of this study is to document indigenous traditional knowledge regarding the medicinal applications and sustainable utilization of mangrove plants in the Sundarbans, focusing mainly on the therapeutic potential of the members of Avicenniaceae family as they are one of the present-day dominant mangrove species in the Indian Sundarbans (Mondal et al. 2012). As contemporary consumers emphasize health, the demand for plant-based remedies is significantly increasing. Delving into the healing properties of these plants, there are auspicious prospects for several marketing sectors like pharmaceuticals, wellness products, and herbal supplements. Thus, the amalgamation of traditional knowledge and scientific

Table 5.1. Therapeutic Uses of Several Mangrove Specimens of the Indian Sundarbans

Family	Scientific Name	Local Name	Parts Used	Traditional Uses
Acanthaceae	*Acanthus illicifolius* L.	Horgoja	Leaves, Roots, Stem	• Leaves treat Tiger bites. Roots treat asthma, paralysis, leucorrhoea, debility, paralysis, osteoblastic activity, snake bite, urinal problem of child, rheumatism, breast and uterine cancer, neurosis.
Avicenniaceae	*Avicennia marina* (Forssk.) Vierh.	Peyara Bain	Fruit	Juice used as concoction to facilitate abortion. Also possesses antiulcer property, can treat rheumatism, smallpox, and other skin diseases.
	Avicennia officinalis L.	Jat Bain	Fruit, Seed, Root, Stem, Leaf, Bark	• Unripe fruits treat boils. Used as anticancer, gastroprotective, astringent, diuretic, antiulcer and skin disorders.
	Avicennia alba Blume	Kalo Bain	Leaves	• Treats rheumatic conditions, smallpox, leprosy, and infertility. Used as contraceptive and against scabies, paralysis treatment, as an aphrodisiac, curing asthma, skin diseases, snake bites, as an analgesic and has antiulcer property.
Rhizophoraceae	*Bruguiera gymnorrhiza* Lamk.	Kakra	Bark	Bark extract controls diarrhea, dysentery. Treats hepatitis, wounds, and skin disease.
	Bruguiera sexangula Poir.	Kakra	Bark	• Bark extract controls diarrhea
	Ceriops decandra (Griff.) Ding Hou	Garan	Bark, Stem	• Used in fencing, to treat skin and digestive disorders, bleeding, leprosy.
	Ceriops tagal (Perr.) Robinson	Mat-garan	Bark	• Stem bark extract stops haemorrhages and treats peptic ulcers, malaria, constipation.
	Kandelia candel (L.) Druce	Goria	Leaf	• Treats frequent urination
	Rhizophora mucronata Lam.	Garjon	Bark, leaves	• Treats eczema, dermatitis, and gastrointestinal issues.
Euphorbiaceae	*Excoecaria agallocha* L.	Genwa	Latex	Poisonous latex applied externally to alleviate pain and swelling. Treats paralysis, leprosy, and is used in abortion.

(*Continued*)

Table 5.1 (Continued)

Family	Scientific Name	Local Name	Parts Used	Traditional Uses
Malvaceae	*Heritiera fomes* Buch-Ham.	Sundari	Bark, seed	Treats ulcers, skin afflictions, acts as astringent. Grounded seed treats dysentery.
	Hibiscus tiliaceus L.	Bhola	Leaf, Bark, Root, Seed	Leaf used as a laxative and Bark mucilage for dysentery. Root treats rheumatism. Seed is used as emetic. Treats boils, headache, fever, wounds and skin disease.
Arecaceae	*Nypa fruticans* Wurmb.	Golpata	Fruit, Roots, Leaves	Alcohol is produced by fermenting fruit pulp. Treats fever and has immense therapeutic benefits. Acts against snake bite, acidity, skin irritation, diabetes, eye problems.
	Phoenix padulosa Roxb.	Hetal	Fruit, Root	The fruit pulp reduces inflammation, fevers, and skin maladies. Roots treat snake bite, rheumatism.
Sonneratiaceae	*Sonneratia apetala* Buch-Ham.	Keora	Fruit, Bark, Leaves	Fruit is used as spice to improve the flavor of cooking. Antimicrobial and anti-inflammatory properties, cures wounds, skin infections, indigestion, haemorrhage, and diarrhea.
	Sonneretia caseolaris Engler.	Chak Keora	Fruit, Root	Edible fruits used to prepare local cuisine due to its sour taste. Fruit extract used as anthelmintic. Cures intestinal problem by parasitic worm, stomachache, indigestion, haemorrhage.
	Sonneretia griffithii Kurz.	Ora	Fruit	Fruit is used as spice to improve the flavor of cooking.
Meliaceae	*Xylocarpus granatum* Koenig.	Dhundul	Bark, Leaves, Fruit	Bark extract treats dysentery. Wood is used for making furniture. Treats viral infections, fever, cholera, dysentery, cholera, gout, and fever.
	Xylocarpus mekongensis Pierre.	Pasur	Bark	Bark extract treats dysentery. Wood is used for making furniture. Treats dysentery.

Source: Saradar et al. 2024, Biswas et al. 2023, Arbiastutie et al. 2021, Chowdhury et al. 2014, Thatoi et al. 2016.

research makes the exploration of medicinal plants in the Sundarbans a field of considerable significance (Patra et al. 2019; Biswas et al. 2023).

Traditional Uses of Indigenous Mangrove Flora

The Sundarbans is the world's largest mangrove ecosystem and a UNESCO World Heritage Site. The mangroves of Sundarban are known for their distinct zonation, with different species of mangroves adapted to different tidal zones. Different species of mangroves grow in different tidal zones. The Sundarbans is home to twenty-six of the world's fifty broad mangrove species. Accordingly, the Indian Sundarbans is mainly famous for the diverse mangrove flora it possesses and has been used traditionally by the local people for therapeutic purposes. Each plant part of these indigenous mangrove species, beginning from their leaves, fruits, seeds, bark, and even their roots, has healing potentials that address a wide range of ailments (Arbiastutie, Diba, and Masriani 2021). These medicinal properties of the plants shed some light on the invaluable wealth our Indian Sundarbans hold. The major mangrove plants that have good medicinal uses are Sundari (*Heritiera fomes*), Garan (*Ceriops decandra*), Matgoran (*Ceriops tagal*), Genwa (*Excoecaria agallocha*), Garjan (*Rhizophora apiculata*), Dhundal (*Xylocarpus granatum*), Keora (*Sonneratia apetala*), Golpata (*Nypa fruticans*), Kankra (*Bruguiera sexangula*), and so on. Table 5.1 shows the traditional therapeutic uses of some famous mangrove specimens residing in the Indian Sundarbans along with the specific plant part bearing such medicinal properties.

The Sundarbans mangrove forest is a habitat of mangrove trees in the delta of the Ganges, Brahmaputra, and Meghna rivers in the Bay of Bengal. The Sundarbans is the world's largest contiguous mangrove forest. The habitat of mangroves is distributed geographically based on the salinity levels as each one of them has an optimal salt-tolerance range. The once-dominated freshwater-loving mangrove genera *Heritiera fomes* and *Nypa fruticans* are on the verge of extinction due to extensive sea level rise that is increasing the salinity levels of the water body of Indian Sundarbans with each passing year. Thus, they are considered low salinity indicator species preferably residing in oligohaline to mesohaline zones. *Exoecaria* and *Bruguiera*, on the other hand, are the medium salinity indicator species, being most abundant in the mesohaline zones. Whereas the species of *Avicennia* (one of the modern-day dominant mangroves in the Indian Sundarbans) are acknowledged as high salinity indicator species found to occupy the polyhaline zones (Barik et al. 2018).

This might be attributable to the multiple salt-tolerance mechanisms they possess involving salt-secreting glands in their leaves and the presence of salinome (Natarajan et al. 2021). Salt-tolerant plants have higher antioxidant activity, which helps with leaf water content, leaf growth, and membrane stability. Alongside, *Avicennia* is able to withstand frequent and long-lasting tidal inundations (Akter et al. 2020). In mangrove succession, *Avicennia* acts as a pioneer species and appears first on the newly accreted lands of the Sundarbans, which in turn creates a favorable habitat condition for the next seral species such as *Heritiera fomes*, *Excoecaria agallocha*, *Ceriops decandra*, and so on. They naturally grow along the river banks, causing reduced bank erosion and stabilizing the coastal lands for crop cultivation (Alam et al. 2017). *Avicennia* sp. thus proves to be valuable in various aspects, which makes it an intriguing candidate for deeper exploration and research.

Avicenniaceae Members: Bioactive Components and Therapeutic Potential

Bioactive components are naturally occurring chemical compounds found in plants, animals, and some microorganisms that have evidently positive effects on human health, potentially acting as preventative or therapeutic agents for various diseases, with possible applications in medicine and functional foods due to their antioxidant, anti-inflammatory, anticancer, and immune-modulating properties; examples include polyphenols, flavonoids, carotenoids, omega-3 fatty acids, and certain peptides, depending on the source material. Thus, the bioactive components are clinically evident, naturally produced organic molecules that do not constitute nutrients but have therapeutic properties that promote public health. They enhance the plant's appearance, aroma, and taste in addition to protecting it from illness and environmental damage.

In this context, this particular study has addressed the botanical wealth of the Avicenniaceae members and also revealed the bioactive components present in them (see Figure 5.1), along with a brief action mechanism of each responsible

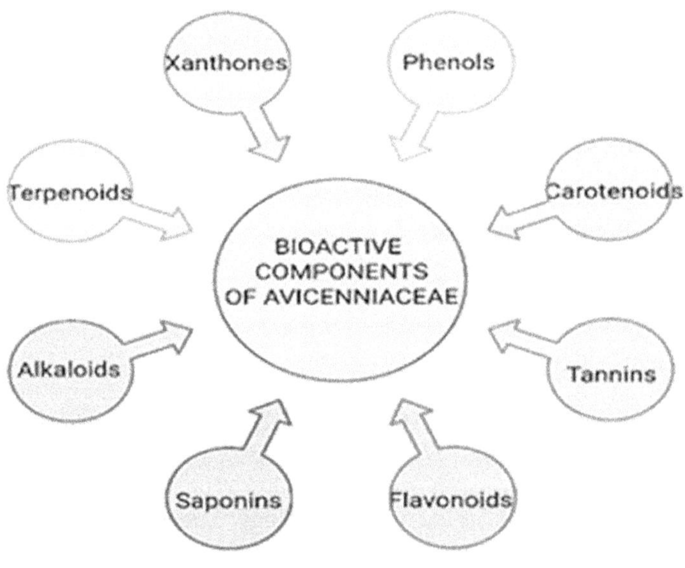

Figure 5.1. Bioactive compounds found in members of Avicenniaceae. *Source*: Author.

compound that contributes to their therapeutic potentials such as antioxidative, anticancer, anti-inflammatory, and antimicrobial benefits (Das 2021). Furthermore, this study has offered medicinal implications of these plants for potential drug discovery that can be beneficial not only to the local settlers of Sundarbans but in general to mankind, as they are currently the most widespread and easily available mangrove genera residing in the Indian Sundarbans. Again, the FTIR (Fourier Transform Infrared) spectrum analysis performed by Mitra et al. of the methanolic and ethanolic extracts of *Avicennia* sp. revealed a diverse array of functional groups. The phenolic compounds in the plant sample have abundant hydroxyl groups, whose enhanced hydroxylation provides toxicity toward microbes, thus resulting in the antibacterial property exhibited by the plants. Also, the carboxylic group helps in C = O stretching renowned for its antimicrobial activities. Moreover, the secondary metabolic LC-MS profiling of the methanol extract of *Avicennia* sp. exposed a range of phytoconstituents which is listed in Table 5.2 that directly contributes to the plant's medicinal benefits (Mitra et al. 2023).

Thus, plants in the Avicenniaceae family have numerous medicinal properties, including antiviral and antibacterial properties. All the medicinal properties, bioactive components, as well as therapeutic potentials such as antioxidative, anticancer, anti-inflammatory, and antimicrobial benefits of Avicenniaceae family members are given in the following points and figures.

(a) **Antioxidative Property:** *Avicennia* sp. is acknowledged for being enriched in certain bioactive components (see Figure 5.2), for instance, tannins, flavonoids, phenols, and carotenoids; an amalgamation of which contributes to their antioxidant capacity (Dahibhate, Roy, and Kumar 2020). Figure 5.2 shows the compounds contributing to the antioxidant potential of *Avicennia* sp.

(b) **Antimicrobial property:** *Avicennia marina* is famous for its potent antimicrobial effects attributable to a widespread array of bioactive elements, including flavonoids, phenols, saponins, and alkaloids (Biswas et al. 2023). Pervasive research by eminent scientists revealed the potency of the abovementioned compounds against a broad spectrum of pathogens, implying their formidable role in preventing microbial infections (Mitra and Pal 2021). Figure 5.3 shows the antimicrobial potentiality of Avicenniaceae members.

(c) **Antibacterial:** As a defense mechanism against stressful and unfavorable environmental conditions, *Avicennia marina* starts accumulating certain phytochemicals like amino acids, phenols, carotenoids, glycosides, and triterpenes in their roots that deciphers antibacterial property to the plant and has proven to be effective against few bacterial strains (Okla et al. 2021). Figure 5.4 shows the antibacterial effect of *Avicennia marina* proven against four renowned bacterial strains.

(d) **Antifungal property:** The roots, fruits, leaves, stem or in another word the entire plant of *Avicennia marina* bears antifungal potential against *Candida albicans* and *Aspergillus fumigatus* (Okla et al. 2021).

Table 5.2.Phytoconstituents Revealed Upon Metabolic Profiling of *Avicennia* sp.

Bioactive Components	Nature of Compound	Medicinal Property	Bioactive Components	Nature of Compound
Metofluthrin	Pyrethroid	Insecticidal property	Metofluthrin	• Pyrethroid
Sec-O-glucosylhamaudol	Natural product	Analgesic	Sec-O-glucosylhamaudol	Natural product
Dimethyldiethanolammonium	Amino-alcohol	Nootropic	Dimethyldiethanolammonium	• Amino-alcohol
Streptonigrin	Amino-quinone	Antitumor and antibacterial property	Streptonigrin	• Amino-quinone
Lofepramine	Tertiary amine	Antidepressant	Lofepramine	Tertiary amine
Sagopilone	Epothilone	Anticancer property	Sagopilone	• Epothilone
Soyasapogenol D				
2-(3,4-Dihydroxyphenyl)-5,7-dihydroxy-4H-chromen-4-on	Triterpenoid saponin	Garan	Soyasapogenol D	• Triterpenoid saponin
4-(3,5-Di-tert-butyl-4-hydroxyphenyl) butyl acrylate	Luteolin	Antioxidative, antitumor and anti-inflammatory properties	2-(3,4-Dihydroxyphenyl)-5,7-dihydroxy-4H-chromen-4-on	• Luteolin
16R,17-dihydroxy-ent-9(11)-kauren-19-al	Phenol	Antioxidant	4-(3,5-Di-tert-butyl-4-hydroxyphenyl) butyl acrylate	• Phenol
	Diterpenoid	Cytotoxic effect	16R,17-dihydroxy-ent-9(11)-kauren-19-al	• Diterpenoid
(4R,5S,8R,9R,10S,13S)-ent-17-hydroxy-16-oxobeyeran-19-al	*Excoecaria agallocha* L.	Genwa	(4R,5S,8R,9R,10S,13S)-ent-17-hydroxy-16-oxobeyeran-19-al	Poisonous latex applied externally to alleviate pain and swelling. Treats paralysis, leprosy and is used in abortion.

Pentadecanoic acid 14-methyl-, methyl ester	Palmitic acid methyl ester	Antioxidant, Antifungal, Antimicrobial	Pentadecanoic acid	Palmitic acid methyl ester
	Hibiscus tiliaceus L.	Bhola	14-methyl-, methyl ester	Leaf used as a laxative and Bark mucilage for dysentery. Root treats rheumatism. Seed is used as emetic. Treats boils, headache, fever, wounds
Bioactive Components	**Nature of Compound**	**Medicinal Property**	**Bioactive Components**	**Nature of Compound**
Metofluthrin	Pyrethroid	Insecticidal property	Metofluthrin	Pyrethroid
Sec-O-glucosylhamaudol	Natural product	Analgesic	Sec-O-glucosylhamaudol	Natural product
Dimethyldiethanolammonium	Amino-alcohol	Nootropic	Dimethyldiethanolammonium	Amino-alcohol
Streptonigrin	Amino-quinone	Antitumor and antibacterial property	Streptonigrin	Amino-quinone
Lofepramine	Tertiary amine	Antidepressant	Lofepramine	Tertiary amine
Sagopilone	Epothilone	Anticancer property	Sagopilone	Epothilone

Source: Mitra et al. 2023, Thatoi et al. 2016.

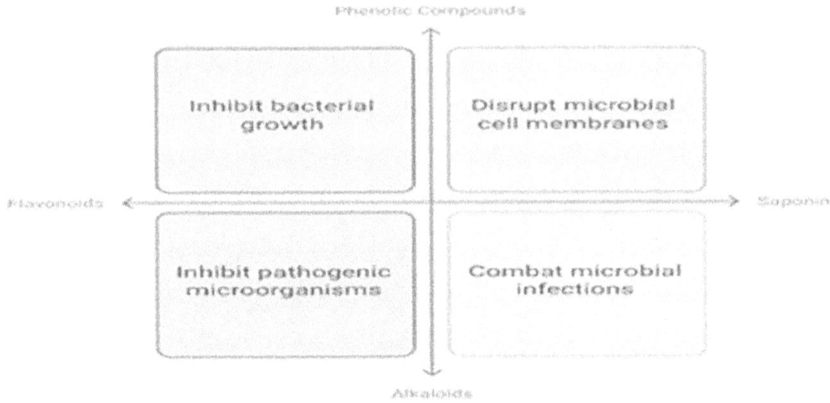

Figure 5.2. Compounds contributing to the antioxidant potential of *Avicennia* sp. Source: Author.

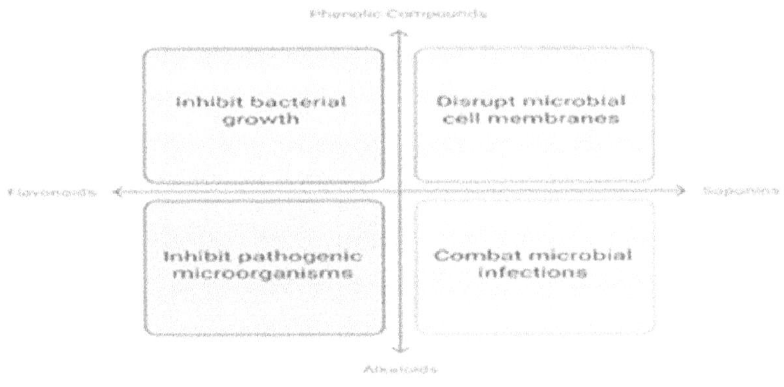

Figure 5.3. Antimicrobial potentialities of Avicenniaceae members. Source: Author.

(e) **Anti-inflammatory property:** Members of Avicenniaceae, especially the leaves of *Avicennia officinalis* and *Avicennia alba*, have a rich repertoire of flavonoids, terpenoids, and phenolic compounds (Mitra et al. 2022). The assortment of these bioactive components in this mangrove family highlights their therapeutic potential against curing inflammation (Sohaib et al. 2022). Figure 5.5 shows the anti-inflammatory property of Avicenniaceae members.

(f) **Anticancer property:** *Avicennia alba* and *Avicennia marina* are recognized for their significant anticancer effects against few cell lines attributable to the presence of flavonoids in them, that upon undergoing apoptosis, kills the human promyelocytic leukemia cells furthermore bringing about the anticancer property in them (Eswaraiah et al. 2020). The leaves of *Avicennia germinans* contain certain important bioactive compounds including 9, 10- anthracenedione which is an aromatic organic compound, and few alkanes: Tetratriacontane and Tetracosane. The latter compound possesses anticancer properties against AGS (human gastric

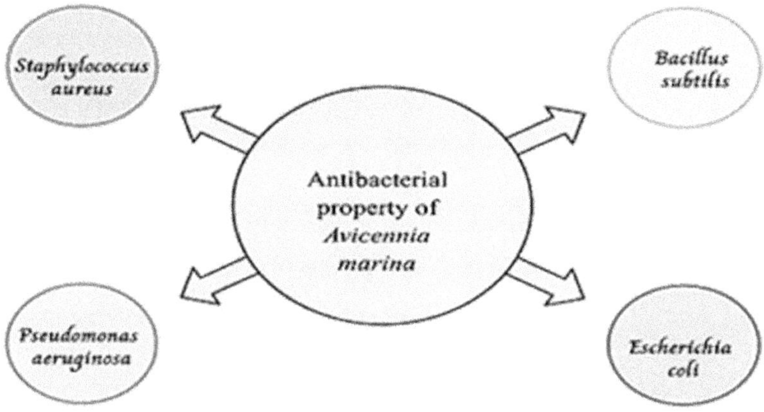

Figure 5.4. Antibacterial effect of *Avicennia marina* proven against four renowned bacterial strains. Source: Author.

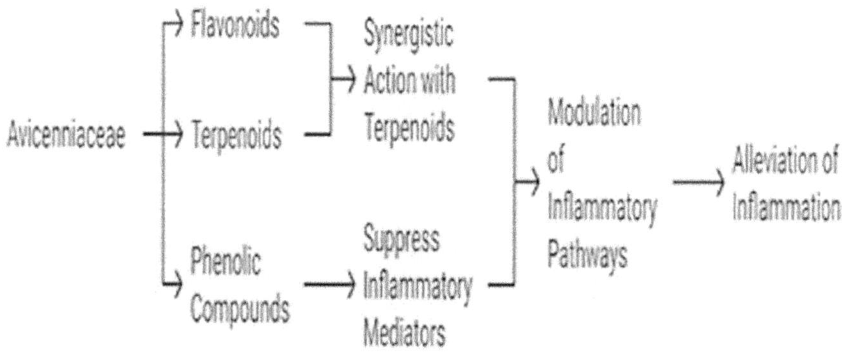

Figure 5.5. Anti-inflammatory properties of Avicenniaceae members. Source: Author.

adenocarcinoma), HT-2918 (parent cell line of human colon adenocarcinoma), and NIH 3T3 (mouse embryonic fibroblast cell line) cell lines (Eswaraiah et al. 2020). Figure 5.6 shows the anticancer property of *Avicennia marina* against five important cancer cell lines.

(g) **Wound healing:** Tannins and phenols, stressing more toward the phenols, in the leaves of *Avicennia* sp. fosters efficient wound-healing properties (Vinoth, Kumaravel, and Ranganathan 2019). Figure 5.7 shows the wound-healing mechanism of *Avicennia* sp.

(h) **Promoting overall skin health:** Carotenoids and xanthones present in those belonging to the Avicenniaceae family suggest significant skin health benefits. Carotenoids, recognized for their antioxidative potential, maintain skin integrity (Sumadri, Basyuni, and Wati 2018). An amalgamation of both these bioactive components implies prospects for skin wellness, thereby providing natural support for various health concerns (Kumar and Pola 2023).

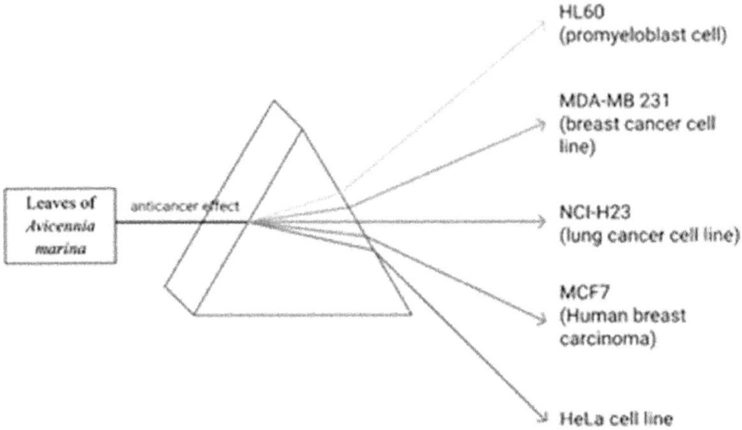

Figure 5.6. Anticancer property of *Avicennia marina* against five important cancer cell lines. Source: Author.

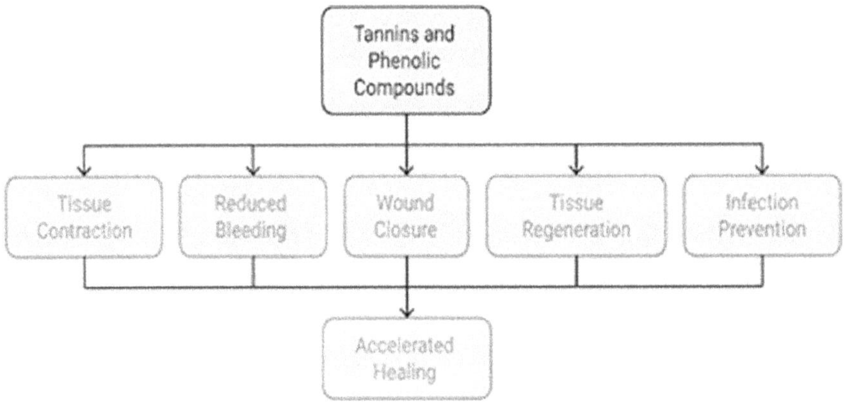

Figure 5.7. Wound-healing mechanism of *Avicennia* sp. Source: Author.

(i) **Antidiuretic:** Leaf extracts of *Avicennia* sp. highlighted diuretic properties as scientists observed that the quantity of Na^+ ions was higher as compared to the K^+ ions excreted. This concluded the plants to act as a potent diuretic causing less hyperkalemic side effects (Sadeer et al. 2022).

Possible Measures to Conserve Ecosystems

Although promising therapeutic potentials are exhibited by the Avicenniaceae family members, their effectiveness and underlying modes of action need to be extensively studied and validated. Their medicinal benefits have been profusely exploited by the local settlers from time immemorial (Chowdhury, Sanyal, and Maiti 2014). Nonetheless, this mangrove-dominated ecosystem suffers from critical threats including climate change caused as an aftermath of sea level rise, cyclonic disturbances, pollution, and anthropogenic load followed by habitat destruction (Biswas et al. 2023). Thus, immediate conservation strategies aiming to manage the ecosystem and pollution levels from industries, engaging in sustainable harvesting toward a more resilient climate are crucial to shield the ethnobotanically rich mangrove flora of the Sundarbans (Nishat, Rahman, and Mahmud 2016). These concomitant efforts will not only maintain the cultural integrity but will also provide invaluable perceptions of sustainable living and traditional healthcare approaches.

The local communities need to be empowered through proper education, motivation, and awareness programs and by adopting eco-friendly approaches for conserving this valuable heritage. The government ruling bodies should plan for alternate modes of income for the local people like local tour guides, cottage industries, and agroforestry that will reduce their dependency on the mangrove forest resources. Anthropological pressure, especially tourist load during the winter season, needs to be regulated by maintaining ecotourism practices based on the carrying capacity of the island. Alongside, commercial hotels and marketplaces in the less vulnerable zones of the Indian Sundarbans and fish processing units will help in improving the economic conditions of the population. Implementing national acts and policies can control poaching practices and habitat loss. The newly unprotected land areas can be recolonized by mangrove afforestation, the size of which needs to be kept under check. Also, nurseries and herbariums need to be constructed for storing seeds and growing mangrove saplings (Nishat, Rahman, and Mahmud 2016).

Conclusion and Recommendation

The divergent group of medicinal plants residing in the Indian Sundarbans constitutes an invaluable asset not only for the local populace but also for the broader medical field. In light of pressing global issues such as antimicrobial resistance and drug efficacy, there is a compelling need to explore and evaluate plant resources for promising solutions. Scientific research and preservation strategies of this ethnobotanical wealth will significantly enhance the pursuit of innovative therapeutic interventions and healthcare solutions. Upon integrating traditional knowledge by utilizing the bioactive components naturally present in the plant pharmacophore with contemporary scientific research, opportunities will arise for unraveling novel pharmaceutical compounds and medicaments with minimal post-therapeutic complications, in turn enriching the global medical cabinet, thereby benefiting human health.

Note

1 The authors are indebted to DBT (Department of Biotechnology)—Boost to University Interdisciplinary Life Science Departments for Education and Research (DBT-BUILDER) for providing all sorts of assistance required for completion of this work.

References

Akter, A., P. Biella, P. Batáry, and J. Klečka. "Changing Pollinator Communities along a Disturbance Gradient in the Sundarbans Mangrove Forest: A Case Study on Acanthus ilicifolius and Avicennia officinalis." *Global Ecology and Conservation* 24, no. e01282 (2020): 1–13.

Alam, M. R., M. Hossain, M. M. Rahman, T. Biswas, S. Nasrin, and M. L. R. Khusi. "Ecological Status and Environmental Protective Role of *Avicennia officinalis* in the Vulnerable Coastal Regions of Bangladesh: An Overview." *Indian Forester* 143, no. 9 (2017): 817–22.

Arbiastutie, Y., F. Diba, and M. Masriani. "Ethnobotanical and Ecological Studies of Medicinal Plants in a Mangrove Forest in Mempawah District, West Kalimantan, Indonesia." *Biodiversitas* 22, no. 6 (2021): 3164–70.

Banerjee, J., S. Biswas, N. R. Madhu, S. R. Karmakar, and S. J. Biswas. "A Better Understanding of Pharmacological Activities and Uses of Phytochemicals of *Lycopodium clavatum*: A Review." *Journal of Pharmacognosy and Phytochemistry* 3, no. 1 (2014): 207–10.

Barik, J., A. Mukhopadhyay, T. Ghosh, S. K. Mukhopadhyay, S. M. Chowdhury, and S. Hazra. "Mangrove Species Distribution and Water Salinity: An Indicator Species Approach to Sundarban." *Journal of Coastal Conservation* 22 (2018): 361–8.

Biswas, G., B. Sarkar, S. R. Sarkar, N. Sharma, S. Sultana, and N. R. Madhu. "Exploring the Ethnobotanical Resources of Indian Sundarbans: An Insight into Medicinal Plants." *IAPH* 2 (2023): 56–71.

Biswas, G. "*Amaranthus spinosus* Linn.: A Common Culinary Herb with Potential Medicinal Value." *IAPH* 1 (2022): 146–54.

Chowdhury, A., P. Sanyal, and S. K. Maiti. "Ethnobotanical Understanding of Mangroves: An Investigation from Central Part of Indian Sundarbans." *International Journal of Botany and Research* 4 (2014): 29–34.

Dahibhate, N. L., U. Roy, and K. Kumar. "Phytochemical Screening, Antimicrobial and Antioxidant Activities of Selected Mangrove Species." *Current Bioactive Compound* 16, no. 2 (2020): 152–63.

Das, S. S. *Mangroves of Indian Sundarban: Ecological, Biochemical and Molecular Aspects*. Lulu Publication, 2021, Raleigh, NC.

Dhakar, S., and H. Tare. "Therapeutic Potential of Polyherbal Tablets: A Comprehensive Assessment of Pharmacological Activity." *International Journal of Experimental Research and Review* 34 (2023): 97–105.

Eswaraiah, G., K. A. Peele, S. Krupanidhi, R. B. Kumar, and T. C. Venkateswarulu. "Identification of Bioactive Compounds in Leaf Extract of *Avicennia alba* by GC-MS Analysis and Evaluation of Its In-vitro Anticancer Potential against MCF7 and HeLa Cell Lines." *Journal of King Saud University–Science* 32, no. 1 (2020): 740–4.

Kassam, K. A., M. Karamkhudoeva, M. Ruelle, and M. Baumflek. "Medicinal Plant Use and Health Sovereignty: Findings from the Tajik and Afghan Pamirs." *Human Ecology* 38 (2010): 817–29.

Kumar, M. K., and S. Pola. "Mangrove Species as a Potential Source of Bioactive Compounds for Diverse Therapeutic Applications." *Marine Antioxidants*, 2023: 249–63.

Labadi, S. "UNESCO World Heritage Convention (1972)." *Springer eBooks*, 2014: 7434–9.

Mitra, A. and Pal, P. K. "A Review on Potential Bioactive Phytochemicals for Novel Therapeutic Applications with special emphasis on Mangrove Species." *Journal of Applied Biology & Biotechnology* 9, no. 4 (2021): 114–121.

Mitra, S., N. Naskar, S. Lahiri, and P. Chaudhuri. "A Study on Phytochemical Profiling of *Avicennia marina* Mangrove Leaves Collected from Indian Sundarbans." *Sustainable Chemistry for the Environment* 4 (2023): 100041.

Mitra, S., F. Islam, R. Das, H. Urmee, A. Akter, A. M. Idris, M. U. Khandaker, Md. A. Almikhlafi, R. Sharma, and T. B. Emran. "Pharmacological Potential of Avicennia alba Leaf Extract: An Experimental Analysis Focusing on Antidiabetic, Anti-inflammatory, Analgesic, and Antidiarrheal Activity." *BioMed Research International* 2022 (2022): 7624189.

Mondal, B. K., and R. Das. "Appliance of Indigenous Knowlege in Mangrove Conservation and Sustaining Livelihood in Indian Sundarban Delta: A Geospatial Analysis." *Traditional Ecological Knowledge of Resource Management in Asia*, 2023: 77–101.

Mondal, B., N. C. Sarkar, C. K. Mondal, R. K. Maiti, and H. G. Rodriguez. "Mangrove Plants and Traditional Ayurvedic Practitioners in Sundarbans Region of West Bengal, India." *ROC* 13, no. 2 (2012): 669–74.

Mullick, R., S. Sinha, and D. Roy. "Role of Phytoplankton in Comprehending the Vulnerabilities Imposed Due to Gangasagar Festival." *IJEES* 50 (2024): 123–9.

Natarajan, P., A. K. Murugesan, G. Govindan, A. Gopalkrishnan, R. Kumar, P. Duraisamy, R. Balaji, Tanuja, P. S. Shyamli, A. K. Parida, and M. Parani. "A Reference-grade Genome Identifies Salt-tolerance Genes from the Salt-secreting Mangrove Species *Avicennia marina*." *Communications Biology* 4 (2021): 851.

Nishat, B., A. J. M. Z. Rahman, and S. Mahmud. "Sundarban Joint Landscape Narrative." *IWA*, 2016.

Okla, M. K., A. A. Alatar, S. S. Al-Amri, W. H. Soufan, A. Ahmad, and M. A. Abdel-Maksoud. "Antibacterial and Antifungal Activity of the Extracts of Different Parts of *Avicennia marina* (Forssk.) Vierh." *Plants (Basel).* 10, no. 2 (2021): 252.

Patra, J. K., G. Das, S. Kumar, and H. Thatoi. *Ethnopharmacology and Biodiversity of Medicinal Plants*. New York: Apple Academic Press, 2019.

Rodriguez, H. G., B. Mondal, N. C. Sarkar, A. Ramaswamy, D. Rajkumar, and R. K. Maiti. "Comparative Morphology and Anatomy of Few Mangrove Species in Sundarbans, West Bengal, India and its Adaptation to Saline Habitat." *International Journal of Stress Management* 3, no. 1 (2012): 1–17.

Sadeer, N. B., and Md. F. Mahomoodally. *Mangroves with Therapeutic Potential for Human Health*. Academic Press, 2022.

Saradar, B., S. Mandal, and S. Kumar. "Ethnobotanical Inventory and Medicinal Potential of Mangrove Flora in the Sundarbans, West Bengal, India." *Journal of Biodiversity and Conservation* 8, no. 1 (2024): 1–6.

Smith-Hall, C., H. O. Larsen, and M. Pouliot. "People, Plants and Health: A Conceptual Framework for Assessing Changes in Medicinal Plant Consumption." *Journal of Ethnobiology and Ethnomedicine* 8 (2012): 1–11.

Sohaib, M., F. N. Al-Barakah, H. M. Migdadi, and F. M. Husain. "Comparative Study among *Avicennia marina*, *Phragmites australis*, and *Moringa oleifera* Based Ethanolic-extracts for Their Antimicrobial, Antioxidant, and Cytotoxic Activities." *Saudi Journal of Biological Sciences* 29, no. 1 (2022): 111–22.

Sumadri, S., M. Basyuni, and R. Wati. "Antimicrobial Activity of Polyisoprenoids of Sixteen Mangrove Species from North Sumatra, Indonesia." *Biodiversitas* 19, no. 4 (2018): 1243–8.

Thatoi, H., D. Samantaray, and S. K. Das. "The Genus *Avicennia*, a Pioneer Group of Dominant Mangrove Plant Species with Potential Medicinal Values: A Review." *Front Life Sciences* 9, no. 4 (2016): 267–91.

Vinoth, R., S. Kumaravel, and R. Ranganathan. "Therapeutic and Traditional Uses of Mangrove Plants." *J. Drug Deliv. Ther.* 9, no. 4 (2019): 849–54.

Mangroves of Indian Sundarbans: A Treasure Trove of Medicinal Properties and Ethnomedicinal Significance

Sreemanti Banerjee,[1*] Chirabrata Sarkar,[2] and Suparna Sardar[1]

[1]Diamond Harbour Women's University, Sarisha, South 24 Parganas, West Bengal, India

[2]West Bengal State University, Barasat, North 24 Parganas, West Bengal, India

*Corresponding Author's Email: sreemantibanerjee@gmail.com

Introduction

The Sundarbans is considered the largest delta and the world's largest continuous mangrove forest, covering 10,000 km^2 of land and water within the Ganges, Brahmaputra, and Meghna River delta (Ghosh et al. 2015). Bangladesh contains 62 percent (6,000 km^2) of the mangrove forest, while India contains 38 percent (Spalding, Kainuma, and Collins 2010). Situated in a unique bioclimatic zone in the coastal region of the Bay of Bengal, it is a significant landmark of ancient heritage, encompassing mythological and historical events. Recognized internationally for its high biodiversity of mangrove flora and fauna on both land and water, the Sundarbans is bestowed with magnificent scenic beauty and natural resources (Ghosh et al. 2015). Here, the mangroves can be categorized into three main groups. True mangroves are typically found in intertidal areas between high water levels of neap and spring tides. There are eighty identified species of true mangroves, with 50–60 species contributing to the functioning of mangrove forests (Bandaranayake 2002). Minor species of mangroves do not form pure communities and have minimal impact on the mangrove ecosystem. The third group, that is, Mangal mangrove associates, are salinity tolerant and are not typically found with true mangroves. Their occurrence is limited to landwards and seawards (Bandaranayake 1998). Ghosh et al. (2002) reported 105 plant species from the Indian Sundarbans, including twenty-five true mangrove species. Of these, eighteen species are dominant, namely *Rhizophora mucronata*, *R. apiculata*, *Bruguiera gymnorrhiza*,

B. sexangula, *B. cylindrica*, *B. parviflora*, *Ceriops decandra*, *C. tagal*, *Kandelia candel*, *Avicennia marina*, *A. alba*, *A. officinalis*, *Sonneratia apetala*, *S. griffithii*, *S. caseolaris*, *Lumnitzera racemosa*, *Phoenix paludosa*, and *Nypa fruticans*, while thirty belong to the mangrove associated species category, thirty-seven are back mangrove species, six are beach flora, and seven are parasites/epiphytes/mistletoes. Certain species, such as *Bruguiera gymnorrhiza*, *Ceriops decandra*, *Avicennia* spp., *Excoecaria agallocha*, *Acanthus ilicifolius*, *Porteresia coarctata*, and *Phoenix paludosa*, are uniformly distributed and abundant throughout the Indian Sundarbans. Others like *Rhizophora apiculata*, *Bruguiera parviflora*, *B.* cylindrica, *B. sexangula*, *Sonneratia caseolaris*, *Ceriops tagal*, *Scyphiphora hydrophyllacea*, *Cynometra ramiflora*, *Acanthus volubilis*, *Cerbera manghas*, and *Dodonea viscosa* have specific and restricted distribution.

However, natural stress factors such as rising salinity, anaerobic conditions due to sea level rise, increased sulfide levels in estuarine sediments, and ongoing erosion caused by high tidal forces, cyclonic storms as well as anthropogenic interferences are significantly degrading the mangrove ecosystem and loss of species (Begam et al. 2020; Chowdhury et al. 2019). In addition to exploring angiosperm diversity, researchers have also investigated algal diversity in the Sundarbans. Satpati, Barman, and Pal (2013) reported thirty-four green algal taxa with *Rhioclonium*, *Lola*, *Cladophora*, and *Chaetomorpha* being the dominant taxa, along with some species of *Spirogyra* and *Trentepohlia*. Barman, Satpati, and Pal (2015) reported thirty-seven cyanobacteria from thirty islands, with *Oscillatora*, *Lyngbya*, and *Leptolyngbya* as the dominant taxa. Banerjee, Singh, and Pal (2024) conducted morphological and molecular characterization of some cyanobacterial taxa from the Sundarbans. Researchers are continuously studying the mangrove ecosystem and there is still uncertainty about the total number of mangrove species in the Indian Sundarbans.

Mangrove plants offer both ecological and economic benefits like acting as carbon sinks, protecting coastlines from erosion, and serving as a nursery for various marine life while also offering economic advantages through fisheries, ecotourism, and potential medicinal uses, making them a valuable ecosystem with both environmental and financial importance. Thus, ecologically, mangrove plants prevent soil erosion, protect coastal land, and provide essential nutrients for estuarine animals through their leaves (Bandaranayake 2002). Additionally, mangrove foliage plays a crucial role in detritus formation, benefiting marine detritivores (Bandaranayake 2002). On the other hand, economically, mangrove plants are used in boat construction, furniture making, tannin production for dyeing and leather, and as folklore medicine due to their rich phytochemical content. These plants contain various bioactive components such as secolabdane diterpenoids, triterpenoids, phytosterols, and other pharmaceutical properties. For example, *Rhizophora* yields rhizophorin A (Adhikari et al. 2016), while *Sonneratia* contains novel sonneratiosides, lupeol, oleanic acid (triterpenoids), β-sitosterol, β-stigmasterol (phytosterol) (Chaiyadej et al. 2004) and *Heritiera* offers procyanidins and other compounds (Stafford 1988). *Bruguiera* and *Avicennia* plants also contribute dammarane triterpenes and pentacyclic triterpenes, respectively (Sharaf, El-Ansari, and Saleh 2000; Jia, Wei, and Xin 2004; Homhual et al. 2006).

Objectives and Methods

Several plant species like *Bruguiera gymnorrhiza*, *Rhizophora mucronata*, *A. ilicifolius* are the most traditionally used medicinal mangroves (Bibi et al. 2019). Several *in vitro* and *in vivo* studies have revealed and confirmed their pharmaceutical properties. Mass spectrometric studies along with advanced techniques confirmed the specific active constituents in the case of many plants. The pharmacological properties of mangrove plants were confirmed through extensive phytochemical screenings. These medicinal plants need to be protected to ensure their ethnomedicinal properties. The tribal communities in the mangrove region relied on the vegetation for timber, fuel wood, and other non-wood forest products (Saenger et al. 2002). It is important to implement conservation measures to safeguard the plants for environmental well-being and to ensure a sustainable supply of other forest products for local people. Promoting self-employment through ecotourism, beekeeping, and fishing industries can help improve the socioeconomic conditions of local communities. The aim of the current study is to explore the ethnobotanical use and phytochemical constituents of mostly true mangrove species in the Indian Sundarbans. Extensive literature review was conducted to identify the active components of the extracts and the pharmacological activities of these plants.

Indian Sundarbans and Ethnomedicinal Plants

A number of authors have presented reports on the medicinal properties of Sundarban mangroves of India and their significance as folklore medicine. Images of some ethnomedical plants are shown in Figure 6.1. In addition, Table 6.1 is representing the ethnomedicinal mangrove plants of the Indian Sundarbans and their uses.

Phytochemical Constituents of the Mangroves

Mangroves contain many phytochemical constituents, including alkaloids, flavonoids, terpenoids, tannins, and phenols. These compounds can be found in the leaves, stems, barks, fruits, and seeds of the mangrove plants. Table 6.1 shows the traditional ethnobotanical usage of forty-three mangrove plants as per the available records. However, extensive characterizations of some mangrove genera were carried out by several researchers, which revealed the active chemical constituents responsible for the pharmacological activities. The following points have focused on the phytochemical constituents of mainly true mangrove genera of Indian Sundarbans like *Acanthus*, *Aegiceras*, *Avicennia*, *Bruguiera*, *Calophyllum*, *Derris*, *Excoecaria*, *Heritiera*, *Lumnitzera*, *Rhizophora*, *Sonneratia*, and *Xylocarpus*.

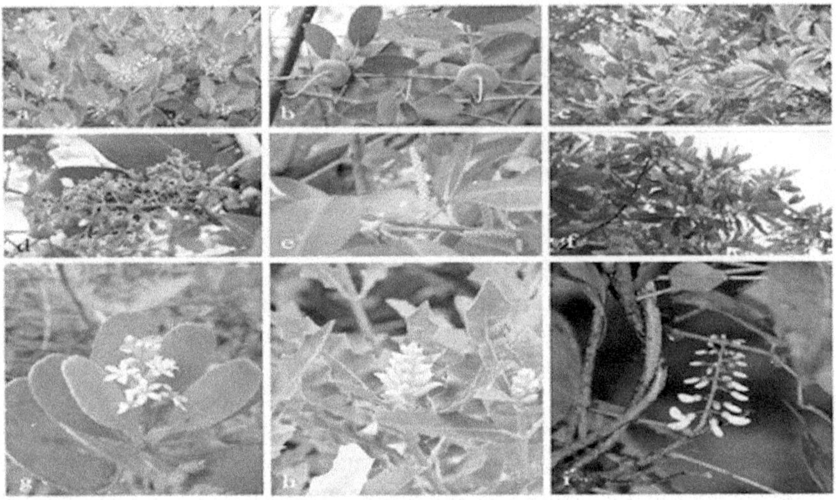

Figure 6.1. Ethnomedicinal plants of Indian Sundarbans. Source: All the images are subject to copyright @ Npark flora and fauna web, reproduced with permission.

(a) ***Acanthus* sp.:** Mainly three species of *Acanthus* have been reported from Indian Sundarbans (see Table 6.1). Ethanolic, methanolic, chloroform, and hexane extracts are obtained from different parts of *A. ilicifolius* like root, leaf, aerial parts, and stem. Pods have been found to contain various chemical compounds: aliphatic glycosides including ilicifolioside B, ilicifolioside C, lignan glycosides like lyoniresinol derivatives, flavonoids (Quercetin and its derivatives), alkaloids (acanthicifoline), trigonellin (Tiwari, Minocha, and Masood 1980; Minocha and Tiwari 1980), 2-Benzoxazolinone (Murty, Wahidulla, and Kamat 1984), and Benzoxazin-3-one (Kokpol, Chittawong, and Miles 1986), lignans, triterpenoid saponins, sterols, fatty acids, and coumaric acid derivatives. Leaf extracts of *A. ebracteatus* also show the presence of polyphenolics and flavonoids. The identified compounds include luteolin, glucocaffeic acid, aesculin, and saponari (Eze et al. 2021). Polyphenolic compounds such as verbascoside, isoverbascoside, magnolenin, vicenin, and apigenin are also found which show several therapeutic properties (Prasansuklab et al. 2018; Ilori, Liew, and Fang 2020). Other ethnomedicinal species of *Acanthus* include *A. volubilis*. However, most publications belong to the species *A. ilicifolius* (Matos, Batista, and Figueirinha 2022).

(b) ***Avicennia* sp.:** Three species of *Avicennia* sp. of Indian Sundarbans have been subjected to investigation by several researchers. As per the reports of Sharaf, El-Ansari, and Saleh (2000) and Jia, Wei, and Xin (2004), *A. marina* contains flavonoids (luteolin derivatives, chrysoeriol 7-O-glucoside, isorhamnetin 3-O-rutinoside, quercetin, kaempferol), naphthalene derivatives (lyoniresinol) (Han et al. 2007), tannins (lapachol) (Bournot 1913), steroid (β-sitosterol) (Jia,

Table 6.1. Ethnomedicinal Plants of Indian Sundarbans

Scientific Name	Family Name	Common Name	Parts Used	Uses	References
Acanthus ilicifolius L.***	Acanthaceae	Horgoja	Leaves, Root	Leaf—Treatment of animal bites Root—After decoction, used for treatment of asthma, leucorrhoea, and rheumatism.	Singh and Aeri 2013; Chowdhury, Sanyal, and Maiti 2014; Ahmed et al. 2021.
Acanthus volubilis L.***	Acanthaceae	Lota Horgoja	Leaves	Remedy for stomach ulcers.	Chowdhury, Sanyal, and Maiti 2014
Acanthus ebracteatus Vahl**	Acanthaceae	Jeruju	Leaves, Fruit, Bark	Fruit—Antiseptic, blood purifier. Treatment of boils, colds. Bark—Extracts are used to treat gangrenous wounds, allergies. Bark, leaf, and fruit extracts can cure snake bite.	Sasidhar 2021
Acrostichum aureum L.**	Pteridaceae	Hudo	Rhizome	Rhizome paste is used to treat boils.	Chowdhury, Sanyal, and Maiti 2014
Aegiceros corniculatum (L.) * * *	Primulaceae	Khalsi	Fruit, Stem, Leaves	Asthma, Arthritis, Cancer, Diabetes	Debnath et al. 2020
Avicennia alba Blume***	Avicenniaceae	Kalo baen	Seed, Leaf	Paste prepared from seeds helps to relieve smallpox ulceration. Wood ash after burning wood is given in dysentery. Plant extract used to treat snake bites.	Ahmed et al. 2021
Avicennia officinalis L.***	Avicenniaceae	Kalo Bani	Fruit, Seed	Unripe fruit is used as a remedy to treat boils.	Chowdhury, Sanyal, and Maiti 2014; Ahmed et al. 2021.
Bruguiera gymnorrhiza (L.) Lam. ex Savigny***	Rhizophoraceae	Kankra	Bark Leaves Roots	Bark extract is useful in controlling diarrhea. Leaf extract—in burns, intestinal worms, and liver disorders. Root extract—Treatment of diabetes.	Chowdhury, Sanyal, and Maiti 2014; Ahmed et al. 2021.
Bacopa monnieri (L.) Wettst.***	Plantaginaceae	Bramhi	Leaves	Used as Nerve tonic.	Sasidhar 2021

(Continued)

Table 6.1 (Continued)

Scientific Name	Family Name	Common Name	Parts Used	Uses	References
Balanites aegyptica (L.) Delile*	Zygophyllaceae	Hing	Leaves	Used in the treatment of abdominal pains, intestinal disorders, malaria, purgative, sleeping sickness, syphilis.	Sasidhar 2021
Borassus flabellifer Linn.	Arecaceae	Tal	Fruit Pulp	Fruit pulp is used as a cooling agent.	Saradar, Mandal, and Kumar 2024
Bruguiera sexangula Poir.***	Rhizophoraceae	Kankra	Bark	Bark is used to treat food poisoning.	Chowdhury, Sanyal, and Maiti 2014
Cassytha filiformis L.	Lauraceae	Akash Bel	Fruit	Fruit extract used to treat sexually transmitted diseases.	Chowdhury, Sanyal, and Maiti 2014
Calophyllum inophyllum L.*	Calophyllaceae	Punnaga	Bark, Leaves, and Fruits	Bark, Leaf—Used as Anticancer agent and disinfectant. Fruit—Treatment of bone fracture. Bark—Treatment of eye diseases.	Sasidhar 2021
Ceriops decandra (Griff.) Ding Hou ***	Rhizophoraceae	Garan	Leaves	Leaves—Used to treat skin infections.	Saradar, Mandal, and Kumar 2024
Ceriops tagal (Perr.) Robinson***	Rhizophoraceae	Mat-Garan	Bark	Stem bark extract used to stop haemorrhages.	Chowdhury, Sanyal, and Maiti 2014
Clerodendrum inerme Gaertn.*	Lamiaceae	Bon-Jui	Leaves	Leaves are used to treat insect bites.	Saradar, Mandal, and Kumar 2024
Clerodendrum infortunatum L.	Lamiaceae	Ghentu	Twig, Flower	Twig and flower decoction is used to kill stomach worm.	Saradar, Mandal, and Kumar 2024
Derris trifoliata Roxb.***	Fabaceae	Chuliakanta	Root	Root is used to treat tuberculosis.	Saradar, Mandal, and Kumar 2024
Derris uliginosa Lour.* * *	Fabaceae	Chuliakanta	Fruit, Bark	Fruit—Arrests haemorrhages. Bark—Used as antispasmodic, stimulant.	Sasidhar 2021
Dolichandrone spathacea (L.f.) K. Schum.	Bignoniaceae	Gorshingiah	Seed	Seed powder paste is used as an antiseptic.	Chowdhury, Sanyal, and Maiti 2014
Excoecaria agallocha L.***	Euphorbiaceae	Genwa	Latex	Latex is used to cure insect bites.	Chowdhury, Sanyal, and Maiti 2014

Heritiera littoralis Aiton* * *	Malvaceae	Sundari	Stem	Used to treat diarrhea.	Ahmed et al. 2021
Heritiera fomes Buch Ham.**	Malvaceae	Sundari	Seed	Seed powder is used to treat diarrhea.	Chowdhury, Sanyal, and Maiti 2014
Hibiscus tiliaceus L.*	Malvaceae	Bhola	Leaves Bark, Root, Seed	Leaf extract used as a laxative. Bark mucilage—treatment of dysentery. Root—used for treatment of rheumatism. Seed—used as antiemetic.	Chowdhury, Sanyal, and Maiti 2014 Chowdhury, Sanyal, and Maiti 2014
Ipomoea pes-caprae (L.) R.Br.*	Convolvulaceae	Chagalkuri	Leaves	Used in the treatment of Jelly fish sting dermatitis.	Sasidhar 2021
Kandelia rheedei Wight & Arn.* * *	Rhizophoraceae	Goria	Bark, Fruit, Leaves	Treatment of diabetes.	Sasidhar 2021
Kandelia candel (L.) Druce***	Rhizophoraceae	Goria	Leaves	Leaf decoction is used to reduce urination in diabetes.	Chowdhury, Sanyal, and Maiti 2014
Lumnitzera racemosa Willd**	Combretaceae	Kripal	Stem	Stem paste is used to treat skin itching.	Chowdhury, Sanyal, and Maiti 2014
*Nypa fruticans*Wurmb***	Arecaceae	Golpata	Fruit	Fruits are edible as tonic.	Saradar, Mandal, and Kumar 2024
Oncosperma tigillarium (Jack) Ridl.* * *	Arecaceae	-	Bark, leaves, Stem	Used in the treatment of Clinical lesions of skin and genitalia.	Sasidhar 2021
Pongamia pinnata (L.) Pierre*	Fabaceae	Karach	Leaves, Bark	Leaf—used in the treatment of Scabies, skin diseases, stomach pain, rheumatism. Bark—used as medicine in intestinal disorders, sinus.	Sasidhar 2021
Pluchea indica Less.**	Asteraceae	Bera Tulsi	Leaf, Root,	Used in the treatment of fever, gangrenous ulcers, rheumatism, scabies.	Sasidhar 2021
Phoenix paludosa Roxb.*	Arecaceae	Hetal	Fruit	The fruit pulp is used to reduce inflammation.	Chowdhury, Sanyal, and Maiti 2014
Rhizophora apiculata Blume* * *	Rhiophoraceae	Gorjon	Bark, Flower, Fruit, Leaves	Used as antiemetic, antiseptic, haemostatic, and also used in the treatment of hepatitis, diarrhea, typhoid.	Sasidhar 2021

(*Continued*)

Table 6.1 (Continued)

Scientific Name	Family Name	Common Name	Parts Used	Uses	References
Rhizophora lamarckii Montrouz.* * *	Rhiophoraceae	Gorjon	Flowers, Leaves	Used for the treatment of Hepatitis.	Sasidhar 2021
Scaevola sericea Vahl.*	Goodeniaceae	Bhadrak, Chhoto redraksha	Bark and Leaves	Used to treat infection, inflammation, coughs, diabetes, eye infections, gastrointestinal disorders, headache, stings, and bites.	Sasidhar 2021
Scyphiphora hydrophyllacea.F. Gaertn**	Rubiaceae	Tagri Bani	Shoot	Shoot is used to treat liver problems.	Chowdhury, Sanyal, and Maiti 2014
Sonneratia apetala Buch Ham.***	Sonneratiaceae	Keora	Fruit	Fruit is used as a spice.	Chowdhury, Sanyal, and Maiti 2014
Sonneratia caseolaris Engler. ***	Sonneratiaceae	Chak Keora	Fruit	Fruits are used to cure stomach worms.	Chowdhury, Sanyal, and Maiti 2014
Sonneratia griffithii Kurz.***	Sonneratiaceae	Ora	Fruit	Fruit is used to treat colds.	Saradar, Mandal, and Kumar 2024
Xylocarpus granatum Koenig.***	Meliaceae	Dhudul	Bark	Bark is used to treat diarrhea.	Chowdhury, Sanyal, and Maiti 2014
Xylocarpus mekongensis Pierre.***	Meliaceae	Pasur	Bark	Bark is used to treat dysentery.	Chowdhury, Sanyal, and Maiti 2014

*** Mangroves;** Mangrove Minors; * Mangrove Associates

Source: Authors.

Wei, and Xin 2004), terpenoid (lupeol) (Mahera et al. 2011), fatty acids (oleic acid, linolenic acid, palmitic acid, stearic acid, lauric acid, and myristic acid) (Manilal et al. 2009). *A. alba* contains naphthalene derivatives: avecenol, avicequinone (Ito et al. 2000), and terpenoid-taraxerol (Mahera et al. 2011). *A. officinalis* contains triterpenoids namely rhizophorin-A, rhizophorin-B, ribenone, excoecarin A, betulin, betulinic acid, taraxerol, taraxerone (Majumdar and Patra 1979; Subrahmanyam, Ratna Kumar, and Damodar Reddy 2006; Mahera et al. 2011), tannins (gallic acids, ellagic acids) (Sura et al. 2011) and naphthalene derivatives (avecenol C) (Anjaneyulu et al. 2003).

(c) ***Bruguiera* sp.:** Both *Bruguiera gymnorrhiza* and *B. sexangula* have been reported from Indian Sundarbans, but *B. gymnorrhiza* is more thoroughly characterized. Bioactive components are isolated from different parts of plants, as reported by earlier researchers. The compounds 3-β-(Z)-coumaroyl lupeol and cyclohexylidene acetonitrile are found in hypocotyls (Yi et al. 2015), dammarane triterpenes (bruguierins) are present in flowers (Homhual et al. 2006), while, brugunins and bruguierols are found in stems (Han et al. 2007). Apart from those, amyrins, lupeols, ursolic acid, taraxerol, gymnorhizol, ellagic acid, and tannins are isolated from different parts of this plant (Sun et al. 2004; Han et al. 2005; Gong et al. 2007; Huang et al. 2009; Zhou et al. 2012). Extracts of different plant parts of *B. sexangula* also show the presence of tannins, flavonoids, terpenoids and cardiac glycosides, but specific compounds are not detected (Machana et al. 2015).

(d) ***Heritiera* sp.:** *H. fomes* and *H. littoralis* are the two common species of *Heritiera* found in Indian Sundarbans. Leaf extract of the *H. fomes* contains reducing sugars, saponins, alkaloids, glycosides, tannins, sterols, and gums. The bark extract shows a high content of proanthocyanidins. Stem bark reveals the presence of procyanidins. Trimeric, pentameric, and hexameric procyanidins are identified from the plant. β-Sitosterol, stigmasterol, and stigmast-4-en-3-one (Stafford et al. 1988; Scalbert et al. 1991). Several bioactive compounds are also detected from *H. littoralis* fruit extracts, which include 2-Naphthalene sulfonic acid and penicillic acid as dominant components (Sá et al. 2001; Black et al. 2013).

(e) ***Rhizophora* sp.:** Both *R. mucronata* and *R. apiculata* plants are true mangroves commonly found in Sundarbans of India and characterized by their pharmaceutical components. The bioactive components are identified from the extract of different plant parts. The presence of secolabdane diterpenoids (rhizophorin A), phomoxanthone, lupeol, β-sitosterol, gallic acid, coumarin, quercetin, and tannins (Adhikari et al. 2016). Methanolic extracts of *Rhizophora apiculata* leaves show the presence of pyrazole, 4-pyrrolidinyl, and ketone derivatives (Prabhu and Guruvayoorappan 2012).

(f) ***Sonneratia* sp.:** Several species of *Sonneratia* are found in Indian Sundarbans namely *S. apetala*, *S. alba*, and S *caseolaris*. The twigs of the *S. alba* plant shows the presence of lupeol, oleanolic acid, betulinic acid (triterpenoids), 2,6-dimethoxy-p-benzoquinone (quinone), a mixture of stigmasterol and β-sitosterol (phytosterol) (Chaiyadej et al. 2004). The leaves of the plant also show the presence of similar compounds. Five novel sonneratiosides A–E and β-D-glucopyranoside (sesquiterpene glycosides), ampelopsisionoside, lauroside A (megastigmane glycosides) and several other ionol glycosides (alangionoside A), flavone (isovitexin), glycosylated hydroquinone (arbutin) are identified by researchers of Japan. *Sonneratia caseolaris* shows the presence of steroids (β-sitosterol, daucosterol, cholesterol) from stem and twigs (Tian et al. 2009), decanoic acid from whole plant (Tian 2007), and luteolin like flavonoids (Sadhu et al. 2006) from leaves. Three anthraquinone compounds (emodin methyl ether, chrysophanol, and emodin) are characterized from the plant for the first time (Chaudhry and Siddiqui 1950).

(g) ***Xylocarpus* sp.:** *X. granatum* is more extensively characterized for its phytochemical constituents than the other species *X. mekongensis*. The bioactive compounds are isolated from leaves, fruits, seeds, barks of stem and roots. It is found that limonoids are the most important group of secondary metabolites reported from the plant. Limonoids are a type of tetranor-tri terpenoid derivative (Dey et al. 2021). Numerous active components are isolated. Limonoids show typical bridges of C_3-O-C_8 and C_1-O-C_8 in mexicanolides, whereas few compounds, which are derivatives of azadirone, show C_1-O-C_{29} bridges (Zhang et al. 2020). Significant pharmacological activities are reported against sundarbanxylogranins B, thaixylogranins A-H, granaxylocarpins A-E, xylomexicanin F, protoxylocarpins F-H isolated from seed, xylomexicanin F, xyloccensin I isolated from stem bark, xylogranin B, xyloccensin S, xylogranatumines A-G from leaves, gedunin, and xyloccensin I from fruits.

(h) ***Ceriops* sp.:** Both *Ceriops decandra* and *C. tagal* are extensively characterized by researchers. The main phytochemical constituent of the plant includes diterpenoids, which are reported from every part of the plant. Ceriopsin A-G, epoxy ent-kaurene, ent-13-Hydroxykaur-16-en-19-oic acid, methyl ent-16β, 17-dihydroxykaur-9(11)-en-19-oate, ent-16β,17-Dihydroxykaur-9(11)-en-19-oic acid are some common diterpenoids, whereas lupeol, lupenone, ursane, ursolic acid, betulin, and betulinic acid are some common triterpenoids isolated from *Ceriops* (Anjaneyulu and Rao 2002; Anjaneyulu et al. 2003; Kumar et al. 2013). The leaves, twigs, roots, fruits, and hypocotyls of *Ceriops tagal* show the presence of diterpenoids of tagalsins and triterpenoids of lupeol, betulinic acid, and cereotagalsins, respectively (Hu et al. 2010; Yang et al. 2015).

(i) ***Lumnitzera racemosa:*** *L. racemosa* contains various macro- and micro-molecules, including organic acids (oxalate, malate, etc.), amino acids (aspartate, proline, etc.), and diverse phytochemicals like tannins (corilagin, castalagin, etc.), terpenoids, and flavonoids (Manohar 2021). Notable compounds include triterpenoids such as lupeol, phytosterols like stigmasterol, and flavonoids such as quercetin and myricetin. The plant also produces punicalagin and triacontanol, with tannin content in the bark ranging from 15–19 percent. The reproductive parts of *L. racemosa* contain mainly triterpenoids (lupeol and betulin), benzoids (methyl salicylate), carotenoids (Oxoisophorone), fatty acid derivatives, and so on.

(j) ***Excoecaria agallocha:*** The main chemical constituents of *E. agallocha* include diterpenoids, triterpenoids, flavonoids, alkaloids, tannins, and some other compounds. Some of the diterpenoids are 3-oxo-ent-13epi-8 (13)-epoxy-15-chloro-14-hydroxylabdane, ent-15-chloro-13,14-dihydroxylabd-8 (9)-en-3-one (Anjaneyulu et al. 2000), ent-15-chloro-labd-8 (9) ene-3α,13,14-triol, excoecarin (S, T1, T2, R1) (Konishi et al. 2003), excoecarin (R2, H, F, G1, G2), excolide A, 11-epi-excolide, 11,13-di-epi-excolide A (Annam et al. 2015), excolide B, agallochaol (D, E, F, A) (Wang et al. 2004; Wang, Li, and Guo 2005), agallochaol B, agallochaexcoerin D-E (Ponnapalli et al. 2013), agallochaexcoerin F, and so on. Triterpenoids include taraxerone, 3-epitaraxerol, taraxerol 3-epilupeol, epi-β-amyrin, epi-α-amyrin, epitaraxerol, epilupeol, and lupenone (Zou et al. 2006; Tian et al. 2008; Liu et al. 2010). Flavonoids 2′,4′,6′,4-tetramethoxychalcone, 3,5,7,3',5'-pentahydroxy-2R,3R-flavanonol, 3-O-α-L-rhamnopyranoside, alkaloid (2,4-dimethoxy-3-ψ,ψ-dimethylallyl-trans-cinnamoyl piperidine), sterols (β–sitostenone and β–sitosterol) (Prakash et al. 1983; Tian et al. 2008) are present along with some other compounds.

(k) ***Calophyllum inophyllum:*** The phytochemical constituents from different parts of the plants have been reported. Stem, bark, and seeds show the presence of inophyllum A, C, E, calophyllolide, calophynic acid, 11,12-anhydroinophyllum A, protocatechuic acid, 1,7-dihydroxy-6-methoxyxanthone, β-sitosterol, gallic acid, and sitosterol-3-O-β-D-glucopyranoside (Zakaria, Ilham, and Muhamad 2014). Caloxanthone N and gerontoxanthone (Xiao et al. 2008), inophinnin (Ee et al. 2011), and many more xanthones (inophinone, pyranojacareubin, rheediaxanthone A, macluraxanthone, 4-hydroxyxanthone, iophinone, rheediaxanthone A, macluraxanthone, and 4-hydroxyxanthone) are present (Mah et al. 2015). Leaves show the presence of fridelin, calophyllic acid, and isocalophyllic acid (Hsieh et al. 2018). Dipyranocoumarins—calophyllolide, inophyllums B, C, G, and P are also detected. These dipyranocoumarins are also present in seeds. Caloxanthone A, calophynic acid, brasiliensic acid, and inophylloidic acid are isolated from roots and nuts.

(l) ***Derris trifoliata:*** Phytochemical screening of stem extracts of *Derris trifoliata* has been reported. The presence of bioactive chemicals with dominance of rotenoids (Mittraphab et al. 2018). However, *D. scandens* is more extensively characterized, but the presence of this species in the Indian Sundarbans is not well confirmed.

m) ***Aegiceras corniculatum:*** The extracts of *A. corniculatum* show the presence of different types of bioactive chemical constituents like flavonoids (kaempferol, quercetin, and isorhamnetin), benzoquinones (such as embelin), tri-terpenes (aegiceradienol, genin-A, proto-primula genin, and aegicerin), polyphenolic acids (gallic acid, coumaric acid, and syringic acid), stilbenes (resveratrol) (Roome et al. 2008; Janmanchi et al. 2017; Bidve, Kadam, and Malpathak 2018).

Pharmacological Actions of the Mangroves

Mangroves are known to possess a range of pharmacological actions, most notably including antioxidant, antimicrobial, antidiabetic, anti-inflammatory, and astringent properties, primarily due to the presence of secondary metabolites like tannins, flavonoids, and phenolic compounds within their bark and leaves, making them valuable in traditional medicine for various ailments like diarrhea, skin infections, and wounds. The following section has focused on the pharmacological activities of the true mangrove genera of Indian Sundarbans like *Acanthus, Aegiceras, Avicennia, Bruguiera, Calophyllum, Derris, Excoecaria, Heritiera, Lumnitzera, Rhizophora, Sonneratia*, and *Xylocarpus*.

(i) **Anti-inflammatory activity:** Anti-inflammatory agents are responsible for reducing inflammation in diverse physiological conditions. Some common non-steroidal anti-inflammatory drugs include ibuprofen and aspirin. Several true mangroves are extensively characterized and anti-inflammatory agents are identified. Researchers identify active components such as 2-Benzoxazolinone (BOA) and benzoxazinoids from *A. ilicifolius* leaves (Kanchanapoom et al. 2001), betulinic acid from *A. alba* and *A. marina* (Sumithra, Kumar, and Kancharana 2011; Hossain et al. 2012), lupeol, which is a dietary triterpene from *C. decandra* (Martelanc, Vovk, and Simonovska 2007), inophinnin from stem bark and calophyllolide from seeds of *C. inophyllum* (Ee et al. 2011; Nguyen et al. 2017), aegiceroside A and two triterpenoid saponins from *A. corniculatum* (Vinh et al. 2019). These compounds show potential as anti-inflammatory agents. While the exact mechanism of their anti-inflammatory action is not fully understood, it is observed that calophyllolide from *Calophyllum* seeds induces an anti-inflammatory response by regulating the expression of cytokines. Additionally, 4-pyrrolidinyl isolated from *Rhizophora apiculata* leaves is found to be an effective antagonist of very-late antigen 4 (VLA4), reducing inflammation by preventing the infiltration of leukocytes into the site of inflammation (Chiba et al. 2006). The ketone derivatives also exhibited anti-inflammatory activities (Insuasty et al. 2010).

(ii) **Antinociceptive activity:** The extracts of the leaf and stem of certain mangrove plants such as *Acanthus, Avicennia, Bruguiera, Heritiera, Excoecaria*, and *Aegiceras* show antinociceptive or analgesic properties. Researchers identify the active biochemical constituents. For example, *A. ilicifolius* contains benzoxazolinone and its derivatives (Sam et al. 1969; Gulcan et al. 2003), *A. alba* contains flavonoids (Kar et al. 2014), *B. gymnorhiza* leaves contain gallic acid, vanillic acid, vanillin, and ellagic acid. Additionally, *B. gymnorhiza* stem contains gallic acid, (+)-catechin, vanillic acid, vanillin, ellagic acid, and benzoic acid (Mahmud et al. 2017). *A. corniculatum* plants are found to contain flavonoids, flavonols, triterpenes, and benzoquinone as responsible compounds for showing analgesic activities. Although crude leaf extracts of *H. fomes* and *E. agallocha* plants also show antinociceptive properties, the active components are not properly detected.

(iii) **Antimicrobial property:** The acetone, ethanol, chloroform, methanol, and ethyl acetate extracts from the plant parts exhibit antimicrobial properties. The bioactive compounds responsible for the antimicrobial effects are extensively studied. Naphthalene derivatives and terpenoids are found in the stem extracts, while fatty acids, flavonoids like quercetin and myricetin, and proanthocyanidins are isolated from leaf and flower extracts of *A. marina*. Flavonoids like quercetin, myricetin, and proanthocyanidins are isolated from twig fractions of *L. racemosa* and *H. fomes* respectively (Stafford et al. 1988). Additionally, triterpenoids (3β-Hydroxy-lup-9(11),12-diene, lupeol, lupan-3β-ol) have been discovered in *Sonneratia alba* (Chaiyadej et al. 2004; Asad et al. 2013), fridelin in leaf extracts of *C. inophyllum* and various benzoquinones (2,5-didehydroxy-6-methyl embelin, embelin, 5-O-ethyl embelin, and 5-O-methyl embelin), polyphenolics and flavonoids from *A. corniculatum* plants show antimicrobial activities against several gram-positive and gram-negative bacteria (Roome et al. 2008; Bidve, Kadam, and Malpathak 2018; Janmanchi et al. 2017). Sundarbanxylogranis B from *Xylocarpus* plant exhibits inhibitory activities against HIV at a concentration of 78.45 ± 1.69 μM (Dai et al. 2017) and granatumin L and their derivatives show inhibitory activities against HIV and influenza virus at concentrations of 15.8 ± 6.87 μM and 14.02 ± 3.54μM respectively (Wu et al. 2008). Furthermore, two compounds namely 5, 7, 4 trihydroxy 6-deprenyl isoflavone and lupalbigenin exhibit inhibitory effects against yeast cells (Sangmalee et al. 2016).

(iv) **Cytotoxic property:** The compounds gedunin, xylogranatumines A-G, protoxylocarpins F-H, xylomexicanin A, granaxylocarpins A-E, xylomexicanin F, thaixylogranins A-H, and xylogranin B, isolated from the *X. granatum* plant, show cytotoxicity against various cancer and human tumor cell lines (Wu et al. 2003; Uddin et al. 2007; Shen et al. 2009; Pudhom et al. 2009; Du et al. 2009; Toume et al. 2013; Zhou et al. 2014). Granaxylocarpins demonstrate the highest cytotoxicity against P388 and A 549 cell lines (Yin et al. 2007). Additionally, caloxanthone N and gerontoxanthone C, isolated from the *C. inophyllum* plant, exhibit cytotoxic effects on chronic myelogenous leukemia cell line (K562). Furthermore, 4-phenylcoumarin isolated from *Calophyllum* shows inhibition of Epstein-Barr virus early antigen activation caused by 12-O-tetradecanoylphorbol-13-acetate. Moreover, various xanthones isolated from stem bark show antiproliferative actions on different cell lines—SNU-1, HeLa, NCI-H34, Hep G2, and K562 (Mah et al. 2015). Additionally, compounds such as calophyllolide, caloxanthone A, calophynic acid, brasiliensic acid, and inophylloidic acid, isolated from roots and nuts of the *Calophyllum* plant, exhibit cytotoxic activity against human epidermoid carcinoma of the nasopharynx cell (Yimdjo et al. 2004). Triterpenoid saponin from the A. corniculatum plant induces apoptosis in B16F10 melanoma cells (Vinh et al. 2020). Furthermore, compounds like sakurasosaponin and sakurasosaponin methyl ester show cytotoxicity against MCF7, A549, and HCT116 cell lines (Vinh et al. 2019), while benzoquinone derivatives exhibited selective cytotoxicity against HL-60, HepG2, BGC-823, and A2780 cell lines (Li et al. 2020). Moreover, compounds such as diosmetin, baicalin, apigenin, and genkwanin detected from leaf extracts of *A. ebracteatus* show anticancer activities (Ning et al. 2021; Zhao et al. 2021). Tagalene A-B and tagalsins A, C, E, and F of *C. tagal* extract show cytotoxic properties (Yang et al. 2015). Furthermore, rotenoids from *Derris trifoliata* exhibit anticancer activities by showing antiangiogenesis (Mittraphab et al. 2018). Luteolin isolated from *Sonneratia caseolaris* shows significant cytotoxic effects. Additionally, the methanolic and ethanolic extracts of *H. fomes* and *L. racemosa* also exhibit cytotoxic properties, although the active constituents are not detected.

(v) **Immunomodulatory activity:** The leaf extract from the *C. decandra* plant is shown to have an immunomodulatory role. Ursolic acid (UA), a pentacyclic triterpenoid carboxylic acid, is found to suppress activation, proliferation, and cytokine secretion in B cells, T cells, and macrophages. It also inhibits the mitogen-induced up-regulation of co-stimulatory molecules and activation markers in B and T cells (Checker et al. 2012).

(vi) **Hepatoprotective activity:** The compound 4-Hydroxy-2(3H) benzoxazolone (HBOA) observed in *A. ilicifolius* leaves has hepatoprotective properties. It works by increasing the antioxidant defense system and protecting hepatic cellular membranes from oxidation (Liu et al. 2013). Additionally, compounds like lyoniresinol and myricetin, which are isolated from the leaves of *Lumnitzera racemosa*, have also shown significant hepatoprotective effects in HepG2 cells, comparable to glycyrrhizin. On the other hand, racemolide exhibits moderate activity (Darwish et al. 2016).

(vii) **Antidiarrheal property:** The methanolic extracts of *A. alba* show the presence of flavonoids, saponins, steroids, alkaloids, and glycosides, which exhibit an antidiarrheal effect. Additionally, the methanolic extracts of *A. officinalis* leaves inhibit the release of autacoids and prostaglandins, thereby preventing the secretion induced by castor oil in a castor oil-induced diarrheal animal model (Ahmed et al. 2007; Rahman et al. 2011).

(viii) **Diuretic property:** The methanolic extracts of *A. officinalis* leaves demonstrate a diuretic effect by reducing the concentration ratio of excreted sodium and potassium ions (Hossain et al. 2012) at a dosage of 200–400 mg/kg.

(ix) **Antiulcerogenic activity:** The anti-ulcerogenic effects of *A. officinalis* leaf extracts are mainly attributed to flavonoids and tannins (Augwa and Nwako, 1988). An aqueous extract of *B. gymnorrhiza* fruit contains a significant concentration of 402.3 mg/g of pinitol, which demonstrates a protective effect against DSS-induced murine experimental colitis. This effect may be due to the attenuation of inflammation by activating the Keap1/Nrf2 signaling pathway and regulating gut microbiota. As a result, it is commonly used to treat dysentery and has the potential to be used as a drug against ulcerative colitis (Lin et al. 2006; Russo et al. 2018; Lin et al. 2020).

(x) **Antioxidative property:** The acetone, ethanol, ethyl acetate, and methanol extracts of *A. marina* fruit and leaf show antioxidative properties as they scavenge the ABTS (2,2-azino-bis(3-ethylbenzothiazoline-6-sulphonic acid)) and CrO_5 (Chromium peroxide). A separate study demonstrates that ethyl acetate, ethanol, and methanol extracts of pneumatophores, as well as aqueous and ethanolic extracts of bark (Lincy, Paulpriya, and Mohan 2013), possessed strong antioxidant activity by scavenging DPPH (2,2-diphenyl-1-picrylhydrazyl), superoxide, and ABTS radicals (Selvasundhari et al. 2014). Methanolic and aqueous extracts of leaves of *L. racemosa* show higher antioxidant activity than stem extracts. Racelactone A, methyl gallate, and myricitrin also show significant inhibition of superoxide anion generation, indicating strong anti-inflammatory activity, which is important in cancer prevention and control. DPPH, superoxide, and hydrogen peroxide scavenging activities are shown by xyloccensin I from *X. granatum* plant (Das et al. 2019). The bark extracts of *S. alba* show the presence of a phenolic compound (3,3'-Di-O-methylellagic acid) which is an antioxidative compound. Proanthocyanidins from *C. decandra* showed antioxidant activities (Rice-Evans, Miller, and Paganga 1996). Other compounds from the leaves of *C. inophyllum* like calophyllic acid and isocalophyllic acid show antioxidant properties (Prasad et al. 2012). The flavonoids and phenolic compounds isolated from the *A. ilicifolius* plant shows high antioxidant activities (Asha, Mathew, and Lakshmanan 2012). The DPPH and ABTS radical-scavenging activities are noticed in the case of leaf extracts of *A. ebracteatus* (Eze et al. 2021). The crude methanolic extracts of *B. sexangula* plant show antioxidant activity (Machana et al. 2015).

(xi) **Osteogenic property:** Calophyllide from the nut of *C. inophyllum* shows osteogenic properties, probably by activating alkaline phosphatase activity (Liu et al. 2015). Acetoside, isoacetoside, and (+)-lyoniresinol 3a-O-β-D-glucopyranoside, isolated from *A. ilicifolius*, facilitate bone formation. The plant is beneficial for osteoporosis treatment (Van Kiem et al. 2008). These active components are actually responsible for the ethnomedicinal uses of the plants in the treatment of rheumatism and bone fractures.

(xii) **Neuropharmacological property:** Different xanthones of *C. inophyllum*, such as euxanthone, mesuaxanthone-A, mesuaxanthone-B, 6-desoxy jacerubin, calophyllin-B, and dehydroxycycloguanandin, are found to reduce motor activity, induce sedation, cause loss of muscle tone, and enhance sleeping time. These xanthones have shown CNS depressant properties (Gopalakrishnan et al. 1980).

(xiii) **Lipid-lowering property:** The leaves of *Calophyllum inophyllum* contain a mixture of diastereomers including calophyllic acid and isocalophyllic acid, 3-oxofriedelin-28-oic acid, canophyllic acid, amentoflavone, shikimic acid, inophyllum C, and inophyllum E. According to Prasad et al. (2012), these compounds have been found to have lipid-lowering effects on plasma cholesterol, triacylglycerol, and phospholipids.

(xiv) **Antidiabetic property:** The active constituents from *X. granatum* exhibit antidiabetic activities. Xyloccensin I, xylogranin B, and xyloccensin S are found to reduce blood sugar levels by inhibiting alpha amylase and alpha glucosidase (Toume et al. 2013; Zhou et al. 2014). Additionally, compounds such as quercetin from *R. mucronata* leaves, orientin, vitexin, and luteolin (which are flavonoids), as well as oleanolic acid (a triterpenoid), and luteolin, apigenin, and diosmetin (flavonoids) from *S. alba* leaves (Asad et al. 2013), show potential in reducing blood glucose levels. Furthermore, HBOA and its derivatives from *Acanthus* also demonstrate the ability to lower blood glucose levels (Liu et al. 2013). Moreover, the diastereomeric mixture of calophyllic acid and isocalophyllic acid isolated from *Calophyllum inophyllum* is found to reduce insulin resistance by enhancing glucose uptake (Jaiswal et al. 2015).

(xv) **Other pharmacological activities:** The compound 2-benzoxazolinone, which is isolated from *A. ilicifolius* leaves, shows anti-leishmanial activity. Stigmasterol is found to reduce intestinal absorption of cholesterol and lower plasma cholesterol levels (Batta et al. 2006; Burg et al. 2013). Punicalagin derived from *L. recemosa* leaves shows an increase in mean arterial blood pressure in Wistar rats, suggesting potential for treating orthostatic hypotension, possibly through norepinephrine release. Additionally, corilagin, chebulinic acid, and castalagin are found to reduce systemic blood pressure in hypertensive rats, with chebulinic acid showing the most promising result (Lin, Hsu, and Cheng 1993). Retroviral infections can be prevented using dipyranocoumarins such as calophyllolide, inophyllums B, C, G, and P, which are isolated from the seeds and leaves of the *C. inophyllum* plant (Patil et al. 1993; Taylor et al. 1994; Spino, Dodier, and Sotheeswaran 1998). Epigallocatechin-3-O-gallate, isolated from *A. corniculatum*, is a catechol analogue that displays strong inhibitory effects on human catechol-O-methyltransferase (COMT), potentially impeding the progression of Parkinson's disease (Zhu et al. 2008; Wei et al. 2012). Tagalsins Q, R, and U of *C. tagal* show antifeedant activity (Hu et al. 2010). The leaves of *B. gymnorrhiza* possess antioxidant and hepatoprotective actions due to the presence of gallic acid, quercetin, and coumarin (Lin et al. 2020). The plant extract is a potential inhibitor of the hepatitis B virus. The extracts of the leaves of *Sonneratia alba* show antibacterial activity. Tyrosinase activity is also shown by the sonneratiosides (Asad et al. 2013; Ragasa et al. 2015; Katsutani et al. 2020).

Conclusion and Future Prospects

Plants are a vital source of essential phytochemical compounds, with mangrove plants standing out for their rich secondary metabolites. This study is dedicated to unveiling the remarkable pharmacological properties of true mangrove plants, particularly their leaves, stems, twigs, roots, and fruit extracts. While these plants have demonstrated significant pharmaceutical potential, most of the research is focused on crude extracts, overlooking the identification of specific components crucial for their medicinal use. However, in-depth studies of plants such as *Acanthus*, *Xylocarpus*, *Avicennia*, and *Calophyllum* have revealed specific components like di and tri terpenoids, flavonoids, xanthones, benzoquinone derivatives, and limonoids, offering promising prospects for new drug discovery. Some properties are commonly found, while specific active components validate the traditional use of these plants. For instance, triterpenoid saponin from *Aegiceras* and 4 phenyl coumarin from *Calophyllum* have been identified as responsible for the anticancer activity of these plants. Similarly, the presence of relevant phytochemicals like acetoside, isoacetoside, and calophylloloid in *A. ilicifolius* and *C. inophyllum* has substantiated their ethnobotanical significance in rheumatism and bone repair. The folklore use of *B. gymnorrhiza* fruit in traditional medicine is also supported by its detected components. Regrettably, few efforts have been made to sustain the ethnobotanical and ethnopharmacological significance of these natural products obtained from the plants. Uncontrolled human activities continue to pose a threat to the habitats of these plants, endangering the *H. fomes* population. It is imperative to comprehensively document the entire checklist of Sundarbans flora, including its ethnobotanical significance, as the traditional knowledge surrounding these plants may vanish with the older generations. It is crucial for skilled individuals to take responsibility for preserving the active components of these plants, laying the foundation for the development of drugs to combat various diseases.

References

Adhikari, A., M. Ray, A. K. Das, and T. K. Sur. "Antidiabetic and Antioxidant Activity of *Rhizophora mucronata* Leaves (Indian Sundarban Mangrove): An *in vitro*: and *in vivo* study." *AYU (An International Quarterly Journal of Research in Ayurveda)* 37, no. 1 (2016): 76–81.

Ahmed, S., S. P. Chakrabarty, S. Zaman, and A.Mitra. "Medicinal Values of the Blue Carbon in Indian Sundarbans." In *Natural Resources and their Ecosystem Services* (Vol. II), edited by M. Abhijit, M. C. Monruskin, and P. C. Shambhu, 169–76. Bangalore: HSRA Publications, 2021.

Ahmed, F., I. Z. Shahid, N. C. Gain, M. S. H. Reza, and S. K. Sadhu. "Antinociceptive and Antidiarrheal Activities of *Bruguiera gymnorrhiza*." *Advances in Traditional Medicine* 7, no. 3 (2007): 280–5.

Anjaneyulu, A. S. R., and V. L. Rao. "Ceriopsins A–D, Diterpenoids from *Ceriops decandra*." *Phytochemistry* 60, no. 8 (2002): 777–82.

Anjaneyulu, A. S. R., and V. L. Rao. "Ceriopsins F and G, Diterpenoids from *Ceriops decandra*." *Phytochemistry* 62, no. 8 (2003): 1207–11.

Anjaneyulu, A. S. R., and V. L. Rao. "Five Diterpenoids (agallochins A–E) from the Mangrove Plant *Excoecaria agallocha* Linn." *Phytochemistry* 55, no. 8 (2000): 891–901.

Anjaneyulu, A. S. R., V. L. Rao, E. Lobkovsky, and J. Clardy. "Ceriopsin E, a New Epoxy ent-Kaurene Diterpenoid from *Ceriops decandra*." *Journal of Natural Products* 65, no. 4 (2002): 592–4.

Annam, S., CH V. Appa Rao, M. Ankireddy, M. B. Sura, M. G. Ponnapalli, and A. V. Sarma. "Epimericexcolides from the Stems of *Excoecaria agallocha* and Structural Revision of Rhizophorin A." *Organic Letters* 17, no. 11 (2015): 2840–3.

Asad, S., Md. Hamiduzzaman, A. T. M. Zafrul Azam, M. Ahsan, and M. M. Masud. "Lupeol, Oleanic Acid & Steroids from *Sonneratia alba* JE Sm (Sonneratiaceae) and Antioxidant, Antibacterial & Cytotoxic Activities of Its Extracts." *International Journal of Advanced Research in Pharmaceutical & BioSciences* 3, no. 1 (2013): 4–10.

Asha, K. K., S. Mathew, and P. T. Lakshmanan. "Flavonoids and Phenolic Compounds in Two Mangrove Species and Their Antioxidant Property." *Indian Journal of Geo-Marine Sciences* 41, no. 3 (2012): 259–64.

Augwa, C. N., and S. O. Nwako. "Preliminary Studies of the Root Extracts of *Nauclea latifolia* Smith, for Antiulcer Properties." *Nigerian Journal of Pharmaceutical Sciences* 4 (1988): 16–23.

Bandaranayake, W. M. "Bioactivities, Bioactive Compounds and Chemical Constituents of Mangrove Plants." *Wetlands Ecology and Management* 10 (2002): 421–52.

Bandaranayake, W. M. "Traditional and Medicinal Uses of Mangroves." *Mangroves and Salt Marshes* 2 (1998): 133–48.

Banerjee, S., A. Singh, and R. Pal. "Taxonomic Interpretation of Non-heterocystous Cyanobacteria (Oscillatoriales) from Eastern India with Particular Emphasis on *Lyngbya Plectonema* Complex." *Revis Bionatura* 9 (2024): 1–22.

Barman, N., G. G. Satpati, and R. Pal. "A Morphotaxonomic Account of Cyanobacterial Diversity of Indian Sundarbans." *Journal of Algal Biomass Utilization* 6, no. 3 (2015): 39–46.

Batta, A. K., G. Xu, A. Honda, T. Miyazaki, and G. Salen. "Stigmasterol Reduces Plasmacholesterol Levels and Inhibits Hepatic Synthesis and Intestinal Absorption in Therat." *Metabolism* 55, no. 3 (2006): 292–9.

Begam, M. M., R. Chowdhury, T. Sutradhar, C. Mukherjee, K. Chatterjee, S. K. Basak, and K. Ray. "Forecasting Mangrove Ecosystem Degradation Utilizing Quantifiable Eco-physiological Resilience-a Study from Indian Sundarbans." *Scientific Reports* 10, no. 1 (2020): 6683.

Bibi, S. N., M. M. Fawzi, Z. Gokhan, J. Rajesh, N. Nadeem, R. R. Rengasamy Kannan, D. G. Albuquerque, and S. K. Pandian. "Ethnopharmacology, Phytochemistry, and Global Distribution of Mangroves-A Comprehensive Review." *Marine Drugs* 17, no. 4 (2019): 231.

Bidve, S. C., V. B. Kadam, and N. P. Malpathak. "Metabolite Profiling and Principle Component Analysis of a Mangrove Plant *Aegiceras corniculatum* L (Blanco)." *Journal of Pharmaceutical Research Science & Technology* 2, no. 1 (2018): 1–9.

Black, C. A. *Soil Fertility Evaluation and Control*. CRC Press, 2013.

Bournot, K. "Gewinnung von Lapachol aus dem Kernholz von *Avicennia tomentosa*." *Archiv der Pharmazie* 251, no. 5 (1913): 351–4.

Burg, V. K., H. S. Grimm, T. L. Rothhaar, S. Grösgen, B. Hundsdörfer, V. J. Haupenthal, V. C. Zimmer, J. Mett, O. Weingärtner, U. Laufs, L. M. Broersen, H. Tanila, T. Vanmierlo, D. Lütjohann, T. Hartmann, and M. O. W. Grimm. "Plant Sterols the Better Cholesterol in Alzheimer's Disease? A Mechanistical Study." *Journal of Neuroscience* 33, no. 41 (2013): 16072–87.

Chaiyadej, K., H. Wongthap, S. Vadhanavikit, and K. Chantrapromma. "Bioactive Constituents from the Twigs of *Sonneratia alba*." *Walailak Journal of Science and Technology (WJST)* 1, no. 1 (2004): 15–22.

Chaudhry, G. R., and S. Siddiqui. "Chemical Examination of Archa (*Sonneratia acida* L.). Part I: Isolation of Three Crystalline Products from the Wood." *Journal of Scientific and Industrial Research* 9B (1950): 118–20.

Chowdhury, R., T. Sutradhar, M. M. Begam, C. Mukherjee, K. Chatterjee, S. K. Basak, and K. Ray. "Effects of Nutrient Limitation, Salinity Increase, and Associated Stressors on Mangrove Forest Cover, Structure, and Zonation across Indian Sundarbans." *Hydrobiologia* 842 (2019): 191–217.

Checker, R., S. K. Sandur, D. Sharma, R. S. Patwardhan, S. Jayakumar, V. Kohli, G. Sethi, B. B. Aggarwal, and K. B. Sainis. "Potent Anti-inflammatory Activity of Ursolic Acid, a Triterpenoid Antioxidant, Is Mediated through Suppression of NF-κB,AP-1andNF-AT." *PloSone* 7, no. 2 (2012): e31318.

Chiba, J., S. Iimura, Y. Yoneda, Y. Sugimoto, T. Horiuchi, F. Muro, Y. Ochiai, T. Ogasawara, M. Tsubokawa, Y. Iigou, G. Takayama, T. Taira, Y. Takata, M. Yokoyama, T. Takashi, A. Nakayama, and N. Machinaga. "4-(Pyrrolidinyl) Methoxybenzoic Acid Derivatives as a Potent, Orally Active VLA-4 Antagonist." *Chemical and Pharmaceutical Bulletin* 54, no. 11 (2006): 1515–29.

Chowdhury, A., P. Sanyal, and S. K. Maiti. "Ethnobotanical Understanding of Mangroves: An Investigation from Central Part of Indian Sundarbans." *International Journal for Botanical Research* 4 (2014): 29–34.

Dai, Y. G., J. Wu, K. P. Padmakumar, and L. Shen. "SundarbanxylograninsA–E, Five New Limonoids from the Sundarban Mangrove, *Xylocarpus granatum*." *Fitoterapia* 122 (2017): 85–9.

Darwish, A. G. G., M. N. Samy, S. Sugimoto, H. Otsuka, H. Abdel-Salam, M. I. Issa, E. S. Shaker, and K. Matsunami. "Bioactive Compounds from the Leaves of *Lumnitzera racemosa* against Acetaminophen-induced Liver Damage in Vitro." *Journal of Arid Land Studies* 26 (2016): 183–6.

Das, S. K., D. Samantaray, S. K. Sahoo, S. K. Pradhan, L. Samanta, and H. Thatoi. "Bioactivity Guided Isolation of Antidiabetic and Antioxidant Compound from *Xylocarpus granatum*. J. Koenigbark." *3Biotech* 9 (2019): 1–9.

Debnath, S. L., P. Kundu, M. Golder, B. Biswas, and S. K. Sadhu. "Phytochemical Characterization and Evaluation of Pharmacological Activities of Leaves of a Mangrove Plant Species-*Aegiceras corniculatum* (L.)" *Tropical Journal of Natural Product Research (TJNPR)* 4, no. 9 (2020): 516–22.

Dey, D., C. Quispe, R. Hossain, D. Jain, R. A. Khan, P. Janmeda, M. T. Islam, H. A. R. Suleria, M. Miquel, S. D. Daştan, M. Kumar, Y. Taheri, A. T. Petkoska, and J. Sharifi-Rad. "Ethnomedicinal Use, Phytochemistry, and Pharmacology of *Xylocarpus granatum* J. Koenig." *Evidence Based Complementary and Alternative Medicine* 2021, no. 1 (2021): 8922196.

Du, S., M. Wang, W. Zhu, and Z. Qin. "A New Fungicidal Lactone from *Xylocarpus granatum* (Meliaceae)." *Natural Product Research* 23, no. 14 (2009): 1316–21.

Ee, G. C. L., S. H. Mah, M. Rahmani, Y. H. Taufiq-Yap, S. S. Teh, and Y. M. Lim. "A New furanoxanthone from the Stem Bark of *Calophyllum inophyllum*." *Journal of Asian Natural Products Research* 13, no. 10 (2011): 956–60.

Eze, F. N., and T. J. Jayeoye. "Chromolaena odorata (Siam Weed): A Natural Reservoir of Bioactive Compounds with Potent Anti-fibrillogenic, Antioxidative, and Cytocompatible Properties." *Biomedicine & Pharmacotherapy* 141 (2021): 111811.

Ghosh, A., S. Mukherjee, N. Sen, M. Dasgupta, and K. R. Naskar. "Check-list of Mangroves and Mangrove Associated Species in the Indian Sundarbans." *Seshaiyana* 10, no. 2 (2002): 211–24.

Ghosh, A., S. Schmidt, T. Fickert, and M. Nusser. "The Indian Sundarban Mangrove Forests: History, Utilization, Conservation Strategies and Local Perception." *Diversity* 7, no. 2 (2015): 149–69.

Gong, J. X., X. Shen, L. G. Yao, H. Jiang, K. Krohn, and Y. W. Guo. "Total Synthesis of Gymnorrhizol, an Unprecedented 15-membered Macrocyclic Polydisulfide from the Chinese Mangrove *Bruguiera gymnorrhiza*." *Organic Letters* 9, no. 9 (2007): 1715–16.

Gopalakrishnan, C., D. Shankaranarayanan, S. K. Nazimudeen, S. Viswanathan, and L. Kameswaran. "Anti-inflammatory and CNS Depressant Activities of Xanthones from *Calophyllum inophyllum* and Mesuaferrea." *Indian Journal of Pharmacology* 12, no. 3 (1980): 181–91.

Gulcan, H. O., E. Kupeli, S. Unlu, E. Yesilada, and M. F. Sahin. "4-(5-chloro-2(3H)-benzoxazolon-3-yl) Butanoic Acid Derivatives: Synthesis, Antinociceptive and Anti-inflammatory Properties." *Archiv der Pharmazie: An International Journal Pharmaceutical and Medicinal Chemistry* 336, no. 10 (2003): 477–82.

Han, L., X. S. Huang, I. Sattler, H. Z. Fu, S. Grabley, and W. H. Lin. "Two New Constituents from Mangrove *Bruguiera gymnorrhiza*." *Journal of Asian Natural Products Research* 9, no. 4 (2007): 327–31.

Han, L., X. Huang, I. Sattler, U. Moellmann, H. Fu, W. Lin, and S. Grabley. "New Aromatic Compounds from the Marine Mangrove *Bruguiera gymnorrhiza*." *Planta Medica* 71, no. 2 (2005): 160–4.

Homhual, S., N. Bunyapraphatsara, T. Kondratyuk, A. Herunsalee, W. Chaukul, J. M. Pezzuto, H. H. Fong, and H. J. Zang. "Bioactive Dammarane Triterpenes from the Mangrove Plant *Bruguiera gymnorrhiza*." *Journal of Natural Products* 69, no. 3 (2006): 421–4.

Hossain, Md H., Md S. I. Howlader, S. K. Dey, A. Hira, and A. Ahmed. "Evaluation of Diuretic and Neuropharmacological Properties of the Methanolic Extract of *Avicennia officinalis* L.leaves from Bangladesh." *International Journal of Pharmaceutical and Phytopharmacological Research* 22 (2012): 121–30.

Hsieh, C., Y. W. Lin, C. H. Chen, W. Ku, F. Ma, H. Yu, and C. Chu. "Yellow and Green Pigments from *Calophyllum inophyllum* L. Seed Oil Induce Cell Death in Colon and Lung Cancer Cells." *Oncology Letters* 15, no. 4 (2018): 5915–23.

Hu, W. M., M. Y. Li, J. Li, Q. Xiao, G. Feng, and J. Wu. "Dolabranes from the Chinese Mangrove, *Ceriops tagal*." *Journal of Natural Products* 73, no. 10 (2010): 1701–5.

Huang, X. Y., Q. Wang, H. L. Liu, Y. Zhang, G. R. Xin, X. Shen, M. L. Dong, and Y. W. Guo. "Diastereoisomeric Macrocyclic Polydisulfides from the Mangrove *Bruguiera gymnorrhiza*." *Phytochemistry* 70, no. 17–18 (2009): 2096–100.

Ilori, N. T. O., C. X. Q. Liew, and C. M. Fang. "The Anti-inflammatory Properties of *Acanthus ebracteatus, Barleria lupulina* and *Clinacanthus nutans*: A Systematic Review." *Molecular Biology Reports* 47, no. 12 (2020): 9883–94.

Insuasty, B., A. Tigreros, F. Orozco, J. Quiroga, R. Abonía, M. Nogueras, A. Sanchez, and J. Cobo. "Synthesis of Novel Pyrazolic Analogues of Chalcones and Their 3-aryl-4-(3-aryl-4, 5-dihydro-1H-pyrazol-5-yl)-1-phenyl-1H-pyrazole Derivatives as Potential Antitumor Agents." *Bioorganic & Medicinal Chemistry* 18, no. 14 (2010): 4965–74.

Ito, C., S. Katsuno, Y. Kondo, H. T. W. Tan, and H. Furukawa. "Chemical Constituents of *Avicennia alba*. Isolation and Structural Elucidation of New Naphthoquinones and Their Analogues." *Chemical and Pharmaceutical Bulletin* 48, no. 3 (2000): 339–43.

Jaiswal, N., N. Gunaganti, C. K. Maurya, T. Narender, and A. K. Tamrakar. "Free Fatty Acid Induced Impairment of Insulin Signaling Is Prevented by the Diastereomeric Mixture of Calophyllic Acid and Isocalophyllic Acid in Skeletal Muscle Cells." *European Journal of Pharmacology* 746 (2015): 70–7.

Janmanchi, H., A. Raju, M. S. Degani, M. K. Ray, and M. G. R. Rajan. "Antituberculosis, Antibacterial and Antioxidant Activities of *Aegiceras corniculatum*, a Mangrove Plant and Effect of Various Extraction Processes on Its Phytoconstituents and Bioactivity." *South African Journal of Botany* 113 (2017): 421–7.

Jia, R., G. Y. Wei, and H. H. Xin. "Studies on the Chemical Constituents from Leaves of *Avicennia marina*." *Sustainable Chemistry for the Environment* 2 (2004): 16–19.

Kanchanapoom, T., M. S. Kamel, R. Kasai, C. Picheansoonthon, Y. Hiraga, and K. Yamasaki. "Benzoxazinoid Glucosides from *Acanthus ilicifolius*." *Phytochemistry* 58, no. 4 (2001): 637–40.

Kar, D. R., G. Ghosh, P. Sudhir Kumar, and P. K. Sahu. "Analgesic and Antipyretic Activities of the Methanolic Extract of Aerial Parts of *Avicennia alba* Blume." *International Journal of Pharm Tech Research* 6, no. 3 (2014): 874–9.

Katsutani, K., S. Sugimoto, Y. Yamano, H. Otsuka, K. Matsunami, and T. Mizuta. "Eudesmane-type Sesquiterpene Glycosides: Sonneratiosides A–E Andeudesmol β-d-Glucopyranoside from the Leaves of *Sonneratia alba*." *Journal of Natural Medicines* 74 (2020): 119–26.

Kiem, P. V., T. H. Quang, T. T. Huong, L. T. H. Nhung, N. X. Cuong, C. V. Minh, E. M. Choi, and Y. H. Kim. "Chemical Constituents of *Acanthus ilicifolius* L. and Effect on Osteoblastic MC3T3E1 Cells." *Archives of Pharmacal Research* 31 (2008): 823–9.

Kokpol, U., V. Chittawong, and D. H. Miles. "Chemical Constituents of the Roots of *Acanthus illicifolius*." *Journal of Natural Products* 49, no. 2 (1986): 355–6.

Konishi, T., K. Yamazoe, T. Konoshima, and Y. Fujiwara. "Seco-labdane Type Diterpenes from *Excoecaria agallocha*." *Phytochemistry* 64, no. 4 (2003): 835–40.

Kumar, V. A., K. Ammani, B. Siddhardha, U. Sreedhar, and G. A. Kumar. "Differential Biological Activities of the Solvent Extracts of *Ceriops decandra* (Griff.) and Their Phytochemical Investigations." *Journal of Pharmacy Research* 7, no. 7 (2013): 654–60.

Li, Y., C. Dong, M. J. Xu, and W. H. Lin. "New Alkylated Benzoquinones from Mangrove Plant *Aegiceras corniculatum* with Anticancer Activity." *Journal of Asian Natural Products Research* 22 (2020): 121–30.

Lin, T. C., F. L. Hsu, and J. T. Cheng. "Antihypertensive Activity of Corilagin and Chebulinic Acid, Tannins from *Lumnitzera racemosa*." *Journal of Natural Products* 56 (1993): 629–32.

Lin, Y. M., J. W. Liu, P. Xiang, P. Lin, G. F. Ye, and L. S. L. Da Sternberg. "Tannin Dynamics of Propagules and Leaves of *Kandelia candel* and *Bruguiera gymnorrhiza* in the Jiulong River Estuary, Fujian, China." *Biogeochemistry* 78 (2006): 343–59.

Lin, Y., X. Zheng, J. Chen, D. Luo, J. Xie, Z. Su, X. Huang, X. Yi, L. Wei, J. Cai, and Z. Sun. "Protective Effect of *Bruguiera gymnorrhiza* (L.) Lam. Fruit On Dextran Sulfate Sodium-induced Ulcerative Colitis in Mice: Role of Keap1/Nrf2 Pathway and Gut Microbiota." *Frontiers in Pharmacology* 10 (2020): 1602.

Lincy, M. P., K. Paulpriya, and V. R. Mohan. "Invitro Antioxidant Activity of *Avicennia marina* (Forssk) Vierh Pneumatophore (Avicenniaceae)." *Science Research Reporter* 3, no. 2 (2013): 106–14.

Liu, L., H. Fan, P. Qi, Y. Mei, L. Zhou, L. Cai, X. Lin, and J. Lin. "Synthesis and Hepatoprotective Properties of Acanthus Ilicifolius Alkaloid A and Its Derivatives." *Experimental and Therapeutic Medicine* 6, no. 3 (2013): 796–802.

Liu, W. H., Y. W. Liu, Z. F. Chen, W. F. Chiou, Y. C. Tsai, and C. C. Chen. "Calophyllolide Content in *Calophyllum inophyllum* at Different Stages of Maturity and Its Osteogenic Activity." *Molecules* 20, no. 7 (2015): 12314–27.

Liu, Z., W. Jiang, Z. W. Deng, and W. H. Lin. "Assignment of the Absolute Stereochemistry of an Unusual Diterpenoid from the Mangrove Plant *Excoecaria agallocha* L." *Journal of Chinese Pharmaceutical Sciences* 19 (2010): 387–92.

Machana, S., B. Vongsak, E. Saifha, T. Ponglumjeak, P. Boonsaem, S. Bupphalun, C. Chonanant, and B. Nuangsaeng. "Phytochemical Screening, Total Phenolic Content and Free Radical Scavenging Activity of *Bruguiera sexangula* and *Connarus semidecandrus* Extracts in Kung Krabaen Bay." *Planta Medica* 81, no. 16 (2015): PW_103.

Mah, S. H., G. C. L. Ee, S. S. Teh, and M. A. Sukari. "*Calophyllum inophyllum* and *Calophyllum soulattri* Source of Anti-proliferative Xanthones and Their Structure–activity Relationships." *Natural Product Research* 29, no. 1 (2015): 98–101.

Mahera, S. A., V. U. Ahmad, S. M. Saifullah, F. V. Mohammad, and K. Ambreen. "Steroids and Triterpenoids from Grey Mangrove Avicennia Marina." *Pakistan Journal of Botany* 43, no. 2 (2011): 1417–22.

Mahmud, I., Md N. H. Zilani, N. N. Biswas, and B. Bokshi. "Bioactivities of *Bruguiera gymnorrhiza* and Profiling of Its Bioactive Polyphenols by HPLC-DAD." *Clinical Phytoscience* 3 (2017): 1–11.

Majumdar, S. G., and G. Patra. "Chemical Investigation on Some Mangrove Species. 1. Genus *Avicennia*." *Journal of the Indian Chemical Society* 56, no. 1 (1979): 111–13.

Manilal, A., S. Sujith, G. S. Kiran, J. Selvin, and C. Shakir. "Biopotentials of Mangroves Collected from the Southwest Coast of India." *Global Journal of Biotechnology and Biochemistry* 4, no. 1 (2009): 59–65.

Manohar, S. M. "A Review of the Botany, Phytochemistry and Pharmacology of Mangrove *Lumnitzera racemosa* Willd." *Pharmacognosy Reviews* 15 (2021): 107–16.

Martelanc, M., I. Vovk, and B. Simonovska. "Determination of Three Major Triterpenoids in Epicuticular Wax of Cabbage (*Brassica oleracea* L.) by High-performance Liquid Chromatography with UV and Mass Spectrometric Detection." *Journal of Chromatography* A1164, no. 1–2 (2007): 145–52.

Matos, P., M. T. Batista, and A. Figueirinha. "A Review of the Ethnomedicinal Uses, Chemistry, and Pharmacological Properties of the Genus *Acanthus* (Acanthaceae)." *Journal of Ethnopharmacology* 293 (2022): 115271.

Minocha, P. K. and K. P. Tiwari. "Chemical Constituents of *Acanthus ilicifolius* Linn." *Polish Journal of Chemistry* 54, no. 10 (1980): 2089–90.

Mittraphab, Y., N. Ngamrojanavanich, K. Shimizu, K. Matsubara, and K. Pudhom. "Anti-angiogenic Activity of Rotenoids from the Stems of *Derris trifoliata*." *Planta Medica* 84, no. 11 (2018): 779–85.

Murty, M. S., S. Wahidulla, and S. Y. Kamat. "Isolation of 2-Benzoxazolinone from *Acanthus ilicifolius*." *Indian Journal of Pharmaceutical Sciences* 46 (1984): 218–19.

Nguyen, V. L., C. T. Truong, B. C. Q. Nguyen, T. N. V. Vo, T. T. Dao, V. D. Nguyen, D. T. T. Trinh, H. K. Huynh, and C. B. Bui. "Anti-inflammatory and Wound Healing Activities of Calophyllolide Isolated from Calophyllum Inophyllum Linn." *PloS one* 12, no. 10 (2017): e0185674.

Ning, R., G. Chen, R. Fang, Y. Zhang, W. Zhao, and F. Qian. "Diosmetin Inhibits Cell Proliferation and Promotes Apoptosis through STAT3/c-Myc Signaling Pathway in Human Osteosarcoma Cells." *Biological Research* 54, no. 1 (2021): 40.

Patil, A. D., A. J. Freyer, D. S. Eggleston, R. C. Haltiwanger, M. F. Bean, P. B. Taylor, M. J. Caranfa, A. L. Breen, and H. R. Bartus. "The Inophyllums, Novel Inhibitors of HIV-1 Reverse Transcriptase Isolated from the Malaysian Tree, *Calophyllum inophyllum* Linn." *Journal of Medicinal Chemistry* 36, no. 26 (1993): 4131–8.

Ponnapalli, M. G., A. Madhu, S. CH. VA. Rao Annam, S. Ravirala, S. Sukki, and V. R. Tuniki. "Unusual Ent-isopimarane-type Diterpenoids from the Wood of *Excoecaria agallocha*." *Tetrahedron Letters* 54, no. 23 (2013): 2942–5.

Prabhu, V. V., and C. Guruvayoorappan. "Anti-inflammatory and Anti-tumor Activity of the Marine Mangrove *Rhizophora apiculata*." *Journal of Immunotoxicology* 9, no. 4 (2012): 341–52.

Prakash, S., M. A. Khan, H. Khan, and A. Zaman. "A Piperidine Alkaloid from *Excoecharia agallocha*." *Phytochemistry* 22, no. 8 (1983): 1836–7.

Prasad, J., A. Shrivastava, A. K. Khanna, G. Bhatia, S. K. Awasthi, and T. Narender. "Antidyslipidemic and Antioxidant Activity of the Constituents Isolated from the Leaves of *Calophyllum inophyllum*." *Phytomedicine* 19, no. 14 (2012): 1245–9.

Prasansuklab, A., and T. Tencomnao. "*Acanthus ebracteatus* Leaf Extract Provides Neuronal Cell Protection against Oxidative Stress Injury Induced by Glutamate." *BMC Complementary and Alternative Medicine* 18 (2018): 1–15.

Pudhom K., D. Sommit, P. Nuclear, N. Ngamrojanavanich, and A. Petsom. "Protoxylocarpins F.–H. Protolimonoids from Seed Kernels of Xylocarpus granatum." *Journal of Natural Products* 72, no. 12 (2009): 2188–91.

Ragasa, C. Y., V. D. Ebajo Jr, M. Mariquit, H. Emelina, R. B. Mandia, and S. Urban. "Triterpenes and Sterols from *Sonneratia alba*." *International Journal of Current Pharmaceutical Research* 6, no. 6 (2015): 256–61.

Rahman, M. A., S. Biswas, V. Balan, A. K. Shill, and U. Bose. "Antidiarrhoeal and Antinociceptive Activities of Leaves *Avicennia alba*." *Pharmacology Online* 1 (2011): 492–500.

Rice-Evans, C. A., N. J. Miller, and G. Paganga. "Structure-antioxidant Activity Relationships of Flavonoids and Phenolic Acids." *Free Radical Biology and Medicine* 20, no. 7 (1996): 933–56.

Roome, T., A. Dar, S. Ali, S. Naqvi, and M. I. Choudhary. "A Study on Antioxidant, Free Radical Scavenging, Anti-inflammatory and Hepatoprotective Actions of *Aegiceras*

corniculatum (stem) Extracts." *Journal of Ethnopharmacology* 118, no. 3 (2008): 514–21.
Russo, M., V. Coppola, E. Giannetti, R. Buonavolontà, A. Piscitelli, and A. Staiano. "Oral Administration of Tannins and Flavonoids in Children with Acute Diarrhea: A Pilot, Randomized, Control-case Study." *Italian Journal of Pediatrics* 44 (2018): 1–6.
Sá, J. C. M., C. C. Cerri, W. A. Dick, R. Lal, S. P. V. Filho, M. C. Piccolo, and B. E. Feigl. "Organic Matter Dynamics and Carbon Sequestration Rates for a Tillage Chronosequence in a Brazilian Oxisol." *Soil Science Society of America Journal* 65, no. 5 (2001): 1486–99.
Sadhu, S. K., F. Ahmed, T. Ohtsuki, and M. Ishibashi. "Flavonoids from *Sonneratia caseolaris*." *Journal of Natural Medicines* 60 (2006): 264–5.
Saenger, P. *Mangrove Ecology, Silviculture and Conservation*. Dordrecht: Kluwer Academic Publishers, 2002.
Sam, J., and J. L. Valentine. "Preparation and Properties of 2-benzoxazolinones." *Journal of Pharmaceutical Sciences* 58, no. 9 (1969): 1043–54.
Sangmalee, S., A. Laorpaksa, B. Sritularak, and S. Sukrong. "Bioassay-guided Isolation of Two Flavonoids from *Derris scandens* with Topoisomerase II Poison Activity." *Biological and Pharmaceutical Bulletin* 39, no. 4 (2016): 631–5.
Saradar, B., S. Mandal, and S. Kumar. "Ethnobotanical Inventory and Medicinal Potential of Mangrove Flora in the Sundarbans, West Bengal, India." *Journal of Biodiversity and Conservation* 8 (2024): 1–6.
Sasidhar, K. "Mangrove Medicinal Plants and Its Chemistry: A Review." *International Journal of Multidisclinary Educational Research* 10, no. 1 (2021): 16–21.
Satpati, G. G., N. Barman, and R. Pal. "A Study on Green Algal Flora of Indian Sundarbans Mangrove Forest with Special Reference to Morphotaxonomy." *Journal of Algal Biomass Utilization* 4, no. 1 (2013): 26–41.
Scalbert, A. "Antimicrobial Properties of Tannins." *Phytochemistry* 30, no. 12 (1991): 3875–83.
Selvasundhari, L., V. Babu, V. Jenifer, S. Jeyasudha, and G. Thiruneelakandan. "Screening of Antioxidant Potential Compounds from *Avicennia marina* Bark." *International Journal of Current Research* 6 (2014): 5490–6.
Sharaf, M., M. A. El-Ansari, and N. A. M. Saleh. "New Flavonoids from *Avicennia marina*." *Fitoterapia* 71, no. 3 (2000): 274–7.
Shen, L. R., M. Dong, B. W. Yin, D. Guo, M. L. Zhang, Q. W. Shi, C. H. Huo, H. Kiyota, N. Suzuki, and B. Cong. "Xylomexicanins A and B, new Δ14, 15-mexicanolides from Seeds of the Chinese Mangrove *Xylocarpus granatum*." *Zeitschrift für Naturforschung C* 64, no. 1–2 (2009): 37–42.
Singh, D. and V. Aeri. "Phytochemical and Pharmacological Potential of *Acanthus ilicifolius*." *Journal of Pharmacy and Bioallied Sciences* 5, no. 1 (2013): 17–20.
Spalding, M., M. Kainuma, and L. Collins. *World Atlas of Mangroves*. London: Earthscan, 2010.
Spino, C., M. Dodier, and S. Sotheeswaran. "Anti-HIV Coumarins from *Calophyllum* Seed Oil." *Bioorganic & Medicinal Chemistry Letters* 8, no. 24 (1998): 3475–8.
Stafford, H. A. "Proanthocyanidins and the Lignin Connection." *Phytochemistry* 27, no. 1 (1988): 1–6.

Subrahmanyam, C., S. Ratna Kumar, and G. Damodar Reddy. "Bioactive Diterpenes from the Mangrove Avicennia Officinalis Linn." *Indian Journal of Chemistry Section B* 45, no. 11 (2006): 2556.

Sumithra, M., J. V. Kumar, and V. S. Kancharana. "Influence of Methanolic Extract of *Avicennia officinalis* Leaves on Acute, Subacute and Chronic Inflammatory Models." *International Journal of PharmTech Research* 3 (2011): 763–8.

Sun, Y. Q., and Y. W. Guo. "Gymnorrhizol, an Unusual Macrocyclic Polydisulfide from the Chinese Mangrove *Bruguiera gymnorrhiza*." *Tetrahedron Letters* 45, no. 28 (2004): 5533–5.

Sura, S., J. Anbu, M. Sultan, and B. Uma. "Antiulcer Effect of Ethanolic Leaf Extract of *Avicennia officinalis*." *Pharmacology Online* 3 (2011): 12–19.

Taylor, P. B., J. S. Culp, C. Debouck, R. K. Johnson, A. D. Patil, D. J. Woolf, I. Brooks, and R. P. Hertzberg. "Kinetic and Mutational Analysis of Human Immunodeficiency Virus Type 1 Reverse Transcriptase Inhibiton by Inophyllums, a Nobel Class of Non-nucleoside Inhibitors." *Journal of Biological Chemistry* 269 (1994): 6325–31.

Tian, M. Q. *Studies on the Chemical Constituents of Two Mangrove Plants Excoecaria agallocha and Sonneratia caseolaris.* Graduate School of Chinese Academy of Sciences (Institute of Oceanography), Qingdao, 2007.

Tian, M. Q., G. M. Bao, N. Y. Ji, X. M. Li, and B. G. Wang. "Triterpenoids and Steroids from *Excoecaria agallocha*." *Zhongguo Zhong yao za zhi= Zhongguozhongyaozazhi= China Journal of Chinese Materia Medica* 33, no. 4 (2008): 405–8.

Tian, M. Q., H. Dai, X. Li, and B. Wang. "Chemical Constituents of Marine Medicinal Mangrove Plant *Sonneratia caseolaris*." *Chinese Journal of Oceanology and Limnology* 27, no. 2 (2009): 288–96.

Tiwari, K. P., P. K. Minocha, and M. Masood. "Acanthicifoline-a New Alkaloid from *Acanthus ilicifolius*." *Polish Journal of Chemistry* 54 (1980): 857–8.

Toume, K., K. Kamiya, M. A. Arai, N. Mori, S. K. Sadhu, F. Ahmed, and M. Ishibashi. "Xylogranin B: A Potent Wnt Signal Inhibitory Limonoid from *Xylocarpus granatum*." *Organic Letters* 15, no. 23 (2013): 6106–9.

Uddin, S. J., L. Nahar, J. A. Shilpi, M. Shoeb, T. Borkowski, S. Gibbons, M. Middleton, M. Byres, and S. D. Sarker. "Gedunin, a Limonoid from *Xylocarpus granatum*, Inhibits the Growth of CaCo-2 Colon Cancer Cell Line in Vitro." *Phytotherapy Research* 21, no. 8 (2007): 757–61.

Vinh, L. B., N. T. M. Nguyet, S. Y. Yang, J. H. Kim, N. V. Thanh, N. X. Cuong, N. H. Nam, C. V. Minh, I. Hwang, and Y. H. Kim. "Cytotoxic Triterpene Saponins from the Mangrove *Aegiceras corniculatum*." *Natural Product Research* 33, no. 5 (2019): 628–34.

Vinh, L. B., N. V. Phong, I. Ali, G. Dan, Y. S. Koh, H. L. T. Anh, D. T. V. Anh, S. Y. Yang, and Y. H. Kim. "Identification of Potential Anti-in3ammatory and Melanoma Cytotoxic Compounds from *Aegiceras corniculatum*," *Medicinal Chemistry Research* 29 (2020): 2020–7.

Wang, J. D., and Y. W. Guo. "Agallochaols A and B, Two New Diterpenes from the Chinese Mangrove *Excoecaria agallocha* L." *Helvetica Chimica Acta* 87, no. 11 (2004): 2829–33.

Wang, J. D., Z. Y. Li, and Y. W. Guo. "Secoatisane and Isopimarane Type Diterpenoids from the Chinese Mangrove *Excoecaria agallocha* L." *Helvetica Chimica Acta* 88, no. 5 (2005): 979–85.

Wei, S. D., Y. M. Lin, M. M. Liao, H. C. Zhou, and Y. Y. Li. "Characterization and Antioxidative Properties of Condensed Tannins from the Mangrove Plant *Aegiceras corniculatum*." *Journal of Applied Polymer Science* 124, no. 3 (2012): 2463–72.

Wu, J., S. Zhang, Q. Xiao, Q. Li, J. Huang, Z. Xiao, and L. Long. "Xyloccensin M and N, Two New B,D-secolimonoids from *Xylocarpus granatum*." *Zeitschriftfür Naturforschung* B 58, no. 12 (2003): 1216–19.

Wu, J., S. Zhang, T. Bruhn, Q. Xiao, H. Ding, and G. Bringmann. "Xylogranatins F–R: Antifeedants from the Chinese Mangrove, *Xylocarpus granatum*, a New Biogenetic Pathway to Tetranortriterpenoids." *Chemistry–A European Journal* 14, no. 4 (2008): 1129–44.

Xiao, Q., Y. B. Zeng, W. L. Mei, Y. X. Zhao, Y. Y. Deng, and H. F. Dai. "Cytotoxic Prenylated Xanthones from *Calophyllum inophyllum*." *Journal of Asian Natural Products Research* 10, no. 10 (2008): 993–7.

Yang, Y., Y. Zhang, D. Liu, M. L. Weber, B. Shao, and W. Lin. "Dolabrane-type Diterpenes from the Mangrove Plant *Ceriops tagal* with Antitumor Activities." *Fitoterapia* 103 (2015): 277–82.

Yi, X. X., J. G. Deng, C. H. Gao, X. T. Hou, F. Li, Z. P. Wang, E. W. Hao, Y. Xie, Z. C. Du, H. X. Huang, and R. M. Huang. "Four New Cyclohexylideneacetonitrile Derivatives from the Hypocotyl of Mangrove (*Bruguiera gymnorrhiza*)." *Molecules* 20, no. 8 (2015): 14565–75.

Yimdjo, M. C., A. G. Azebaze, A. E. Nkengfack, A. Michele Meyer, B. Bodo, and Z. T. Fomum. "Antimicrobial and Cytotoxic Agents from *Calophyllum inophyllum*." *Phytochemistry* 65, no. 20 (2004): 2789–95.

Yin, S., X. N. Wang, C. Q. Fan, L. P. Lin, J. Ding, and J. M. Yue. "Limonoids from the Seeds of the Marine Mangrove *Xylocarpus granatum*." *Journal of Natural Products* 70, no. 4 (2007): 682–5.

Zakaria, M. B., Z. Ilham, and N. A. Muhamad. "Anti-inflammatory Activity of *Calophyllum inophyllum* Fruits Extracts." *Procedia Chemistry* 13 (2014): 218–20.

Zhang, J. C., Q. Liao, L. Shen, and J. Wu. "Twenty-five Limonoids from the Hainan Mangrove, *Xylocarpus granatum*." *Bioorganic Chemistry* 100 (2020): 103903.

Zhao, F., Z. Zhao, Y. Han, S. Li, C. Liu, and K. Jia. "Baicalin Suppresses Lung Cancer Growth Phenotypes via miR-340-5p/NET1 Axis." *Bioengineered* 12, no. 1 (2021): 1699–707.

Zhou, Z. F. and Y. W. Guo. "Bioactive Natural Products from Chinese Marine Flora and Fauna." *Acta Pharmacologica Sinica* 33, no. 9 (2012): 1159–69.

Zhou, Z. F., L. Y. Kong, T. Kurtán, H. L. Liu, A. Mándi, J. Li, Y. C. Gu, and Y. W. Guo. "Four Phragmalin Orthoesters from the Chinese Mangrove *Xylocarpus granatum*." *Planta Medica* 80, no. 11 (2014): 949–54.

Zhu, B. T., J. Y. Shim, M. Nagai, and H. W. Bai. "Molecular Modelling Study of the Mechanism of High-potency Inhibition of Human Catechol-o-methyltransferase by (–)-epigallocatechin-3-O-gallate." *Xenobiotica* 38, no. 2 (2008): 130–46.

Zou, J. H., J. Dai, X. Chen, and J. Q. Yuan. "Pentacyclic Triterpenoids from Leaves of *Excoecaria agallocha*." *Chemical and Pharmaceutical Bulletin* 54, no. 6 (2006): 920–1.

Possible Application and Ethnomedicinal Use of Aquatic and Semiaquatic Plants

Kankana De[1] and Arun Makal[2]

[*1]Department of Anthropology, Vidyasagar University, West Bengal, India

[2]Department of Anthropology, Bangabasi Evening College, University of Calcutta, Kolkata, India

*Corresponding Author's Email: arunmakal6@gmail.com

Introduction

Medicinal plants and herbs have been discovered and used in traditional practices since prehistoric times. Many great civilizations, including the Mesopotamians, Romans, Greeks, and Indus Valley people, have shown that humans always favored living near plants, streams, lakes, and different types of water bodies to get their foods and shelters. Thus, plants are a primary source of nutrients and medicine for humans and animals since ancient times (Ganchev, Kuneva, and Stoyanova 2019; Tagde et al. 2021; Manokari, Subramanian, and Sorna 2019; Arya et al. 2022). Also, humans consume many parts of plants, including fruits, flowers, leaves, stems, roots, and seeds. Plants produce hundreds of chemical compounds for various functions, including defense and protection against insects, fungi, diseases, and herbivorous mammals. Various plants, like aquatic and semiaquatic, are also significant for human health and well-being. These aquatic and semiaquatic medicinal plants and herbs have biological, pharmacological, nutraceutical, and commercial uses (Swapna et al. 2011; Cronk and Fennessy 2016; Heidi and Smith 2018; Aasim et al. 2019).

Aquatic and semiaquatic plants are found in many ecological zones, including wetlands, lakes, rivers, and coastal zones. Aquatic plants are mainly adapted to live in water environments, such as freshwater marshes, streams, lakes, and salt marshes. They can be floating, fixed, or submerged like algae. These plants provide food and habitat for many animals, including fish, waterfowl, and moose. On the other hand, semiaquatic plants are adapted to live with their roots partially or entirely in water. These semiaquatic plants include mangroves, reeds, water spinach, pond cypress, and so on. On the basis of medicinal uses and physicochemical effects, the aquatic and semiaquatic plants may be classified into two categories: major and minor. Major aquatic and semiaquatic medicinal plants have very high medicinal and economic values and are readily available for commercial purposes for different human well-being. Conversely, the minor aquatic and semiaquatic medicinal plants are those plants that still contain healing qualities against multiple illnesses.

In addition, the major and minor aquatic and semiaquatic plants are highly rich in diversified secondary metabolites due to their association with water bodies and weather conditions. But due to lack of availability of these plant resources and having little knowledge regarding their pharmacological properties, the regional and economic value of these major and minor aquatic and semiaquatic plants are unobserved, overlooked, and neglected by researchers. For that reason, in this current era of traditional medicinal uses, the research on aquatic and semiaquatic plants is very significant because of their phytochemicals, bioactive compounds, and nutritional value as well as biological and pharmacological activities.

Objectives and Methods

From the above understandings, it is revealed that the aquatic and semiaquatic medicinal plants play a vital role in humans' lives, including the biological, pharmacological, and economic uses. This particular chapter aims to explore the current evidence on ethnomedicinal and pharmacological uses of aquatic and semiaquatic medicinal plants. Aquatic and semiaquatic plants belonging to various families like Acanthaceae, Apiaceae, Araceae, Asteraceae, Ceratophyllaceae, Convolvulaceae, Hydrocharitaceae, Marsileaceae, Nymphaeaceae, Oxalidaceae, Plantaginaceae, Polygonaceae, Scrophulariaceae, Trapaceae, and Typhaceae of some lakes, wetland areas of the Midnapore Sadar block of the district Paschim Medinipur of Indian state of West Bengal were selected for this study by applying purposive sampling. This study reveals that the various parts of these aquatic and semiaquatic plants are used as dietary supplements. Besides, these plants are also famous for their profitable value and are used as components in some pharmaceutical industries.

Study Area and People

This study selected many aquatic and semiaquatic medicinal plants belonging to various families of different wetland areas of the Midnapore Sadar block of the district Paschim Medinipur of Indian state of West Bengal. The Midnapore Sadar block forms an administrative division in Medinipur Sadar subdivision of Paschim Medinipur district in the Indian state of West Bengal. Geographically, the Midnapore Sadar block is bounded by Salboni and Keshpur blocks in the north, Kharagpur II block in the east, Kharagpur I and Jhargram blocks in the south, and Binpur-I block in the west. The Midnapore Sadar block has an area of 323.64 km^2. It has 1 panchayat samity, 9 gram panchayats, 129 gram sansads (village councils), 271 mouzas, and 232 inhabited villages. The Medinipur police station serves this block. The headquarters of this block is at Barapathar Cantonment. Midnapore Sadar block had a forest cover of 5,940 hectares, against a total geographical area of 33,300 hectares in 2005–6. The Gram panchayats of Midnapore Sadar block/panchayat samiti are Bonpura, Chandra, Dherua, Kankabati (Tantigeria), Monidaha, Panchkhuri I, Panchkhuri II, Pathra, and Siromoni.

The drainage network of the Midnapore Sadar block of the district Paschim Medinipur is dominated by rivers like the Shilabati, Kangsabati, and Subarnarekha. This block has many wetlands. These wetlands of this block are affected by the behavior of the Ganga River and are prone to degradation. Most wetlands are fragmented into smaller patches, with only 10 percent being core wetlands. These wetlands are vulnerable to degradation due to hydrological instability, fragmentation, and overdependence on floods. The uses of these wetlands in this region are dynamic in nature in terms of space and time. The wetlands of this block are the source of a variety of plants including floating plants, water spinach, medicinal plants or herbs, ferns, and moss. The village people of the Midnapore Sadar block are closely connected with the plant wealth of their surroundings for day-to-day requirements, mostly medicines for their illnesses. They believe that they have a significant level of understanding and experience about the application and practices of the plants and their products (Pandit 2011; Ghosh et al. 2021) (Figure 7.1).

The village people of the Midnapore Sadar block use a variety of plants, including aquatic and semiaquatic, for consumption and to cure various diseases. This study has mainly identified various aquatic and semiaquatic medicinal plants used by the local communities of the Midnapore Sadar block. They use different local or regional names for these aquatic and semiaquatic medicinal plants. The local names of some of the famous aquatic and semiaquatic medicinal plants in the region of Midnapore Sadar block are *Brhami-shak*, *Hinche* or *Helencha*, *Kulkhara*, *Thankuni*, *Shaluk*, *Kolmi-shak*, *Paniphol*, and so on. Among these, the *Brhami-shak* is a herb found in marshes and moist soils in the Midnapore Sadar region. It has many therapeutic uses, including as an astringent, laxative, and bronchodilator. The leaves can be used to increase memory and cure colds and coughs. Besides, the *Kolmi-shak* is a semiaquatic plant that is grown as a vegetable for its tender shoots. It is a perennial plant that grows in moist soil along the margins of freshwater in ditches, marshes, and wet rice fields. This *Kolmi-shak*, also known as Water Spinach, is widely cultivated in Southeast Asia, East Asia, and South Asia. It is generally believed to have been first domesticated in Southeast Asia. The village people of Midnapore Sadar use these aquatic and semiaquatic medicinal plants and herbs in their daily diet and try to eat them on a regular basis. Besides, some of the village people collect these aquatic and semiaquatic medicinal plants daily and sell them in the nearby local markets for their survival. This is another significant consideration for the selection of Midnapore Sadar block for this study.

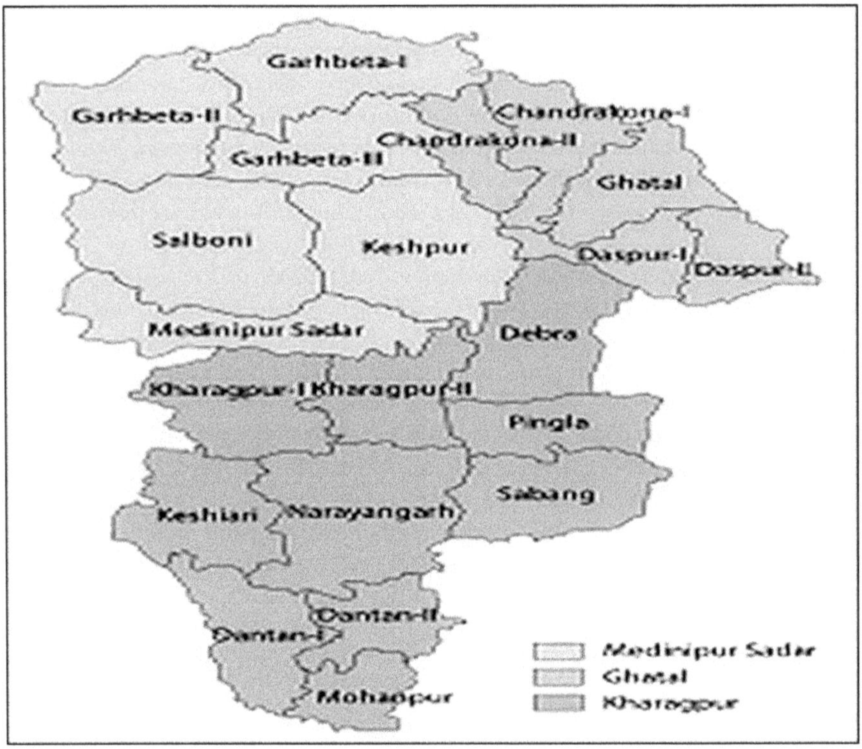

Figure 7.1. Midnapore Sadar block of the district Paschim Medinipur of West Bengal, India. Source: Author.

Aquatic/Semiaquatic Plants: Medicinal Importance

Nowadays, the use of plants in modern medicine is in high demand. Among the different types of plants, aquatic and semiaquatic plants categorically show significant ecological roles as the dominant primary producers of shallow water ecosystems. They are also called hydrophytes or macrophytes, which have rich economic prominence to mankind. The aquatic and semiaquatic plants directly serve as the major source of energy for a greater diversity of biota besides conserving the aquatic environment. These aquatic and semiaquatic medicinal plants are rich in bioactive compounds and show various commercial and nutraceutical uses. Besides, these plants have many unique biological features and are important for their agricultural, horticultural, ornamental, and medicinal significance. Various plant species of aquatic and semiaquatic origin are reported to have valuable folklore utilization in traditional medicine and are used in phytoremediation (Krishnasamy et al. 2014; Dhir et al. 2009; Saravanakumar and Prabhakaran 2013). Accordingly, the aquatic and semiaquatic medicinal plants are important for a number of reasons, including bioactive compounds, traditional medicine, nutritional value, antimicrobial properties, antioxidant activity, antidiabetic activity, herbal medicines, and wastewater treatment. Thus, aquatic and semiaquatic plants produce bioactive compounds that can be used to protect human and livestock health. Second, these plants have been used in traditional medicine worldwide. Next, aquatic plants are high in nutritional value. On the other hand, the phytochemicals of aquatic and semiaquatic plants have antimicrobial properties. In addition, some plants have antioxidant activity, which can be used to treat skin infections and wound dressings. Again, some aquatic plants have antidiabetic properties. Moreover, herbal medicines can promote growth and strengthen the metabolism of aquatic animals. As a final point, aquatic plants can also play a role in wastewater treatment.

In our country like India, aquatic and semiaquatic plants are broadly used for a variety of purposes since ancient times and are even used today mostly for food, fodder, and fiber (Bornette 2011; Pareek and Kumar 2013). But not much work has been done to quantify their medicinal use. A few studies have been done on the ethno-medicinal uses, economic significance, as well as edible characteristics of aquatic and semiaquatic plants (Maya et al. 2003; Jain et al. 2007; Swapna et al. 2011). The people of the study region mostly use the aquatic and semiaquatic plants as a food source. For example, *Brahmi-shak*, or *Bacopa monnieri*, also known as water hyssop, is a medicinal plant used for a variety of health benefits, including improving memory, reducing stress, and treating inflammation. Here, this *Brahmi-shak* is eaten in a variety of ways, such as in salads, curries, or chutneys. It is also eaten with ghee or clarified butter. Another example shows that the *Helencha*, also known as fried buffalo spinach, is a common recipe in the study region. This traditional recipe is an age-old remedy for boosting digestive health and improving gut health. The botanical name for *Helencha* is *Enhydra fluctuans*. The leaves of *Helencha* are also used to make chops with other ingredients like flour, rice flour, ginger paste, turmeric powder, cumin powder, and chili powder. *Helencha* leaves are said to have medicinal properties and can help with diarrhea, constipation, and other health issues. Helencha leaves are said to be good for the liver. They can help increase hemoglobin levels in the blood. They can help with pain. Other examples express that *Kulekhara*, also known as *Hyrophila auriculata*, is a medicinal plant with many uses. It is a common herb in the study region and is used in cooking and traditional medicine. *Kulekhara* leaves are used in salads and *saag* dishes. It is used as a replacement for fresh methi. Kulekhara leaves have anti-inflammatory properties and help to cure arthritis, joint pain, and inflammatory bowel diseases. Besides, these leaves have analgesic properties and help with curing headaches, menstrual cramps, and muscle aches. The leaves of *Kulekhara* also have diuretic properties and help with kidney health and water retention. Again, *Kulekhara* leaves can help with digestive health, constipation, indigestion, and bloating. In addition, the *Kulekhara* seeds can help with blood disorders and urinary problems. *Kulekhara* oil has antibacterial properties and can help with various illnesses. *Kulekhara* has been used to treat pain, jaundice, malaria, and as an aphrodisiac. In this way, a large number of aquatic and semiaquatic plants in the study region are very significant for food, fodder, fiber, and medicine among local communities of the Midnapore Sadar block of the district Paschim Medinipur of Indian state of West Bengal.

Aquatic/Semiaquatic Plants in the Study Region

Nowadays, the aquatic and semiaquatic plants are extensively used for different practices globally such as consumption, medicinal, ornamental, and religious offering. Similarly, in a country like India, 50 to 60 percent of people live near the water bodies and use the aquatic and semiaquatic plants of various species as traditional food and medicine. The present study has enlisted a number of aquatic and semiaquatic plants of the Midnapore Sadar block of the district Paschim Medinipur which have medicinal properties. The people of this region use these aquatic and semiaquatic plants for their daily consumption and use them as medicine to treat a variety of diseases (see Table 7.1 and Table 7.2). Several study reports show that these aquatic and semiaquatic plants possess high nutritional values, medicinal uses, and many biological and pharmacological functions due to the presence of their bioactive combinations. This study has classified aquatic and semiaquatic medicinal plants according to the local people of the Midnapore Sadar block. The people of this block consume a large number of aquatic and semiaquatic medicinal plants. This study has enlisted ten aquatic medicinal plants belonging to various families like Araceae, Ceratophyllaceae, Hydrocharitaceae, Nymphaeaceae, Plantaginaceae, Polygonaceae, Trapaceae, and Typhaceae as well as ten semiaquatic medicinal plants belonging to various families like Acanthaceae, Apiaceae, Araceae, Asteraceae, Convolvulaceae, Marsileaceae, Oxalidaceae, Polygonaceae, and Scrophulariaceae of some lakes, wetland areas of the Midnapore Sadar block (see Figure 7.2 and Figure 7.3).

Aquatic Plants: Remedial and Lucrative Uses

This study has revealed that local people of the Midnapore Sadar block of the district Paschim Medinipur extremely use ten aquatic plants which have consumption and medicinal properties. The local name of these ten aquatic medicinal plants are *Bekh-unjuber*, *Dubia-shak*, *Hogla*, *Jaljhangi*, *Karpur*, *Paniphol*, *Shaluk*, *Topopana*, *Water-lily*, and *Water-thyme*. The detailed uses of these ten aquatic plants, such as their consumption, lucrative, and medicinal properties, are given here.

1. ***Bekh-unjuber*:** The scientific name of the plant *Bekh-unjuber* is *Polygonum barbatum* and the family belongs to the Polygonaceae. It is grown in the irrigated low land and tidal rice fields. It is also grown in the marshy grasslands. This plant is also called knotgrass, joint weed, or smart weed. This plant is used for treating ulcers, colic, and scabies. It also has anticancer and anti-inflammatory properties. *Polygonum barbatum* extract is used to reduce the growth, migration, and invasion of colorectal cancer cells. It may also induce apoptosis in these cells. The seeds of *P. barbatum* are used to relieve colic pain. A paste made from the root of *P. barbatum* is used externally to treat scabies. *P. barbatum* root extract has been used to treat ulcers. *P. barbatum* root extract is astringent and cooling. *P. barbatum* is also shown to have antioxidant, antimicrobial, anti-inflammatory, and other properties.

Table 7.1. Aquatic Medicinal Plants Used by the Local People of Midnapore Sadar Block

Local Name	Scientific Name	Family Name	Parts Used	Medicinal Uses
Bekh-unjuber	*Polygonum barbatum*	Polygonaceae	Leaves, root, and seed	For the treatment of ulcer, and root extract as astringent and as carminative agent.
Dubia-shak	*Polygonum plebeium R. Br.*	Polygonaceae	Seeds	For the treatment of diarrhea, eczema, inflammation, liver illness, and ringworm.
Hogla	*Typha lephantine Roxb*	Typhaceae	Rhizomes, pollen, and flowers	Astringent and diuretic, used to treat dysentery, gonorrhea, and measles.
Jaljhangi	*Ceratophyllum demersum*	Ceratophyllaceae	Whole plant	It is applied as a pain reliever and also used as an anti-inflammatory.
Karpur	*Limnophila indica*	Plantaginaceae	Leaves	The leaves of the plant are used to treat fevers, dysentery, and elephantiasis. It is also considered an antiseptic and carminative.
Paniphol	*Trapa bispinosa Roxb*	Trapaceae	Plant, nut, and rootstock	Plants have antimicrobial activity and fresh nuts help to cure stomach and heart burning. Rootstock used as a diuretic and astringent.
Shaluk	*Nymphaea nouchali*	Nymphaeaceae	Root, stem, leaves, and flowers	Root is used as a demulcent for piles and dyspepsia. The stem is used to treat, blood vomiting, and leprosy. The tender leaves are used for burning sensation of the body. The flower is used to cure cough and skin eruptions.
Topopana	*Pistia stratiotes*	Araceae	Leaves	Leaf extracts helps to reduce inflammation in allergic reactions, arthritis, and fevers.
Water-lily	*Nymphaea odorata*	Nymphaeaceae	Roots, Leaves, Rhizomes, and Flowers	Dried roots help to treat gastrointestinal and bronchial conditions. Leaves helps to treat inflammation associated with mucous membranes. Flowers help to protect the body from possible injury.
Water-thyme	*Hydrilla verticillata*	Hydrocharitaceae	Stem, leaves, and flowers	Thyme tea helps to reduce coughs, sore throats, and congestion.

Source: Author.

Table 7.2. Semiaquatic Medicinal Plants Used by the Local People of Midnapore Sadar Block

Local Name	Scientific Name	Family Name	Parts Used	Medicinal Uses
Amrul-shak	*Oxalis corniculata*	Oxalidaceae	Whole plant and Leaves	Amrul-shak helps to treat indigestion, constipation, and diarrhea. It also treat skin diseases and skin eruptions
Bhrami-shakh	*Bacopa monnieri*	Scrophulariaceae	Leaves	Fried leaves help improve brain development
Bon-palong	*Rumex maritimus*	Polygonaceae	Leaves, seeds, and roots	The seeds are used as sex stimulants and aphrodisiac. The leaves are used to cure external burns and ringworm. The roots are used to cure skin diseases.
Hinche	*Enydra fluctuans*	Asteraceae	Leaves	Helencha leaves help reduce acidity, heartburn, and inflammation. They also help with indigestion, muscle relaxation, and diarrhea
Keshutte	*Eclipta prostrata*	Asteraceae	Whole plant, leaves, and flower	Used to treat diseases of the skin, liver, stomach, asthma and other respiratory illnesses
Kolmi-shak	*Ipomoea aquatic*	Convolvulaceae	Whole plant	Kolmi-shak helps to treat metal poisoning, diabetes, and constipation. It can strengthen liver function
Kulekhara	*Hygrophila auriculata*	Acanthaceae	Whole plant and Leaves	Kulekhara is rich in iron that helps to increase hemoglobin levels in people with anemia. It helps to reduce blood glucose levels. It can improve digestion.
Sushni-shak	*Marsilea quadrifolia*	Marsileaceae	Whole plant and Leaves	This plant is used to treat coughs, bronchitis, snake bites, and abscesses.
Taro	Colocasia esculenta	Araceae	Leaves	Taro leaves help to boost immunity. It is high in fiber that also help improve heart health
Thankuni	*Centella asiatica*	Apiaceae	Leaves	The leaf juice helps relieve hypertension. It boosts the immune system and treats skin conditions.

Source: Author.

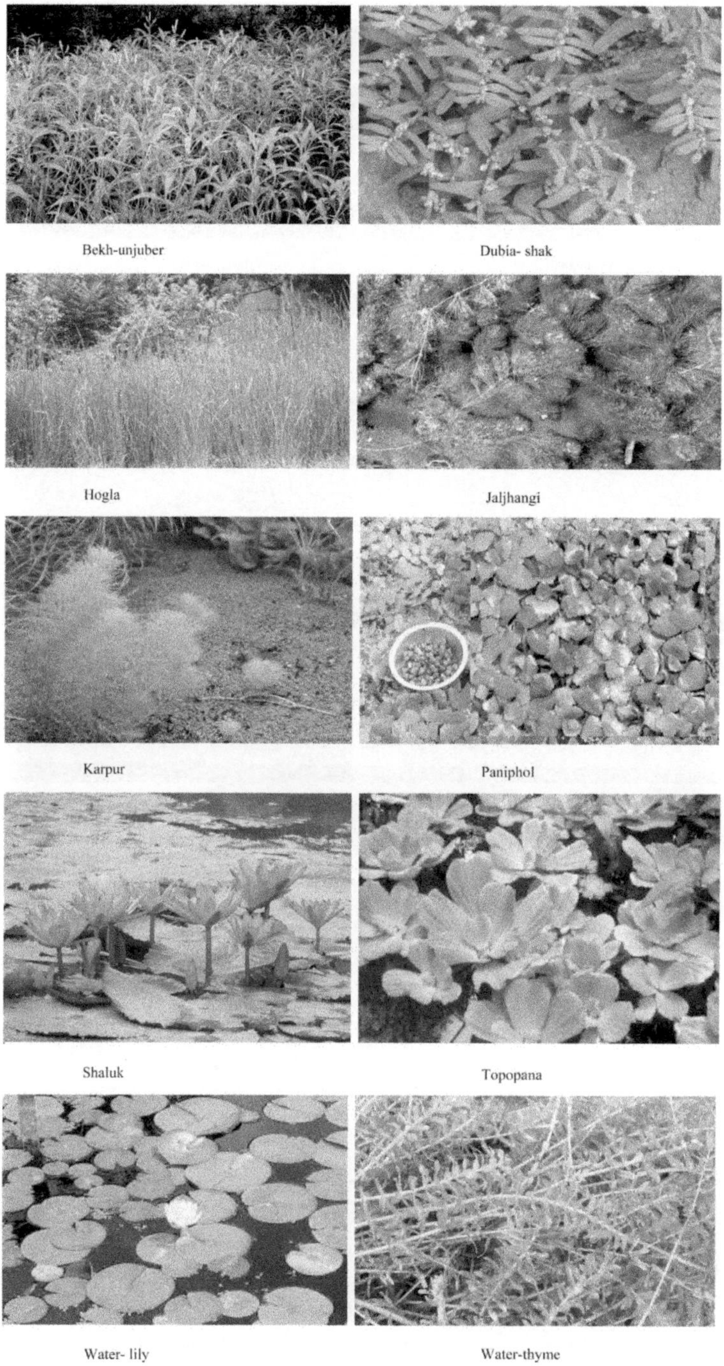

Figure 7.2. Aquatic medicinal plants of the Midnapore Sadar block. Source: Author.

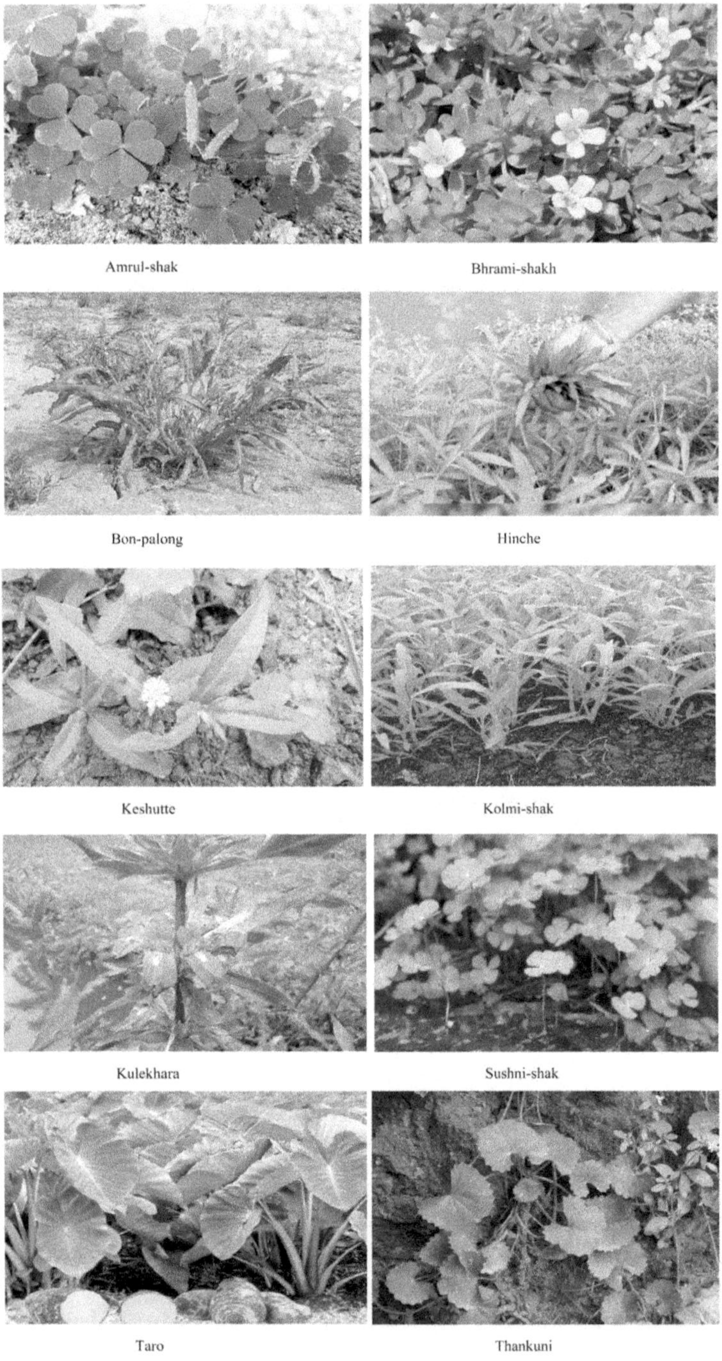

Figure 7.3. Semiaquatic medicinal plants of the Midnapore Sadar block. Source: Author.

2. ***Dubia-shak*:** The scientific name of the plant *Dubia-shak* is *Polygonum plebeium R. Br.* and the family belongs to the Polygonaceae. It is also termed as common knotweed. It is a flowering plant and grows in full sun to partial shade and in moist and well-drained soil. The leaves, stem, and root of this plant are used for medicinal purposes. This plant has many pharmacological properties like anticancer, anti-inflammatory, antioxidant, antinociceptive, cytoprotective, and neuroprotective. This perennial herb is used as traditional medicine to treat a variety of purposes like liver disease, inflammation, and gastrointestinal disorders. Hence, it is used to treat liver disorders like jaundice and hepatitis. Besides, it is used to treat diarrhea, dysentery, bowel complaints, eczema, ringworm, and other inflammatory conditions. It is also used to treat pneumonia, urinary infections, and to treat dandruff.
3. ***Hogla*:** The scientific name of the plant *Hogla* is *Typha elephantina Roxb* and the family belongs to the Typhaceae. This plant is grown in wetlands, sedge meadows, along slow-moving streams, riverbanks, and lake shores. It is also found in areas of widely fluctuating water levels such as roadside ditches, reservoirs, and other disturbed wet soil areas. This plant is also known as *Cattail* and is used traditionally to treat many diseases. The female flowers of this plant are used to treat wounds, burns, and bleeding. Besides, the plant is used to treat bacterial infections, blood clotting disorders, cystitis, leprosy, strangury, and splenic enlargement. In addition, many parts of this *Hogla* plant are edible. The seeds can be used to feed cattle and chickens. This plant is also used by the local people of the Midnapore Sadar block for making small huts. This plant can be used to make paper, fiber, and biofuel.
4. ***Jaljhangi*:** The scientific name of the plant *Jaljhangi* is *Ceratophyllum demersum* and the family belongs to the Ceratophyllaceae. This plant is grown in lakes, ponds, and slow-moving streams. This plant is also known as *Coontail* or Hornwort. It is used to treat a variety of conditions, including fevers, sunburn, and scorpion stings. This *C. demersum* is used as a pain reliever and to treat inflammation, infections, and wounds. It is used as an antioxidant and as a chemopreventive agent, as well as to treat ulcers and diarrhea. It is also used to improve water quality.
5. ***Karpur*:** The scientific name of the plant *Karpur* is *Limnophila indica and the* family belongs to the Plantaginaceae. This plant is grown in the mud of river banks and rice fields. *L. indica* is also known as *Marshweed*. It is used in traditional medicine to treat fevers, dysentery, and elephantiasis. It is also considered an antiseptic and carminative. The leaves of the plant are used in infusions to treat dysentery. The juice of the plant is rubbed on the body to treat fevers. A liniment made from this plant and coconut oil is used to treat elephantiasis. The extracts of the plant are shown to inhibit the growth of bacteria. This plant is also considered antiseptic and carminative.
6. ***Paniphol*:** The scientific name of the plant *Paniphol* is *Trapa bispinosa Roxb*, and the family belongs to the Trapaceae. This plant is grown in shallow bodies of water, such as ponds, marshes, and slow-moving streams. It is an aquatic

plant that floats freely on the water. The other names of this *Paniphal* are water chestnut and *Singhara*. This water chestnut is used in traditional medicine for many purposes, including treating heart disease, digestive issues, and skin conditions. Water chestnuts contain potassium, which helps to lower blood pressure and reduce the risk of stroke. On the other hand, these water chestnuts are natural diuretics which help to eliminate salt and lower blood pressure. These chestnuts are high in fiber, which can help with digestion and weight loss. Its flour is used as a substitute for wheat flour. It also can help keep skin hydrated and protect it from pigmentation. It helps to purify the blood by removing toxins. These water chestnuts contain iodine which is important for normal thyroid function.

7. ***Shaluk*:** The scientific name of the plant *Shaluk* is *Nymphaea nouchali* and the family belongs to the Nymphaeaceae. This plant is grown in ponds, canals, and lakes in many villages of the Midnapore Sadar block of the district Paschim Medinipur. This *Shaluk* is also known as the Indian red water lily. It has many medicinal uses as a digestive aid, anti-inflammatory, and antioxidant. The tannins in *Shaluk* help to treat diarrhea. On the other hand, the fiber and vitamins in *Shaluk* help to soothe stomachaches and help to relieve flatulence. The anti-inflammatory properties of *Shaluk* help to relieve joint swelling and stiffness. Moreover, Shaluks are a good source of natural antioxidants, which protect the body from damage caused by free radicals.
8. ***Topopana*:** The scientific name of the plant *Topopana* is *Pistia stratiotes* and it belongs to the family Araceae. This floating aquatic plant is grown in slow-moving water bodies like ponds, lakes, and canals. This plant is also called water lettuce or water cabbage. This plant is used to treat a variety of conditions, including fevers, blood diseases, and skin infections. The dried leaves are powdered and applied to wounds and sores to disinfect them. The powdered leaves are also used to treat syphilitic eruptions. Besides, the leaves are infused in water to create an eyewash to treat allergic conjunctivitis. The leaves are burned into ash and used to treat ringworm infections of the scalp. In addition, the leaves of this plant are also used to treat various conditions of eczema, leprosy, ulcers, and piles. Furthermore, the leaf infusions are used to treat bladder complaints, kidney afflictions, hematuria, dysentery, and anemia. Moreover, this plant has diuretic, antidiabetic, antidermatophytic, antifungal, and antimicrobial properties. It has the potential to absorb heavy metals without developing toxicity or reduction in growth. It is used for water purification and to combat water pollution. Again, the leaves and roots of this plant have potential nutritional uses. The leaves have high values of mineral elements and antioxidants.
9. ***Water-lily*:** The scientific name of the plant *Water-lily* is *Nymphaea odorata* and the family belongs to the Nymphaeaceae. This plant is grown in shallow lakes, ponds, and slow-moving streams. This *N. odorata* is also called the white water lily. It is used in folk medicine to treat a variety of conditions. The root, bulb, flowers, seeds, and rhizomes of this plant are used for medicinal purposes. The

root can be boiled into a liquid for gargling. Besides, the root can be boiled into a liquid for drinking. In case of vaginal conditions, the plant can be applied directly to the affected area. Furthermore, this plant is applied directly to the affected area in case of throat and mouth diseases. Conversely, in case of burns and boils, this plant can be used as a warm compress. Moreover, this is used in skin lotions to treat boils, ulcers, tumors, baldness, and inflammation. It is used to treat cramps, irregular periods, or excessive menstrual bleeding. This plant helps to relieve irritating skin conditions as well as eczema, acne, and dry skin. Again, the seeds, flowers, and rhizomes of this plant may be eaten raw or cooked. The rhizomes of this *N. odorata* help to treat coughs and colds. The stem of this plant may be placed directly on teeth to treat a toothache.

10. ***Water-thyme*:** The scientific name of the plant *Water-thyme* is *Hydrilla verticillata* and it belongs to the family Hydrocharitaceae. This plant is grown in fresh or brackish bodies of water, such as lakes, ponds, rivers, streams, and marshes. Water-thyme can grow in deep or shallow water. This plant has many medicinal uses, including treating respiratory issues, digestive problems, and skin conditions. It is also used as a food preservative. This *Water-thyme* can help with bronchitis, asthma, congestion, colds, flu, sore throat, and seasonal allergies. The anti-inflammatory properties of this plant help to relieve coughing and nasal congestion. It can help with colic, diarrhea, flatulence, and intestinal pain. Thyme can help improve digestion. It can help with acne, eczema, and other skin conditions. Thyme oil is used as a toner to tighten skin. Beside, this thyme oil is applied to the scalp to treat baldness. Furthermore, this *Water-thyme* helps with the treatment of menstrual pain, blood pressure, and weight control, and can help with immunity and bone health. This *Water-thyme* is also used as a food preservative because it has antibacterial properties.

Semiaquatic Plants: Remedial and Lucrative Uses

Beside revealing aquatic medicinal plants, this study has also explored that local people of the Midnapore Sadar block tremendously use ten semiaquatic plants which have consumption and medicinal properties. The local name of these ten semiaquatic medicinal plants are *Amrul-shak*, *Bhrami-shakh*, *Bon-palong*, *Hinche*, *Keshutte*, *Kolmi-shak*, *Kulekhara*, *Sushni-shak*, *Taro*, and *Thankuni*. The details of these ten semiaquatic medicinal plants are given here.

1. ***Amrul-shak*:** The scientific name of the plant *Yellow Oxalis* is *Oxalis corniculata* and family belongs to the family Oxalidaceae. This plant is grown in moist areas, near water, and in shade. It can be found in gardens, fields, and along roadsides. This herb is also known as *Amrul-shak* or Indian sorrel. This *Amrul-shak* has a wide range of medicinal uses in the study region, serving as an astringent, vermifuge, emmenagogue, and antiseptic. This herb has antibacterial, anti-

inflammatory, and antidiabetic properties. It is eaten as a vegetable by the local people of the study area. This *Amrul-shak* helps in the treatment of indigestion, constipation, and diarrhea. It also helps to treat skin diseases and skin eruptions. Besides, this *Amrul-shak* helps to treat fevers and biliousness. It can help in the treatment of vitamin C deficiency, anorexia, and act as an appetite stimulant. Moreover, this plant is used to help in the treatment of wounds, burns, sprains, and snake bites. This herb is used to treat urinary tract infections and helps to treat influenza.

2. ***Bhrami-shakh*:** The scientific name of the plant *Bhrami-shakh* is *Bacopa monnieri* and it belongs to the family Scrophulariaceae. It is grown in wet environments such as canals and marshy areas. It can also grow in shallow waters and freshwater. This plant is also called water hyssop, thyme-leaved gratiola, and herb of grace. *B. monnieri* is a perennial herb with medicinal uses. It is commonly used in Ayurvedic medicine to improve memory, reduce stress, and treat insomnia. The brain tonic made from the *Brahmi-shak* plant improves memory, concentration, and learning ability. It has adaptogenic properties that help to reduce anxiety and stress. Its coolant action helps to promote good quality sleep. It can also lower blood pressure by releasing nitric oxide. The leaves of *B. monnieri* help to improve insulin sensitivity and lower blood glucose levels. Besides, the *Brahmi* oil can help prevent hair loss and improve the quality of hair strands. This oil can be used as a neuralgic to treat joint pain. Furthermore, *Brahmi* can be used as a head rub to treat headaches. In addition, the *Brahmi* tea can help manage colds, chest congestion, and bronchitis. It has anti-inflammatory properties that can help reduce inflammation in the throat and respiratory tracts.
3. ***Bon-palong*:** The scientific name of the plant *Bon-palong* is *Rumex maritimus* and it belongs to the Polygonaceae family. This plant is grown in wet and saline environments such as marshes and coastal areas. This plant is also called golden dock. Most parts of this plant are used for medical purposes. The leaves are applied to treat external burns and ringworm. The seeds are used as aphrodisiacs and sex stimulants, as well as to relieve pain in the back and lumbar region. The roots of *R. maritimus* are used to cure skin diseases. In addition, an infusion of *R. maritimus* is used to treat bloat. It is used as a purgative to cleanse the bowels and to relieve itching.
4. ***Hinche*:** The *Hinche* is a semiaquatic herb. The scientific name of this herb is *Enhydra fluctuans* and it belongs to the Asteraceae family. It is grown in marshy areas, ponds, and lakes. The popular name of *Hinche* is *Helencha*. This herb has many medicinal properties like anti-inflammatory, antimicrobial, antioxidant, antidiabetic, antidiarrheal, and hepatoprotective. It is used by the local people of the Midnapore Sadar block as a traditional medicine to treat a variety of conditions, including diarrhea, indigestion, and inflammation. The leaves of *Helencha* are effective against bacteria like *Escherichia coli*, *Pseudomonas aeruginosa*, *Staphylococcus aureus*, and *Micrococcus luteus*. *Hinche* leaves can be used to treat skin conditions. They can also be used to treat nervous system

conditions. These *Hinche* leaves are used as a demulcent in cases of gonorrhea and are used as a cooling agent by making a paste and applying it to the head.

5. ***Keshuti:*** The scientific name of the plant *Keshutte is Eclipta prostrata* and the family belongs to the *Asteraceae*. This plant is grown in moist, poorly drained wet areas, ditches, and near rivers and swamps. This plant is also known as *Bhringraj*, *Keshut*, *Keshutte*, *Keshuti*, *Keshraj*, *Kalkeshi*, *Keshari*, and *Kalsatar*. This *E. prostrata* is a medicinal plant with white flowers that is also known as the false daisy. This plant is used by the local people to treat a variety of diseases as traditional medicine. It is used to treat diseases of the skin, liver, and stomach. Besides, this plant is also used to treat tumors and hepatitis C virus. Apart from these, this plant is used to treat burns, dermatitis, wounds, and vitiligo. It is used to treat asthma, bronchitis, and cough. Furthermore, it is used to treat liver and spleen enlargement, jaundice, and liver deficiency. Specifically, this plant is used to promote hair growth and is used to treat hair loss and graying of hair. Moreover, this plant is used to treat hemoptysis, hematemesis, hematuria, epistaxis, and uterine bleeding. It is used to treat snake bites, inflammation, diabetes, and cancer.
6. ***Kolmi-shak:*** The scientific name of the plant *Kolmi-shak* is *Ipomoea aquatica* and it belongs to the family Convolvulaceae. This plant is grown in water areas and in soil. The local people of the Midnapore Sadar block cultivate this plant in their kitchen garden. It is popularly known as water spinach. It is used to treat a variety of conditions, including metal poisoning, liver function, constipation, inflammation, and digestion. Accordingly, this water spinach helps to treat metal poisoning and heavy metal toxicity. It also helps to strengthen liver function and metabolism. It helps to treat diabetes and constipation. It helps to treat inflammation, fever, jaundice, bronchitis, and biliousness. It is rich in fiber and can help with digestion. Other medicinal uses include piles, ringworm, and opium poisoning. This water spinach is a nutritious vegetable that is rich in vitamins and minerals, including vitamin C, iron, manganese, and magnesium. It is also a good source of food protein.
7. ***Kulekhara:*** The scientific name of the plant *Kulekhara* is *Hygrophila auriculata* and it belongs to the family Acanthaceae. This plant is grown in marshy regions and also in the ground where it can spread and grow naturally. The other names of this *Kulekhara* are Marsh pennywort, *Kokilaksha*, *Gokulakanta*, *Neeramulli*, and *Nirmulli*. This *Kulekhara* plant has a variety of medicinal uses including anemia, digestion, blood sugar, pain relief, anti-inflammatory, antibacterial, and antioxidant. Accordingly, the Kulekhara leaves can increase hemoglobin levels and help treat anemia. It helps to improve digestion and stomach and liver function. It also helps to reduce blood glucose levels in people with diabetes. Besides, these *Kulekhara* leaves can act as an analgesic to relieve pain. They have anti-inflammatory properties. In addition, these *Kulekhara* leaves have antibacterial properties and support the immune system. These *Kulekhara* leaves also have antioxidant properties that protect the body from damage caused by free radicals. They can support liver and kidney health. These *Kulekhara* leaves

help to relieve respiratory issues. Moreover, the *Kulekhara* seeds are also used to treat blood disorders and urinary problems.

8. ***Sushni-shak*:** The scientific name of the plant *Sushni-shak* is Marsilea quadrifolia and it belongs to the family Marsileaceae. This plant is an herbaceous, aquatic fern that can grow in wet, sandy, or medium soil. This plant is also called water clover. It has several medicinal uses. It is used to treat coughs, bronchitis, snake bites, abscesses, and other conditions. It is also used as a vegetable. This *Sushni-shak* is used as an anti-inflammatory. It is used as a diuretic, depurative, and to treat fevers, coughs, and other respiratory troubles. This *Sushni-shak* is also used as a vegetable and helps to improve brain power. This plant is used to induce sleep as well as to balance blood pressure and to relieve unusual skin burning.
9. ***Taro*:** The scientific name of the plant *Taro* is *Colocasia esculenta* and it belongs to the family *Araceae*. This plant is grown in a wide range of soil types, but it does best in deep, well-drained, friable loams. The local people call this *Taro* as *Kochu*. Besides, the root of *Taro* is called *Maan-Kochu*. Again, the leaves of the *Taro* plant are called *Kachu-pata* or *Kachu-shak*. This *Taro* contains bioactive molecules that may help treat cancer and cancer-related risk factors. It is also beneficial for treating cancers of the lungs and oral cavity. This plant part is low in cholesterol and high in potassium, which helps to regulate blood pressure and reduce the risk of cardiovascular diseases. The fiber of *this* plant also helps to promote a healthy heart and helps to clean the digestive system. It helps with the treatment of blood sugar control, weight loss, and digestive health. Its vitamins A, C, and E help to maintain a healthy immune system and promote healthy skin. Its antioxidants help to strengthen eyesight. It helps to treat skin rashes, nausea, and cold and flu. Moreover, it is a good source of carbohydrates, protein, and other micronutrients. Its root is an excellent source of dietary fiber and good carbohydrates that both improve the function of the digestive system and contribute to healthy weight loss. Its high levels of vitamin C, vitamin B6, and vitamin E also help to maintain a healthy immune system and may eliminate free radicals.
10. ***Thankuni*:** The scientific name of the plant *Thankuni* is *Centella asiatica* and it belongs to the family *Apiaceae*. This plant is grown in wetland, marshy, and shady areas with well-drained soil. This plant is also known as *Gotu-kola*. This plant has been used for thousands of years to treat a variety of conditions, including wound healing, skin health, and cognitive function. This plant is used to improve blood circulation and collagen production that can help wounds heal. This plant also has anti-inflammatory and antioxidant properties that help to reduce inflammation and oxidative stress in the skin. *Thankuni* is also called a brain tonic and is believed to improve cognitive function, memory, and concentration. It may also help with anxiety and stress. *Thankuni* may help with digestive health, respiratory health, and hypertension. It may also have anticancer properties. The local people of the Midnapore Sadar block said that they regularly consume the raw leaves of this *Thankuni* plant.

Conclusion and Recommendation

Aquatic and semiaquatic plants play a significant role in maintaining the health and stability of aquatic ecosystems by providing habitats for various organisms, improving water quality through nutrient absorption, producing oxygen through photosynthesis, and serving as a food source for aquatic animals; essentially acting as a key component of the food chain within the water body. From the present study, it is revealed that aquatic and semiaquatic plants play a significant role in human life also by providing food, medicine, and raw materials. They also help to clean the environment by removing pollutants from water. Humans use various aquatic and semiaquatic plants for medicinal purposes besides using different other types of plant resources. As a result, aquatic and semiaquatic medicinal plants play an essential role in human well-being to fulfill their daily needs. These aquatic and semiaquatic plants also have biological, pharmacological, nutraceutical, and economic uses. In other words, they are also referred to as hydrophytes or macrophytes and play countless economic significance to mankind. In our country, aquatic and semiaquatic plants have been extensively used for a diversity of purposes since ancient times and are used or cultivated even today particularly for food, fodder, fiber, and medicine.

Keeping the understandings and significance of aquatic and semiaquatic plants in mind, this particular chapter explored ten aquatic medicinal plants belonging to various families like Araceae, Ceratophyllaceae, Hydrocharitaceae, Nymphaeaceae, Plantaginaceae, Polygonaceae, Trapaceae, and Typhaceae as well as ten semiaquatic medicinal plants belonging to various families like Acanthaceae, Apiaceae, Araceae, Asteraceae, Convolvulaceae, Marsileaceae, Oxalidaceae, Polygonaceae, and Scrophulariaceae of some lakes, wetland areas of the Midnapore Sadar block of the district Paschim Medinipur of Indian state of West Bengal. These studied aquatic and semiaquatic medicinal plants are rich in alkaloids, flavonoids, terpenoids, phenolics, saponins, tannins, dietary fiber, glycosidic derivatives, carbohydrates, and proteins. These phytochemicals have been used for their antimicrobial, antioxidant, hepatoprotective, sedative, anticonvulsant, cytotoxic, antiparasitic, and antidiabetic activities. Apart from this, various parts of these aquatic and semiaquatic plants are used as dietary supplements and in the synthesis of green nanoparticles. These plants are also known for their economic value and are used as an ingredient in some pharmaceutical industries.

This research study has only enlisted ten aquatic and ten semiaquatic medicinal plants in the study area. But a variety of aquatic and semiaquatic medicinal plant species are found in this area which have many differences between them and genetic variations within them. In addition, these unknown aquatic and semiaquatic medicinal plant species may have a wide range of phytochemicals with potential bioactive properties. Thus, sufficient research work on these aquatic and semiaquatic medicinal plants of the Midnapore Sadar block of the district Paschim Medinipur is done. In other words, many aquatic and semiaquatic plants of this region are still unexplored and unidentified. Therefore, more extensive and specific research works on these aquatic and semiaquatic medicinal plant species are required to examine the natural phytochemicals and bioactive compounds for their agricultural, horticultural, nutraceutical, ornamental, medicinal, and economic importance. Accordingly, it is recommended that the qualitative and quantitative study on these aquatic and semiaquatic plants and their uninterrupted observation and protection are very important in the present time to explore their richness for the development and discovery of pharmaceutical drugs. Finally, the present study can be taken as a reference for future studies to conduct research on the ethnomedicinal use, phytochemistry, and other possible applications of aquatic and semiaquatic medicinal plants.

References

Aasim, M., K. M. Khawar, S. I. Ahmed, and M. Karataş. "Multiple Uses of Some Important Aquatic and Semiaquatic Medicinal Plants." In *Plant and Human Health, Volume 2: Phytochemistry and Molecular Aspects*, edited by M. Ozturk, and K. R. Hakeem, 541–78. Switzerland AG: Springer Nature, 2019.

Arya, A. K., M. Durgapal, A. Bachheti, Deepti, K. K. Joshi, Y. H. Gonfa, R. K. Bachheti, and A. Husen. "Ethnomedicinal Use, Phytochemistry, and Other Potential Application of Aquatic and Semiaquatic Medicinal Plants." *Evidence-Based Complementary and Alternative Medicine* 2022 (2022): 1–19.

Bornette, G., and S. Puijalon. "Response of Aquatic Plants to Abiotic Factors: A Review." *Aquatic Sciences* 73, no. 1 (2011): 1–14.

Cronk, J. K., and M. S. Fennessy. *Wetland Plants: Biology and Ecology.* Boca Raton, FL: CRC Press, Taylor and Francis, 2016.

Dhir, B., Sharmila, P., and P. Pardha Saradhi. "Potential of Aquatic Macrophytes for Removing Contaminants from the Environment." *Critical Reviews in Environmental Science and Technology* 39, no. 9 (2009): 754–81.

Ganchev, G., V. Kuneva, and A. Stoyanova. "Nutritional and Energy Value of Two Wheat Varieties." *Bulgarian Journal of Agricultural Science* 25, no. 3 (2019): 47–52.

Ghosh, S., M. Jana, J. Duary, B. R. Das, and S. Bhaumik. "Floristic Study of Perennial Flora and Ethnomedicinal Uses in Annual Ground Fire Affected Part of Dry Deciduous Forest, Godapiyasal Paschim Medinipur, West Bengal, India." *The Journal of Phytopharmacology* 10, no. 6 (2021): 484–9.

Heidi, V. D., and A. L. Smith. *National Biodiversity Assessment: Progress on the Inland Aquatic Component.* Pretoria: National Biodiversity Assessment Freshwater-component, 2018.

Jain, A., et al. "Aquatic/Semi-Aquatic Plants Used in Herbal Remedies in the Wetlands of Manipur, Northeastern India." *Indian Journal of Traditional Knowledge* 6, no. 2 (2007): 346–51.

Krishnasamy, J., R. Arumugam, and S. Ariyan. "Ornamental Aquatic and Semi-Aquatic Plants in Coimbatore District." *Biolife* 2, no. 2 (2014): 557–71.

Manokari, M., M. Subramanian, and P. Sorna. "Herbal Remedies from Aquatic and Semi-aquatic Plants Conserved at Siddha Medicinal Plants Garden (CCRS), Mettur Dam, Salem District, Tamil Nadu." *Journal of Research in Siddha Medicine* 2, no. 2 (2019): 74–87.

Maya, S., V. Sarojini Menon, and G. Sreekandan Nair. "Economic Importance of River Vegetation of Kerala – A Case Study." *Journal of Economic and Taxonomic Botany* 27 (2003): 796–803.

Pandit, P. K. "Conservation and Cultural Dimensions of Sacred Groves in Paschim Medinipur District, West Bengal, India." *The Indian Forester* 137, no. 5 (2011): 571–88.

Pareek, A., and A. Kumar. "Aquatic Plants of Rajasthan, India with Medicinal Value." *The Journal of Ethnobiology and Traditional Medicine, Photon* 119 (2013): 434–8.

Saravanakumar, K., and J. Prabhakaran. "Aquatic Floral Populations in Veeranamlake Command Area, Tamil Nadu, India." *International Journal of Current Biotechnology* 1, no. 1 (2013): 18–26.

Swapna, M. M., R. Prakashkumar, K. P. Anoop, C. N. Manju, and N. P. Rajith. "A Review on the Medicinal and Edible Aspects of Aquatic and Wetland Plants of India." *Journal of Medicinal Plants Research* 5, no. 33 (2011): 7163–76.

Tagde, P., P. Tagde, and F. Islam, et al. "The Multifaceted Role of Curcumin in Advanced Nanocurcumin Form in the Treatment and Management of Chronic Disorders." *Molecules* 26, no. 23 (2021): 7109–33.

Part III

Medicinal Plants

Phytochemical Analysis and Antimicrobial Activities

8

Use of Ethnomedicines as an Elixir of Life: Phytochemical Analysis of Traditional Medicinal Plants in India

Sutibra Narayan Mondal, Souhardya Ray, Dola Boral, and Sandip More*

PG Department of Botany, Murshidabad University, Murshidabad, West Bengal, India

*Corresponding author's email: smbot@msduniv.ac.in

Introduction

Ethnomedicines are the knowledge of traditional medicines or the interdisciplinary sciences used by various ethnic groups, especially among the indigenous groups of society (Kumar and Ashaq 2021). The knowledge about the ethnomedicines is important because they have been used since time immemorial for the treatment of various diseases, and the knowledge about them is transferred orally across generations, but they are still documented in various ancient literatures like that of Ayurveda, Unani, Siddha, and Amchi (Pushpangadan et al. 2018). Many sections of today's society, especially among developing nations, use traditional or the ethnomedicines, as they are still popular because they are cheap and easily available to them. More than 60 percent of the world population and more than 80 percent of people from developing nations use traditional medicines for the treatment of various human diseases (Shrestha and Dhillion 2003).

Among the practices in ethnomedicines, plants form the major source for the treatment of various human ailments due to the presence of various bioactive compounds in them (Manandhar 1995). Many plant species are used as the source of traditional medicines, and more than 8000 plant species are known to be used in the treatment of various diseases (Mukherjee, Venkatesh, and Ponnusankar 2010). So, plants ranging from the lower groups like the thallophytes to the more advanced phanerogams are all included in the use of ethnomedicines. Ethnomedicines and the use of plants are the link of biocultural activity, which is connected to the various cultures of different parts of society. Therefore, the knowledge about this medicinal system should be preserved and properly documented (Lepcha et al. 2019).

The knowledge about the ethnomedicines has been documented in the ancient medical literature like Ayurveda, Homeopathy, Unani, and Siddha, which are associated with various cultures of society (Borins 1987). Among the traditional medical sciences, Ayurveda is one of the oldest, and it shows how plants are used in the Ayurveda system for the proper and holistic treatment of any disease. Much more documentation and proper research in the field of exploration of various bioactive compounds can lead to the proper growth and development of traditional medical science (Dua Pradeep and Dua Pamila 2012). Plants are the main component in this alternative medical system (Rajendran 2016). These traditional medicines are used due to economic viability and low toxicity, and they can be available to various underprivileged sections of society. Indian *materia medica* contains a plethora of information about the various plants used in various folklore medicines, which have been used since ancient times for the treatment of various human ailments (Basu et al. 2023).

Medicinal plants form the major formulations for the production of herbal drugs. These plants form the base for the source of the indigenous medicines and are used as nutraceuticals and dietary supplements. Medicinal plants are used all over the world both in allopathic and traditional medicines. Not only in the traditional medicinal system, but these medicinal plants form 20–25 percent of the drug component of allopathic medicines all over the world. The proper documentation and knowledge about medicinal plants are important to distinguish the poisonous plants from those that are useful to healthcare and that can be further used for better drug development (Rates 2001). Plants form the base of ethnobotanical knowledge, and these are used by local communities for the treatment of many human diseases; thus, the knowledge about ethnobotany and medicinal plants provides essential information on the medicinal plants used as drugs (Sheng-Ji 2001). The demand for medicinally important plants is increasing because they are more economical and far less toxic products are obtained from them (Lipp 1996).

The knowledge of the use of medicinal plants ranges from the local household level to the international levels. Better assessment of the medicinal plants for proper use and drug discovery is necessary, as the drugs derived from the medicinal plants treat diseases in a holistic way and are more economical and have less toxicity than other chemicals. The benefits of using medicinal plants are obtained from three different levels: producers, consumers, and the society-wide use of these plants (Smith-Hall, Larsen, and Pouliot 2012). With the ever-increasing population, there is pressure to meet the demands of the people for the supply of medicinal plants for the treatment of diseases with the help of the traditional medical system. Proper bioprospecting with a view to the sustainable utilization of medicinal plants can be harvested for proper drug discovery and further use in both traditional and modern medicine (McGaw et al. 2005). Plants ranging from the lower cryptogams to the more advanced phanerogams have been used in the treatment of various diseases, and their information has been mentioned in various literatures. Moreover, their importance is increasing because the trend of herbal medicines is rising in today's society, as they are far less toxic than the synthetic drugs used.

Plants are the source of many medicines because they contain various bioactive compounds. These compounds range from the primary to the secondary metabolites. The concept of secondary metabolites was first described by the Nobel Prize winner in Physiology or Medicine in 1910, Albrecht Kossel (Jones 1953). The secondary metabolites present in them are not used in their daily functioning, but they have been developed in them as a result of coevolution or the red queen hypothesis to survive in nature. These secondary metabolites are a source of major components used in the preparation of many herbal medicines for the treatment of various diseases in humans (Mandal et al. 2023). Plant secondary metabolites help them survive in nature; they protect against herbivores and also attract pollinators. These secondary metabolites can be extracted and used as the source of many drugs (Pagare et al. 2015).

Plant secondary metabolites can be classified into three broad major groups which are Terpenoids, Phenolics, and the Nitrogen-containing compounds. These classes of compounds play a major role in drug development and the treatment of various diseases (Chinou 2008). Different classes of secondary metabolites obtained and separated from the plants are Alkaloids, Phenylpropanoids, and Terpenoids, which are essential in many pharmaceutical industries. These chemically active natural products are useful for the treatment of various ailments like hypertension, ulcers, and antimicrobial activity (Sharma 2018). Few examples of medicinally important terpenes isolated are Azadirachtin which is a triterpene obtained from *Azadirachta indica* L. and is used in insect pest control. One of the most widely used diterpenes is Taxol, isolated from *Taxus brevifolia* Nutt, which is used as an anticancer agent. Paclitaxel is a taxane-based drug used in the treatment of breast cancer (De Laurentiis et al. 2008).

Another group of the plant secondary metabolites is the phenolics, which are considered the largest group of plant secondary metabolites. Phenols can be further classified into divisions based on their structures like Simple phenolics, Tannins, Coumarins, Flavonoids, Lignans, Chromones and Xanthones and Stilbens (Hussein and El-Anssary 2019). Phenolic groups, mainly Flavonoids obtained from the medicinal plants, are used as antioxidants (Padmaja, Sravanthi, and Hemalatha 2011). Alkaloids are another important class of secondary metabolites obtained from various groups of plants. Alkaloids are of various types, and among them, Indole alkaloids are important because they have served therapeutic purposes since ancient times. Another group of secondary metabolites is Saponins which have certain medicinal properties like antimicrobial activity (Haralampidis, Trojanowska, and Osbourn 2002). They are mostly derived from triterpenoid compounds or from the cyclization of steroidal compounds. Saponins have the properties of surfactants, and they have tremendous medicinal importance (Osbourn 2003).

Due to these various secondary metabolites present in them, plants are considered as nature's biosynthetic laboratories, which serve as the source for the formulations of many herbal drugs (Rungsung et al. 2015). Secondary metabolites are also known as natural products; plants produce them via various biosynthetic pathways, and each of the secondary metabolites is unique in certain groups of plants, and they help in curing various diseases in humans and animals. This is the reason the phytochemical analysis of some medicinally important plants is carried out for both the quantitative and qualitative estimation (Santhi 2011). In addition, the crude plant extracts are used for analysis of the different secondary metabolites present in them (Nandagoapalan, Doss, and Marimuthu 2016). These phytochemical extracts are bioactive, and they contribute to the treatment of various ailments (Yadav and Agarwala 2011). Thus, the phytochemical analysis of the medicinal plants used in the traditional medicinal system provides detailed answers about the important secondary metabolites present in them. These medicinal plants are used in the treatment of diseases in a holistic manner (Ganjhu et al. 2015).

Objectives

Identification of the ethnomedicinal plants is mandatory in the traditional medical system to form proper documentation. On the other hand, the analysis of the different phytochemical constituents of the ethnomedicinally important plants by qualitative and quantitative analysis of both primary and secondary metabolites is also essential. Various parts of the medicinal plants are used in the treatment of different diseases. These medicinal plants are mentioned in certain literature and are less documented. Thus, the proper documentation, conservation, as well as proper sustainable utilization of these medicinal plants is required. This proper documentation cum conservation will help in promoting the knowledge of these plants to far more sectors of contemporary society. Besides, the phytochemical analysis of these medicinal plants can lead to further improvement in new drug development in the pharmaceutical industry. Therefore, the proper analysis of the phytochemicals and uses of these significant medicinal plants can help to build a strong document which can serve as the purpose to impart knowledge about the ethnomedicinal drugs and their uses among various sections of the society.

Methodology

Twenty different ethnomedicinally important plants mentioned in various traditional medical systems have been considered in this study. After identification of these plants, proper documentation has been prepared based on the plant parts used for the treatment of different diseases. The phytochemical study has also been carried out to identify the various compounds present in these plants. The phytochemical screening has been done for the analysis of both the primary and secondary metabolites in them. Besides, different methods have been applied for the qualitative analysis of the phytochemicals. The qualitative estimation for the determination of the primary metabolites from the plant extracts has been carried out. Also, the qualitative estimation of the secondary metabolites present in them has been done by proper extraction from different parts of the plants. Moreover, a number of methods for the estimation of different secondary metabolites have been incorporated.

i. **Test for Alkaloids:** The Dragendorff's test is a color test that detects the presence of alkaloids in a sample. Mix 1 ml of the reagent with 2 ml of the plant extract. The presence of alkaloids is indicated by a reddish-brown precipitate (Harborne 1998).
ii. **Test for Flavonoids:** The Shinoda test is a qualitative test for the presence of flavonoids in a sample. Mix 2 ml of plant extract, add a few magnesium turnings, and two to three drops of strong hydrochloric acid. The presence of flavonoids is indicated by a pink or red coloring (Bohm and Koupai-Abyazani 1994).
iii. **Tannins Test:** The Ferric Chloride test is a way to detect the presence of tannins in a sample. Add a few drops of 5 percent ferric chloride solution to 2 ml of the plant extract. A dark blue or greenish-black coloration indicates the presence of tannins (Evans 2002).
iv. **Saponins Test:** The Foam test is a qualitative test for the presence of saponins in a plant sample. The test involves shaking a plant extract with water to create foam, and then observing whether the foam is stable. In a test tube, agitate 2 ml of the plant extract with 5 ml of distilled water. Saponins are indicated by persistent froths (Sofowora 1996).
v. **Terpenoids Test:** The Salkowski test is a chemical test commonly used to detect the presence of terpenoids in a plant extract. Add 2 ml of chloroform and 1 ml of concentrated sulfuric acid to 2 ml of the plant extract. A reddish-brown coloration at the interface indicates the presence of terpenoids (Edeoga, Okwu, and Mbaebie 2005).
vi. **Steroids Test:** The Liebermann-Burchard test is a chemical test commonly used to detect the presence of steroids, particularly cholesterol, by observing a color change when a sample is mixed with acetic anhydride and concentrated sulfuric acid; a positive result typically shows a green color development, indicating the presence of a sterol compound like cholesterol. Add 2 ml of acetic anhydride and 1 ml of concentrated sulfuric acid to 2 ml of the plant extract. A blue or green coloration indicates the presence of steroids (Harborne 1998).
vii. **Phenols Test:** Phenols test typically refers to the Ferric Chloride Test, which is a chemical test used to identify the presence of phenol functional groups in an organic compound by adding a few drops of neutral ferric chloride solution to the sample, resulting in a color change like red, blue, green, or purple if phenols are present. A few drops of 5 percent ferric chloride solution are added to 2 ml of the plant extract. A deep blue or black coloration indicates the presence of phenols (Singleton, Orthofer, and Lamuela-Raventóset al. 1999).
viii. **Glycosides Test:** Glycosides test is a general term for any chemical test used to detect the presence of glycosides (molecules containing a sugar unit attached to another compound), while the "Keller-Kiliani test" is a specific chemical test used to identify the presence of cardiac glycosides, which are a type of glycoside characterized by the presence of deoxysugars like digitoxose; it is considered the

most reliable test for detecting cardiac glycosides within a plant extract. Add 2 ml of glacial acetic acid containing one drop of ferric chloride solution to 2 ml of the plant extract. Add 1 ml of concentrated sulfuric acid. A brown ring at the interface indicates the presence of glycosides (Evans 2002).

These different methods have been employed for the detection of the different phytochemicals from the different parts of the medicinal plants that are used in the treatment of various diseases. The specific phytochemicals present in the plants used in the treatment of certain human ailments have been studied from various literatures and mentioned here in tabular format. Various literature and ancient texts have been followed for this study of the ethnomedicinally significant plants. In addition, various parts of the plants which are used in the treatment of different diseases have been documented in this particular chapter.

Findings

Qualitative phytochemical analysis of medicinal plants in India involves identifying the presence of phytochemicals, which are compounds that give plants their color and fragrance. These phytochemicals are responsible for the plant's antimicrobial and antioxidant properties. Table 8.1 shows the qualitative study of different phytochemicals of twenty different plant samples. From this table, we can see the qualitative estimation of the various secondary metabolites present in them. Conversely, Table 8.2 shows the different exact phytochemicals present in the plants that are essential for the treatment of various diseases. Lastly, Table 8.3 points out the different parts of the plants which are used in the treatment of human ailments.

Discussions

Medicinal plants have been used since time immemorial for curing various diseases, and they still serve as the primary aid in mostly developing parts of the world (Hoareau and DaSilva 1999). These plants due to their multifaceted use have great importance in the traditional medical system (Tandon and Yadav 2017). Different phytochemicals have been studied in this research. Mostly, the secondary metabolites have been studied from the twenty different ethnomedicinally important plants available from India. The plant parts have been taken, and after making the extracts, they have been analyzed using different methods for the determination of the different secondary metabolites present in them.

Table 8.1 shows the different qualitative estimation of the various secondary metabolites present in the above-studied plants. It shows the presence or the absence of the various important secondary metabolites like alkaloids, phenolics, tannins, terpenoids, saponins, glycosides, and anthraquinones. Furthermore, Table 8.2 shows

Table 8.1. Qualitative Study of Different Phytochemicals of Twenty Different Plant Samples

Sl. No.	Plant Name	Alkaloids	Flavonoid	Tannins	Saponons	Terpenoids	Steroids	Phenols	Glycosides
1	*Adhatoda vasica Nees*	+	+	+	+	+	+	+	+
2	*Allium sativum* L.	–	+	+	+	+	+	+	–
3	*Aloe vera* (L.) Burm.f.	+	+	+	+	+	+	+	+
4	*Andrographis paniculata* (Burm.f.) Nees	+	+	+	+	+	+	+	+
5	*Azadirachta indica* A. Juss.	+	+	+	+	+	+	+	+
6	*Bacopa monnieri* (L.) Wettst.	+	+	+	+	+	–	+	–
7	*Camellia sinensis* L. (Kuntze)	+	+	+	+	+	+	+	+
8	*Catharanthus roseus* (L.) G. Don	+	+	+	+	+	–	+	–
9	*Centella asiatica* (L.) Urb.	+	+	–	+	+	–	+	–
10	*Curcuma longa* L.	–	+	+	+	+	+	+	+
11	*Mentha piperita* L.	+	+	+	+	+	–	+	+
12	*Mentha spicata* L.	+	+	+	+	+	–	+	+
13	*Moringa oleifera* Lam.	+	+	+	+	+	+	+	+
14	*Ocimum basilicum* L.	+	+	–	+	+	–	+	–
15	*Ocimum sanctum L.*	+	+	–	+	+	–	+	–
16	*Phyllanthus emblica* L.	+	+	+	+	+	+	+	+
17	*Piper nigrum* L.	+	+	+	+	+	+	+	+
18	*Tinospora cordifolia* (Willd.) Hook.f. & Thomson	+	+	–	–	+	+	+	+
19	*Withania somnifera* (L.) Dunal	+	+	+	+	+	+	+	+
20	*Zingiber officinale* Roscoe	+	+	+	+	+	–	+	+

Table 8.2. List of Studied Plant Taxa along with the Major Phytochemicals and Their Medicinal Uses

Plant Name	Major Phytochemicals	References
Adhatoda vasica Nees	It contains several biologically active phytochemical compounds. Some of the key compounds include alkaloids (vasicine, vasicol, vasicinone, peganine), phenolics, flavonoids, tannins, saponins, and phytosterols.	Singh, Singh, and Singh 2023
Allium sativum L.	Some of the key compounds include alliin, allicin, ajoene, vinyldithiin, diallyl sulfide, S-allyl-cysteine, and flavonoids such as quercetin.	Lidiková et al. 2022
Aloe vera (L.) Burm.f.	It contains over 200 bioactive chemical constituents. Some of the key phytochemical compounds include vitamins, enzymes, minerals, sugars, lignin, saponins, salicylic acids, amino acids, phenolic acids, flavonoids, tannins, and anthraquinones.	Nalimu et al. 2021
Andrographis paniculata (Burm.f.) Nees	It contains a variety of phytochemical compounds. Some of the key compounds include diterpenoids, flavonoids, polyphenols, alkaloids, tannins, saponins, and phlobatannin.	Intharuksa et al. 2022
Azadirachta indica A. Juss.	It contains a wide range of phytochemical compounds. Some of the key compounds include azadirachtin, nimbidin, nimbolide, olichinolide-B, azadiradione, desacetyl and deacetyl nimbin.	Bhagwat and Kadam 2020
Bacopa monnieri (L.) Wettst.	Some of the key compounds include bacosides A, B, and C, alkaloids (brahmine, nicotinine, herpestine), saponins, triterpenoid saponins, stigmastanol, β-sitosterol, betulinic acid, D-mannitol, stigmasterol, amino acids (α-alanine, aspartic acid, glutamic acid, serine), and pseudojujubogenin glycoside.	Jeyasri et al. 2022
Camellia sinensis L. (Kuntze)	Some of the key compounds include polyphenols (mainly catechins), flavonoids, alkaloids (caffeine), amino acids (theanine), and methylxanthines.	Roychoudhury and Chakraborty 2022
Catharanthus roseus (L.) G. Don	It contains a variety of phytochemical compounds. Some of the key compounds include alkaloids (vinblastine, vincristine), flavonoids, phenols, steroids, glycosides, tannins, and saponins.	Singh and Singh 2023a
Centella asiatica (L.) Urb.	Some of the key compounds include triterpenoids (asiaticoside, madecassoside), flavonoids, tannins, saponins, and phenolic acids.	Konwar et al. 2021
Curcuma longa L.	It includes compounds like curcuminoids (curcumin, desmethoxycurcumin, bisdemethoxycurcumin), volatile oils (tumerone, atlantone, zingiberone), sugars, proteins, and resins.	Rajesh and Reddy 2020

(Continued)

Table 8.2 (Continued)

Plant Name	Major Phytochemicals	References
Mentha piperita L.	Major phytochemicals include flavonoids, tannins, alkaloids, steroids, saponins, anthocyanins, and volatile oils (menthol, menthone).	Chakraborty, Ray Chakravarti, and Bhattacharjee 2022
Mentha spicata L.	Phenolic acids like rosmarinic acid, cryptochlorogenic acid, m-coumaric acid, chlorogenic acid), flavonoids, terpenes, quinines, and polysaccharides.	Li, Tian, and Li 2018
Moringa oleifera Lam.	Some of the key compounds include tannins, alkaloids, steroids, reducing sugars, phenols, glucosinolates, tocopherols, carotenoids, ascorbic acid, minerals, and polyunsaturated fatty acids.	Saini, Sivanesan, and Keum 2016
Ocimum basilicum L.	It includes alkaloids, phenolics, flavonoids, tannins, saponins, reducing sugars, cardiac glycosides, steroids, and glycosides.	Nadeem et al. 2021
Ocimum sanctum L.	Key compounds include eugenol, caryophyllene, luteolin, apigenin, rosmarinic acid, chlorogenic acid, caffeic acid, quercetin, and their derivatives.	Mahmoud, El-Gendy, and El-Khateeb 2020
Phyllanthus emblica L.	Some of the key compounds include polyphenols, tannins, ascorbic acid (vitamin C), gallic acid, ellagic acid, flavonoids, and alkaloids.	Prananda et al. 2023
Piper nigrum L.	Key compounds include alkaloids, phenolic compounds, flavonoids, carotenoids, terpenoids, tannins, and glycosides.	Ashokkumar et al. 2021
Tinospora cordifolia (Willd.) Hook.f. & Thomson	It includes alkaloids (berberine, jatrorrhizine, magnoflorine, tembetarine), diterpenoid lactones, furanolactone, tinosporine, and steroids.	Singh and Singh, 2023
Withania somnifera (L.) Dunal	It contains a variety of phytochemical compounds. Some of the key compounds include withanolides, sitoindosides, alkaloids (anaferine, anahygrine), flavonoids, tannins, saponins, phenolic compounds, and steroidal lactones.	Saleem, Ahmad, and Dar 2020
Zingiber officinale Roscoe	Some of the key compounds include gingerols, shogaols, paradols, zingerols, flavonoids, phenolic compounds, and essential oils (sesquiterpenes like zingiberene, bisabolene, zingiberol, sesquiphellandrene, and curcumene).	Mao et al. 2022

the different exact phytochemicals present in the plants like the presence of vasicine and vasicinol from *Adhatoda vasica* (L.) Nees and the presence of important allicin and alliin from *Allium sativum* L. Indole alkaloids like reserpine obtained from *Rauvolfia serpentina* L. are used in the treatment of various respiratory diseases (Sagi et al. 2016). Another indole alkaloid is vinblastine, and vincristine obtained from *Catharanthus*

Table 8.3. Ethnomedicinally Used Plants along with the Parts Used in Treatment of Human Diseases

Plant Species	Family Name	Parts Used	Medicinal Value	References
Adhatoda vasica Nees	Acanthaceae	Leaves, Roots	Used for respiratory issues, expectorant, and anti-inflammatory properties	Sharma 2020a
Allium sativum L.	Amaryllidaceae	Bulb	Antibacterial, antiviral, and cardiovascular benefits	Johnson 2020
Aloe vera (L.) Burm.f.	Asphodelaceae	Leaves	Used for skin conditions, burns, and digestive issues	Smith 2020
Andrographis paniculata (Burm.f.) Nees	Acanthaceae	Leaves, Stems	Used for immune support, anti-inflammatory, and hepatoprotective properties	Verma 2021
Azadirachta indica A. Juss.	Meliaceae	Leaves, Bark, Seeds	Antibacterial, antifungal, and anti-inflammatory properties	Kumar 2021
Bacopa monnieri (L.) Wettst.	Plantaginaceae	Whole plant	Cognitive enhancer, used for memory and brain health	Rao 2020
Camellia sinensis (L.) Kuntze	Theaceae	Leaves	Used for antioxidant, anti-inflammatory, and cognitive function	Patel 2021a
Catharanthus roseus (L.) G. Don	Apocynaceae	Leaves, Roots	Used for cancer treatment, antidiabetic, and antimicrobial properties	Rao 2019
Centella asiatica (L.) Urb.	Apiaceae	Leaves, Stems	Used for wound healing, cognitive enhancement, and skin health	Das 2019b
	Zingiberaceae	Rhizome	Anti-inflammatory, antioxidant, and antimicrobial properties	Brown 2019

Mentha piperita L.	Lamiaceae	Leaves	Used for digestive issues, antispasmodic, and antimicrobial properties	Green 2019
Moringa oleifera Lam.	Moringaceae	Leaves, Seeds, Pods	Nutrient-rich, used for immune support and anti-inflammatory purposes	Patel 2021b
Mentha spicata L.	Lamiaceae	Leaves	Used for digestive issues, antispasmodic, and antimicrobial properties	Das 2019a
	Lamiaceae	Leaves, Seeds	Used for digestive health, anti-inflammatory, and antimicrobial properties	White 2020
Ocimum sanctum L.	Lamiaceae	Leaves, Seeds	Adaptogen, used for stress relief and immune support	White 2018
Phyllanthus emblica L.	Phyllanthaceae	Fruit	Rich in vitamin C, used for immune support and digestive health	Patel 2019
Piper nigrum L.	Piperaceae	Fruit	Used for digestive health, anti-inflammatory, and antioxidant properties	Verma 2020
Tinospora cordifolia (Willd.) Hook.f. & Thomson	Menispermaceae	Stem, Leaves	Immunomodulatory, antipyretic, and anti-inflammatory properties	Sharma 2020b
Withania somnifera (L.) Dunal	Solanaceae	Roots	Used for stress relief, energy boost, and immune support	Pushpakaran2023
Zingiber officinale Roscoe	Zingiberaceae	Rhizome	Used for nausea, digestive issues, and anti-inflammatory purposes	Green 2021

roseus L. is also used in the treatment of lung diseases (Mohammadgholi, Rabbani-Chadegani, and Fallah 2013). Different types of saponins and terpenoids have been studied from various literatures and are also mentioned in this research.

In addition, Table 8.3 shows the different ethnomedicinal plants and their parts used for the treatment of various human diseases. Different parts like the leaves, stem, root, and rhizomes are used in the treatment of various diseases like diabetes and hypertension. These plant parts also have immunomodulatory effects, anticancer activity, and anti-inflammatory properties, which are mentioned in Table 8.3. This knowledge about the medicines and plant resources is very significant. As a result, various steps have been taken for the proper documentation of these plants. These medicinal plants have great potential for the treatment of various human ailments (Mukherjee et al. 2014). This research provides a comprehensive study about the most important twenty different ethnomedicinally important plant species along with their uses for the treatment of various human diseases and also the important phytochemicals present in them. These important phytochemicals are mostly the secondary metabolites which are useful to human society for the treatment of various diseases.

Conclusion

This study has documented different traditionally used plants in a proper way. Particularly, twenty different ethnomedicinally important plants of our country have been considered in this study. These plants are commonly used by traditional healers and other practitioners in India. The uses of these plants for the treatment of various human ailments are recognized in various ancient literatures. Plants are used for the treatment of human diseases owing to the variety of different phytochemicals present in them. These phytochemicals are mostly secondary metabolites which are used in the treatment of various ailments. With modern techniques like HPLC (High Pressure Liquid Chromatography), NMR (Nuclear Magnetic Resonance), and GC-MS (Gas Chromatography-Mass Spectrometry), the extraction of specific phytochemicals from these plants has been possible.

In this study, the specific phytochemicals of twenty medicinal plants have been documented by reviewing various literatures. Thus, this documentation of twenty medicinal plants provides the specific phytochemicals present in them. It also highlights the details of the plants and their parts used for the treatment of human diseases. In addition, it is renowned that different phytochemicals present in the studied twenty medicinal plants serve as a treasure trove in medicinal efficacy. Moreover, this study contributes a contemporary aspect about linking the traditional practices of medicine and the modern scientific methods by identifying the specific phytochemicals in the studied plants for the betterment of human society.

Yet again, this study helps in linking both the traditional medical sciences in India and the modern scientific advances for the better protection of the plants, proper bioprospecting, and proper new drug discovery from the ethnomedicinally important plant species. Therefore, the phytochemical analysis of ethnomedicinally important plants acts as a crucial foundation for new pharmacological research, as it helps identify the active chemical compounds within the plant, providing key insights into potential therapeutic mechanisms and allowing researchers to target specific bioactive molecules for further investigation and drug development. Consequently, this phytochemical analysis of twenty ethnomedicinally important plant species provides the important accessories for a better understanding of new pharmacological research and also helps to maintain a connection between nature and human society in an interwoven way.

References

Ashokkumar, K., M. Murugan, M. K. Dhanya, A. Pandian, and T. D. Warkentin. "Phytochemistry and Therapeutic Potential of Black Pepper [Piper nigrum (L.)] Essential Oil and Piperine: A Review." *Clinical Phytoscience* 7, no. 52 (2021): 1–11.

Basu, R., S. Dasgupta, S. N. Babu, and A. Noor. "Medicinal Plants in the Indian Traditional Medicine and Current Practices." In *Bioprospecting of Tropical Medicinal Plants*, edited by A. Karuppusamy, S. P. Sasidharan, and X. Yang, 235–86. Springer Nature: Switzerland, 2023.

Bhagwat, V. C., and V. B. Kadam. "Studies on Phytochemical Constituents of *Azadirachta indica* A. Juss. and Melia azedarach Linn." *Plant Archives* 20, no. 1 (2020): 2505–8.

Bohm, B. A., and M. R. Koupai-Abyazani. "Flavonoids and Condensed Tannins from Leaves of Hawaiian *Vaccinium reticulatum* and *V. calycinum* (Ericaceae)." *Pacific Science* 48, no. 4 (1994): 458–63.

Borins, M. "Traditional Medicine in India." *Canadian Family Physician* 33, no. 1061 (1987): 1063–5.

Brown, A. "The Medicinal Properties of Turmeric." *Herbal Medicine Journal* 10, no. 4 (2019): 45–52.

Chakraborty, K., A. Ray Chakravarti, and S. Bhattacharjee. "Bioactive Components of Peppermint (*Mentha piperita* L.), Their Pharmacological and Ameliorative Potential and Ethnomedicinal Benefits: A Review." *Journal of Pharmacognosy and Phytochemistry* 11, no. 1 (2022): 109–14.

Chinou, I. "Primary and Secondary Metabolites and Their Biological Activity." In *TLC in Phytochemistry*, vol. 99, edited by M. Waksmundzka-Hajnos, J. Sherma, and T. Kowalska, 59–76. Boca Raton: CRC Press, 2008.

Das, R. "Spearmint: Benefits and Uses." *Journal of Medicinal Plants* 12, no. 2 (2019a): 78–85.

Das, S. "Gotu Kola: A Review of Its Medicinal Properties." *Journal of Medicinal Plants* 12, no. 2 (2019b): 78–85.

De Laurentiis, M., G. Cancello, D. D'Agostino, M. Giuliano, A. Giordano, E. Montagna, and S. De Placido. "Taxane-based Combinations as Adjuvant Chemotherapy of Early Breast Cancer: A Meta-analysis of Randomized Trials." *Journal of Clinical Oncology* 26, no. 1 (2008): 44–53.

Dua Pradeep, D. P., and D. P. Dua Pamila. "Research in Ayurveda: Challenges and Way Forward." *International Journal of Research in Ayurveda and Pharmacy* 3, no. 1 (2012): 23–6.

Edeoga, H. O., D. E. Okwu, and B. O. Mbaebie. "Phytochemical Constituents of Some Nigerian Medicinal Plants." *African Journal of Biotechnology* 4, no. 7 (2005): 685–8.

Evans, W. C. *Trease and Evans Pharmacognosy*. London: Saunders Publishers, 2002.

Ganjhu, R. K., P. P. Mudgal, H. Maity, D. Dowarha, S. Devadiga, S. Nag, and G. Arunkumar. "Herbal Plants and Plant Preparations as Remedial Approach for Viral Diseases." *Virus Disease* 26, no. 4 (2015): 225–36.

Green, B. "Ginger: A Natural Remedy." *Journal of Herbal Medicine* 12, no. 3 (2021): 78–85.

Green, C. "Peppermint: Benefits and Uses." *Journal of Medicinal Plants* 11, no. 2 (2019): 67–74.

Haralampidis, K., M. Trojanowska, and A. E. Osbourn. "Biosynthesis of Triterpenoid Saponins in Plants." *Advances in Biochemical Engineering Biotechnology* 75 (2002): 31–49.

Harborne, J. B. "Phytochemical Methods: A Guide to Modern Techniques of Plant Analysis." 3rd ed., Chapman and Hall, 1998.

Hoareau, L., and E. J. DaSilva. "Medicinal Plants: A Re-emerging Health Aid." *Electronic Journal of Biotechnology* 2, no. 2 (1999): 3–4.

Hussein, R. A., and A. A. El-Anssary. "Plants Secondary Metabolites: The Key Drivers of the Pharmacological Actions of Medicinal Plants." *Herbal Medicine* 1, no. 3 (2019): 11–30.

Intharuksa, A., W. Arunotayanun, W. Yooin, and P. Sirisa-ard. "A Comprehensive Review of *Andrographis paniculata* (Burm. f.) Nees and Its Constituents as Potential Lead Compounds for COVID-19 Drug Discovery." *Molecules* 27, no. 14 (2022): 4479.

Jeyasri, R., P. Muthuramalingam, V. Suba, M. Ramesh, and J. T. Chen. "*Bacopa monnieri* and their Bioactive Compounds Inferred Multi-Target Treatment Strategy for Neurological Diseases: A Cheminformatics and System Pharmacology Approach." *Biomolecules* 10, no. 4 (2022): 536.

Johnson, M. "Garlic: A Natural Antibiotic." *Journal of Herbal Medicine* 15, no. 3 (2020): 123–30.

Jones, M. E. "Albrecht Kossel, a Biographical Sketch." *The Yale Journal of Biology and Medicine* 26, no. 1 (1953): 80.

Konwar, M., M. P. Sarma, D. P. Parasar, D. Saikia, and P. Bhagawati. "Phytochemical Analysis of Leaves of *Centella Asiatica* (L)." *Research Journal of Agricultural Sciences, An International Journal Journal* 10, no. 3 (2021): 1–8.

Kumar, N., and M. Ashaq. "Study of Ethnomedicinal Plants of Tehsil Akhnoor, Jammu and Kashmir." *International Journal of Research and Analytical Reviews* 8 (2021): 67–78.

Kumar, R. "Neem: A Versatile Medicinal Plant." *Journal of Herbal Medicine* 13, no. 1 (2021): 55–62.

Lepcha, T. T., P. Pradhan, K. S. Gaira, H. K. Badola, M. Shahid, and M. Singh. "Ethnomedicinal Use of Plants by Bhutia Tribe in Sikkim Himalaya." *Proceedings of the Ist Himalayan Researchers Consortium* 1 (2019): 71–78.

Li, X., T. Tian, and X. Li. "Phytochemical Characterization of *Mentha spicata* L. Under Differential Dried-Conditions and Associated Nephrotoxicity Screening of Main Compound with Organ-on-a-Chip." *Frontiers in Pharmacology* 9 (2018): 1067.

Lidiková, J., N. Čeryová, T. Tóth, J. Musilová, A. Vollmannová, K. Mammadova, and E. Ivanišová. "Garlic (Allium sativum L.): Characterization of Bioactive Compounds and Related Health Benefits." In *Herbs and Spices – New Advances,* edited by E. Ivanišová. IntechOpen, London, 2022.

Lipp, F. J. "The Efficacy, History, and Politics of Medicinal Plants." *Alternative Therapies in Health and Medicine* 2 (1996): 36–41.

Mahmoud, Y. I., A. M. El-Gendy, and S. A. El-Khateeb. "Phytochemical and Antioxidant Profiling of Ocimum Sanctum." *Journal of Food Science and Technology* 57, no. 5 (2020): 1723–32.

Manandhar, N. P. "A Survey of Medicinal Plants of Jajarkot District, Nepal." *Journal of Ethnopharmacology* 48, no. 1 (1995): 1–6.

Mandal, A., S. More, M. Biswas, S. N. Mondal, S. Ray, and S. Ghosh. "Study on Secondary Metabolites of Some Ethnomedicinally Important Plants of Murshidabad District, West Bengal, India." *Journal of Plant Science Research* 39, no. 2 (2023): 31–8.

Mao, Q. Q., X. Y. Xu, S. Y. Cao, R. Y. Gan, H. Corke, and H. B. Li. "Bioactive Compounds and Bioactivities of Ginger (*Zingiber officinale* Roscoe)." *Foods* 8, no. 6 (2022): 185.

McGaw, L., A. Jäger, O. Grace, C. Fennel, and J. van Staden. "Medicinal Plants." In *Ethics in Agriculture — An African Perspective*, edited by A. Van Niekerk, 67–83. Dordrecht: Springer, 2005.

Mohammadgholi, A., A. Rabbani-Chadegani, and S. Fallah. "Mechanism of the Interaction of Plant Alkaloid Vincristine with DNA and Chromatin: Spectroscopic Study." *DNA and Cell Biology* 32, no. 5 (2013): 228–35.

Mukherjee, P. K., S. Bahadur, R. K. Harwansh, and S. K. Chaudhary. "Shifting Paradigm for Validation of Medicinal Plants in Indian Traditional Medicine." *Indian Drugs* 51 (2014): 5–14.

Mukherjee, P. K., P. Venkatesh, and S. Ponnusankar. "Ethnopharmacology and Integrative Medicine - Let the History Tell the Future." *Journal of Ayurveda and Integrative Medicine* 1, no. 2 (2010): 100–9.

Nadeem, H. R., S. Akhtar, P. Sestili, T. Ismail, S. Neugart, and T. Esatbeyoglu. "Toxicity, Antioxidant Activity, and Phytochemicals of Basil (*Ocimum basilicum* L.) Leaves Cultivated in Southern Punjab, Pakistan." *Foods* 11, no. 9 (2021): 1239.

Nalimu, F., J. Oloro, I. Kahwa, and P. E. Ogwang. "Review on the Phytochemistry and Toxicological Profiles of *Aloe vera* and *Aloe ferox*." *Future Journal of Pharmaceutical Sciences* 7, no. 1 (2021): 145.

Nandagoapalan, V., A. Doss, and C. Marimuthu. "Phytochemical Analysis of Some Traditional Medicinal Plants." *Bioscience Discovery* 7, no. 1 (2016): 17–20.

Osbourn, A. E. "Saponins in Cereals." *Phytochemistry* 62, no. 1 (2003): 1–4.

Padmaja, M., M. Sravanthi, and K. P. J. Hemalatha. "Evaluation of Antioxidant Activity of Two Indian Medicinal Plants." *Journal of Phytology* 3, no. 3 (2011).

Pagare, S., M. Bhatia, N. Tripathi, S. Pagare, and Y. K. Bansal. "Secondary Metabolites of Plants and Their Role: Overview." *Current Trends in Biotechnology and Pharmacy* 9, no. 3 (2015): 293–304.

Patel, M. "Moringa: The Miracle Tree." *Journal of Herbal Medicine* 14, no. 3 (2021a): 33–40.

Patel, S. "Amla: A Powerhouse of Nutrients." *Journal of Medicinal Plants* 11, no. 3 (2019): 67–74.

Patel, T. "Green Tea: Health Benefits." *Journal of Herbal Medicine* 14, no. 3 (2021b): 33–40.

Prananda, A. T., A. Dalimunthe, U. Harahap, Y. Simanjuntak, E. Peronika, N. E. Karosekali, P. A. Z. Hasibuan, R. A. Syahputra, and P. C. Situmorang. "*Phyllanthus emblica*: A Comprehensive Review of Its Phytochemical Composition and Pharmacological Properties." *Frontiers in Pharmacology* 14 (2023): 1–20.

Pushpakaran, Arun M. K. "Health Benefits of Ashwagandha (Withania somnifera): A Comprehensive Review of Its Therapeutic Potential." *The Pharma Innovation Journal* 12, no. 7 (2023): 645–52.

Pushpangadan, P., V. George, T. Ijinu, and M. A. Chithra. "Ethnomedicine, Health Food and Nutraceuticals-traditional Wisdom of Maternal and Child Health in India." *Edelweiss Applied Science and Technology* 2, no. 1 (2018): 113–17.

Rajendran, T. P. "Biological Resource Base for Traditional Medicines." *Health, Nature and Quality of Life* 41 (2016): 46–68.

Rajesh, M., and P. Reddy. "Review on *Curcuma longa*: Ethnomedicinal Uses, Pharmacological Properties, and Phytochemistry." *Research Journal of Pharmacy and Technology* 13, no. 8 (2020): 3753–60.

Rao, N. "Brahmi: Enhancing Cognitive Function." *Journal of Ayurveda* 10, no. 1 (2020): 45–52.

Rao, S. "Periwinkle: A Medicinal Plant with Diverse Uses." *Journal of Medicinal Plants* 12, no. 1 (2019): 78–85.

Rates, S. M. K. "Plants as Source of Drugs." *Toxicon* 39, no. 5 (2001): 603–13.

Roychoudhury, S., and S. Chakraborty. "Phytochemical Composition and Biological Activities of *Camellia sinensis* (L.) Kuntze." *Journal of Agricultural and Food Chemistry* 70, no. 5 (2022): 1234–45.

Rungsung, W., K. K. Ratha, S. Dutta, A. K. Dixit, and J. Hazra. "Secondary Metabolites of Plants in Drugs Discovery." *World Journal of Pharmaceutical Research* 4, no. 7 (2015): 604–13.

Sagi, S., B. Avula, Y. H. Wang, and I. A. Khan. "Quantification and Characterization of Alkaloids from Roots of *Rauwolfia serpentina* Using Ultra-high Performance Liquid Chromatography-photo Diode Array-mass Spectrometry." *Analytical and Bioanalytical Chemistry* 408 (2016): 177–90.

Saini, R. K., I. Sivanesan, and Y. S. Keum. "Phytochemicals of *Moringa oleifera*: A Review of Their Nutritional, Therapeutic and Industrial Significance." *3 Biotech* 6, no. 3 (2016): 203.

Saleem, M., A. Ahmad, and B. A. Dar. "An Updated Review on Phytochemistry and Molecular Targets of *Withania somnifera* (L.) Dunal." *Frontiers in Pharmacology* 11 (2020): 1049332.

Santhi, R. "Phytochemical Screening of Nerium Oleander Leaves." *International Research Journal of Pharmacy* 2, no. 1 (2011): 131–5.

Sharma, A. "Gene Expression Analysis in Medicinal Plants under Abiotic Stress Conditions." In *Plant Metabolites and Regulation under Environmental Stress*, edited by P. Ahmad, M. A. Ahanger, V. P. Singh, D. K. Tripathi, P. Alam, and M. N. Alyemeni, 407–14. London: Academic Press, 2018.

Sharma, K. "Vasaka: A Traditional Remedy for Respiratory Health." *Journal of Ayurveda* 10, no. 2 (2020a): 45–52.

Sharma, P. "Giloy: The Wonder Herb." *Journal of Ayurveda* 9, no. 2 (2020b): 88–95.

Sheng-Ji, P. "Ethnobotanical Approaches of Traditional Medicine Studies: Some Experiences from Asia." *Pharmaceutical Biology* 39, no. 1 (2001): 74–9.

Shrestha, P. M., and S. S. Dhillion. "Medicinal Plant Diversity and Use in the Highlands of Dolakha District, Nepal." *Journal of Ethnopharmacology* 86, no. 1 (2003): 81–96.

Singh, H. B., and S. K. Singh. "Phytochemistry and Pharmacology of *Tinospora cordifolia*: A Review." *Journal of Ethnopharmacology* 30, no. 2 (2023a): 123–35.

Singh, S. K., and H. B. Singh. "Phytochemistry and Pharmacology of *Catharanthus roseus* (L.) G. Don and *Rauvolfia serpentina* (L.) Benth. ex Kurz." In *Bioprospecting of Tropical Medicinal Plants*, edited by K. Arunachalam, X. Yang, and S. P. Sasidharan. Switzerland AG: Springer Nature, 2023b.

Singh, T., O. M. Singh, and H. B. Singh. "*Adhatoda vasica* Nees: Phytochemical and Pharmacological Profile." *International Journal of Research in Pharmaceutical Sciences* 12, no. 3 (2023): 123–35.

Singleton, V. L., R. Orthofer, and R. M. Lamuela-Raventós. "Analysis of Total Phenols and Other Oxidation Substrates and Antioxidants by Means of Folin-Ciocalteu Reagent." *Methods in Enzymology* 299 (1999): 152–78.

Smith, J. "Aloe Vera: A Comprehensive Review." *Journal of Medicinal Plants* 15, no. 2 (2020): 123–30.

Smith-Hall, C., H. O. Larsen, and M. Pouliot. "People, Plants and Health: A Conceptual Framework for Assessing Changes in Medicinal Plant Consumption." *Journal of Ethnobiology and Ethnomedicine* 8 (2012): 1–11.

Sofowora, A. "Research on Medicinal Plants and Traditional Medicine in Africa." *The Journal of Alternative and Complementary Medicine* 2, no. 3 (1996): 365–72.

Tandon, N., and S. S. Yadav. "Contributions of Indian Council of Medical Research (ICMR) in the Area of Medicinal Plants/Traditional Medicine." *Journal of Ethnopharmacology* 197 (2017): 39–45.

Verma, R. "Black Pepper: A Spice with Medicinal Benefits." *Journal of Ayurveda* 9, no. 3 (2020): 88–95.

Verma, S. "Kalmegh: A Potent Medicinal Herb." *Journal of Herbal Medicine* 13, no. 1 (2021): 55–62.

White, C. "Holy Basil: Benefits and Uses." *International Journal of Ayurveda* 8, no. 1 (2018): 33–40.

White, D. "Basil: A Culinary and Medicinal Herb." *Journal of Ayurveda* 9, no. 1 (2020): 88–95.

Yadav, R. N. S., and M. Agarwala. "Phytochemical Analysis of Some Medicinal Plants." *Journal of Phytology* 3, no. 12 (2011): 10–14.

An Exploration into the Phytochemical Enrichment of *Lawsonia inermis* L. and Its Medicinal Implications

Debapriya Das,[1] Debleena Roy,[1] and Dipu Samanta[2*]

[1]PG Department of Botany, Lady Brabourne College, Kolkata, West Bengal, India

[2]Department of Botany, Dr. Kanailal Bhattacharyya College, Howrah, West Bengal, India

*Corresponding Author's Email: Dipusamanta2010@gmail.com[2]

Introduction

Humans have been directly and indirectly dependent on plants for food, raw materials, medicines, and much more for a very long time. With the advancement of science, the exploration of the intricate workings of plants, optimizing and manipulating the plant's resources for societal benefit becomes very necessary (Chaachouay and Zidane 2024). With each passing day, more and more plants are coming into the light for their beneficial role in the medicinal and commercial sector (Fayiah et al. 2024). For plants to be useful in the industrial front, the secondary metabolite pool of the plants must be utilized and manipulated properly (Marchev, Zhenya, and Milen 2020). "Secondary metabolites" refer to organic compounds produced by plants, not directly involved in the normal growth and development of the plant but helping the plant adapt to various biotic and abiotic stresses by mediating ecological interactions, playing to the advantage of the organism by increasing its probability forof survival (Barberis et al. 2020). Humans use plants and their secondary metabolites as sources of medicines, flavoring agents, pigments, and food (Kaushik et al. 2021). One such plant is *Lawsonia inermis*. *L. inermis* or *Mehendi* has established its role as a commercially important plant and is the only source of dye, mehendi, and is also used to make perfumes and cosmetics. Apart from the commercial sector, the plant extends its dominance in the medicinal field (Das et al. 2023). There has been mention of *L. inermis* in the Ayurvedic texts containing important medicinal properties like antioxidant, anticarcinogenic, antidiabetic, antimicrobial, wound healing, antiproliferative properties, and many more (Adiga, Gandhi, and Prakash 2022).

Previous research on *L. inermis* mainly pertains to the phytochemical profiling and its medicinal importance, which makes it important to the medicinal industries and commercial industries. Some of the important secondary metabolites include lawsone, chlorogenic acid, caffeic acid, apigenin, rutin, kaempferol, and various other polyphenols and flavonoids (Moutawalli et al. 2024). Not much research, however, has been conducted in the area of optimal manipulation of the plant's resources by enhancing the secondary metabolite content of the plant (*L. inermis* L.). This can be successfully achieved in various ways, but one such efficient and economic method is elicitation. In this process, this study has tried to enhance the phytochemicals by subjecting it to various stress factors (biotic and abiotic) through a fixed period of time (Halder, Sarkar, and Jha 2019). This study has also tried to discuss and explore the secondary metabolites present in the plant and the pathways from which they are derived, along with possible ways for augmenting the phytochemicals of the plant, paving the way for future research. Thus, this research study can also benefit human society in innumerable ways (Youl et al. 2024).

Medicinal Attributes of *Lawsonia inermis* L.

L. inermis is renowned for being the only source of the dye locally called *mehendi*. In other words, *Lawsonia inermis*, also known as *henna*, has many medicinal attributes, including antioxidant, antibacterial, and anti-inflammatory properties. This *henna* contains substances that might help fight certain infections. There is also some information that henna might decrease the growth of tumors, prevent or reduce spasms, decrease inflammation, and relieve pain. The Ayurvedic texts mention this plant as an important remedy in curing many diseases like cancer, microbial infections, and arthritis (Adiga, Gandhi, and Prakash 2022). Ayurveda values *henna* for its cooling, anti-inflammatory, and antimicrobial properties. It is often used to reduce *pitta* imbalances such as skin irritation, inflammation, or excessive body heat. The *henna*'s ability to pacify the body makes it ideal during warm seasons or when the mind and body are overheated.

Hence, it becomes necessary to discuss the various medicinal properties of the *L. inermis* plant and the compounds that are responsible for imparting the plant its medicinal characteristics. Morphologically, the plant is a small tree or shrub. This *L. inermis* is cultivated for roots, flowers, stem bark, and seeds for their medicinal uses. Proteins, carbohydrates, and fatty acids are primary metabolites along with secondary metabolites such as tannins, quinones, terpenoids, and coumarins which are present in the *L. inermis* plant. The phytochemical constituents of *L. inermis* are responsible for its analgesic, anti-inflammatory, hepatoprotective, and hypoglycemic properties. Thus, this plant has also been reported for antibacterial, antifungal, immunostimulatory, antioxidant, and cytotoxic activity. The presence of these properties in the *L. inermis* plant develops it as medicine against various pathogenic organisms and diseases. Table 9.1 highlights the various medicinal properties of the plant parts and the types of phytochemicals responsible for the same.

Table 9.1. Medicinal Properties of *L. inermis* L. Respecting Nature of Phytochemicals

Sl. No.	Medicinal Property	Plant Part	Phytochemical Responsible for the Medicinal Attribute
1.	Anticarcinogenic	Leaf, Stem	Phenols
2.	Antifungal	Leaf	Flavonoids, Glycosides, Naphthoquinone
3.	Antibacterial	Leaf	Alkaloids, Steroids, Naphthoquinones, Flavonoids, Terpenoids, Saponins
4.	Antiulcer	Leaf	Glycosides, Alkaloids, Naphthoquinones, Terpenoids, Tannins, Phenolic Compounds
5.	Analgesic	Leaf	Tannins, Flavonoids
6.	Anti-arthritic	Leaf	Phenols
7.	Antidiabetic	Leaf	Phenols, Flavonoids
8.	Anti-dengue	Leaf	Flavonoids And Phenols
9.	Hepatoprotective	Leaf	Coumarins, Monoterpenoids, Essential Oils, Diterpenoids, Steroids, Alkaloids, Polyphenols
10.	Immunostimulatory	Leaf	Essential Oils, Terpenoids, Steroids, Phenols

Source: Pradhan et al. 2012.

Pathway Analysis of *Lawsonia inermis*

The *Lawsonia inermis*, commonly known as *henna*, belongs to the family of Lythraceae. This *L. inermis* plant includes many phytochemicals that contribute to its healing properties and commercial importance. Thus, the *henna* plant (Lawsonia inermis) contains many phytochemicals, including flavonoids, tannins, and polyphenols. Some of the phytochemical constituents that can be derived from this plant are flavonoids, tannins, and naphthoquinone derivatives. In detail, this *Lawsonia inermis* contains a variety of bioactive compounds like flavonoids, coumarins, triterpenoids, steroids, xanthones, polyphenols, fatty acids, alkaloids, quinones, tannins, leucocyanidin, epicatechin, catechin, and quercetin. Specifically, the ethanol extract of leaves of *L. inermis* (AL-Fetaehab sample) shows D-allose (17.61 percent), lawsone (12.87 percent), beta-D-glucopyranoside, methyl (12.74 percent), phytol (10.78 percent), 1-isobutoxy-1-methoxypropane (9.18 percent), as well as n-hexadecanoic acid.

The *henna* plant (Lawsonia inermis) is used in the cosmetics, cloth, and wood protection industries due to its antimicrobial, antioxidant, and UV protective properties. Among different phytochemicals of *L. inermis*, flavonoids are found in the leaves, including flavonols, flavones, and isoflavones; tannins are found in the leaves, including condensed and hydrolysable tannins; polyphenols are found in all parts of the plant, including epicatechin, catechin, and quercetin; steroids are found in the leaves including oleanane, ursane, and lupine types; triterpenoids are found in the leaves; alkaloids are found in the leaves; saponins are found in the leaves, particularly in ethanol extracts; glycosides are found in the leaves, particularly in ethyl acetate and n-hexane extracts; coumarins are found in the plant; xanthones are found in the plant and quinones are found in the plant.

Table 9.2 explores in detail the main phytochemicals and their corresponding pathways from which they are derived. From Table 9.2, it is very clear that the plant is rich in phenylpropanoid and shikimic acid pathways. The main phytochemical

Table 9.2. Main Phytochemicals and Their Associative Pathways

Sl. No.	Phytochemicals	Pathway
1.	Lawsone	Naphthoquinone pathway (derivative of the shikimic acid pathway)
2.	Flavonoids	Derived from the phenylpropanoid pathway, which is involved in the biosynthesis of flavonoids.
3.	Tannins	Phenylpropanoid pathway (Formed from the polymerization of flavonoids and other phenolic compounds.)
4.	Essential oils	Terpene biosynthetic pathway
5.	Alkaloids	Generally synthesized from amino acids through various biosynthetic routes.
6.	Saponins	Terpenoid biosynthetic pathway.
7.	Phenolic Acids	Phenylpropanoid pathway

Source: Gull et al. 2013.

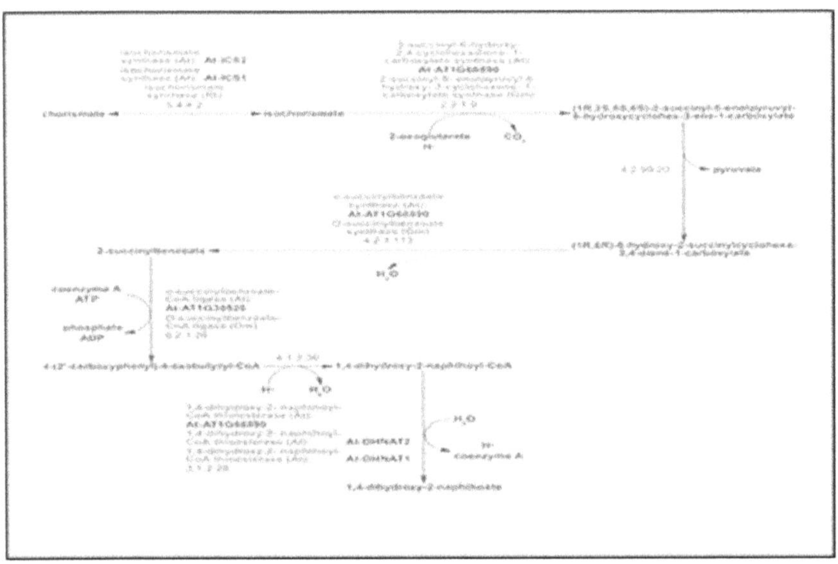

Figure 9.1. Lawsone Biosynthesis Pathway found in the Plant Metabolic Network (PMN) Database. Source: Author.

lawsone is responsible for the dyeing properties of the plant and is also derived from the naphthoquinone pathway which is formed through the shikimic acid pathway (Widhalm and Rhodes 2016). In addition, Figure 9.1 represents a naphthoquinone pathway from the PMN database which has its precursor from the shikimic acid pathway considered as the epicenter in producing aromatic compounds from which the naphthoquinones are derived. The pathway leading to lawsone involves a number of modifications (hydroxylation and oxidation) of the precursors derived from the shikimic acid pathway. Hence, it can be correlated that augmentation of the shikimic acid pathway can increase the phytochemical pool of the plant and can also increase its medicinal and commercial properties.

Elicitation: Effective in Augmentation of Plant Phytochemicals

The elicitation of phytochemicals is a process where various techniques are used to enhance their production in plants, in a rapid and cost-effective manner. This can be done through various ways, including chemical, abiotic, and biotic factors. Understanding the mechanism of elicitation of phytochemicals and the role of stimuli that initiate it is necessary for various fields of study, including agriculture, food science, and pharmacology (Piechowiak 2024). This process helps to generate plants with a greater accumulation of secondary metabolites, which can in turn increase the economic value of the plant. With the growing scientific techniques and development in biotechnology, including the variety of tissue culture techniques, the process of elicitation has become very easy and less cumbersome (Ramirez-Estrada et al. 2016). This introduction sets the tone for discussing the various elicitors present and their action mechanism.

(i) **Mechanism of Action of Elicitors:** Any substance that stimulates a specific response in an organism related to defense mechanisms and physiological processes is termed an elicitor. In broader contexts, elicitors can refer to an agent that provokes a response in an organism (Thakur and Sohal 2013; Thakur et al. 2024). In plants, elicitors can be pathogens, chemicals, or even physical agents that can trigger the production of defense compounds, enhancing the plant's adaptability to the stimuli. They play a crucial role in regulating the plant's metabolism and involve the production of organic compounds. Again, they are not directly involved in growth or reproduction but serve in helping the plant perform certain ecological functions like defense and adaptation (see Figure 9.2).

(ii) **Elicitor Categorization and their Effects:** It is very important to select the correct elicitor for the proper augmentation of plant secondary metabolites. The elicitor used and its concentration can vary from one plant to another. The duration through which the elicitor is applied is also a key regulatory factor for the proper functioning of plants. Prolonged application of elicitor in excess concentration can lead to toxicities in the plant and can kill the plant eventually (Malik, Ilakiya, and Kalaivani 2020). Taking into consideration the variety, elicitors can be classified into biotic and abiotic elicitors (see Figure 9.3).

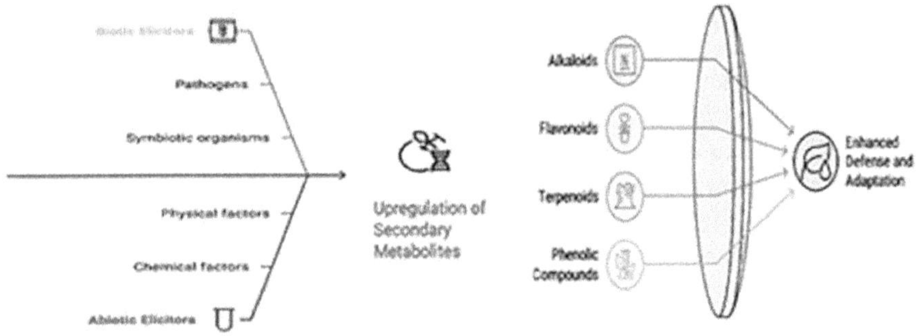

Figure 9.2. Mechanism of action of elicitors. Source: Author.

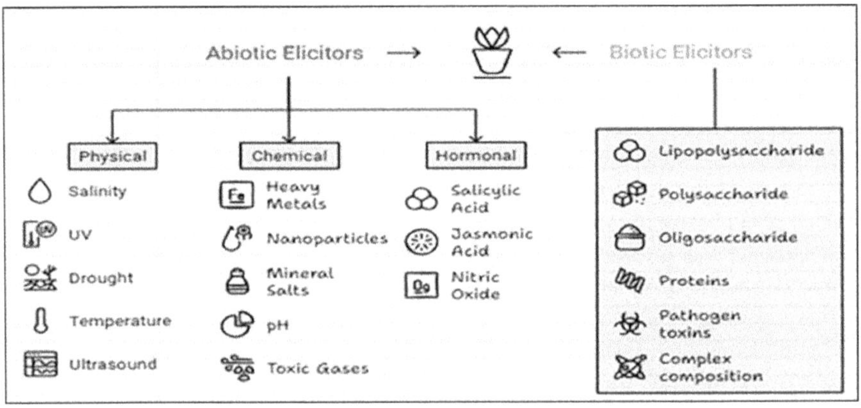

Figure 9.3. A pictorial presentation of elicitor classification. Source: Author.

As the name suggests, any substances of non-biological origin which can elicit a plant's defenses and production of secondary metabolites are referred to as abiotic elicitors. They can be physical in nature like drought, salinity, temperature, radiation which can induce a stress response in the plant, leading to an enhanced production of plant secondary metabolites (Petrova, Kamelia, and Maria 2024). The plant *Salvia virgata* when exposed to salinity (NaCl) stress, zinc oxide nanoparticles (ZnONP), salicylic acid (SA), and their combination showed an enhanced production of plant secondary metabolites. Salinity stress reduced the levels of chlorophyll a, chlorophyll b, and carotenoid pigments, and increased the content of all three pigments, in plants treated with the combination of SA, ZnONP, and the SA + ZnONP. Salt stress has also shown to elevate the levels of phenolics, flavonoids, and proline (Bozaba and Kuru 2024). Similarly, the effect of various combinations of salinity levels on the traits of *Alcea rosea* (hollyhock) varieties has shown that salt stress can lead to an increase in total phenolic content and total flavonoid content, while it decreased these levels in certain varieties. The Saman variety has exhibited the highest secondary metabolites under severe salt stress indicating that it is the most salt-tolerant variety among those studied (Sadeghi et al. 2024).

Certain chemicals can also act as elicitors like nanoparticles, heavy metals, and minerals signaling the plant to use secondary metabolites to enhance its adaptability. Researchers have become intrigued by nanomaterials because their small size allows for easier penetration and manipulation of cellular metabolism leading to increased production of phytochemicals. The effects of selenium nanoparticles on tomato plants grown in cadmium-contaminated soil when examined have shown a positive effect on plant growth. After the addition of the selenium nanoparticles, an enhanced level of ascorbic acid, phenolic compounds, flavonoids, and proline is seen, while also boosting the activities of stress-related enzymes (Ahmad et al. 2024). The impact of foliar application of Zn–Al and Mg–Al LDH nanoparticles (10 ppm) on Geranium plants has shown an enhanced dry biomass and increase in the uptake of Zn and Mg. The secondary metabolic pathways are also enriched in treated plants resulting in more levels of tocopherols and polyphenolics (Hashem et al. 2024).

When phytohormones and their chemical derivatives are applied in regulated amounts for a certain time frame, an induction of stress conditions can lead to an enhanced production of phytochemicals. Plants tend to modify their metabolism in response to the intensity of environmental signals. The plant *Hypericum perforatum* treated with chitosan, selenium, salicylic acid, and a mixture of these compounds has shown changes in the levels of phytochemicals. Selenium and salicylic acid are found to be more effective in increasing the phenolic compounds like neochlorogenic acid (Stasińska-Jakubas et al. 2024). On the other hand, a well-known herb namely *Salvia verticillata* L. is famous for its rosmarinic acid (RA) content; when treated with methyl jasmonate (MJ) and multi-walled carbon nanotubes, a significant increase in stress hormones like jasmonic acid, abscisic acid, and salicylic acid levels is observed along with an increase in RA content, suggesting that the changes in hormones can increase the accumulation of phenolic acids in *S. verticillata* (Rahmani and Radjabian 2024). Co-treatment with jasmonic acid and salicylic acid has also been shown to boost the production of phenolic compounds significantly in medicinal plants (Jeyasri et al. 2023).

Biotic elicitors, as the name suggests, have a biological origin which can include bacterial, algal, or fungal remains or organisms like proteins, cell wall components, or complexes of organisms. These microbes can play an important role in this process by inducing the plants to respond to the biotic stressors (Kumari et al. 2024). For instance, therapeutic potential of *Valeriana jatamansi* lies in its bioactive secondary metabolites like valepotriates and sesquiterpenoids. When leaf-cell suspension cultures are subjected to endophytes, significant increases in the fresh and dry cell biomasses as well as the production of key metabolites are observed, indicating their potential as biotic elicitors (Thakur et al. 2024). When over five weeks old callus of *Catharanthus* roseus is subjected to different concentrations of *Ascophyllum nodosum* seaweed extract, significant increases in callus growth are observed with the highest average fresh weight of 739.3 mg and alkaloid levels, including Vinblastine,

Vincristine, Vindoline, and Catharanthine, serving as an excellent example of an algal elicitor (Zamil, Salim, and Zubaida 2023). Enhanced biosynthesis of the alkaloids aervine and methylaervine in callus-derived cell suspension cultures of *Aerva javanica* is seen using various biotic and abiotic elicitors over twenty days. The callus derived when subjected to *Agrobacterium rhizogenes* increased aervine and methylaervine levels, suggesting that elicitor stimulation can improve both the quantity and quality of alkaloids (Selvakumar et al. 2024).

Other Conditions of Elicitation Process

Optimal elicitation in plants involves using substances called elicitors to stimulate the production of secondary metabolites. This process helps plants survive in adverse conditions. Various conditions of the elicitation process include ensuring user involvement, addressing incomplete requirements, prioritizing requirements, considering stakeholder biases, managing complex systems, facilitating open communication, addressing cultural differences, adapting to changing project needs, reviewing existing documentation, and utilizing appropriate elicitation techniques based on the project context; essentially, making sure the process actively engages relevant users, gathers comprehensive information, and navigates potential challenges to effectively identify project requirements. Consequently, some important factors need to be kept in mind for optimal elicitation; those are described in the following points.

(a) **Elicitor concentration:** The concentration of the elicitor and application duration can determine the metabolic response. Too much of an elicitor can lead to toxicity rather than stimulation. The secondary metabolite induction requires an optimal level of elicitors which, when exceeded, stimulates a hypersensitive response in plants and leads to cell death (Naik and Jameel 2016). When various concentrations of methyl jasmonate and salicylic acid (50, 100, 150, 200, and 250 μM) were added to the suspension culture of *Gymnema sylvestre*, it was found that gymnemic acid increased with the use of 150 μM and 200 μM of each elicitor individually (Chodisetti et al. 2014).

(b) **Medium Composition:** Growth conditions and medium composition can enhance the production of desired compounds, regulating which is very necessary from the industrial point of view (VanderMolen et al. 2013). Several studies indicate that more nitrate availability can lead to suppression in the secondary metabolite production in *Arabidopsis thaliana*, *Nicotiana tabacum*, and *Hordeum vulgare* (Wang, Xiujuan, and Crawford 2007). In *Taxus globosa*, callus cultures of leaves and young shoots in Gamborg's B5 medium with growth regulators elevated taxane production across different media and inoculum sizes, revealing that Gamborg's B5 yielded the highest taxol production (Tapia et al. 2013). But these greatly depend on the plant's secondary metabolite makeup and composition.

(c) **Cultural Practices:** Plant growth conditions, especially cultural practices like fertilization, irrigation, soil type, and plant density can affect the overall health and metabolism in plants. The availability of nutrients, especially potassium, nitrogen, and phosphorus, can affect the secondary metabolite production. Excessive nitrogen is seen to suppress and reduce the production of phenols and flavonoids in plants like *Nicotiana tabacum* and *Sorghum bicolor* (Ibrahim et al. 2011). Drought conditions have been shown to increase the levels of phenols and flavonoids in plants along with other secondary metabolites and ROS (Yadav et al. 2021). An increase in plant density has also been shown to alter the secondary metabolites due to increased competition for resources, as seen in *Cannabis sativa* (Zhang et al. 2022). Some studies also show that intercropping with legumes can increase soil health, leading to an increase in phenolic content of the plant (Wolyn 2018).

(d) **Timing of Elicitation:** The duration of the elicitor application can affect the yield of secondary metabolites in plants. It also affects the time period of expression of the specific biosynthetic pathway. Early elicitation often leads to a quicker and more robust accumulation of metabolites. Few studies indicate that eliciting with jasmonic acid at specific developmental stages can maximize flavonoid production (Sohn et al. 2022).

When considering elicitation in plants, several factors beyond the type of elicitor must be taken into account to optimize secondary metabolite production. Additionally, the plant species and genetic variations play an important role in determining the metabolic pathways during elicitation. Finally, the mode of application of the elicitor and time span can also have a significant impact on the effectiveness of the elicitation process (Sohn et al. 2022).

Study in Contexts

The shikimic acid pathway is essentially used to synthesize basic amino acids by plants and lower organisms such as bacteria, fungi, and algae. Thus, the aromatic phytochemicals such as phenols, naphthoquinones, and anthraquinones are derivatives of the shikimic acid pathway. The shikimic acid pathway is a metabolic route that produces aromatic amino acids and other secondary metabolites in plants, bacteria, and fungi. This particular study has addressed the phytochemicals which are derivatives of the shikimic acid pathway. Table 9.3 provides a concise view of some of the effective elicitors of this shikimic acid and naphthoquinone pathway.

Table 9.3. Elicitors of Shikimic Acid and Naphthoquinones in Plants

Sl. No.	Plant	Elicitors	Compounds and Pathway
1.	*Carthamus tinctorius* shoot	Methyl jasmonate (Liu et al. 2024)	Chlorogenic Acid, Shikimic Acid Pathway
2.	*Inula crithmoides* shoot culture	NaCl, (Rodrigues, Nuno, and Custódio 2024)	Chlorogenic Acid, Hydroxybenzoic Acid, Luteolin-7-O-Glucoside, And Naringenin-7-O-Glucoside; Gentisic Acid, Shikimic Acid Pathway
3.	*Hyoscyamus niger* root culture	Epibrassinolide and methyl jasmonate, (Albayrak, Tunahan, and Nilgün 2024)	Gallic Acid, Epicatechin, Cinnamic Acid And Chlorogenic Acid; Shikimic Acid Pathway
4.	Hairy root cultures of *Plumbago ariculata*	Methyl Jasmonate (Li et al. 2024)	Shikimic Acid And Methylvaleric Acid Pathway
5.	Root culture of *Rhinacanthus nasutus*	Salicylic acid, methyl jasmonate, chitosan and *Trichoderma harzianum* extract (Suksawat and Panichayupakaranant 2024)	Rhinacanthin; Naphthoquinone Pathway
6.	*In vitro* regenerated shoots of *Plumbago zeylanica*	Silver nanoparticles (Santra, Chakraborty, and Ghosh 2024)	Plumbagin; Naphthoquinone Pathway
7.	*Plumbago indica* regenerated shoots	Methyl jasmonate, salicylic acid, yeast extract (Jirakiattikul et al. 2024)	Plumbagin; Naphthoquinone Pathway
8.	Root culture of *Impatiens balsamea*	Methyl jasmonate (Sakunphueak and Panichayupakaranant 2010)	Naphthoquinones
9.	*Rindera graeca* transgenic roots	Silica xerogel (Wierzchowski et al. 2024)	Naphthoquinones
10.	Callus cultures of *Salvia*	Synthetic auxin with salicylic acid (Szymczyk et al. 2021)	Tanshinone, Terpenoid Pathway

Source: Authors.

Proposed Possible Elicitors for *Lawsonia inermis*

A detailed careful examination and in-depth analysis into the phytochemicals and pathways elicited up to date reveal that very little research has been made into the avenue of elicitation of naphthoquinones and its derivatives. The aspect of elicitation of *Lawsonia inermis* also remains ambiguous as no other previous work has been done in this field. However, closely meticulous inspection into the phytochemical composition of the plant and the pathways as depicted in Table 9.1 and Table 9.2, salicylic acid, yeast extract, and methyl jasmonate can serve as possible candidates for elicitation of secondary metabolites of *Lawsonia inermis*, especially the main pigment lawsone. Besides, some previous studies have revealed that chitosan is not a very effective elicitor and had negligible effects on the naphthoquinone content of *Drosera capensis* (Krolicka et al. 2010). Chitosan can trigger plant defense responses by mimicking a pathogen attack, leading to increased production of secondary metabolites like phytoalexins, which help plants combat pathogens. Different plant species may respond differently to chitosan application. If these elicitors can be used efficiently and optimized, they can lead to enhanced lawsone content of *Lawsonia inermis*, which can benefit the medicinal and commercial sectors, in turn benefiting society at large.

Conclusion and Future Prospects

Proper manipulation and optimized utilization of plants and their secondary metabolites can benefit society. Synthetic medicines have an infamous name for the harmful side effects they induce. Shifting to plant-based alternatives can not only be rewarding but also save us from long-term health problems. The plant *Lawsonia inermis*, even though it is famous commercially, stores a repository of important bioactive compounds which, if manipulated, can help to heal many diseases. The importance of these phytochemicals, as already discussed, throws light on the medicinal potential of the plant. Besides, increasing the phytochemical potential of the plant can lead to medicinal and agricultural gains which can help in boosting the economy, providing an additional source of income to the farmers and encouraging local entrepreneurship. Finally, the plant stands out as a rich resource to the country that can effectively impact the commercial and medicinal sectors. By investing more in research and agricultural practices which focus on the optimal utilization of the plant's rich metabolic pool, the *Henna* plant can be effectively used for the benefit of society.

References

Adiga, A., A. Gandhi, and L. H. P. Prakash. "Comprehensive Review on Madayantika (*Lawsonia inermis* L.)." *JAIMS* 7 (2022): 204–10.

Ahmad, A., J. Sumera, I. Sumera, S. Kiran, K. G. Mansour, and J. Talha. "Alleviation Potential of Green-synthesized Selenium Nanoparticles for Cadmium Stress in *Solanum lycopersicum* L: Modulation of Secondary Metabolites and Physiochemical Attributes." *Plant Cell Reports* 43 (2024).

Albayrak, İ., D. Tunahan, and G. B. Nilgün. "Enhancement of *in vitro* Production of Tropane Alkaloids and Phenolic Compounds in *Hyoscyamus niger* by Culture Types and Elicitor Treatments." *PCTOC* 156 (2024).

Barberis, M., C. Daniele, G. Marta, and N. Massimo. "Secondary Metabolites in Nectar-mediated Plant-pollinator Relationships." *Plants* 12 (2020): 550.

Bozaba, T. O., and İ. S. Kuru. "The Effect of the Combined Application of Elicitors to *Salvia virgata* Jacq. under Salinity Stress on Physiological and Antioxidant Defense." *BMC Plant Biology* 24 (2024): 788.

Chaachouay, N., and L. Zidane. "Plant-derived Natural Products: A Source for Drug Discovery and Development." *Drugs and Drug Candidates* 3 (2024): 184–207.

Chodisetti, B., K. Rao, S. Gandi, and A. G. Giri. "Gymnemic Acid Enhancement in the Suspension Cultures of *Gymnema sylvestre* by Using the Signalling Molecules—Methyl Jasmonate and Salicylic Acid." *IVP* 51 (2014): 88–92.

Das, D., B. Mallick, S. Sinha, S. Ganguli, D. Samanta, R. Banerjee, and D. Roy. "Unearthing the Inhibitory Potential of Phytochemicals from *Lawsonia inermis* L. and Some Drugs against Dengue Virus Protein NS1: An *in silico* Approach." *Journal of Biomolecular Structure and Dynamics* 43, no. 7 (2023): 3449–66.

Fayiah, M., S. F. Muloma, S. Salimatu, and K. K. Mohamed. "Value of Herbal Medicine to Sustainable Development." In (Eds.), *Phytochemistry*. Reference Series in Phytochemistry, edited by S. C. Izah, M. C. Ogwu, and M. Akram, 1429–56. Cham: Springer, 2024.

Gull, I., S. Maria, A. Muhammad, and A. Muhammad. "Phytochemical, Toxicological and Antimicrobial Evaluation of *Lawsonia inermis* Extracts against Clinical Isolates of Pathogenic Bacteria." *Annals of Clinical Microbiology and Antimicrobials* 12 (2013): 36.

Halder, M., S. Sarkar, and S. Jha. "Elicitation: A Biotechnological Tool for Enhanced Production of Secondary Metabolites in Hairy Root Cultures." *Engineering in Life Sciences* 19 (2019): 880–95.

Hashem, S., A. Hamada, M. Fatma, M. H. Momtaz, M. A. Amal, K. O. Mohammad, and S. Mona "Zn–Al and Mg–Al Layered Double Hydroxide Nanoparticles Improved Primary and Secondary Metabolism of Geranium Plants." *RSC Advances* 14 (2024): 28376–89.

Ibrahim, M. H., Z. E. J. Hawa, R. Asmah, and A. R. Zaharah. "Involvement of Nitrogen on Flavonoids, Glutathione, Anthocyanin, Ascorbic Acid and Antioxidant Activities of Malaysian Medicinal Plant *Labisia pumila* Blume (Kacip Fatimah)." *International Journal of Molecular Sciences* 13 (2011): 393–408.

Jeyasri, R., M. Pandiyan, K. Kannan, S. Hyunsuk, H. C. Sung, and R. Manikandan. "Methyl Jasmonate and Salicylic Acid as Powerful Elicitors for Enhancing the Production of Secondary Metabolites in Medicinal Plants: An Updated Review." *PCTOC* 153, no. 3 (2023): 447–58.

Jirakiattikul, Y., R. Srisopa, S. Kanokwan, C. Kornkanok, and R. Panumart. "Enhancement of Plumbagin Production through Elicitation in *in vitro*-regenerated Shoots of *Plumbago indica* L." *Plants* 13, no. 11 (2024): 1450.

Kaushik, B., S. Jatin, Y. Keshav, K. Prithik, and A. Shourie. "Phytochemical Properties and Pharmacological Role of Plants: Secondary Metabolites." *Biosci Biotechnol Res Asia* 18 (2021): 23–35.

Krolicka, A., S. Anna, S. Krzysztof, B. Rafal, A. Gwizdek-Wisniewska, A. Skrzypczak, M. Kaminski, and E. Lojkowska. "Teratomas of *Drosera capensis* var. *alba* as a Source of Naphthoquinone: Ramentaceone." *PCTOC* 103, no. 3 (2010): 285–92.

Kumari, H. K., D. Vijaysri, T. Chethan, Swati, and V. Mamtha. "Impact of Microbial Inoculants on the Secondary Metabolites Production of Medicinal Plants." In *Microbes-*

Based Approaches for the Management of Hazardous Contaminants, edited by A. Kumar, L. Shukla, J. Singh, and L. F. R. Ferreira. Hoboken, NJ: John Wiley & Sons, Inc., 2024.

Li, Y., Z. Zi-An, H. Ju, L. Ting, C. Qibing, L. Jiani, Y. Lijuan, H. Di, and S. Gao. "MeJA-induced Hairy Roots in *Plumbago auriculata* L. by RNA-seq Profiling and Key Synthase Provided New Insights into the Sustainable Production of Plumbagin and Saponins." *Frontiers in Plant Science* 15 (2024).

Liu, Z., Z. Xiaofeng, M. Ali, S. Huijie, D. Linxiao, Y. Zhongping, Z. Yingping, and G. Meijin. "Uncovering the Role of Hydroxycinnamoyl Transferase in Boosting Chlorogenic Acid Accumulation in *Carthamus Tinctorius* Cells under Methyl Jasmonate Elicitation." *International Journal of Molecular Sciences* 25 (2024): 2710.

Malik, N. A. A., S. K. Ilakiya, and N. Kalaivani. "Elicitor and Receptor Molecules: Orchestrators of Plant Defense and Immunity." *International Journal of Molecular Sciences* 21 (2020): 963.

Marchev, A. S., P. Y. Zhenya, and I. G. Milen. "Green (Cell) Factories for Advanced Production of Plant Secondary Metabolites." *Critical Reviews in Biotechnology* 40 (2020): 443–58.

Moutawalli, A., Z. B. Fatima, O. Lahcen, E. F. Elmostafa, B. Hanane, D. Anass, and Z. Ahmed. "Quantitative Phytochemical, Antioxidant and Antimicrobial Properties of the Seeds of *Lawsonia inermis* L." *Plant Science Today* 11 (2024).

Naik, P. M., and M. A. K. Jameel. "Abiotic and Biotic Elicitors–role in Secondary Metabolites Production through *in vitro* Culture of Medicinal Plants." In *Abiotic and Biotic Stress in Plants - Recent Advances and Future Perspectives*, edited by Arun K. Shanker and C. Shanker. London: Intechopen.com, 2016.

Petrova, M., M. G. Kamelia, and G. Maria. "Influence of Abiotic and Biotic Elicitors on Organogenesis, Biomass Accumulation, and Production of Key Secondary Metabolites in Asteraceae Plants." *International Journal of Molecular Sciences* 25 (2024): 4197.

Piechowiak, T. "Elucidation of the Mechanism of Elicitation of Edible Sprouts Using UV-C Radiation." *Biocatalysis and Agricultural Biotechnology* 57 (2024): 103081.

Pradhan, R., D. Prasad, V. Alok, S. Padhye, B. Bernhard, S. Rainer, A. Ahmad, and H. S. Fazlul. "From Body Art to Anticancer Activities: Perspectives on Medicinal Properties of Henna." *Current Drug Targets* 13, no. 14 (2012): 1777–98.

Rahmani, N., and T. Radjabian. "Integrative Effects of Phytohormones in the Phenolic Acids Production in *Salvia verticillata* L. under Multi-walled Carbon Nanotubes and Methyl Jasmonate Elicitation." *BMC Plant Biology* 24, no. 56 (2024).

Ramirez-Estrada, K., V. L. Heriberto, H. Diego, M. Elisabeth, G. Marta, R. Cusidó, and J. Palazon. "Elicitation, an Effective Strategy for the Biotechnological Production of Bioactive High-added Value Compounds in Plant Cell Factories." *Molecules* 21 (2016): 182.

Rodrigues, M. J., N. Nuno, and L. Custódio. "NaCl Elicitation Enhances Metabolite Accumulation and Stress Resilience in *Inula crithmoides* L. Shoot Cultures: Implications for Its Nutritional and Medicinal Value." *PCTOC* 157 (2024).

Sadeghi, A., R. Jamshid, K. Hassan, and T. C. Baldwin. "Differential Responses of Hollyhock (*Alcea Rosea* L.) Varieties to Salt Stress in Relation to Physiological and Biochemical Parameters." *Science Reports* 14 (2024): 8105.

Sakunphueak, A., and P. Panichayupakaranant. "Increased Production of Naphthoquinones in Impatiens Balsamina Root Cultures by Elicitation with Methyl Jasmonate." *Bioresource Technology* 101 (2010): 8777–83.

Santra, I., A. Chakraborty, and B. Ghosh. "Evaluation of Plumbagin Synthesis: Mimicking *in vivo* Plant Systems through the Application of Elicitors Inducing Stress on *in vitro* Regenerated *Plumbago zeylanica* L." *PCTOC* 157 (2024).

Selvakumar, B., et al. "Enhancing the Aervine and Methylaervine Production in In Vitro Cultures of Aerva javanica (Burm. F.) Schult via Elicitors and Agrobacterium rhizogenes-Mediated Hairy Root Cultures." *Journal of Plant Biochemistry and Biotechnology* 33 (2024): 353–66.

Sohn, S. I., P. Subramani, R. Kasinathan, J. V. L. Muthiah, K. T. Senthil, S. Balaji, Y. A. B. Zoclanclounon, S. Jayabalan, and R. Manikandan. "Jasmonates in Plant Growth and Development and Elicitation of Secondary Metabolites: An Updated Overview." *Frontiers Plant Science* 13 (2022).

Stasińska-Jakubas, M., D. Sławomir, M. Strzemski, K. Rubinowska, and B. Hawrylak-Nowak. "Differentiated Response of *Hypericum perforatum* to Foliar Application of Selected Metabolic Modulators: Elicitation Potential of Chitosan, Selenium, and Salicylic Acid Mediated by Redox Imbalance." *Phytochemistry* 227 (2024): 114231.

Suksawat, T., and P. Panichayupakaranant. "Enhanced Rhinacanthin Production in *Rhinacanthus nasutus* Roots Using a Hydroponics and Elicitation System." *Journal of Young Pharmacists* 16, no. 2 (2024): 216–22.

Szymczyk, P., G. Szymańska, E. Kochan, J. Szemraj, and R. Grąbkowska. "Elicitation of Solid Callus Cultures of *Salvia miltiorrhiza* Bunge with Salicylic Acid and a Synthetic Auxin (1-naphthaleneacetic Acid)." *PCTOC* 147 (2021): 491–502.

Tapia, N., Z. Alejandro, M. Bonfill, E. Ventura, D. Cruz-Vega, A. D. Villar, F. Cruz-Sosa, and L. Osuna. "Effect of the Culture Medium and Biotic Stimulation on Taxane Production in *Taxus globosa* Schltdl *in vitro* Cultures." *Acta Physiologie Plantarum* 35 (2013): 3447–55.

Thakur, A., K. Thakur, A. Kumar, A. Rambhau Warghat, D. Kumar, and S. S. Pandey. "Endophyte-based Fungal Elicitors for Enhanced Production of Valepotriates and Sesquiterpenoids in Leaf Cell Suspension Cultures of *Valeriana jatamansi* Jones." *Journal of Applied Microbiology* 135, no. 9 (2024): lxae242.

Thakur, M., and B. S. Sohal. "Role of Elicitors in Inducing Resistance in Plants against Pathogen Infection: A Review." *ISRN Biochemistry* 2013 (2013): 1–10.

VanderMolen, K. M., A. R. Huzefa, T. El-Elimat, and N. H. Oberlies. "Evaluation of Culture Media for the Production of Secondary Metabolites in a Natural Products Screening Program." *AMB Express* 3 (2013).

Wang, R., X. Xiujuan, and N. Crawford. "Nitrite Acts as a Transcriptome Signal at Micromolar Concentrations in *Arabidopsis* Roots." *Plant Physiol* 145, no. 4 (2007): 1735–45.

Widhalm, J. R., and D. Rhodes. "Biosynthesis and Molecular Actions of Specialized 1,4-naphthoquinone Natural Products Produced by Horticultural Plants." *Horticulture Research* 3 (2016).

Wierzchowski, K., B. Nowak, K. Mateusz, K. Sykłowska-Baranek, and M. Pilarek. "Effect of Silica Xerogel Functionalization on Intensification of *Rindera graeca* Transgenic Roots Proliferation and Boosting Naphthoquinone Production." *Life* 14, no. 1 (2024): 159.

Wolyn, D. J. "Adaptation of Asparagus to Overwinter in Cold Climates." *Acta Horticulturae* 1223 (2018): 135–44.
Yadav, B., A. Jogawat, M. S. Rahman, and O. P. Narayan. "Secondary Metabolites in the Drought Stress Tolerance of Crop Plants: A Review." *Gene Reports* 23 (2021): 101040.
Youl, O., S. Konaté, N. Ernest, R. B. Sombié, K. Boukaré, M. Koala, A. Zoungrana. "Phytochemical Analysis and Antimicrobial Activity of *Lawsonia inermis* Leaf Extracts from Burkina Faso." *American Journal of Plant Sciences* 15 (2024): 552–76.
Zamil, H. A., A. S. Salim, and A. I. Zubaida. "Enhancement of Secondary Metabolite Production from Callus of *Catharanthus roseus* (L.) G. Don. through Elicitation with Seaweed Extract." *The Pharma Innovation Journal*, SP-12, no. 9 (2023): 2198–208.
Zhang, H., Y. Wen-Qiang, W. Yunxuan, Z. Jian-Bing, and L. Yi-Dong. "Morphological Control and Interfacial Compatibilization of Fully Biobased PLA/ENR Blends via Partial Crosslinking ENR with Sebacic Acid." *Industrial Crops and Products* 180 (2022): 114707.

10

Antimicrobial Activity of Some Ethnomedicinal Plants of India and Their Potential Application in Modern Medicine

Camellia Nandi*

Department of Botany, Scottish Church College, Kolkata, West Bengal, India

*Corresponding Author's Email: camellia.nandi@scottishchurch.ac.in

Introduction

Ethnomedicinal plants have been used traditionally in various cultures for their healing properties, including antimicrobial effects. Many of these plants contain bioactive compounds that can inhibit the growth of bacteria, fungi, and viruses. India is home to a large number of medicinal plants. Our traditional knowledge of medicinal plants used to treat diseases is one of the oldest in the world (Tiwary et al. 2024). Owing to their applicability as ethnomedicine, several plants have been exploited to develop modern medicines ever since. Ethnomedicine deals with the utilization of traditional knowledge of plants, folk beliefs, methods, and techniques of utilizing them for the treatment of infections and diseases (Atnafu et al. 2018; Faye, Birhanu, and Belete 2021). Due to the cultural acceptability of ethnomedicines and their effectiveness against several infections and diseases, cheaper cost, and local availability, it enables the development of modern medications.

India's diverse biodiversity and deep cultural traditions have contributed to a wealth of ethnomedicinal knowledge, particularly in the use of plants with antimicrobial effects. Traditional medical systems like Ayurveda, Siddha, and Unani have long relied on these plants to address infections caused by bacteria, fungi, and viruses. As antibiotic resistance becomes an escalating concern, there is an increasing interest in exploring these traditional remedies as potential alternatives or adjuncts to synthetic drugs. Although herbal medicines are less potent in comparison to synthetic drugs in some cases, they are still considered less toxic or having fewer side effects in contrast to synthetic drugs (Pandey, Rastogi, and Rawat 2013).

On the other hand, Antimicrobial resistance (AMR) has become a major public health issue globally, and the World Health Organization (WHO) has highlighted it as a serious threat to international health security. In reality, antimicrobial resistance occurs when bacteria and fungi develop ways to survive drugs that are designed to kill them. These mechanisms include (i) altering the drug target, (ii) inactivating the drug, (iii) changing membrane permeability, (iv) expelling the drug, and (v) acquiring new genetic material. In this context, the traditional medicine systems, particularly those that incorporate the use of ethnomedicinal plants, offer a promising avenue for discovering new antimicrobial agents. India is a country which is rich in biodiversity, and numerous plants have been identified for their therapeutic potential, specifically for their ability to combat microbial infections. Further, India is recognized as one of the world's "megadiverse" countries, harboring a vast array of plant species. Ayurveda, a traditional Indian medical system, heavily relies on medicinal plants and has documented the use of thousands of plant species for various ailments. Again, India's varied topography and climate contribute to a wide range of plant species with potential medicinal properties. Scientists are actively studying Indian plants to identify and isolate bioactive compounds with antimicrobial properties.

Objectives and Methods

India's ethnomedicinal flora includes over 7,500 species of plants used in traditional medicine (Chibuzo 2019). In other words, in India, of the 17,000 species of higher plants, 7,500 are known for medicinal uses. This proportion of medicinal plants is the highest proportion of plants known for their medical purposes in any country in the world for the existing flora of that respective country. The knowledge of these medicinal plants has been passed down through generations with significant contributions from various cultural and regional practices. In addition, this knowledge has been mainly passed on orally and through traditional healers. The traditional healers have passed down their knowledge of medicinal plants from generation to generation. In some cases, families specialize in specific treatments. This knowledge has helped people find medications to alleviate pain and cure different illnesses. Besides, this knowledge has helped upgrade old properties, discover new ones, and improve the processing and usage of medicinal plants. Moreover, this knowledge could bring a new revolution in the treatment of diseases.

In this regard, this particular research comprehensively explores the antimicrobial activities of key ethnomedicinal plants in India by discussing their traditional uses, bioactive compounds, and modes of action. Because the ethnomedicinal plants are plants traditionally used by local communities to treat various ailments, with their therapeutic properties stemming from bioactive compounds like alkaloids, flavonoids, terpenes, and phenolic acids, which act through diverse mechanisms like antioxidant, anti-inflammatory, antimicrobial, and anticancer activities, often targeting specific cellular pathways depending on the plant and its bioactive constituents, this allows them to be used for conditions ranging from pain relief to wound healing and infectious disease management. On the other hand, by highlighting both scientific studies and traditional knowledge, this study aims to underline the significance of these plants in addressing global health challenges, particularly antibiotic resistance. Because antibiotic resistance occurs when bacteria develop defenses against the antibiotics designed to kill them. Once resistance develops to one antibiotic, different antibiotics, which can be less effective or have more side effects, are needed for treatment.

Ethnomedicinal Plants and Their Antimicrobial Properties

Numerous traditional medicinal plants found across different regions of India have been scientifically proven to possess antimicrobial properties, meaning they can inhibit the growth of bacteria and fungi, which is why they are often used in traditional medicine to treat infections. Thus, many ethnomedicinal plants in various regions of India have antimicrobial properties including Tulsi *(Ocimum tenuiflorum)*, Garlic *(Allium sativum)*, Turmeric *(Curcuma longa)*, Ginger *(Zingiber officinale)*, Neem *(Azadirachta indica)*, Ghrito-kumari or Aloe vera *(Aloe barbadensis)*, Chotra *(Lantana camara)*, and Ashoka *(Saraca asoca)*. The key points and detailed examination of these ethnomedicinal plants like their traditional uses, bioactive compounds, and modes of action are given here.

(A) Tulsi (*Ocimum tenuiflorum*, Family: Lamiaceae)

Ocimum tenuiflorum, (syn. *O. sanctum*) commonly termed as Holy Basil or Tulsi or Tulasi, is a revered plant in traditional medicine, particularly in Ayurvedic practices. Native to the Indian subcontinent, Tulsi is widely cultivated across India and other tropical and subtropical regions of the world. Belonging to the Lamiaceae family which also includes other aromatic plants such as sage, mint, and oregano, *Ocimum tenuiflorum* is a herbaceous shrub known for its distinctive, aromatic leaves. The plant has been an integral part of Ayurvedic medicine for several thousand years and is regarded as one of the most potent medicinal herbs in traditional Indian healthcare systems (Saha, Bandyopadhyay, and Ghosh 2018). The name "Tulsi" is derived from the Sanskrit word "tulasi," which means "the incomparable one," reflecting its revered status in Hinduism and its widespread use in ritualistic practices. In addition to its sacred and spiritual significance, it is planted around temples or in homes to promote harmony and spiritual well-being. Tulsi is also used in folk medicine across different cultures for a variety of ailments. Tulsi is believed to help the body cope with physical and mental stress, promoting overall balance and health (Chaudhary, Pal, and Gupta 2018).

The therapeutic value of *Ocimum tenuiflorum* is attributed to the numerous bioactive compounds found within its leaves, seeds, and essential oil. Among the most important are eugenol, caryophyllene, flavonoids, terpenoids, and phenolic acids. These compounds are responsible for the plant's broad spectrum of pharmacological activities, which include antimicrobial, anti-inflammatory, antioxidant, antidiabetic, and anticancer effects (Mishra, Singh, and Pandey 2016). The antimicrobial properties of Tulsi are particularly notable, as it has been shown to exhibit antibacterial, antifungal, antiviral, and even antiprotozoal effects, making it a valuable plant for combating infections (Jain et al. 2022). Some of the important bioactive compounds of Tulsi are mentioned below:

(i) **Eugenol ($C_{10}H_{12}O_2$):** Eugenol is the primary active component of *Ocimum tenuiflorum*, known for its potent antimicrobial properties. Although the primary source of eugenol is clove, tulsi is a potent source as well with concentrations ranging between 4.2–4.97 mg/g tissue (Ulanowska and Olas 2021). Research has demonstrated that eugenol exhibits antibacterial activity against various pathogens, including *E. coli ATCC29213, K. pneumoniae MTCC39, S. aureus ATCC25922, C. albicans MTCC277, ATCC90028* strains (Sharma et al. 2024). It is antibacterial, antifungal, and even acts against a number of parasites like *Fasciola gigantica, Giardia lamblia*, and *Haemonchus contortus* (Ulanowska and Olas 2021). The mechanism of action involves damaging the bacterial cell membrane, which causes the leakage of intracellular components and ultimately results in cell death (Figure 10.1).

(ii) **Rosmarinic Acid ($C_{18}H_{16}O_8$):** Rosmarinic acid is another significant compound found in *Ocimum tenuiflorum*. This phenolic compound has shown antimicrobial activity against a range of bacteria, particularly those associated with foodborne illnesses. Studies indicate that rosmarinic acid can inhibit the growth of *Salmonella* spp. and *E. coli* (Kernou et al. 2023). It also inhibits the growth of *Listeria monocytogenes* by disrupting their metabolic processes (Elafify et al. 2022).

(iii) **Linalool ($C_{10}H_{18}O$):** Linalool, a terpene alcohol, is also present in *Ocimum tenuiflorum*. It exhibits antibacterial effects and has been shown to be effective against strains of *P. aeruginosa* by reducing biofilm production (Lahiri et al. 2021). The antibacterial action of linalool is attributed to its capacity to penetrate through the bacterial membranes and interfere with their cellular functions.

(iv) **Caryophyllene ($C_{15}H_{24}$):** Caryophyllene or β-caryophyllene is a sesquiterpene that demonstrates significant antibacterial activity. Research has indicated that it is effective against both gram-positive and gram-negative bacteria (Xiao et al. 2012).

Tulsi essential oil has proved to be antimicrobial against a host of pathogens like *Staphylococcus aureus, E. coli, Pseudomonas aeruginosa*, all of which cause skin infections (Yamani et al. 2016). Tulsi extract shows antibacterial effects against bacteria like *P. aeruginosa, S. aureus*, and *Bacillus pumilus*. Tulsi extract and tulsi oil have also shown inhibitory effects against the pathogen *Mycobacterium tuberculosis* (Jain et al. 2022). Tulsi exhibits notable antimicrobial properties against a variety of pathogens, supported by a rich phytochemical profile and multiple mechanisms of action. Its potential as a natural alternative to conventional antimicrobials is promising, particularly in light of increasing antibiotic resistance. Future research should focus on clinical applications, optimal extraction methods, and the synergistic effects of combining Tulsi with other therapeutic agents to enhance its antimicrobial efficacy (Table 10.1).

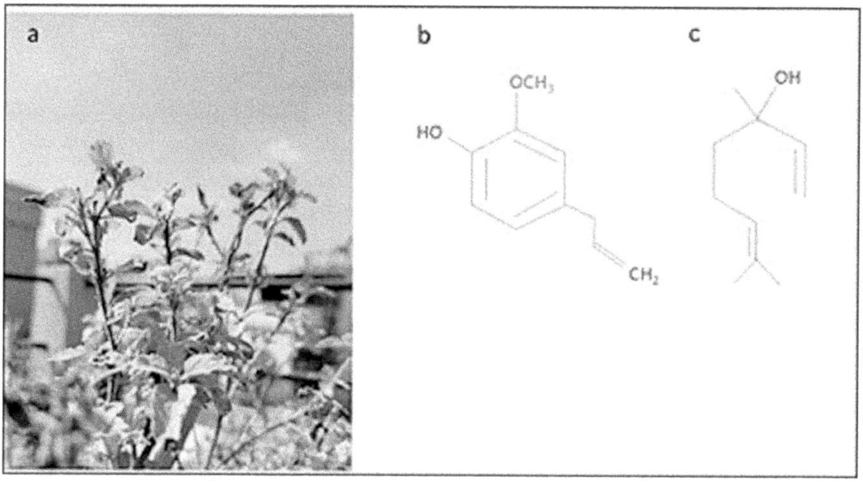

Figure 10.1. a. Ocimum tenuiflorum plant, b. Chemical structure of Eugenol, c. Chemical structure of Linalool. Source: Author.

Table 10.1. Antimicrobial Activity of Tulsi

Source	Antimicrobial Activity	References
Tulsi essential oil	Inhibits growth of *E. coli, P. aeruginosa, S. aureus.*	Mahmood et al. 2008; Yamani et al. 2011
Tulsi essential oil	Inhibits growth of Methicillin-resistant *S. aureus* (MRSA). *E. coli, P. aeruginosa*, and *S. aureus.*	Yamani et al. 2016
Tulsi extract	Tulsi extract at 5% and 10% concentrations was effective against *Aggregatibacter actinomycetemcomitans.*	Mallikarjun et al. 2016
Tulsi extract and Tulsi oil	Inhibitory effects was observed against the pathogen *Mycobacterium tuberculosis.*	Jain et al. 2022

Source: Authors.

In Indian traditional medicinal system, different parts of *Ocimum tenuiflorum* like the leaves, stem, root, flower, seeds, and even the entire plant have been recommended for the treatment of diseases like bronchitis, bronchial asthma, malaria, dysentery, diarrhea, skin diseases, and chronic fever (Prakash and Gupta 2005). In conclusion, *Ocimum tenuiflorum* is a plant of considerable therapeutic potential with extensive evidence supporting its antimicrobial, adaptogenic, and antioxidant properties. As both a medicinal herb and a cultural icon, Tulsi continues to play a vital role in promoting health and wellness. Given the growing interest in natural remedies and the limitations of modern pharmaceuticals, Tulsi's diverse bioactive compounds and its long history of use make it a promising candidate for further research and development in the context of modern healthcare.

(B) Garlic (*Allium sativum*, Family: Amaryllidaceae)

Garlic, scientifically known as *Allium sativum*, has long been valued not only for its role in cooking but also for its therapeutic benefits. It is widely recognized in traditional medicine systems like Ayurveda, Traditional Chinese Medicine, and among various indigenous healing practices around the world. Known for its distinctive pungent odor, garlic has been revered for its flavoring properties as well as for its extensive health benefits, which have been documented for thousands of years. It is particularly noted for its antimicrobial, cardiovascular, anti-inflammatory, and anticancer effects, which have made it a cornerstone of ethnobotanical practices. Garlic contains several bioactive compounds, including:

(a) **Allicin ($C_6H_{10}OS_2$):** The primary active compound formed when garlic is chopped or crushed. It's a thiosulfinate and is synthesized from allin (S-allyl-l-cysteine sulfoxide), a non-proteinogenic amino acid (Borlinghaus et al. 2014). Allicin is active against a broad range of different gram-positive and gram-negative bacteria. Its effectiveness is comparable to β-lactam antibiotics like penicillin and ampicillin and even glycosidic antibiotics such as kanamycin (Fujisawa et al. 2009; Borlinghaus et al. 2014). However, unlike penicillin, allicin is active against both gram-positive and gram-negative bacteria whereas penicillin is mostly not active against gram-negative bacteria. It is also active against multidrug-resistant bacteria. One such example includes methicillin-resistant *Staphylococcus aureus* (MRSA) resistant to methicillin (Cutler and Wilson 2004; Nakamoto et al. 2020). Allicin is active against gram-positive bacteria like *Bacillus* spp., *Streptococcus* spp., methicillin-sensitive and methicillin-resistant *Staphylococcus aureus* strains (Borlinghaus et al. 2014). It also shows antiviral, antifungal, and antiparasitic properties (Nakamoto et al. 2020). Allicin modifies proteins with thiol groups in bacteria leading to inactivation of several bacterial enzymes and aggregation of proteins (Müller et al. 2016) (Figure 10.2).

(b) **Diallyl polysulfides ($C_6H_{10}S_n$, where n = 1-9):** They contribute to the characteristic odor and have antimicrobial properties. These constitute garlic oil, which is obtained through steam distillation. The higher the value of sulfur atoms, the more potent their antimicrobial property (Nakamoto et al. 2020).

(c) **Ajoene ($C_9H_{14}OS_3$):** It is a compound derived from allicin with demonstrated antifungal and antibacterial effects. Both ajoenes, *Z*-ajoene and *E*-ajoene, are obtained from garlic oil macerate products (Block 1985). Ajoene is potent against *H. pylori* (Ohta et al. 1999). They also show antifungal activities against *Aspergillus niger* and *Candida albicans* (Nakamoto et al. 2020).

Garlic has been found to exhibit potent antibacterial properties, particularly against gram-positive pathogens such as *Staphylococcus aureus* and *Bacillus cereus*. Research suggests that allicin, a key bioactive compound in garlic, exerts its antimicrobial effect

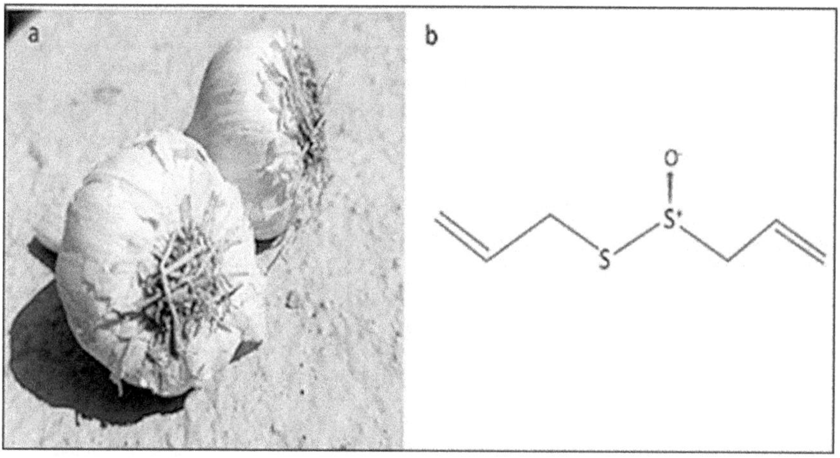

Figure 10.2. a. Allium sativum bulb, b. Chemical structure of Allicin. Source: Author.

by compromising the integrity of the bacterial cell wall and impeding protein synthesis (Bae et al. 2004). Furthermore, garlic has also demonstrated efficacy in combating gram-negative bacteria, including *Escherichia coli* and *Pseudomonas aeruginosa*, highlighting its broad-spectrum antibacterial potential. Research indicates that the lipid bilayer of the bacterial membrane is compromised by allicin, leading to cell lysis (Ryu et al. 2004). Garlic's antifungal properties have been extensively documented. It has shown effectiveness against various fungi, including *Candida albicans* and *Aspergillus niger*. Ajoene, in particular, has been noted for its ability to inhibit fungal growth by interfering with cell membrane integrity (Borchers et al. 2004).

Emerging research suggests that garlic may also possess antiviral properties. Studies have reported its efficacy against viruses such as the influenza virus and herpes simplex virus. These effects are attributed to the immune-modulating effects of garlic (Moulin et al. 2010). Allicin and DAS disrupt bacterial cell membranes, leading to leakage of cellular contents. Garlic compounds inhibit the synthesis of bacterial proteins, effectively stunting microbial growth. Garlic can induce oxidative stress in microorganisms, leading to cell death (Cohen et al. 2017). Garlic has been found to enhance the effectiveness of conventional antibiotics. This synergy is particularly important in combating antibiotic-resistant strains. For instance, studies have shown that combining garlic extract with antibiotics like amoxicillin improves their effectiveness against resistant strains of bacteria (Vogt et al. 2016) (Table 10.2).

In India, garlic is used to treat a wide range of ailments. In Ayurvedic medicine, garlic is considered a powerful remedy to balance the body's doshas, treat respiratory issues, digestive disorders, and alleviate hypertension (Agarwal, Gupta, and Singh 2007). It has been used to treat cough and cold by consuming it in the form of powder or raw with salt by the tribes of Upper Dibang Valley, Arunachal Pradesh and Bellary district, Karnataka, India (Devi, Rakshit, and Sarania 2014; Murthy and Vidyasagar 2013). The Gond tribes of Bhandara district of Maharashtra have been known to treat

Table 10.2. Antibacterial Activity of Compounds and Secondary Metabolites of Garlic

Source	Antimicrobial Activity	References
Allicin	Growth inhibition of *Streptococcus* spp., *Vibrio cholerae, Helicobacter pylori, Enterococci* spp., *Escherichia coli, Bacillus* spp.	Cavallito and Bailey 1944; Small et al. 1947; Jonkers et al. 1999; Bhatwalkar et al. 2021
Diallyl polysulfide	Growth inhibition of *Staphylococcus aureus, Klebsiella pneumoniae, Helicobacter pylori.*	Bhatwalkar et al. 2021
Ajoene	Growth inhibition of *Streptomyces griseus, Bacillus subtilis, Escherichia coli.*	Bhatwalkar et al. 2021
Garlic extract	Growth inhibition of Methicillin sensitive *Staphylococcus aureus* NBRC 12732, Methicillin-resistant *Staphylococcus aureus, Pseudomonas syringae, Agrobacterium tumefaciens, E. coli* K12, *B. subtilis, S. typhi.*	Fujisawa et al. 2009; Cutler and Wilson 2004; Curtis et al. 2004; Bhatwalkar et al. 2021
Garlic paste	Inhibition of *Escherichia coli* O157:H7.	Gupta and Ravisankar 2005; Bhatwalkar et al. 2021
Garlic powder	Inhibition of *Escherichia coli, Vibrio* sp., *Bacillus subtilis, Helicobacter pylori.*	Bhatwalkar et al. 2021

Source: Authors.

cuts and external wounds with garlic along with fruits of *Semecarpus anacardium* and the resin from *Gardenia tubifera* which is then warmed with castor oil (Gupta et al. 2010). The Sahariya tribe of Jhansi district, Uttar Pradesh, uses garlic with onion to treat bronchitis (Nigam and Sharma 2010). Today, with a growing interest in natural remedies and herbal medicine, garlic continues to be widely used and studied for its therapeutic potential. Modern science has validated many of its traditional applications, and garlic is now recognized as a valuable functional food and a potential adjunct in the treatment of various diseases, particularly those related to infection and cardiovascular health.

(C) Turmeric (*Curcuma longa*, Family: Zingiberaceae)

Curcuma longa, widely known as turmeric, has garnered considerable interest in both traditional and contemporary medical fields, owing to its abundant array of bioactive constituents, with curcumin being the most prominent. Turmeric is a rhizomatous plant that is native to India, which contributes to the largest production of turmeric in the world (Velayudhan et al. 2012). It has been widely used as traditional medicine in the country and is a popular condiment. Turmeric has the active ingredient curcumin, which renders it antimicrobial and anti-inflammatory in nature. This review examines the antimicrobial properties of turmeric, focusing on its active compounds, their underlying mechanisms of action, and their prospective therapeutic applications. We will explore the effectiveness of these compounds against a diverse spectrum of pathogens, including bacteria, fungi, viruses, and parasites, while considering their potential impact on health and their role in the management of various diseases. Turmeric contains several bioactive compounds, including:

a) **Curcumin ($C_{21}H_{20}O_6$):** Curcumin (diferuloylmethane) is the most studied active compound in *Curcuma longa*, accounting for approximately 2–5 percent of the rhizome's weight. Its chemical structure consists of two aromatic rings connected by a methylene bridge, contributing to its diverse biological activities (Anand et al. 2008). Curcumin has shown broad-spectrum antibacterial activity against both gram-positive and gram-negative bacteria (Figure 10.3).
b) **Turmerones ($C_{15}H_{20}O_6$):** Turmerones are essential oil components derived from turmeric. They include α-turmerone, β-turmerone, and ar-turmerone. These compounds contribute to turmeric's aroma and also possess notable antimicrobial properties (Figure 10.4).

Curcumin integrates into bacterial membranes, altering their permeability and leading to leakage of cytoplasmic contents (Rana et al. 2015). Curcumin is known to inhibit the formation of biofilms (protective structures produced by bacteria) that contribute to chronic infections (Shome et al. 2023). Studies have demonstrated its effectiveness against *Staphylococcus aureus*. Curcumin inhibits the growth of this pathogenic

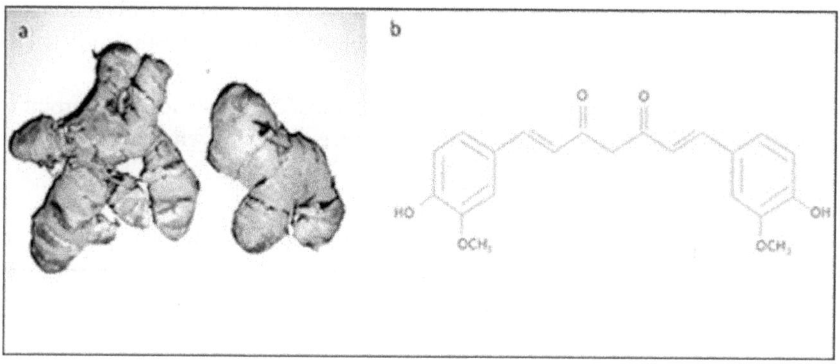

Figure 10.3. a. Curcuma longa rhizome, b. Chemical structure of Curcumin. Source: Author.

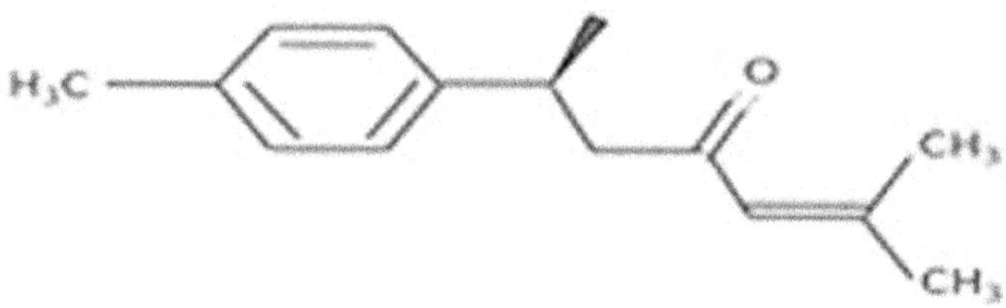

Figure 10.4. a. Chemical structure of Turmerones. Source: Author.

bacterium, which is associated with various infections, including skin and respiratory infections (Teow and Ali 2017). Curcumin also disrupts the cell membrane integrity of *E. coli*, leading to increased permeability and eventual cell death (Sadeghi et al. 2020). Curcumin has been found to exhibit significant activity against *H. pylori*, a bacterium linked to peptic ulcers and gastric cancer. It acts by inhibiting bacterial adhesion and reducing inflammation (Nabavi et al. 2015).

Curcuma longa exhibits antifungal properties against various fungal pathogens: Curcumin demonstrates significant antifungal activity against *Candida albicans* by disrupting the integrity of the fungal cell wall and impairing its growth (Kumar et al. 2016). Curcumin inhibits the growth of *Aspergillus niger*, a common mold that can cause food spoilage and opportunistic infections in immunocompromised individuals (Srinivasan, Chandran, and Sujatha 2014). Curcumin alters the structural integrity of fungal cell walls, resulting in cell lysis (Narasimhan et al. 2017). It triggers apoptotic pathways in fungal cells, leading to programmed cell death (Ranjbar et al. 2019).

Turmerones have been found to be active against *Staphylococcus aureus* ATCC 25923, *Bacillus subtilis* ATCC 14931, and *Escherichia coli* ATCC 25922 (Kheira et al. 2023). In addition to curcumin and turmerones, *Curcuma longa* contains various flavonoids, phenolic compounds, and essential oils that may also exhibit antimicrobial activities. These include eugenol, bisdemethoxycurcumin, and multiple terpenes (Satyajit, Latif, and Gray 2010; Kheira et al. 2023). Metabolites like borneol, 1,8-cineole, sabinene, and turmerone derived from *Curcuma longa* were found to be antimicrobial in nature (Kim, Choi, and Lee 2003; Iweala et al. 2023). Table 10.3 enumerates the antibacterial activity of turmeric.

In Ayurveda, turmeric is considered a "rasayana," a substance that promotes longevity and rejuvenation. It is believed to balance the body's energies or "doshas"

Table 10.3. Antibacterial Activity of Compounds and Secondary Metabolites of Turmeric

Source	**Antimicrobial Activity**	**References**
Curcumin	Bacterial growth inhibition of *Bacillus subtilis* 168, *Escherichia coli* BL21, K12 MG1655 strains.	Rai et al. 2010
	Elimination of *Helicobacter pylori* from stomach of mice.	De et al. 2009
Curcuma longa fractions with antibiotics	Bacterial growth reduction of Pseudomonas aeruginosa, *Vibrio cholerae, S. aureus, B. subtilis, Escherechia coli.*	Sasidharan et al. 2014
Curcumin and α-methyl cinnamaldehyde	Growth inhibition and haemolysis of *Candida* (38 isolates).	Khan et al. 2012
Turmeric extract (@100, 50, 25, and 12.5 mg/mL) in water and ethanol solvents	Growth inhibition was observed for *Bacillus* sp., *Staphylococcus aureus, E. coli* using disc diffusion method.	Odo et al. 2023

Source: Authors.

(Vata, Pitta, and Kapha), and its uses span a variety of conditions such as digestive issues, respiratory infections, liver problems, and inflammatory conditions (Patwardhan, Vaidya, and Chorghade 2004). In India, turmeric has been used as ethnomedicine for treating various ailments like pneumonia, bronchial ailments, dysentery, and infectious wounds (Jacob 2016). Turmeric paste has been traditionally used by Nepal for treating infected wounds, cuts, and injuries (Singh et al. 2010). In India, it is a common practice to mix turmeric with milk (referred to as "golden milk") or other medicinal herbs to aid in digestion, promote liver detoxification, and relieve symptoms of arthritis and joint pain (Ali, Ali, and Lall 2008). The rising interest in natural remedies, coupled with turmeric's rich ethnobotanical history, has led to its growing incorporation in both dietary supplements and pharmaceutical formulations aimed at promoting health and preventing disease.

(D) Ginger (*Zingiber officinale*, Family: Zingiberaceae)

It is a herbaceous plant with a fleshy articulated rhizome, with a brown epidermis. The rhizome of ginger is used as a condiment all over the world. It is also used in the pharmaceutical industry and traditional medicine (Teles et al. 2019). The term ginger is derived from the Sanskrit word, "śṛṅgavera" meaning horn-shaped body (Uchibayashi 2001). In Ayurveda, ginger is considered the "Universal Medicine" because it helps with many health problems. The plant has been utilized in China for approximately 2,500 years to address ailments such as colds, nausea, and headaches. Today, it is well-regarded in herbal medicine, particularly for alleviating muscular pain, rheumatological disorders, and arthritis (Das, Nadar, and Rathod 2021). Ginger plays a significant role in lowering the incidence of cancers (Mao et al. 2019). It is commonly used to alleviate symptoms associated with inflammation, rheumatic conditions, and digestive issues. The root possesses carminative, digestive, perspiration-inducing, anti-influenza, and stimulating effects (Pfeiffer et al. 2006; Soares 2009). The antimicrobial properties of ginger are largely attributed to its rich content of bioactive compounds, which include:

i. **Gingerol ($C_{17}H_{26}O_4$) and Shogaol ($C_{17}H_{24}O_3$):** These are the primary phenolic compounds in ginger, with gingerol being the major bioactive constituent in fresh ginger, while shogaol is more abundant in dried ginger. Both compounds exhibit significant anti-inflammatory, anticancer, and antimicrobial properties (Maghraby et al. 2023). Gingerols are generally a blend of volatile phenolic compounds, with 6-gingerol being the predominant form, while 4-, 8-, 10-, and 12-gingerols are present in smaller amounts (Maghraby et al. 2023). 6-, 8-, and 10-gingerol change to shogaols through dehydration. The pungent and sweet aroma in dry ginger is attributed to shogaols (Shukla and Singh 2007). 6-gingerol, 8-gingerol, and 6-shogaol effectively inhibit the biofilm formation in *Candida albicans* (Lee et al. 2018). 6-gingerol also showed antibacterial activity against *Pseudomonas aeruginosa, Acinetobacter baumannii, Klebsiella pneumoniae*, and *Staphylococcus aureus* (Elfaky et al. 2024) (Figure 10.5).

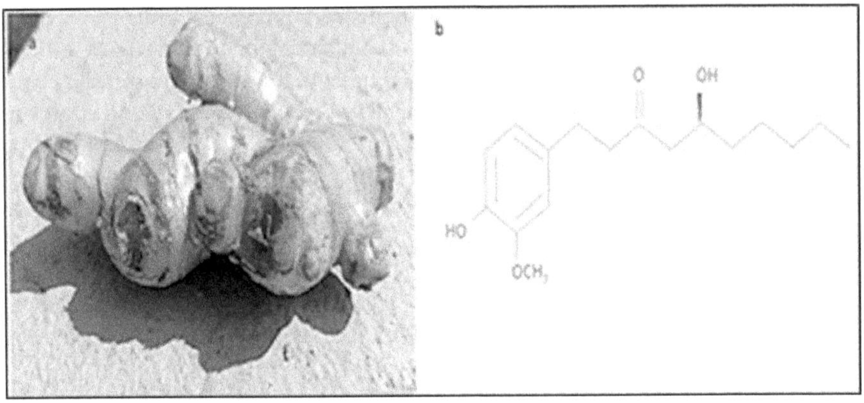

Figure 10.5. a. Zingiber officinale rhizome, b. Chemical structure of Gingerol. Source: Author.

ii. **Zingerone ($C_{11}H_{14}O_3$):** This is a volatile compound formed during the drying process of ginger. When gingerols are subjected to thermal treatment, they are converted into zingerone (also known as vanillylacetone), which is the primary compound responsible for the pungency of ginger (Das, Nadar, and Rathod 2021). Zingerone has been shown to possess antimicrobial activity, particularly against certain bacterial strains. Zingerone, raffinose, 6-gingerol, and analogs of 6- and 8-gingerol have shown activity against *P. aeruginosa* (Lee et al. 2018).
iii. **Ginger essential oil**, which contains compounds such as β-phellandrene, zingiberene, and ar-curcumene, also contributes to the antimicrobial effects of ginger against bacteria like *P. vulgaris*, *E. coli*, *B. cereus*, and so on (Teles et al. 2019).

Ginger has antimicrobial properties due to its bioactive compounds. It can be used to prevent microbial growth and has been studied against pathogenic and spoilage microorganisms in foods. It has been shown to be effective against *E. coli*, *Salmonella typhi*, and *Bacillus subtilis*. It has been shown to have antifungal properties. Ginger has been shown to have antibacterial activity against periodontal bacteria. Ginger has been shown to have inhibitory activities against *Candida albicans*. Ginger's antimicrobial properties may be useful in replacing synthetic antimicrobials in food products. Ginger's antimicrobial properties may improve against different illnesses. Thus, ginger shows antimicrobial activity against a wide range of pathogens. Table 10.4 summarizes the antimicrobial activities of Ginger:

Ginger has been utilized for millennia across diverse cultures as a therapeutic agent for a wide array of ailments, ranging from respiratory issues like coughs and colds to digestive disturbances such as nausea, as well as conditions like arthritis, migraines, and hypertension (Bode and Dong 2011). Its medicinal properties have been extensively acknowledged in numerous traditional medical systems, including Traditional Chinese Medicine, Ayurveda, Unani medicine, and Iranian Traditional Medicine (Rahmawati et al. 2024).

Table 10.4. Antimicrobial Activities of Ginger

Source	Antimicrobial Activity	References
Rhizome extract	Ethanolic extract of rhizome shows antibacterial activity against *E. coli, P. aeruginosa, S. aureus, Enterobacter sp., Klebsiella sp., Proteus sp., and Bacillus sp.*	Karuppiah and Rajaram 2012
Gingerol and Shogaol	6-gingerol, 8-gingerol, and 6-shogaol effectively inhibit the biofilm formation in *Candida albicans.*	Lee et al. 2018
	6-gingerol also showed antibacterial activity against *Acinetobacter baumannii, Klebsiella pneumoniae, Pseudomonas aeruginosa*, and *Staphylococcus aureus.*	Elfaky et al. 2024
	6-gingerol also showed effective antibacterial activity against *M. tuberculosis* strains H37Rv, the multidrug-resistant MDR (JAL-2261), the drug-resistant XDR (MYC-431).	Bhaskar et al. 2020
6-Dehydrogingerdione, 6-shogaol, 10-gingerol, and 6-gingerol	Effective against drug-resistant *A. baumannii.*	Wang et al. 2010
Zingerone, raffinose, 6-gingerol and analogs of 6- and 8-gingerol	Antibacterial activity against *P. aeruginosa.*	Lee et al. 2018
Ginger essential oil	Antibacterial activity against *P. vulgaris, K. pneumoniae* where it formed an inhibition halo of 18.4 mm and 20.5 mm.	Singh et al. 2008
	Antimicrobial effect against *B. cereus, L. monocytogenes, S. aureus, E. coli, S. typhimurium.*	Bag and Chattopadhyay 2015
	Ginger essential oil with 6-, 8-, and 10-shogaol when used at a concentration of 100 µg/mL, it shows antifungal activity against *C. albicans* (25 mm halo), *G. candidum* (21 mm halo), *F. oxysporum* (22 mm halo), *A. flavus* (20 mm halo).	Ghasemzadeh et al. 2018

Source: Authors.

(E) Neem (*Azadirachta indica*, Family: Meliaceae)

Neem is one of the most widely used plants, known for its antibacterial and antifungal effects, particularly in treating skin infections. It's an evergreen tree which has been extensively used in Ayurveda, Unani, and traditional Chinese medications for several centuries for treating various infections and diseases (Herrera-Calderon et al. 2019). In India, they have been used for over 4,000 years since Vedic times (Mandal and Mandal 2011). *Azadirachta indica* is native to India and Myanmar and revered as the "Divine tree" or "The village pharmacy" for its innumerable health benefits (Islas et al. 2020). Neem and its extract have been used as insect repellent, as antibacterial agents, for health supplements, for combating inflammation, diabetes, and even cancer. The various parts of the neem tree have different medicinal properties. The different plant parts like bark, leaves, flowers, fruits, seeds, and oil have insecticidal, larvicidal, antifungal, antimalarial, antibacterial, anti-inflammatory, antiulcer, antiallergic, hypolipidemic, hypotensive, and hyperglycaemic activities (Aslam et al. 2009; Campos et al. 2016). There are thirty-five biologically active constituents that show antimicrobial activity (Herrera-Calderon et al. 2019).

a. **Azadirachtin ($C_{35}H_{44}O_{16}$):** It is a tetranortriterpenoid (limonoids), obtained from seeds, fruits, leaves, and callus of neem, with the highest concentration being in the neem seed. Azadirachtin has antimalarial and antimicrobial properties.
b. **Nimbin ($C_{30}H_{36}O_9$):** Nimbin is a bitter triterpenoid compound obtained from neem oil. It has anti-inflammatory, fungicidal, and antibacterial potential (Gupta et al. 2017). When extracted and dissolved with chloroform, nimbin shows activity against *E. coli* (Usman, Fitzsimmons-Thoss, and Tawfike 2020). Nimbin,

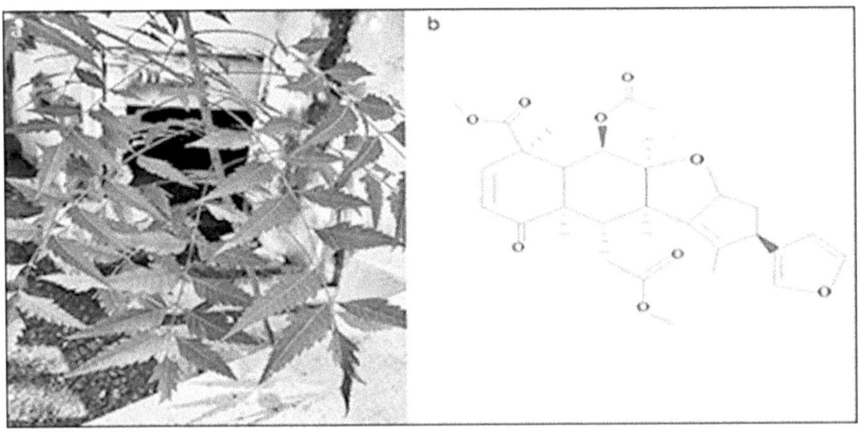

Figure 10.6. a. *Azadirachta indica* plant, b. Chemical structure of Nimbin. Source: Author.

nimbinin, and nimbidin found in neem leaves are together responsible for disrupting the cell membrane of different bacteria and their metabolic processes (Wylie and Merrell 2022). Some other potent antimicrobial phytochemicals include azadiradione, azadirone, nimbolide, and gedunin (Gupta et al. 2017) (Figure 10.6).

Neem exhibits broad-spectrum antimicrobial activity against a diverse array of pathogens, including *Staphylococcus aureus*, *Enterococcus faecalis*, *Candida albicans*, and *Streptococcus mutans* (Mistry et al. 2014; Singh et al. 2020; Wylie and Merrell 2022). Research has demonstrated that neem-based toothpaste effectively reduces the presence of *S. mutans* in the oral cavity, while also serving as a preventive measure against gingivitis and plaque buildup (Selvaraj et al. 2020; Nimbulkar et al. 2020) (Table 10.5).

Traditionally Neem leaves are used for treating several diseases like malaria, dental and gastrointestinal disorders, fevers, and skin diseases in India (Sujarwo et al. 2016). Neem-based products are traditionally used in pest control in gardening and agriculture in India (Habluetzel, Lucantoni, and Esposito 2009). Neem oil is applied during skin diseases like furuncles and eczema, and for relieving intestinal worm infections (Forster and Moser 2000). The use of neem is mentioned in ancient Ayurvedic scriptures, "Charaka Samhita" and "Sushruta Samhita," where it is mentioned how neem was used traditionally in the form of decoction, infusion, extract, powders, and medicated oil. Neem has the potential in curing diseases like ulcers (vrna), vomiting (vami), worms (krimi), and swelling (sopha). It reduces the bad effects of poisonous bites (Srirangarayan, Ramasamy, Thangam 2020).

(F) **Ghrito-kumari or Aloe vera (*Aloe barbadensis*, Family: Asphodelaceae)**

Aloe vera is widely known for its soothing properties, especially for skin conditions, but it also possesses significant antimicrobial activity. The gel from Aloe vera leaves contains compounds such as anthraquinones, saponins, and lectins, which contribute to its antibacterial and antifungal properties. Aloe vera has been shown to be effective against a variety of pathogens, including *Staphylococcus aureus*, *Escherichia coli*, and *Candida albicans* (Surjushe et al. 2008). The antimicrobial effects of Aloe vera are attributed to its ability to inhibit bacterial growth and reduce inflammation at the site of infection. Additionally, Aloe vera is used in traditional medicine for treating skin infections, wounds, and burns, where its antimicrobial properties play a key role in preventing infection and promoting healing.

(G) Chotra (*Lantana camara*, Family: Verbenaceae)

Lantana camara, a plant often used in folk medicine for its anti-inflammatory and antimicrobial effects, has shown promising results against various bacterial and fungal pathogens. Extracts from its leaves, flowers, and stems have demonstrated activity against *Staphylococcus aureus*, *Escherichia coli*, and *Candida albicans* (Dua,

Table 10.5. Antimicrobial Activity of Neem

Source	Antimicrobial Activity	References
Neem leaf and bark extract	Inhibition of *Escherichia coli* O157:H7 from cultured specimen of cow manure. This has application in farms and orchards that are adjacent to cattle.	Ravva and Korn 2015
Neem leaf extract	The extract containing tannins, saponins, terpenoids, alkaloids showed antibacterial activity against *E. coli* concentration of 58.77%.	Sahrawat et al. 2018
	Active against *Acinetobacter baumannii. Citrobacter* spp, *E. coli, Proteus* spp, *K. pneumoniae, P. aeruginosa, and Enterobacter* spp.	Faujdar, Bisht, and Sharma 2020
	Neem leaf extract is effective in improving the CD4+ T cell counts in HIV infected patients when administered regularly.	Mbah et al. 2007
Neem extract	Active against different biofilm-forming bacteria like *Porphyromonas gingivalis, Streptococcus viridans, S. aureus*, and fungi like *Candida albicans*.	Anand et al. 2016; Bansal et al. 2019; Andonissamy et al. 2019; Tasanarong, Patntirapong, and Aupaphong 2021; Wylie and Merrell 2022
	Active against the biofilm-forming bacteria *Enterococcus faecalis* that affects the human body.	Mustafa 2016; Bhardwaj et al. 2017
	An aqueous neem extract is effective against *Vibrio parahaemolyticus* that affects shrimp quality thereby improving survival rate of shrimp by 76%.	Morales-Covarrubias et al. 2016
Neem cake extract	Ethyl acetate extract of neem cake is active against different bacteria that affect meat quality like *Campylobacter jejuni, Lactobacillus curvatus, Carnobacterium* sp, and *Leuconostoc* sp.	Del Serrone, Failla, and Nicoletti 2015
Neem bark, leaf, and twig extract	Effective against the bacteria *Streptococcus mutans* with an inhibition zone of 11.81 mm.	Kumari et al. 2019
Methanolic, ethanolic, and aqueous neem extracts from stem, leaf, and bark	These have shown significant antimalarial activity against different *Plasmodium falciparum* and *Plasmodium berghei* strains.	Tepongning et al. 2018; Wylie and Merrell 2022
Neem polysaccharides (P1 and P2) and their sulphated derivatives (P1S and P2S)	They can inhibit HSV-1 nucleic acid synthesis. Antiviral activity is due to interference in the early stages of HSV-1 replication.	Faccin-Galhardi et al. 2019
Azadirachtin	Azadirachtin is effective against cerebral malaria.	Okoh et al. 2021
Nimbin	It is effective against the envelope protein of all 4 types of Dengue virus.	Lavanya, Ramaiah, Anbarasu 2015
Nimbocinol	It binds to papain-like protease of SARS-CoV-2 and is capable of hindering viral replication.	Balkrishna, Mittal, Arya 2021

Source: Authors.

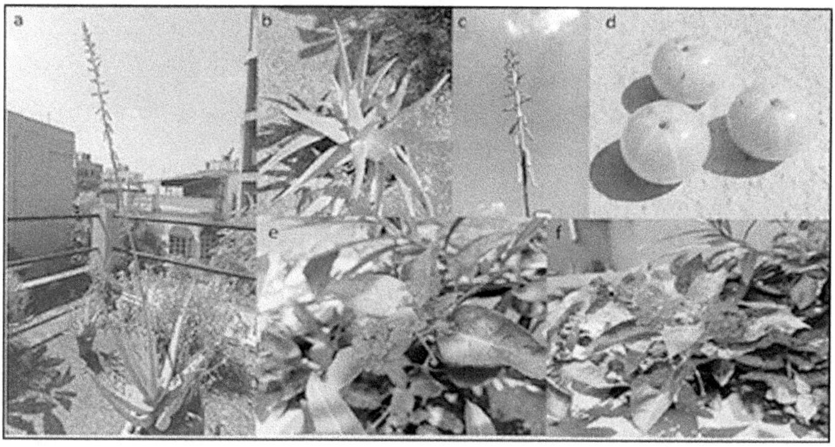

Figure 10.7. a–b. Aloe vera plant, c. Inflorescence of Aloe vera, d. *Phyllanthus emblica*, e–f. *Lantana camara*. Source: Author.

Kumar, and Suman 2010). The antimicrobial properties of *Lantana camara* are thought to be due to its rich composition of flavonoids, terpenoids, and phenolic compounds, which interfere with microbial cell wall synthesis and disrupt cellular function. *Lantana camara's* ability to combat a wide range of infections makes it a valuable plant in traditional medicine, especially for treating topical infections and wounds (Figure 10.7).

Discussion and Conclusion

The antimicrobial activities of ethnomedicinal plants such as ginger (*Zingiber officinale*), tulsi (*Ocimum tenuiflorum*), turmeric (*Curcuma longa*), neem (*Azadirachta indica*), garlic (*Allium sativum*), aloe vera, *Lantana camara*, and so on, provide compelling evidence for their long-standing use in traditional medicine systems around the world. These plants have been extensively utilized for their ability to combat a variety of infectious agents, including bacteria, fungi, and viruses, thus playing an essential role in maintaining human health and well-being. The antimicrobial properties of these plants are attributed to their diverse array of bioactive compounds such as gingerols, curcumin, allicin, eugenol, nimbin, flavonoids, and saponins, which have demonstrated efficacy against common and drug-resistant pathogens. For instance, ginger has shown significant antibacterial and antifungal effects, particularly against gastrointestinal pathogens, while tulsi has proven antiviral and antibacterial benefits, particularly in respiratory and skin infections. Turmeric is a well-known anti-inflammatory and antimicrobial agent, with curcumin exerting antibacterial and antifungal actions. Similarly, garlic contains allicin, a powerful compound that is particularly effective against both gram-positive and gram-negative bacteria. Neem,

Table 10.6. Antimicrobial Activity of Some Other Ethnomedicinal Plants

Taxa	Source of Antimicrobial Activity	Antimicrobial Activity	Ethnobotanical Importance	References
Aloe vera Family: *Asphodelaceae*	*Aloe vera* gel extract	Significant activity against *Klebsiella pneumoniae* and *E.coli* and fungi like *Aspergillus niger* and *Candida*.	Used to treat wounds and cuts. Also used for treating sunburns, burns, inflammatory skin problems.	Kedarnath et al. 2013; Dal'Belo, Gaspar, and Campos 2006
		The gel extracts showed effective antimicrobial activity against skin infection pathogens like *Salmonella* spp., *Escherichia coli*, *Shigella*, and *Staphylococcus aureus*.		Arbab et al. 2021
Lantana camara Family: Verbenaceae	Leaf, flower extract	Water extract is most effective against a host of pathogens like *E. coli*, *P. aeruginosa*, *S. aureus*, *B. cereus*, *S. typhi*, *K. aerogenes*, *P. vulgaris*, *S. boydii*, *A. fumigatus*; *A. flavus*; *A. niger*; *C. albicans*.	Leaf extract is used as antimicrobial agent in skin diseases.	Dabur et al. 2007
		Ethanolic leaf extract was active against *P. vulgaris and V. cholerae* while the root extract was active against *P. vulgaris* and *P. aeruginosa*.		Barreto et al. 2010

Ashoka (*Saraca asoca*) Family: Fabaceae	Bark extract	Water extract is most effective against a host of pathogens like *E. coli*; *S. typhi*, *P. aeruginosa*; *S. aureus*; *B. cereus*; *K. aerogenes*, *P. vulgaris*, *Shigella boydii*, *A. fumigatus*; *A. flavus*; *A. niger*; *C. albicans*.	Bark is used for treatment of pimple, bowel related diseases.	Dabur et al. 2007
Amla (*Phyllanthus emblica*) Family: Euphorbiaceae	Fruit and Seed extract	Water extract is most effective against a host of pathogens like *S. typhi*, *P. aeruginosa*; *S. aureus*; *B. cereus*; *K. aerogenes*, *P. vulgaris*, *Shigella boydii*.	Used in treatment of asthma, bronchitis.	Dabur et al. 2007
		Methanolic extract showed activity against *Bacillus subtilis*, *Staphylococcus aureus*, and *Shigella dysenteriae*. In another study, it was effective against *S. typhi* and *S. enteritidis*.		Tjipta et al. 2023
Bael *(Aegle marmelos)* Family: Rutaceae	Fruit extract	Methanolic extract is effective against pathogens like *E. coli*; *S. typhi*, *P. aeruginosa*; *S. aureus*; *B. cereus*; *K. aerogenes*, *P. vulgaris*, *Shigella boydii*.	It is used in the treatment of diarrhea and dysentery.	Dabur et al. 2007

Source: Authors.

with its broad spectrum of antimicrobial activity, has been used in treating skin diseases, and aloe vera is particularly noted for its ability to address skin infections, wounds, and burns. Aloe vera and *Lantana camara* further expand the range of natural antimicrobial agents, particularly for skin and topical infections. Amla and *Aegle marmelos* contribute antioxidant and antimicrobial benefits, promoting both immune health and infection prevention.

These ethnomedicinal plants are traditionally used for medicinal purposes in different cultures and serve as potential alternatives to synthetic antibiotics because they offer a diverse range of bioactive compounds with antimicrobial properties, often acting through multiple mechanisms, while also potentially addressing the whole body system rather than just targeting a single pathogen, leading to a more holistic approach to healthcare. Thus, these studied ethnomedicinal plants not only offer potential alternatives to synthetic antibiotics but also present a more holistic approach to infection prevention and treatment. Their ability to combat infections, reduce inflammation, and modulate immune responses places them in a unique position to be used both preventively and therapeutically. Furthermore, the increasing prevalence of antibiotic resistance underscores the need for continued exploration and integration of these natural antimicrobial agents into modern medical practices.

The growing body of research into the mechanisms underlying the antimicrobial properties of these plants highlights their therapeutic potential, suggesting that their bioactive compounds may serve as templates for developing novel antimicrobial drugs. However, while promising, further clinical studies are needed to confirm their efficacy, optimize dosages, and evaluate any potential side effects or interactions with conventional medicines. Additionally, research into the synergistic effects of these plants, either with one another or with existing antibiotics, could lead to enhanced therapeutic strategies. In conclusion, the antimicrobial properties of ethnomedicinal plants like ginger, tulsi, turmeric, neem, garlic, and aloe vera are well-documented and represent a rich source of natural compounds that could significantly contribute to combating infectious diseases. With the growing concerns about antibiotic resistance and the global push toward sustainable healthcare practices, these plants offer valuable, cost-effective, and accessible alternatives or adjuncts to conventional antimicrobial therapies.

References

Agarwal, R., S. Gupta, and R. Singh. "Garlic and Its Medicinal Properties in Ayurveda." *International Journal of Pharmacology* 3, no. 1 (2007): 1–8.

Ali, S. S., M. A. Ali, and N. Lall. "Curcuma Longa L. (Turmeric) and Its Medicinal Applications: A Review." *Phytotherapy Research* 22, no. 5 (2008): 635–49.

Anand, P., S. G. Thomas, A. B. Kunnumakkara, C. Sundaram, K. B. Harikumar, B. Sung, S. T. Tharakan, K. Misra, I. K. Priyadarsini, K. N. Rajasekharan, and B. B. Aggarwal. "Biological Activities of Curcumin and Its Analogues (Congeners) Made by Man and Mother Nature." *Biochemical Pharmacology* 76 (2008): 1590–611.

Anand, P. J., A. S. Athira, S. Chandramohan, K. Ranjith, V. V. Raj, and V. D. Manjula. "Comparison of Efficacy of Herbal Disinfectants with Chlorhexidine Mouthwash on Decontamination of Toothbrushes: An Experimental Trial." *Journal of the International Society of Preventive and Community Dentistry* 6, no. 1 (2016): 22–7.

Andonissamy, L., S. Karthigeyan, S. A. Ali, and J. W. Felix. "Effect of Chemical Denture Disinfectants and Tree Extracts on Biofilm-Forming *Staphylococcus aureus* and *Viridans Streptococcus* Species Isolated from Complete Denture." *Journal of Contemporary Dental Practice* 20, no. 11 (2019): 1307–14.

Arbab, S., H. Ullah, W. Weiwei, X. Wei, S. U. Ahmad, L. Wu, and J. Zhang. "Comparative Study of Antimicrobial Action of Aloe Vera and Antibiotics against Different Bacterial Isolates from Skin Infection." *Veterinary Medicine and Science* 7, no. 5 (2021): 2061–7.

Aslam, F., K. U. Rehman, M. Asghar, and M. Sarwar. "Antibacterial Activity of Various Phytoconstituents of Neem." *Pakistan Journal of Agricultural Sciences* 46, no. 3 (2009): 209–13.

Atnafu, H., T. Awas, S. Alemu, and S. Wube. "Ethnobotanical Study of Medicinal Plants in Selale Mountain Ridges, North Shewa Zone, Ethiopia." *Biodiversity International Journal* 2, no. 6 (2018): 567–77.

Bae, H., et al. "Antibacterial Activity of Garlic Extract Against *Staphylococcus aureus*." *Journal of Antimicrobial Chemotherapy* 54, no. 2 (2004): 209–15.

Bag, A., and R. R. Chattopadhyay. "Evaluation of Synergistic Antibacterial and Antioxidant Efficacy of Essential Oils of Spices and Herbs in Combination." *PLoS ONE* 10, no. 7 (2015): e0131321.

Balkrishna, A., R. Mittal, and V. Arya. "Computational Evidences of Phytochemical Mediated Disruption of PLpro Driven Replication of SARS-CoV-2: A Therapeutic Approach Against COVID-19." *Current Pharmaceutical Biotechnology* 22, no. 10 (2021): 1350–9.

Bansal, V., M. Gupta, T. Bhaduri, S. A. Shaikh, F. R. Sayed, and V. Bansal. "Assessment of Antimicrobial Effectiveness of Neem and Clove Extract Against *Streptococcus mutans* and *Candida albicans*: An In Vitro Study." *Nigerian Medical Journal* 60, no. 6 (2019): 285–9.

Barreto, F., E. Sousa, A. Campos, J. Costa, and F. Rodrigues. "Antibacterial Activity of *Lantana camara* Linn and *Lantana montevidensis* Brig Extracts from Cariri-Ceará, Brazil." *Journal of Young Pharmacists* 2, no. 1 (2010): 42–4.

Bhardwaj, A., N. Srivastava, V. Rana, V. K. Adlakha, and A. K. Asthana. "How Efficacious Are Neem, Tulsi, Guduchi Extracts and Chlorhexidine as Intracanal Disinfectants? A Comparative Ex Vivo Study." *Ayu* 38, no. 1–2 (2017): 70–5.

Bhaskar, A., A. Kumari, M. Singh, S. Kumar, S. Kumar, A. Dabla, S. Chaturvedi, V. Yadav, D. Chattopadhyay, and D. V. Prakash. "[6]-Gingerol Exhibits Potent Anti-Mycobacterial and Immunomodulatory Activity Against Tuberculosis." *International Immunopharmacology* 87 (2020): 106809.

Bhatwalkar, S. B., et al. "Antibacterial Properties of Organosulfur Compounds of Garlic (Allium sativum)." *Frontiers in Microbiology* 12 (2021): 1–20.

Block, E. "The Chemistry of Garlic and Onions." *Scientific American* 252 (1985): 114–19.

Bode, A. M., and Z. Dong. "The Amazing and Mighty Ginger." In *Herbal Medicine: Biomolecular and Clinical Aspects*, 2nd ed., Chapter 7, edited by I. F. F. Benzie and S. Wachtel-Galor, 133–47. Boca Raton: CRC Press, 2011.

Borchers, A. T., et al. "Garlic (*Allium sativum*): A Review of Its Protective Effects Against Cancer and Cardiovascular Disease." *Alternative Medicine Review* 9, no. 2 (2004): 104–12.

Borlinghaus, J., F. Albrecht, M. C. H. Gruhlke, I. D. Nwachukwu, and A. J. Slusarenko. "Allicin: Chemistry and Biological Properties." *Molecules* 19, no. 8 (2014): 12591–618.

Campos, E. V., J. L. de Oliveira, M. Pascoli, R. de Lima, and L. F. Fraceto. "Neem Oil and Crop Protection: From Now to the Future." *Frontiers in Plant Science* 7 (2016): 1494.

Cavallito, C., and J. Bailey. "Allicin, the Antibacterial Principle of *Allium sativum*. I. Isolation, Physical Properties, and Antibacterial Action." *Journal of the American Chemical Society* 66 (1944): 1950–1.

Chaudhary, P., A. Pal, and M. Gupta. "Ocimum tenuiflorum (Tulsi): A Review of Its Antimicrobial and Therapeutic Potentials." *Phytochemical Reviews* 17, no. 3 (2018): 745–62.

Chibuzo, U. C. "Antimicrobial Activity of Azadirachta indica (Neem) Leaf Extract on Some Bacteria." International Journal of Current Microbiology and Applied Sciences 8, no. 7 (2019): 431–7.

Cohen, M. M., et al. "Garlic: A Review of Its Antimicrobial Properties." *International Journal of Medicinal Plants* 5, no. 2 (2017): 44–50.

Curtis, H., U. Noll, J. Störmann, and A. J. Slusarenko. "Broad-Spectrum Activity of the Volatile Phytoanticipin Allicin in Extracts of Garlic (*Allium sativum* L.) Against Plant Pathogenic Bacteria, Fungi, and Oomycetes." *Physiological and Molecular Plant Pathology* 65 (2004): 79–89.

Cutler, R. R., and P. Wilson. "Antibacterial Activity of a New, Stable, Aqueous Extract of Allicin Against Methicillin-Resistant *Staphylococcus aureus*." *British Journal of Biomedical Science* 61 (2004): 71–4.

Dabur, R., A. Gupta, T. K. Mandal, D. D. Singh, V. Bajpai, A. M. Gurav, and G. S. Lavekar. "Antimicrobial Activity of Some Indian Medicinal Plants." *African Journal of Traditional, Complementary, and Alternative Medicines* 4, no. 3 (2007): 313–18.

Dal'Belo, S. E., L. R. Gaspar, and P. M. B. G. M. Campos. "Moisturizing Effect of Cosmetic Formulations Containing Aloe Vera Extract in Different Concentrations Assessed by Skin Bioengineering Techniques." *Skin Research and Technology* 12 (2006): 241–6.

Das, S., S. S. Nadar, and V. K. Rathod. "Integrated Strategies for Enzyme-Assisted Extraction of Bioactive Molecules: A Review." *International Journal of Biological Macromolecules* 191 (2021): 899–917.

Devi, A., K. Rakshit, and B. Sarania. "Ethnobotanical Notes on *Allium* Species of Arunachal Pradesh, India." *Indian Journal of Traditional Knowledge* 13 (2014): 606–12.

De, R., P. Kundu, S. Swarnakar, T. Ramamurthy, A. Chowdhury, G. B. Nair, and A. K. Mukhopadhyay. "Antimicrobial Activity of Curcumin Against *Helicobacter pylori* Isolates from India and During Infections in Mice." *Antimicrobial Agents and Chemotherapy* 53, no. 4 (2009): 159.

Del Serrone, P., S. Failla, and M. Nicoletti. "Natural Control of Bacteria Affecting Meat Quality by a Neem (*Azadirachta indica* A. Juss) Cake Extract." *Natural Product Research* 29, no. 10 (2015): 985–7.

Dua, V. K., S. Kumar, and R. Suman. "Antimicrobial Activity of *Lantana camara* Linn." *Indian Journal of Experimental Biology* 48 (2010): 1083–7.

Elafify, M., M. T. Elabbasy, R. Samir, E. Ali, W. Fathy, W. Eldin, W. Darwish, E. Eldrehmy, and R. Reda. "Prevalence of Multidrug-Resistant *Listeria monocytogenes* in Dairy

Products with Reduction Trials Using Rosmarinic Acid, Ascorbic Acid, Clove, and Thyme Essential Oils." *Journal of Food Quality* 2022, no. 1 (2022): 1–12.

Elfaky, M. A., Okairy, H. M., Abdallah, H. M., Koshak, A. E., Mohamed, G. A., Ibrahim, S. R. M., Alzain, A. A., Hegazy, W. A. H., Khafagy, E. S., & Seleem, N. M. "Assessing the Antibacterial Potential of 6-gingerol: Combined Experimental and Computational Approaches." Saudi Pharmaceutical Journal 32, no. 5 (2024): 1–13.

Faccin-Galhardi, L. C., S. Ray, N. Lopes, I. Ali, S. F. Espada, J. P. Dos Santos, et al. "Assessment of Antiherpetic Activity of Nonsulfated and Sulfated Polysaccharides from *Azadirachta indica*." *International Journal of Biological Macromolecules* 137 (2019): 54–61.

Faujdar, S., D. Bisht, and A. Sharma. "Antibacterial Potential of Neem (*Azadirachta indica*) Against Uropathogens Producing Beta-Lactamase Enzymes: A Clue to Future Antibacterial Agent?" *Biomedicine and Biotechnology Research Journal* 4, no. 3 (2020): 232–8.

Faye, G., T. Birhanu, and T. Belete. "Survey and Antimicrobial Activity Study of Ethnomedicinal Plants in Selected Districts of North Shewa Zone, Oromia, Ethiopia." *Infection and Drug Resistance* 14 (2021): 2619–31.

Forster, P., and G. Moser. *Status Report on Global Neem Usage*. Deutsche Gesellschaft für Technische Zusammenarbeit (GTZ), 2000.

Fujisawa, H., K. Watanabe, K. Suma, K. Origuchi, H. Matsufuji, T. Seki, and T. Ariga. "Antibacterial Potential of Garlic-Derived Allicin and Its Cancellation by Sulfhydryl Compounds." *Bioscience, Biotechnology, and Biochemistry* 73 (2009): 1948–55.

Ghasemzadeh, A., H. Jaafar, A. Baghdadi, and A. Tayebi-Meigooni. "Formation of 6-, 8-, and 10-Shogaol in Ginger Through Application of Different Drying Methods: Altered Antioxidant and Antimicrobial Activity." *Molecules* 23, no. 7 (2018): 1646.

Gupta, R., M. G. Vairale, R. R. Deshmukh, P. R. Chaudhary, and S. R. Wate. "Ethnomedicinal Uses of Some Plants Used by Gond Tribe of Bhandara District, Maharashtra." *Indian Journal of Traditional Knowledge* 9 (2010): 713–17.

Gupta, S., and S. Ravishankar. "A Comparison of the Antimicrobial Activity of Garlic, Ginger, Carrot, and Turmeric Paste against Escherichia coli O157:H7 in Laboratory Buffer and Ground Beef." *Foodborne Pathogens and Disease* 2, no. 4 (2005): 330–40.

Gupta, S. C., S. Prasad, A. K. Tyagi, A. B. Kunnumakkara, and B. B. Aggarwal. "Neem (*Azadirachta indica*): An Indian Traditional Panacea with Modern Molecular Basis." *Phytomedicine* 34 (2017): 14–20.

Habluetzel, A., L. Lucantoni, and F. Esposito. "Azadirachta indica as a Public Health Tool for the Control of Malaria and Other Vector-Borne Diseases." *Indian Journal of Medical Research* 130, no. 2 (2009): 112–14.

Herrera-Calderon, O., K. Ejaz, M. Wajid, M. Shehzad, J. A. Tinco-Jayo, E. Enciso-Roca, et al. "Azadirachta indica: Antibacterial Activity of Neem Against Different Strains of Bacteria and Their Active Constituents as Preventive in Various Diseases." *Pharmacognosy Journal* 11, no. 6 (2019): 1597–604.

Islas, J. F., E. Acosta, Z. G. Buentello, J. L. Delgado-Gallegos, M. G. Moreno-Treviño, B. Escalante, J. E. Moreno-Cuevas. "An Overview of Neem (*Azadirachta indica*) and Its Potential Impact on Health." *Journal of Functional Foods* 74 (2020): 104171.

Iweala, E. J., M. E. Uche, E. D. Dike, and E. A. Ugbogu. "Curcuma longa (Turmeric): Ethnomedicinal Uses, Phytochemistry, Pharmacological Activities, and Toxicity

Profiles-A Review." In *Natural Products with Pharmacological Potential*, edited by O. O. Olatunji, vol. 2. Bentham Science Publishers, 2023.

Jacob, J. "Comparative Studies in Relation to the Structure and Biochemical Properties of the Active Compounds in the Volatile and Non-Volatile Fractions of *Turmeric* (*Curcuma longa*) and *Ginger* (Zingiber officinale)." *Studies in Natural Products Chemistry* 48 (2016): 101–35.

Jain, A., A. Mehta, S. Jain, and G. Saxena. "Antimicrobial Activity of Tulsi (*Ocimum sanctum* Linn): A Systematic Review." *International Journal of Research in Ayurveda and Pharmacy* 13, no. 4 (2022): 111.

Jonkers, D., et al. "Antimicrobial Properties of allicin from Garlic." *Microbes and Infection* 1, no. 2 (1999): 125–9.

Karuppiah, P., and S. Rajaram. "Antibacterial Effect of *Allium sativum* Cloves and *Zingiber officinale* Rhizomes Against Multiple-Drug Resistant Clinical Pathogens." *Asian Pacific Journal of Tropical Biomedicine* 2, no. 8 (2012): 597–601.

Kedarnath, K., Dr. Kaveri, V. Chimkod, and C. Patil. "Antimicrobial Activity of Aloe Vera Leaf Extract." *International Journal of Applied Biology and Pharmaceutical Technology* 4, no. 4 (2013): 286–90.

Kernou, O. N., Z. Azzouz, K. Madani, and P. Rijo. "Application of Rosmarinic Acid with Its Derivatives in the Treatment of Microbial Pathogens." *Molecules* 28, no. 10 (2023): 4243.

Khan, R., A. Malik, J. Ahmad, and M. M. A. Rizvi. "Anticandidal Activity of Curcumin and Methyl Cinnamaldehyde." *Fitoterapia* 83, no. 4 (2012): 643–9.

Kheira, M., M. Boumediene, T. T. Aicha, and P. Sonnet. "Chemical Composition and Antioxidant and Antimicrobial Activities of Curcuma longa L. Essential Oils." *Egyptian Journal of Chemistry* 66, no. 7 (2023): 283–95.

Kim, M.-K., G.-J. Choi, and H.-S. Lee. "Fungicidal Property of *Curcuma longa* L. Rhizome-Derived Curcumin Against Phytopathogenic Fungi in a Greenhouse." *Journal of Agricultural and Food Chemistry* 51 (2003): 1578–81.

Kumar, A., S. Dhamgaye, I. K. Maurya, A. Singh, M. Sharma, and R. Prasad. "Curcumin Targets Cell Wall Integrity via Calcineurin-mediated Signaling in *Candida albicans*." *Antimicrobial Agents and Chemotherapy* 58, no. 1 (2016): 167–75.

Kumari, D. P., S. M. Shenoy, S. Khijmatgar, A. Chowdhury, E. Lynch, and C. R. Chowdhury. "Antibacterial Activity of New Atraumatic Restorative Treatment Materials Incorporated with Azadirachta indica (Neem) against Streptococcus mutans." *Journal of Oral Biology and Craniofacial Research* 9, no. 4 (2019): 321–5.

Lahiri, D., M. Nag, B. Dutta, S. Dey, D. Mukherjee, S. J. Joshi, and R. R. Ray. "Antibiofilm and Anti-Quorum Sensing Activities of Eugenol and Linalool from *Ocimum tenuiflorum* Against *Pseudomonas aeruginosa* Biofilm." *Journal of Applied Microbiology* 131, no. 6 (2021): 2821–37.

Lavanya, P., S. Ramaiah, and A. Anbarasu. "Computational Analysis Reveals Inhibitory Action of Nimbin Against Dengue Viral Envelope Protein." *Virus Disease* 26, no. 4 (2015): 243–54.

Lee, J. H., Y. G. Kim, P. Choi, J. Ham, J. G. Park, and J. Lee. "Antibiofilm and Antivirulence Activities of 6-Gingerol and 6-Shogaol Against *Candida albicans* Due to Hyphal Inhibition." *Frontiers in Cellular and Infection Microbiology* 8 (2018): 299.

Maghraby, Y. R., R. M. Labib, M. Sobeh, and M. A. Farag. "Gingerols and Shogaols: A Multi-Faceted Review of Their Extraction, Formulation, and Analysis in Drugs and

Biofluids to Maximize Their Nutraceutical and Pharmaceutical Applications." *Food Chemistry: X* 20 (2023): 100947.

Mahmood, Z., H. Tabassum, and K. Javed. "Antimicrobial Activity of Ocimum sanctum L. (Tulsi) Essential Oil against Clinical Isolates of Escherichia coli, Pseudomonas aeruginosa, and Staphylococcus aureus." *Indian Journal of Pharmaceutical Sciences* 70, no. 6 (2008): 837–40.

Mallikarjun, S., A. Rao, G. Rajesh, R. Shenoy, and M. Pai. "Antimicrobial Efficacy of Tulsi Leaf (*Ocimum sanctum*) Extract on Periodontal Pathogens: An In Vitro Study." *Journal of Indian Society of Periodontology* 20, no. 2 (2016): 145–50.

Mandal, S., and M. Mandal. "The Ayurvedic, Unani, and modern scientific perspectives of neem (Azadirachta indica)." *The Internet Journal of Alternative Medicine* 10, no. 1 (2011): 1–6.

Mao, Y.-F., Y.-Z. Li, J.-X. Wang, K. Xiong, and J.-X. Li. "Cooling Ability/Capacity and Exergy Penalty Analysis of Each Heat Sink of Modern Supersonic Aircraft." *Entropy* 21, no. 3 (2019): 223.

Mbah, A. U., I. J. Udeinya, E. N. Shu, C. P. Chijioke, T. Nubila, F. Udeinya, et al. "Fractionated Neem Leaf Extract Is Safe and Increases CD4+ Cell Levels in HIV/AIDS Patients." *American Journal of Therapeutics* 14, no. 4 (2007): 369–74.

Mistry, K. S., Z. Sanghvi, G. Parmar, and S. Shah. "The Antimicrobial Activity of *Azadirachta indica, Mimusops elengi, Tinospora cordifolia, Ocimum sanctum* and 2% Chlorhexidine Gluconate on Common Endodontic Pathogens: An In Vitro Study." *European Journal of Dentistry* 8, no. 2 (2014): 172–7.

Mishra, S., P. Singh, and P. Pandey. "Medicinal Properties of *Ocimum tenuiflorum* (Tulsi): A Review." *Journal of Medicinal Plants Studies* 4, no. 5 (2016): 177–82.

Morales-Covarrubias, M. S., N. García-Aguilar, M. D. Bolan-Mejía, and A. C. Puello-Cruz. "Evaluation of Medicinal Plants and Colloidal Silver Efficiency Against *Vibrio parahaemolyticus* Infection in *Litopenaeus vannamei* Cultured at Low Salinity." *Diseases of Aquatic Organisms* 122, no. 1 (2016): 57–65.

Moulin, T., et al. "Influence of Garlic on the Immune Response." *Journal of Ethnopharmacology* 130, no. 2 (2010): 406–15.

Müller, A., J. Eller, F. Albrecht, P. Prochnow, K. Kuhlmann, J. E. Bandow, A. J. Slusarenko, and L. I. Leichert. "Allicin Induces Thiol Stress in Bacteria Through S-Alylmercapto Modification of Protein Cysteines." *Journal of Biological Chemistry* 291 (2016): 11477–90.

Mustafa, M. "Antibacterial Efficacy of Neem (*Azadirachta indica*) Extract Against *Enterococcus faecalis*: An In Vitro Study." *Journal of Contemporary Dental Practice* 17, no. 10 (2016): 791–4.

Murthy, S. M., and G. M. Vidyasagar. "Traditional Knowledge on Medicinal Plants Used in the Treatment of Respiratory Disorders in Bellary District, Karnataka, India." *Indian Journal of Natural Products and Resources* 4 (2013): 189–93.

Nabavi, S. F., A. Sureda, M. Daglia, E. Sobarzo-Sánchez, and S. M. Nabavi. "Curcumin: A Natural Product for Pharmacological Applications." *Journal of Pharmacy and Pharmacology* 67, no. 2 (2015): 200–25.

Nakamoto, M., K. Kunimura, J. I. Suzuki, and Y. Kodera. "Antimicrobial Properties of Hydrophobic Compounds in Garlic: Allicin, Vinyldithiin, Ajoene, and Diallyl Polysulfides." *Experimental and Therapeutic Medicine* 19, no. 2 (2020): 1550–3.

Narasimhan, M., S. Maheshwaran, I. A. Abu-Yousef, A. F. Majdalawieh, J. Rethavathi, P. E. Das, and P. Poltronieri. "Anti-Bacterial and Anti-Fungal Activity of Xanthones Obtained via Semi-Synthetic Modification of α-Mangostin from Garcinia mangostana." *Molecules* 22, no. 2 (2017): 275.

Nigam, G., and N. K. Sharma. "Ethnoveterinary Plants of Jhansi District, Uttar Pradesh." *Indian Journal of Traditional Knowledge*, 9 (2010): 664–7.

Nimbulkar, K. A., S. T. Gajbhiye, and R. H. Deshpande. "Neem-based Toothpaste for Prevention of Oral Diseases." *Journal of Indian Dental Association* 14, no. 4 (2020): 69–72.

Odo, E. O., J. A. Ikwuegbu, E. I. Obeagu, S. A. Chibueze, and R. E. Ochiaka. "Analysis of the Antibacterial Effects of Turmeric on Particular Bacteria." *Medicine (Baltimore)*, 102, no. 48 (2023): e36492.

Ohta, R., N. Yamada, H. Kaneko, K. Ishikawa, H. Fukuda, T. Fujino, and A. Suzuki. "In Vitro Inhibition of the Growth of *Helicobacter pylori* by Oil-Macerated Garlic Constituents." *Antimicrobial Agents and Chemotherapy* 43 (1999): 1811–12.

Okoh, M. P., R. K. Singla, C. Madu, O. Soremekun, J. Adejoh, L. A. Alli, et al. "Phytomedicine in Disease Management: In-Silico Analysis of the Binding Affinity of Artesunate and Azadirachtin for Malaria Treatment." *Frontiers in Pharmacology* 12 (2021): 751032.

Pandey, M. M., S. Rastogi, and A. K. Rawat. "Indian Traditional Ayurvedic System of Medicine and Nutritional Supplementation." *Evidence-Based Complementary and Alternative Medicine* 2013 (2013): 376327.

Patwardhan, B., A. D. B. Vaidya, and M. Chorghade. "Ayurveda and Natural Products Drug Discovery." *Current Science* 86, no. 6 (2004): 789–99.

Pfeiffer, E., F. F. Heuschmid, S. Kranz, and M. Metzler. "Microsomal Hydroxylation and Glucuronidation of [6]-Gingerol." *Journal of Agricultural and Food Chemistry* 54, no. 23 (2006): 8769–74.

Prakash, P., and N. Gupta. "Therapeutic Uses of Ocimum sanctum Linn (Tulsi) with a Note on Eugenol and Its Pharmacological Actions: A Review." *Indian Journal of Physiology and Pharmacology* 49, no. 2 (2005): 125–31.

Rahmawati, N., M. Sholikhah, I. Y. Subositi, F. I. Mustofa, S. Haryanti, H. Widodo, R. Mujahid, A. Maruzy, and Y. Widiyastuti. "Traditional Uses of Ginger (*Zingiber officinale Roscoe*) Based on Ethnomedicine Study in 254 Indonesian Ethnic Groups." *Indian Journal of Traditional Knowledge* 23, no. 5 (2024): 464–72.

Rai, P., D. Jaiswal, S. Mehta, D. Rai, B. Sharma, and G. Watal. "Effect of *Curcuma longa* Freeze-Dried Rhizome Powder with Milk in STZ-Induced Diabetic Rats." *Indian Journal of Clinical Biochemistry* 25 (2010): 175–81.

Rana, C., H. Piplani, V. Vaish, B. Nehru, and S. N. Sanyal. "Downregulation of PI3-K/Akt/PTEN Pathway and Activation of Mitochondrial Intrinsic Apoptosis by Diclofenac and Curcumin in Colon Cancer." *Molecular and Cellular Biochemistry* 402, no. 1–2 (2015): 225–41.

Ranjbar, M. E., M. R. Zamani, and J. Khara. "The Effects of Iron-enrichment on the Antioxidant Properties of Wheat Flour and Bread." *Journal of Agricultural Science and Technology* 21, no. 3 (2019): 855–66.

Ravva, S. V., and A. Korn. "Effect of Neem (*Azadirachta indica*) on the Survival of *Escherichia coli* O157 in Dairy Manure." *International Journal of Environmental Research and Public Health* 12, no. 7 (2015): 7794–803.

Ryu, S. Y., et al. "Antibacterial Activity of Garlic and Its Mechanism of Action." *Microbiology and Immunology* 48, no. 3 (2004): 223–30.

Sadeghi, N., M. Mansourian, A. Khosravi, and M. Ghorbani. "Curcumin Nanoemulsion Improves Antibacterial Activity against Escherichia coli by Disrupting Membrane Integrity." *Journal of Applied Microbiology* 129, no. 6 (2020): 1424–32.

Saha, R., A. Bandyopadhyay, and A. Ghosh. "Ocimum tenuiflorum (Tulsi): A Holistic Medicinal Herb." *Journal of Ethnopharmacology* 225 (2018): 38–50.

Sahrawat, A., J. Sharma, R. N. S. Rahul, S. Tiwari, M. D. Joshi, A. Pundhir, et al. "Phytochemical Analysis and Antibacterial Properties of *Azadirachta indica* (Neem) Leaves Extract Against *E. coli*." *Journal of Pharmacognosy and Phytochemistry* 7, no. 4 (2018): 1368–71.

Sasidharan, N. K., S. R. Sreekala, J. Jacob, and B. Nambisan. "In Vitro Synergistic Effect of Curcumin in Combination with Third Generation Cephalosporins Against Bacteria Associated with Infectious Diarrhea." *Biomedical Research International* (2014): 1–9.

Satyajit, D. S., Z. Latif, and A. I. Gray. *Natural Products Isolation*, 2nd ed. New Jersey: Humana Press, 2010.

Selvaraj, K., N. Bharath, R. Natarajan, S. Dinesh, S. Murugesan, and S. Selvaraj. "Comparative Evaluation of Antimicrobial Efficacy of Toothpastes Containing Probiotic and Neem as Primary Ingredient on Salivary *Streptococcus mutans* in Melmaruvathur Population: An In Vivo Study." *Journal of Pharmacy and Bioallied Sciences* 12, Suppl. 1 (2020): S595–600.

Sharma, S., R. Rolta, D. Salaria, and K. Dev. "In Vitro Antibacterial and Antifungal Potentials of *Ocimum tenuiflorum* and *Ocimum gratissimum* Essential Oil." *Pharmacological Research - Natural Products* 4 (2024): 100065.

Shome, S., A. D. Talukdar, R. Nath, and S. Tewari. "Curcumin-ZnO Nanocomposite Mediated Inhibition of *Pseudomonas aeruginosa* Biofilm and Its Mechanism of Action." *Journal of Drug Delivery Science and Technology* 81 (2023): 104301.

Shukla, Y., and M. Singh. "Cancer Preventive Properties of Ginger: A Brief Review." *Food and Chemical Toxicology* 45, no. 4 (2007): 683–90.

Singh, G., I. P. S. Kapoor, P. Singh, C. S. de Heluani, M. P. de Lampasona, and C. A. Catalán. "Chemistry, Antioxidant and Antimicrobial Investigations on Essential Oil and Oleoresins of Zingiber Officinale." *Food and Chemical Toxicology* 46, no. 12 (2008): 3296–302.

Singh, G., I. Kapoor, P. Singh, C. S. de Heluani, M. P. de Lampasona, and C. A. Catalan. "Comparative Study of Chemical Composition and Antioxidant Activity of Fresh and Dry Rhizomes of *Turmeric* (*Curcuma longa* Linn)." *Food and Chemical Toxicology* 48 (2010): 1026–31.

Singh, M., D. Sharma, D. Kumar, G. Singh, G. Swami, and M. S. Rathore. "Formulation, Development, and Evaluation of Herbal Effervescent Mouthwash Tablet Containing *Azadirachta indica* (Neem) and Curcumin for the Maintenance of Oral Hygiene." *Recent Patents on Drug Delivery & Formulation* 14, no. 2 (2020): 145–61.

Small, E., R. R. Bailey, and A. M. M. M. M. Bailey. "A Study of the Antibacterial Activity of Allium sativum (Garlic)." *Canadian Journal of Public Health* 38, no. 1 (1947): 49–56.

Soares, F. *Naturais: Cultivo e Uso Medicinal (Naturals: Cultivation and Medicinal Use).* Editora Europa, 2009.

Srirangarayan, R. S., M. Ramasamy, and R. P. Thangam. "Hidden Elixir in Indian Sub-Continent – *Azadirachta indica* Linn." *SSRN Electronic Journal* (2020): 1–4.

Srinivasan, M., P. K. Chandran, and N. Sujatha. "The Inhibitory Effects of Curcuma *longa* L. Essential Oil and Curcumin on *Aspergillus flavus* Link Growth and Morphology." *Journal of Essential Oil-Bearing Plants* 17, no. 5 (2014): 1011–23.

Sujarwo, W., A. P. Keim, G. Caneva, C. Toniolo, and M. Nicoletti. "Ethnobotanical Uses of Neem (*Azadirachta indica* A. Juss.; Meliaceae) Leaves in Bali (Indonesia) and the Indian Subcontinent in Relation with Historical Background and Phytochemical Properties." *Journal of Ethnopharmacology* 189 (2016): 186–93.

Surjushe, A., R. Vasani, and D. G. Saple. "Aloe Vera: A Short Review." *Indian Journal of Dermatology* 53, no. 4 (2008): 163–6.

Tasanarong, T., S. Patntirapong, and V. Aupaphong. "The Inhibitory Effect of a Novel Neem Paste Against Cariogenic Bacteria." *Journal of Clinical and Experimental Dentistry* 13, no. 11 (2021): e1083–8.

Teles, A. M., B. A. dos Santos, C. G. Ferreira, A. N. Mouchreck, K. S. Calabrese, A. L. Abreu-Silva, and F. Almeida-Souza. "Ginger (Zingiber officinale) Antimicrobial Potential: A Review." In *Ginger Cultivation and Its Antimicrobial and Pharmacological Potentials*, edited by Haiping Wang. IntechOpen, 2019.

Teow, S. Y., and S. A. Ali. "Altered Antibacterial Activity of Curcumin in the Presence of Serum Albumin, Plasma and Whole Blood." Pakistan Journal of Pharmaceutical Sciences 30, no. 2 (2017): 449–57.

Tepongning, R. N., J. N. Mbah, F. L. Avoulou, M. M. Jerme, E. K. Ndanga, and F. B. Fekam. "Hydroethanolic Extracts of *Erigeron floribundus* and *Azadirachta indica* Reduced *Plasmodium berghei* Parasitemia in Balb/c Mice." *Evidence-Based Complementary and Alternative Medicine* (2018): 5156710.

Tiwary, R. K., et al. "Ethnobotanical Study of Medicinal Plants Used by the Indigenous Community of the Western Region of Mizoram, India." *Journal of Ethnobiology and Ethnomedicine* 20, no. 2 (2024): 1–18.

Tjipta, P. A., D. Aminah, H. Urip, Y. Simanjuntak, P. Epina, K. Natasya Elsa, H. P. A. Zaitun, S. R. Abdi, S. P. Cahaya, and N. Fahrul. "Phyllanthus emblica: A Comprehensive Review of Its Phytochemical Composition and Pharmacological Properties." *Frontiers in Pharmacology* 14 (2023): 1288618.

Uchibayashi, M. "Etymology of Ginger." *Yakushigaku Zassh: The Journal of Japanese History of Pharmacy* 36, no. 1 (2001): 58–60.

Ulanowska, M., and B. Olas. Biological Properties and Prospects for the Application of Eugenol—A Review. *International Journal of Molecular Sciences* 22, no. 7 (2021): 3671.

Usman, A., V. Fitzsimmons-Thoss, and A. Tawfike. "Anti-Bacterial, Anti-Oxidant and Cytotoxic Activities of Nimbin Isolated from African *Azadirachta indica* Seed Oil." *Advanced Journal of Chemistry, Section B: Natural Products and Medical Chemistry* 2, no. 2 (2020): 81–90.

Vogt, M., et al. "Synergistic Effects of Garlic and Antibiotics Against Resistant Bacterial Strains." *Clinical Microbiology and Infection* 22, no. 8 (2016): 740–6.

Wang, H. M., C. Y. Chen, H. A. Chen, W. C. Huang, W. R. Lin, T. C. Chen, C. Y. Lin, H. J. Chien, P. L. Lu, C. M. Lin, and Y. H. Chen. "Zingiber officinale (Ginger) Compounds Have Tetracycline-Resistance Modifying Effects against Clinical Extensively Drug-Resistant *Acinetobacter baumannii*." *Phytotherapy Research* 24, no. 12 (2010): 1825–30.

Wylie, M. R., and D. S. Merrell. "The Antimicrobial Potential of the Neem Tree *Azadirachta indica*." *Frontiers in Pharmacology* 13 (2022): 891535.

Xiao, W., Y. Yang, Z. Xie, and J. Shi. "Chemical Composition and Antimicrobial Activities of Essential Oils of *Ocimum* Species." *Journal of Medicinal Plants Research* 6, no. 8 (2012): 1496–501.

Yamani, H. A., E. C. Pang, N. Mantri, and M. A. Deighton. "Antimicrobial Activity of Tulsi (Ocimum tenuiflorum) Essential Oil and Their Major Constituents against Three Species of Bacteria." *Indian Journal of Microbiology* 51, no. 3 (2011): 327–35.

Yamani, H. A., E. C. Pang, N. Mantri, and M. A. Deighton. "Antimicrobial Activity of Tulsi (*Ocimum tenuiflorum*) Essential Oil and Their Major Constituents Against Three Species of Bacteria." *Frontiers in Microbiology* 7 (2016): 681.

11

Utilization of Ethnomedicinal Plants for Their Potential Antimicrobial Activity

Shreeya Purkait[1, 2], Jit Sarkar[3], Sunanda Halder[4], Sudipta Mukherjee[3, 5], Abhishek Mukherjee[2], and Krishnendu Acharya[3]

[*1]Agricultural and Ecological Research Unit, Indian Statistical Institute, Giridih, Jharkhand, India

[2]School of Materials Science and Nanotechnology, Jadavpur University, Kolkata, India

[3]Molecular and Applied Mycology and Plant Pathology Laboratory, Department of Botany, University of Calcutta, Kolkata, West Bengal, India

[4]Department of Botany, Bethune College, University of Calcutta, Kolkata, West Bengal, India

[5] West Bengal Biodiversity Board, Department of Environment, Government of West Bengal, Kolkata, West Bengal, India

*Corresponding Author's Email: krish_paper@yahoo.com

Introduction

The interaction between human civilizations and their plant environments is the primary objective of ethnobotany (Tiwari and Yadav 2003). Indigenous knowledge on the use of natural resources is frequently documented using ethnobotanical studies (Farnsworth 1990; Jain 1994; Palit and Gurung 2008; Prance 1991). In a sociocultural setting, traditional knowledge is location specific, time tested, and practiced by ethnic communities worldwide based on the use of natural resources for everyday survival, such as nutrition, habitation, medical care, and fodder (Anas et al. 2024; Bhat, Kumar, and Bussmann 2013; Ferrari, Zank, and Hanazaki 2024; Haq and Singh 2020; Kumar et al. 2021a; Raj et al. 2018; Reyes-García 2010; Signorini, Piredda, Bruschi 2009; Sreedevi et al. 2013; Syed et al. 2024; Upasana 2015; Vitalini et al. 2013). The Botanical Survey of India (BSI) reports that among the 45,000 listed plant species, roughly 30,000 species or two-thirds are of significant interest due to their potential therapeutic applications

(Nautiyal, Nautiyal, and Prakash 2015). The use of herbs or plants for traditional or folk medicine is a common practice among many rural or indigenous people in many developing nations (Ait Bouzid et al. 2024; Banerjee 2024; Bhadra and Manjunath 2024; Izah et al. 2024; Ralte, Sailo, and Singh 2024; Vineeta et al. 2022).

The World Health Organization (WHO) estimates that 80 percent of people worldwide have to rely on traditional or folk medicine (Vineeta et al. 2022). Additionally, during the past few years, the usage of herbal supplements has grown from 2.5 percent to 12.0 percent worldwide (Stickel and Schuppan 2007). Ayurveda, Siddha, and Unani are traditional as well as primary rural healthcare systems for a large population in India. The country's traditional medical system is also a collection of local and folk traditions based on an extensive repository of information about numerous plants (Jamshidi-Kia, Lorigooini, and Amini-Khoei 2017; Nishteswar 2019; Pandey, Rastogi, and Rawat 2013; J. Sharma et al. 2012). In India, over 3,000 plant species have been documented to have therapeutic characteristics, of which 90 percent being wild (Chakraborty et al. 2012). Medicinal plants are becoming increasingly important globally due to their economic, social, ecological, nutraceutical, and therapeutic advantages (Fitzgerald, Heinrich, and Booker 2019; Howes et al. 2020; Li et al. 2020; Negi, Maikhuri, and Rawat 2011; Pammi, Suresh, and Giri 2023; Pant, Pandey, and Dall'Acqua 2021; Shahrajabian et al. 2023; A. Sharma et al. 2021; Theodoridis et al. 2023; Vaou et al. 2021).

Plant-based natural products consist of phytochemicals that exhibit diverse physical, chemical, and biological properties (Goyal, Sasmal, and Nagori 2011). Phytochemicals comprise a mixture of primary and secondary metabolites, including proteins, carbohydrates, alkaloids, glycosides, terpenoids, phenolics, and flavonoids (Ayaz et al. 2019). Natural compounds may enhance the interaction of an antimicrobial agent with its target within the pathogen, hence mitigating the development of resistance. This technique can mitigate toxicity by using lower amounts of both drugs (Sanhueza, Faundez, and Paz 2017). Meanwhile, scientists have expressed increasing concern regarding the efficacy of existing antibiotics in treating various infectious diseases. Numerous studies have focused on identifying new alternative medications to address resistance issues. Nature serves as a potential resource for drug discovery.

Objectives and Methods

For decades, the phytochemicals of plants have drawn the attention of scientists due to their diverse structures, fewer side effects, and greater acceptability among individuals (Ferrazzano et al. 2015). Many of these phytochemicals exhibit antimicrobial properties (Dah-Nouvlessounon et al. 2023). Approximately 80 percent of the world's developing countries rely on plant-derived medicines as their primary treatment option (Shewamene, Dune, and Smith 2020). Furthermore, plants constitute the foundation of various medical practices including Ayurveda and Traditional Chinese Medicine (Cheesman et al., 2017). Therefore, in this research, an effort has been made to present current knowledge on ethnomedicinal plants, particularly in the Indian context, utilized in traditional medicine systems for their antibacterial properties with specific emphasis on characterized bioactive compounds and their efficacy against various microorganisms.

Indian Tribes and Medicinal Plants

A significant portion of India is made up of tribal groups. The Government of India's 2011 census data indicates that around 8.6 percent of India's population constitutes tribes. It is commonly observed throughout India that this group of people suffers from extreme poverty and economic regression, frequently with inadequate access to modern healthcare and education. They mostly use traditional medicines for healthcare, which are reliant only on the availability of local medicinal plants (Sharma et al. 2016). In the underdeveloped world, traditional medical knowledge plays a significant role in the primary healthcare system. The majority of rural residents rely on subsistence farming to survive, and they have extensive cultural wisdom about forest resources for treating various ailments (Uniyal 2003). Traditional knowledge based on plants is now widely used to find new sources of medications and nutraceuticals (Kosalge and Fursule 2009). Even though allopathic medicine has made tremendous advancements in helping millions of people worldwide suffering from a wide range of illnesses, traditional medical systems, also referred to as alternative or complementary medical systems, have seen a rise in popularity in recent years.

In ancient age, people used plant-based treatments for their survival; whereas, due to a lack of medicinal knowledge, plant-based treatments could not be properly utilized, resulting in the development of alternative traditional medicines. Out of eighteen states in India, tribes of nine states have mostly utilized plants against serious microbial diseases like leprosy, tuberculosis, and influenza. The tribal communities like Apatani, Mongpa, and Singpo (tribes of Arunachal Pradesh) have utilized *Bidens pilosa* L. against serious ear and eye infection (Khongsai, Yadav, and Singh 2011). Similarly Jaintia, a tribe of Assam, uses different parts of various plants against pneumonia, tuberculosis, and some other microbial diseases (Sajem and Gosai 2006). The knowledge of plant source medicines is described in Table 11.1, which is a small dataset of ethnomedicinal plants for the development of traditional medicines from a tribal base. This is due to a variety of circumstances, including the emergence of drug resistance to different allopathic medications and the negative side effects linked to several allopathic medications (Md. Hossan et al. 2012). Ethnomedicinal plants have been an integral part of traditional healthcare systems across India, with each state having its own rich repository of plant knowledge.

Table 11.1. Name of the Tribes and Parts of Plants They Use for Particular Microbial Disease

Region	Tribes Name	Name of the Plants	Disease	Part Used	References
Arunachal Pradesh	Apatani, Mongpa, Singpo, Tangsa, Padam, Nyishi,	*Ageratum conyzoides* L.	Stomach disorder	Leaves/ Paste of leaf	Khongsai, Yadav, and Singh 2011
		Andrographis paniculata (Burm. f.) Wall. ex Nees.			
		Carica papaya L.		Fruit latex	
		Bidens pilosa L.	Ear, Eye disease	Leaves/ Leaf of juice with water are applied	
		Centella asiatica (L.) Urb.	Blood dysentery, Leprosy, Tuberculosis	Leaves/ Extract of Leaf	
		Oroxylum indicum Vent.			
		Costus speciosus (Koen.) Smith	Respiratory blockage, Urination Burning	Roots, Stems	
		Houttuynia cordata Thunb.	Gonorrhea, Dysentery	Leaves, Stem/ Extract	
		Syzygium cumini (L.) Skeels.			
		Mentha arvensis L.	Stomach disorder, Influenza,	Leaf decoction	
		Ocimum sanctum L.	Bronchitis, Stomachache	Leaves, seeds/ Extract of leaf, seed powder with honey effective for cold	
		Piper brachystachyum Wall.			
		Zanthoxylum armatum Skeels DC Roxb.			
		Solanum khasianum Clarke	Toothache	Fruits / Utilized the smoke of dried fruit burn	
		Spilanthes paniculata DC.			

Assam	Jaintia	*Ageratum conyzoides* L.	Stomach disorder	Leaves/ Paste of leaf	Sajem and Gosai 2006
		Alstonia scholaris L. R. Br.			
		Coriandrum sativum L.			
		Centella asiatica (L.) Urb.	Blood dysentery, Leprosy, Tuberculosis	Leaves/ Extract of Leaf	
		Scoparia dulcis L.			
		Justicia adhatoda L.	Pneumonia		
		Spilanthes paniculata DC.	Toothache	Flowers	
		Tabernaemontana divaricata (L.) R. Br.		Root, Bark/ Extract	
Central Himalayas	Tolchhas (Bhotiya), Marchhas (Bhotiya), Jadhs (Bhotiya)	*Saussurea obvallata* (DC.) Edgew.	UTI	Roots, Leaves / Decoction	Maikhuri and Rao 2000
		Nepata discolor Royle ex Benth	Tuberculosis	Leaf decoction	
		Megacarpaea polyandra Benth.	Stomach disorder, Dysentery	Leaves, Root/ Decoction of Root	
		Berberis aristata DC.	Eye disease	Root /Root decoction (juice)	
Madhya Pradesh	Bheel, Sahariya	*Aegle marmelos* L. Correa.	Digestive problem, Cholera	Root, leaves, fruit / Ripe fruit pulp is used to improve digestive disorder	Prakash 2015
		Syzygium cumini (L.) Skeels.			
		Azadirachta indica A. JUSS.	Tuberculosis	Leaves, Fruit	
		Cassia fistula Linn	Leprosy,	Leaves, Stem, Root/ Extract of leaf	
		Centella asiatica (L.) Urb.	Blood dysentery, Tuberculosis	Leaves/ Extract of Leaf	
		Dalbergia sissoo Roxb.			
		Ficus religiosa Linn.	Gonorrhea.	Bark/ Powder of bark	
Maharashtra	Dhangars, Gowlis	*Argemone mexicana* L.	Dysentery	Tuber, Root, Latex, leaves	Bhosle et al. 2009
		Justicia adhatoda L.			
		Mangifera indica L.			
		Syzygium cumini (L.) Skeels.			
		Azadirachta indica A. JUSS.	Tuberculosis	Leaves, Fruit	
		Ficus religiosa Linn.	Gonorrhea	Bark/ Powder of bark	
		Lawsonia inermis L.	Mouth ulcer	Leaves / paste	

(*Continued*)

Table 11.1 (Continued)

Region	Tribes Name	Name of the Plants	Disease	Part Used	References
North Orissa	Moroda, Hatikote	*Aegle marmelos* L. Correa.	Digestive problem, Cholera	Root, leaves, fruit / Ripe fruit pulp is used to improve digestive disorder	Rout, Panda, and Mishra 2009
		Andrographis paniculata (Burm. f.) Wall. ex Nees.	Stomach disorder	Leaves/ Extract of leaf	
		Cassia fistula Linn.	Leprosy	Leaves, Stem, Root/ Extract of leaf	
Tamil Nadu	Irula	*Andrographis paniculata* (Burm. f.) Wall. ex Nees.	Stomach disorder	Leaves/ Extract of leaf	Rasingam 2012
		Caesalpinia sepiaria Roxb.			
		Argemone mexicana L.	Dysentery	Tuber, Root, Latex, leaves	
		Jatropha curcas L.	Toothache	Bark, Latex/ Decoction prepared from bark mixed with water	
		Justicia adhatoda L.	Pneumonia, Dysentery,	Leaves /Decoction of leaf	
		Lawsonia inermis L.	Mouth ulcer	Leaves / paste	
		Syzygium cumini (L.) Skeels.	Stomach disorder, Dysentery, Diarrhea	Fruit, Seed, Bark/ Bark decoction, fruit eaten raw	
Tripura	Reang	*Ageratum conyzoides* L.	Stomach disorder	Leaves/ Paste of leaf	Shil, Choudhury, and Das 2014
		Mentha arvensis L.			
		Homalomena aromatica (Spreng.) Schott.	White spot in eyes	Rhizome/ Decoction	
		Jatropha gossypifolia L.	Toothache	Stem extract	
		Tabernaemontana divaricata (L.) R. Br.			
		Justicia adhatoda L.	Pneumonia, Dysentery	Leaves /Decoction of leaf	

Uttarakhand	Tharu	*Alstonia scholaris* L. R. Br.	Stomach disorder	Bark, leaves/ Extract of leaf	Prakash 2015
		Aegle marmelos L. Correa.	Digestive problem, Cholera	Root, leaves, fruit / Ripe fruit pulp is used to improve digestive disorder	
		Saussurea obvallata (DC.) Edgew.	UTI	Roots, Leaves / Decoction	
West Bengal	Santhal, Kora, Oraon	*Andrographis paniculata* (Burm. f.) Wall. ex Nees.	stomach disorder	Leaves/ Extract of leaf	Begum and Mandal 2016
		Argemone mexicana L.	Dysentery	Tuber, Root, Latex, Leaves, Seeds	
		Justicia adhatoda L.			
		Mangifera indica L.			
		Scoparia dulcis L.			
		Azadirachta indica A. JUSS.	Tuberculosis	Leaves, Fruit	
		Centella asiatica (L.) Urb.	Blood dysentery, Leprosy, Tuberculosis	Leaves/ Extract of Leaf	
		Jatropha curcas L.	Toothache	Bark, Latex/ Decoction prepared from bark mixed with water	

Source: Authors.

Ethnomedicinal Plants in India

Traditional medicine continues to be widely used in developing countries and is seeing a growing adoption rate even in industrialized nations, where people are increasingly turning to alternative therapies alongside conventional medicine. For many people in our country like India, traditional medicine is the most readily available healthcare option due to limited access to modern medical facilities. Here, traditional medicine is deeply rooted in social-cultural practices and is seen as a natural and holistic approach to health. People in various regions of India are increasingly interested in natural remedies, the potential benefits of herbal medicine, and a focus on preventative healthcare, which contributes to the rising popularity of traditional medicine practices.

Thus, approximately every country in the world has traditional medical systems, and it is believed that these systems treat a wide range of illnesses by using over 80,000 plant species (Md. Hossan et al. 2012). Communities of ancient ethnic groups all over the world have learned to use the abundance of local herbs for medicinal purposes. Previous studies have described the potency of traditional plant-based materials in bacterial diseases. Each plant part has effective roles in fighting against gram-positive and gram-negative bacteria, but also the plant family has a differentiation in the effectiveness against bacteria (Mohagheghzadeh et al. 2007). A large number of plants from Fabaceae and Lamiaceae have effective work against *Bacillus subtilis*, *Staphylococcus aureus*, and *Escherichia coli* (Kumar 2017). In Table 11.2, the traditional plants with their families are described along with their effectiveness as antimicrobial material.

Major Bioactive Compounds in Ethnomedicinal Plant Extracts

The bioactive compounds of plants are mostly secondary metabolites which have an aromatic ring with at least one hydroxyl group. The secondary metabolites control primary pathways like coenzymes and hormones. They function as antibiotics and poisons during stress. They play a vital role in plants, but their numerous pharmacological properties also make them relevant for human health. The major bioactive compounds, which are found in the extracts of various plant parts that combat diseases include:

(a) Alkaloid

The alkaloids are nitrogen-containing heterocyclic chemicals that often have a bitter flavor and strong action. Within the kingdom of plants, they are not widely distributed. Different groups have specific clinical properties.

i. **Tropane Alkaloid:** These substances, which are muscarinic receptor antagonists with anticholinergic activity, are used medicinally to lessen discomfort,

Table 11.2 Name of the Ethnomedicinal Plants with Their Family and Their Parts Used Against Bacteria

Family	Plants Name	Part Used/Extract/Fraction	Antimicrobial Activity against Bacteria	References
Ranunculaceae	*Nigella sativa* Linn.	Seeds	*Shigella dysenteriae, Staphylococcus aureus*	Zahin et al. 2010
Meliaceae	*Azadirachta indica* A. Juss.	Aqueous, ethanolic, methanolic extract of Leaves/Bark	*Campylobacter jejuni, Pseudomonas aeruginosa, Staphylococcus aureus, Escherichia coli*	Kumar 2017 Zahin et al. 2010
Anacardiaceae	*Mangifera indica* Linn.	Leaves	*P. aeruginosa, S. aureus, E. coli*	Bbosa et al. 2007
	Pistacia integerrima Stew ex Brandis	Stem	Gram-positive and gram-negative bacteria	Ansari, Ali, and Najmi 1998
Rutaceae	*Citrus sinensis* Linn.	Rind	*Staphylococcus aureus, S. paratyphi, E. coli*	Ahmad and Beg 2001 Stange et al. 1993
	Murraya koenigii Spreng.	Leaves	Gram-positive bacteria	Zahin et al. 2010
Fabaceae	*Acacia arabica* Wild.	Fruit	*Pseudomonas aeruginosa, Klebsiella pneumoniae, E. coli*	Eldeen, Elgorashi, and van Staden 2005
	Acacia catechu Wild.	Bark	*E. coli, Bacillus subtilis*	Gupta et al. 2004
	Caesalpinia bonducella Linn.	Seeds	*S. aureus, Micrococcus flavus*	Dickson et al. 2007
	Cassia angustifolia Vahl.	Aqueous extract of Seeds/leaves	*Staphylococcus aureus*	Kumar 2017
	Cassia fistula Linn.	Fruit	*Bacillus mycoides, Bacillus subtilis, E. coli, Mycobacterium smegmatis*	Rizvi et al. 2009
	Delonix regia Gamble	Flowers	*S. aureus*	Parekh and Chanda 2007
Moraceae	*Morus alba* Linn.	Fruit	*Streptococcus sobrinus, S. sanguis, Porphyromonas gingivalis*	Park et al. 2003
Cannabaceae	*Cannabis sativa* Linn.	Leaves	Gram-positive and gram-negative bacteria	Grange and Snell 1996

(*Continued*)

Table 11.2 (Continued)

Family	Plants Name	Part Used/Extract/Fraction	Antimicrobial Activity against Bacteria	References
Myrtaceae	*Eucalyptus globulus* Labile	Leaves	Gram-positive and gram-negative bacteria	Takahashi, Kokubo and Sakaino 2004
	Syzygium aromaticum Linn.	Aqueous, ethanolic, methanolic extract of Flower bud	*S. aureus*	Cai and Wu 1996
	Syzygium cumini Linn.	Seeds/ Bark/ Leaves	*S. aureus*	Zahin et al. 2010 Oliveira et al. 2007
Apiaceae	*Carum copticum* Benth and Hook.	Fruit	Gram-positive and gram-negative bacteria	Mohagheghzadeh et al. 2007
	Centella asiatica Linn. Urb.	Methanolic and aqueous extract of Leaves	*M. leprae, S. aureus*	Ahmad and Beg 2001
Asteraceae	*Cichorium intybus* Linn.	Root	Gram-positive and gram-negative bacteria	Nishimura and Satoh 2006
Apocynaceae	*Calotropis gigantea* (L.) R. Br	Petroleum ether fraction from the Root/Bark	*Sarcina lutea, Shigella sonnei*	Fuster, Kaiser-Bunbury, and Olesen 2020
	Holarrhena antidysenterica Wall.	Bark	*S. dysenteriae, C. albicans, Staphylococcus aureus, S. paratyphi*	Rani and Khullar 2004
Solanaceae	*Solanum nigrum* Linn.	Ethanolic and methanolic extract of Fruit	Gram-positive and gram-negative bacteria	Gurib-Fakim 2006
	Datura alba L.	Ethanolic extract from leaves	*Staphylococcus sp., klebsiella sp.*	Kumar 2017
Acanthaceae	*Adhatoda vasica* Nees.	Whole plant	Gram-positive and gram-negative bacteria	Grange and Snell 1996

Lamiaceae	*Mentha arvensis* Linn.	Leaves	*Bacillus subtilis*	Schelz, Molnar, and Hohmann 2006
	Mentha piperita L.	Ethanol, methanol, ethyl acetate extract of Leaves	*B. subtilis, E. coli, S. aureus*	Kumar 2017
	Ocimum sanctum Linn.	Whole plant/Methanolic extract of leaves	*S. aureus, S. dysenteriae, E. coli*	Norajit et al. 2007
	Satureja montana L.	Leaves/Stem	*Salmonella typhimurium*	Kumar 2017
Euphorbiaceae	*Emblica officinalis* Gaertn	Fruit	*Staphylococcus aureus, S. paratyphi*	Zahin et al. 2010 Ahmad and Beg 2001
Zingiberaceae	*Zingiber officinale* Rosc.	Ethanolic and aqueous extract of Rhizome	*B. cereus, L. monocytogenes*	Norajit et al. 2007
	Zizyphus jujube Lam	Bark/leaves	Gram-positive and gram-negative bacteria	Li, Li, and Lockington 2005
	Curcuma longa L.	Methanol and water extract Root	Gram-positive and gram-negative bacteria	Apisariyakul, Vanittanakom, and Buddhasukh 1995
Liliaceae	*Allium sativum* Linn.	Methanolic and aqueous extract of Bulb/leaves	*Campylobacter jejuni, S. paratyphi, S. dysenteriae, E. coli*	Kumar 2017 Zahin et al. 2010 Ahmad and Beg 2001
	Aloe barbadensis Mill.	Whole plant	*Corynebacterium sp., Salmonella sp., S. aureus*	Martínez et al. 1996
Poaceae	*Podophyllum emodi* Wall ex Hook	Root	Gram-positive and gram-negative bacteria	Moraes et al. 2002

Source: Authors.

hypersecretion, and smooth muscular spasms. Tropane alkaloids are found in the Solanaceae (nightshade family), including *Datura* spp. (thorn apples), *Atropa belladonna* (deadly nightshade), and Hyoscyamus *niger* (Henbane) (Griffin and Lin 2000).

ii. **Pyrrolizidine Alkaloid:** Hepatotoxicity upon bioactivation is one of its negative effects in both humans and animals. Asteraceae (daisy family), especially *Senecio* spp. (ragworts) and Boraginaceae (borage family), generate pyrrolizidine alkaloids (Casado, Morante-Zarcero, and Sierra 2022).

iii. **Isoquinoline Alkaloid:** These alkaloids exhibit a variety of biochemical properties that are pertinent to medical application, such as stimulating bone marrow leukocytes and myocardial contractility and inhibiting a variety of diseases like pain, cancer cells, and germs. Isoquinoline alkaloids are mostly produced by the Papaveraceae (poppy family) and Berberidaceae (barberry family) (Chrzanowska, Grajewska, and Rozwado 2016).

iv. **Methylxanthine Alkaloid:** In both humans and animals, methylxanthines bind to the adenosine receptor by varying degrees and produce neurological effects, at low to moderate ingestion that may be considered stimulating. High methylxanthine intake in rodents results in testicular atrophy and decreased sperm production. *Theobroma cacao* (cacao) and *Coffea arabica* (coffee) are the primary sources of methylxanthine alkaloids (Tokusoglu 2019).

v. **Pseudo Alkaloid:** Pseudoalkaloids are substances with similar chemical characteristics to alkaloids. The central nervous system is affected by pseudoalkaloids. Pseudoalkaloids can be extracted from species in the Taxaceae (yew family), such as *Taxus baccata* (yew), and Apiaceae (carrot family), such as *Cicuta virosa* (cowbane) and *Conium maculatum* (hemlock) (J. X. Wang et al. 2020).

(b) Glycosides

The different types of secondary metabolites that are attached to uronic acid or a mono- or oligosaccharide make up glycosides. Glycone is the term for the uronic acid or saccharide portion, while aglycone is the term for the other portion. Groups of glycosides are described below:

(a) **Cardiac Glycosides:** Cardiac glycoside aglycones are steroidal in structure. They have the effect of inhibiting the cell membrane's Na+/K+-ATPase pumps. These pumps are found in the heart cells and are essential to their operation. These substances have highly noticeable effects on the heart, increasing contractility and decreasing pace. Plants belonging to the Scrophulariaceae (figwort family), specifically *Digitalis purpurea* (foxglove) and the Convallariaceae (convall family), of which *Convallaria majalis* (lily of the valley) is a classic example, contain cardiac glycosides (Prassas and Diamandis 2008).

(b) **Cyanogenic Glycosides:** The aglycones in cyanogenic glycosides are made from amino acids. Rosaceae (rose family) species, especially *Prunus* spp., contain cyanogenic glycosides (Gleadow and Woodrow 2002).
(c) **Glucosinolates:** Glucosinolates are sulfur-containing pungent amino acid-derived aglycones. The substances seem to reduce the hepatic bioactivation of environmental procarcinogens and exhibit a diverse range of actions on cytochrome P450 isoforms in different cells. The Brassicaceae (*Brassica* family) is the key producer of glucosinolates (Tripathi and Mishra 2007).
(d) **Saponins:** Saponins have antitumor and immune-modulating properties. A variety of plant families contain saponins. They include the significant sheep poisonous plant *Narthecium ossifragum* (bog asphodel) and the Liliaceae (lily family) (Oakenfull 1981).
(e) **Anthraquinone Glycosides:** Anthraquinone glycosides can stimulate colon peristalsis and produce water and electrolytes. The distribution of anthraquinone glycosides in the kingdom of plants is comparatively rare. They are found in the Polygonaceae (dock family), such as *Rheum* spp. (rhubarb) and *Rumex crispus* (curly dock) (Sakulpanich and Gritsanapan 2009).

(c) Resins

Resins are lipid-soluble combinations consisting of both volatile and nonvolatile chemicals. Mono- and sesquiterpenoids dominate the volatile fraction, while diterpenoid and triterpenoid molecules may make up the nonvolatile fraction. Resins can be used as a carrier of drug delivery or sometimes they can act as an active drug ingredient (Anand, Kandarapu, and Garg 2001).

(d) Flavonoids

A core three-ring structure makes up flavonoids. Proanthocyanidins are flavonoid oligomers. Phenol groups are present in all substances and have a general antioxidant action. Different structures have different other activities, such as lowering inflammation or carcinogenicity. Phytoestrogens are the main name for the isoflavone group. A wide variety of plant families include pigments called flavonoids and proanthocyanidins. Fabaceae (bean family) species produce isoflavones (Morris and Zhang 2006).

(e) Terpenoids

Isoprene, a five-carbon building block, is used to compose the terpenoids. There are four types of terpenoids: Monoterpenoid, Diterpenoid, Sesqui-terpenoid, and Phenylpropanoid. They have a wide range of effects, some of which have been used in herbal medicines. In addition to gastrointestinal stimulation, antiviral, antibacterial, and antitumor actions are particularly significant. They do not, however, have a toxicity level unless they are concentrated as volatile oils. Although they are found in

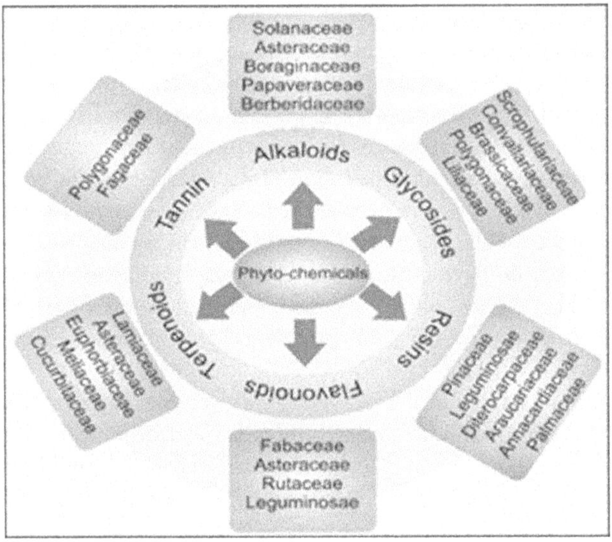

Figure 11.1. Names of bioactive compounds and their family. Source: Author.

many different families, the Lamiaceae (thyme family) is the most well-known plant family for these chemicals (Ajikumar et al. 2008).

(f) Tannin

Tannins bind to proteins indiscriminately; larger tannins are employed as astringents to treat transudates, skin bleeding, and diarrhea. In the kingdom of plants, tannins are found in great abundance. Polygonaceae (knotweed family) and Fagaceae (beech family) are the families linked to the presence of tannins (Pizzi 2021) (Figure 11.1).

Extraction Methods

In pharmaceuticals, the phrase "extraction" refers to the process of employing certain solvents in typical extraction processes to separate the medicinally active parts of plant or animal tissues from the inactive or inert components. Separating the easily soluble plant metabolites from the insoluble cellular debris (residue) is the aim of all extraction processes. Below is a discussion of some well-known extraction techniques (both traditional and contemporary) from medicinal plants.

(i) **Maceration:** A very simple extraction method, known as maceration, is utilized in drug development to extract bioactive substances from plant sources. This increases concentration and extraction yield by facilitating the diffusion and surface release of bioactive chemicals (Mohammadi et al. 2020).

(ii) **Percolation:** When making tinctures and fluid extracts, this is the method most commonly employed to extract the active components (Wang et al. 2023). Percolation can be conducted through a percolator.

(iii) **Reflux:** A boiling solvent is used to treat the material in this hot extraction procedure. A condenser is installed on top of the round-bottomed flask to recycle the solvent vapor. The extraction of thermolabile natural compounds is not possible with it (Zhang, Lin, and Ye 2018).

(iv) **Digestion:** This type of maceration involves applying temperature (between 40° and 60°C) while the extraction process is underway (Bitwell et al. 2023).

(v) **Tincture:** It is an alcohol-based plant material extract. Fresh plant material and ethyl alcohol are mixed at 1:5 ratios. The tincture's alcohol content allows it to be kept without decomposition at room temperature (Yunusova, Turdieva, and Ilkhamova 2022).

(vi) **Infusion:** The plant material is macerated with either cold or boiling water for a brief amount of time during this extraction procedure. It is a diluted mixture of the crude drugs' easily soluble ingredients (Majekodunmi 2015).

(vii) **Decoction:** This method involves boiling the plant powder in a specific amount of water for a standardized time, cooling it, and then straining or filtering it. This process works well for extracting components that are heat-stable and soluble in water. Usually, this method is employed to make the Ayurvedic extracts known as "quath" or "kwath" (Gao et al. 2022).

(viii) **Steam Distillation:** It is the typical procedure used to separate volatile oil from unfiltered plant parts. Steam distillation is a straightforward vaporization process that involves running steam through the substance (Masango 2005).

(ix) **Hydro-distillation:** This method is commonly employed to separate essential oils and other bioactive compounds from plant materials. A heating mantle is used to boil the plant material after it has been soaked in water. Because of the impact of hot water, the essential oil travels with the steam after being released from the plant tissues' oil glands. A common glass device called a clevenger apparatus is used to condense the steam-oil mixture, separate the oil from the water, and recycle the condensed water (Mejri, Abderrabba, and Mejri 2010).

(x) **Soxhlet Extraction:** This technique, named for the German agricultural chemist Franz Ritter von Soxhlet, is the most effective way to continuously extract a solid using a heated solvent. A specialized glass refluxing unit called a Soxhlet apparatus is primarily utilized for the extraction of organic solvents (Zhang, Lin, and Ye 2018).

(xi) **Pressurized Liquid Extraction (PLE):** The technique makes use of high pressure and temperature, where a higher temperature speeds up the extraction process by making the solvent more diffusive, while a higher pressure keeps the organic solvent liquid without boiling and compels it to enter the matrix pores. It is also known as enhanced solvent extraction system (ESE) or accelerated solvent extraction system (ASE) (Mustafa and Turner 2011).

(xii) **Supercritical Fluid Extraction (SFE):** In Supercritical Fluid Extraction (SFE), gases, typically CO_2, are used and compressed into a dense liquid. After that, the liquid is forced through a cylinder that holds the substance that has to be removed. The liquid containing the extract is then pushed into a separation chamber, where the gas is collected for further use and the extract is separated from it. By altering the temperature and pressure, the solvent characteristics of CO_2 can be controlled. One benefit of SFE is that it totally evaporates CO_2, leaving no solvent residues behind (Cabeza et al. 2017).

(xiii) **Ultrasonic Extraction:** In pharmaceutical engineering, this method is used to separate bioactive substances from plants, including vitamins, polyphenols, and polysaccharides. High-frequency sound causes natural chemicals to be released from the plant tissues during this process, damaging the cell wall (Shen et al. 2023).

(xiv) **Microwave-Assisted Extraction (MAE):** By this method, a compound is extracted from a sample matrix into solvent by microwave energy (Sparr Eskilsson and Björklund 2000). Several drugs, such as antiviral, anticancer, and antibacterial medicines, can be made via microwave-assisted synthesis.

(xv) **Solid Phase Extraction (SPE):** In drug development, solid phase extraction (SPE) is a method used to separate and purify analytes from a liquid sample prior to chromatographic analysis (Zhou et al. 2024) (Figure 11.2).

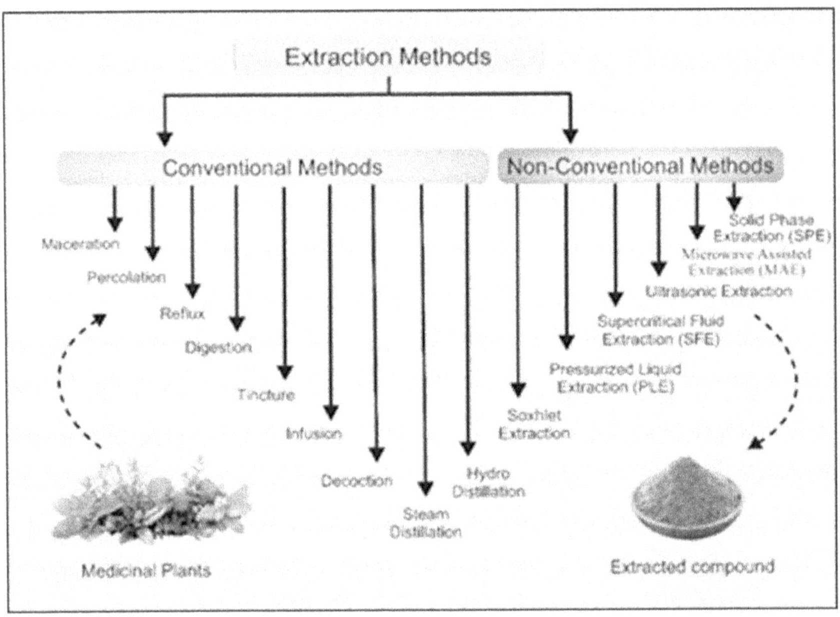

Figure 11.2. Extraction methods of bio-active compounds. Source: Author.

Techniques for Assessment of Antibacterial Efficiency

Numerous antimicrobal susceptibility testing (AST) methods are available to identify bacterial sensitivity to antibiotics. Practicality, adaptability, automation, affordability, repeatability, accuracy, and whether the data will be used for clinical or research objectives are just a few of the many factors that affect technique selection. The primary and widely recognized methods include the disk-diffusion and broth or agar dilution techniques. Alternative methods, such as the poisoned food technique, are employed specifically for antifungal testing. To investigate the antimicrobial effect of an agent comprehensively, time-kill tests and flow cytofluorometric methods are advised. These methods yield insights into the nature of the inhibitory effect, distinguishing between bactericidal and bacteriostatic actions, as well as identifying whether the effect is time-dependent or concentration-dependent, along with the extent of cell damage to the test microorganism. Moreover, the AST methods must yield trustworthy results in routine laboratory analysis in order to be compared to a recognized "gold standard" reference methodology.

Gram-positive *Staphylococcus aureus* (ATCC 29213) and *Enterococcus faecalis* (ATCC 29212) as well as gram-negative *Pseudomonas aeruginosa* (ATCC 25922) and *Escherichia coli* (ATCC 27853) are recommended by the Committee for Clinical Laboratory Standards (CLSI) for the preliminary test for antibacterial activity (Sarkar et al. 2024). The CLSI guidelines and the European Committee on Antimicrobial Susceptibility Testing (EUCAST) are available to standardize in vitro AST procedures pertinent to clinical testing; these guidelines are also used for biologically active substances since they lack their own standards (Humphries et al. 2018). Many studies depend on the minimum inhibitory concentration (MIC). MIC values for antibiotics range from 0.01 to 10 μg/mL while plant extracts are classified as antimicrobials if their MICs fall between 100 and 1000 μg/mL (Silva et al. 2013). Certain authors propose varying cutoffs based on the specific compound. For instance, a concentration of 1000 μg/mL is identified as the breakpoint for a polyphenol. However, because they are a complex collection of chemicals, natural extracts could not perform as expected in the test system. There are numerous obstacles to overcome when implementing clinical advice for natural extracts.

Antimicrobial Mechanisms of Ethnomedicinal Plants

Synthetic antimicrobial agents have received approval in numerous countries; however, the application of natural compounds derived from ethnomedicinal plants remains a major concern for many researchers (Moloney 2016). Ethnomedicinal plants possess significant potential for the identification of novel bioactive compounds capable of combating resistant microorganisms (Verpoorte 1998; Wright 2017). Chemicals derived from ethnomedicinal plants constitute a diverse array of compounds that occur naturally within these organisms. Restoration of the clinical application of older antibiotics can be achieved by enhancing their potency, thereby mitigating the issue of resistance (Barbieri et al. 2017; Lewis and Ausubel 2006). Bioactive compounds derived from plants, known as phytochemicals, are primarily secondary metabolites utilized for therapeutic applications. Secondary metabolites result from secondary plant metabolism and may manifest as either intermediate or end products (Serda et al. 2012). Their antimicrobial activity varies significantly based on the structure, quantity, and positioning of substituent groups, the presence of glycosidic linkages, alkylation of hydroxyl groups, and the geographic and climatic conditions of the country of origin. Variations in the quality and quantity of bioactive secondary metabolites influence their antimicrobial activity against various microbial strains (Arima and Danno 2002; Assob et al. 2011; Merkl et al., 2010).

Bioactive plant extracts typically comprise complex mixtures of components, and their synergistic interactions may produce an amplified effect (Cowan 1999). These compounds can influence the microbial cell through various mechanisms. Bioactive compounds primarily target the cytoplasmic membrane, influencing its structure, integrity, permeability, and functionality in various manners (Radulovic et al. 2013; Saleem, Saeed, and Ahmad 2010; Savoia 2012). Research indicates that plant extracts may comprise inhibitors of efflux pump (EP) (Savoia 2012). Furthermore, the inhibition of normal cell communication, specifically quorum sensing (QS), has been identified as a promising mechanism of action for bioactive compounds targeting multidrug-resistant (MDR) pathogens. QS-inhibitors must effectively reduce the expression of QS-controlled genes while maintaining chemical stability to withstand the metabolic and disposal processes of the host organism (Radulovic et al. 2013; Savoia 2012). Some compounds can alter or inhibit protein-protein interactions, thereby serving as effective modulators of immune response, mitosis, and apoptosis (Anand et al. 2019). Furthermore, they can disrupt intermediary metabolism (Anandhi et al. 2014), induce the coagulation of cytoplasmic constituents (Mogosanu et al. 2015), and inhibit or disrupt biofilm formation, which provides a protective advantage to pathogens during infection (Quave et al. 2012; Talekar, Choudhury, and Choudhury 2014).

Conclusion and Future Prospects

Ethnomedicinal research is the study of unique information about plant wealth and the pursuit of new resources for the production of herbal remedies, consumable plants, and other plant-related products (Kumar et al. 2021b). Throughout history, people have utilized plants to improve their physical health, and even in the present day, ethnomedicinal plants are becoming more and more popular due to their fewer side effects and availability. According to the data recorded by the World Health Organization around 65–80 percent of people worldwide, especially in developing nations, rely on plants for their medical treatment, and this is widely recognized in traditional cultures. Herbal medicine continues to be used extensively to treat and manage a wide range of illnesses, especially in rural and isolated parts of India. The market for herbal medications is currently valued at forty billion and is predicted to grow by 16 percent over the next three to four years. Nevertheless, the market demand for many plants exceeds output, which encourages adulteration in Ayurvedic medications (Semwal et al. 2019). However, subsequent research should focus on structural modifications of compounds to enhance pharmacokinetics and pharmacodynamics, as well as analyses of structure-activity relationships. Further studies are needed to investigate the synergistic interactions within ethnomedicinal plant extracts and between compounds and antibiotics, aiming to elucidate the mechanisms underlying the antimicrobial activity of these compounds and to identify multiple pathways for potential targeting. The interactions between ethnomedicinal plant extracts and antimicrobial agents can be either beneficial, as in synergism, or detrimental, as in antagonism. Consequently, additional research is necessary, particularly in vivo studies and investigations into the toxicity of these products, for them to be acknowledged as biomedical agents.

The advancement of effective antimicrobial susceptibility tests (ASTs) that provide benefits over traditional methods for the extraction, isolation, and analysis of bioactive compounds is expected to significantly enhance the quality of plant antimicrobials. Additional research is necessary for the determination of the minimum inhibitory concentration (MIC) of ethnomedicinal plant extracts to obtain results that can be compared with those of currently utilized antibiotics. Existing in vitro antimicrobial susceptibility tests require enhancement through the establishment of validated in vivo antimicrobial susceptibility tests. Enhancements in the efficiency of ASTs may depend not solely on the advancement of more intricate techniques but also on the application of best practices across all phases of the production and supply chain of ethnomedicinal plant medicines. Advanced techniques in biotechnology, genomics, proteomics, and metabolomics are currently utilized in ethnomedicinal plant research, contributing to the development of alternative natural antimicrobials. Technologies that can simultaneously identify active mixture compounds, characterize their interactions, and elucidate potential mechanisms of action have yet to be developed. The integration of assessment technologies with advancements in instrument automation presents significant opportunities to utilize the chemical diversity of bioactive compounds from ethnomedicinal plants in the search for novel antimicrobial drugs.

The antimicrobial activity of ethnomedicinal plants presents a promising approach to address the growing challenges associated with antimicrobial resistance. Consequently, it is imperative to identify and isolate novel bioactive compounds from ethnomedicinal plants that remain insufficiently investigated. The extensive variety of these compounds has demonstrated therapeutic potential as antimicrobials and as modifiers of antimicrobial resistance. The prospective application of novel bioactive compounds remains complex. Extensive in vitro and in vivo tests are essential to ensure the selection of active and nontoxic antimicrobial compounds derived from plants. Exploiting the potential synergistic or antagonistic effects of compounds within and between ethnomedicinal plant extracts presents a significant challenge. With advancements in biotechnology, it is evident that we will enhance our ability to investigate the chemical composition of ethnomedicinal plants and refine techniques for the extraction, fractionation, and identification of bioactive compounds, which exhibit varied chemical structures and mechanisms of action.

Standardizing extraction methods and in vitro testing would enhance the systematic nature of the search and facilitate the interpretation of results. Furthermore, reference models have not been utilized in the investigation of plant extract mixtures, and subsequent research will determine their relevance for this methodology. Research focusing on the mechanisms of action, interactions with antibiotics or other ethnomedicinal plants or compounds, as well as the pharmacokinetic and pharmacodynamic profiles of the extracts, should be prioritized. This work aims to address the primary challenges identified in the field, facilitating the adoption of more efficient and effective methods for the expedited utilization of new therapeutic ethnomedicinal plants against microbes.

References

Ahmad, I., and A. Z. Beg. "Antimicrobial and Phytochemical Studies on 45 Indian Medicinal Plants against Multi-drug Resistant Human Pathogens." *Journal of Ethnopharmacology* 74, no. 2 (2001): 113–23.

Ait Bouzid, H., M. Ibourki, A. Hamdouch, S. Oubannin, A. Asbbane, O. Hallouch, L. Bijla, J. Koubachi, K. Majourhat, and S. Gharby. "Moroccan Aromatic and Medicinal Plants: A Review of Economy, Ethnobotany, Chemical Composition, and Biological Activities of Commonly Used Plants." *Food and Humanity* 2 (2024): 100259.

Ajikumar, P. K., K. Tyo, S. Carlsen, O. Mucha, T. H. Phon, and G. Stephanopoulos. "Terpenoids: Opportunities for Biosynthesis of Natural Product Drugs Using Engineered Microorganisms." *Molecular Pharmaceutics* 5, no. 2 (2008): 167–90.

Anand, U., R. Bulusu, B. McMahon, O. Newman, L. O'Driscoll, and F. M. Lyng. "Protein–protein Interaction Modulators: Advances, Successes and Challenges." *Future Medicinal Chemistry* 11, no. 13 (2019): 1521–42.

Anand, V., R. Kandarapu, and S. Garg. "Ion-exchange Resins: Carrying Drug Delivery Forward." *Drug Discovery Today* 6, no. 17 (2001): 905–14.

Anandhi, M., M. S. Josephine, V. Jeyabalaraja, and S. Satthiyaraj. "A Novel Approach on Network Security Using Edge Detection Techniques in Biometric Applications." International Journal of Applied Engineering Research 9, no. 21 (2014): 8673–80.

Anas, E. M., K Mohamed, B. Said, N. Mourad, S. Chaimae, L. Boutaina, N. Abderrahman, C. Essediya, B. Taha, R. Chaimae, C. El, and M. Anas. "Traditional Knowledge and Biodiversity of Medicinal Plants in the Taounate Region for Treating Human Diseases: An Ethnobotanical Perspective." *Ethnobotany Research and Applications* 29 (2024): 1–22.

Ansari, S. H., M. Ali, and A. K. Najmi. "Antibacterial Activity of Pistacia Integerrima Stem Extracts against Gram-positive and Gram-negative Bacteria." *Journal of Ethnopharmacology* 63, no. 3 (1998): 247–9.

Apisariyakul, A., Y. Vanittanakom, and D. Buddhasukh. "Antifungal Activity of Turmeric Oil Extracted from Curcuma longa (Zingiberaceae)." *Journal of Ethnopharmacology* 49, no. 3 (1995): 163–9.

Arima, H., and G. Danno. "Isolation of Antimicrobial Compounds from Guava (Psidium guajava L.) and Their Structural Elucidation." *Bioscience, Biotechnology, and Biochemistry* 66, no. 8 (2002): 1727–30.

Assob, J. C. N., H. L. F. Kamga, D. S. Nsagha, A. L. Njunda, P. F. Nde, E. A. Asongalem, A. J. Njouendou, B. Sandjon, and V. B. Penlap "Antimicrobial and Toxicological Activities of Five Medicinal Plant Species from Cameroon Traditional Medicine." *BMC Complementary and Alternative Medicine* 11 (2011): 1–11.

Ayaz, M., F. Ullah, A. Sadiq, F. Ullah, M. Ovais, J. Ahmed, and H. P. Devkota. "Synergistic Interactions of Phytochemicals with Antimicrobial Agents: Potential Strategy to Counteract Drug Resistance." *Chemico-Biological Interactions* 308 (2019): 294–303.

Banerjee, S. *Introduction to Ethnobotany and Traditional Medicine.* Singapore: Springer, 2024.

Barbieri, R., E. Coppo, A. Marchese, M. Daglia, E. Sobarzo-Sánchez, S. F. Nabavi, et al. "Phytochemicals for Human Disease: An Update on Plant-Derived Compounds Antibacterial Activity." *Microbiological Research* 196 (2017): 44–68.

Bbosa, G. S., D. B. Kyegombe, J. Ogwal-Okeng, R. Bukenya-Ziraba, O. Odyek, and P. Waako. "Antibacterial Activity of Mangifera indica (L.)." *African Journal of Ecology* 45 (2007): 13–16.

Begum, N., and S. Mandal. "A Contribution to the Medicinal Plants Used by the Tribal People of Lateritic Belt of West Bengal." *World Journal of Pharmacy and Pharmaceutical Sciences* 5, no. 8 (2016): 1420–31.

Bhadra, A., and B. T. Manjunath. "Herbal Healing Traditions: A Study of Folk Medicines Used by Traditional Healers of Sonamukhi Block, Bankura District, West Bengal, India." *Plant Science Today* 11, no. 1 (2024): 1–9.

Bhat, J. A., M. Kumar, and R. W. Bussmann. "Ecological Status and Traditional Knowledge of Medicinal Plants in Kedarnath Wildlife Sanctuary of Garhwal Himalaya, India." *Journal of Ethnobiology and Ethnomedicine* 9, no. 1 (2013): 1–18.

Bhosle, S. V., V. P. Ghule, D. J. Aundhe, and S. D. Jagtap. "Ethnomedical Knowledge of Plants Used by the Tribal People of Purandhar in Maharashtra, India." *Ethnobotanical Leaflets* 13 (2009): 1353–61.

Bitwell, C., S. Indra, Sen, C. Luke, and M. K. Kakoma. "A Review of Modern and Conventional Extraction Techniques and Their Applications for Extracting Phytochemicals from Plants." *Scientific African* 19 (2023): e01585.

Cabeza, L. F., A. de Gracia, A. I. Fernández, and M. M. Farid. "Supercritical CO2 as Heat Transfer Fluid: A Review." *Applied Thermal Engineering* 125 (2017): 799–810.

Cai, L., and C. D. Wu. "Antimicrobial Activity of the Extracts and Compounds from Syzygium aromaticum and Psidium guajava Leaves against Streptococcus mutans." *Journal of Dental Research* 75 (1996): 203.

Casado, N., S. Morante-Zarcero, and I. Sierra. "The Concerning Food Safety Issue of Pyrrolizidine Alkaloids: An Overview." *Trends in Food Science & Technology* 120 (2022): 123–39.

Chakraborty, R., B. K. De, N. Devanna, and S. Sen. "North East India an Ethnic Storehouse of Unexplored Medicinal Plants." *Journal of Natural Product and Plant Resources* 2, no. 1 (2012): 143–52.

Cheesman, M. J., A. Ilanko, B. Blonk, and I. E. Cock. "Developing New Antimicrobial Therapies: Are Synergistic Combinations of Plant Extracts/Compounds with

Conventional Antibiotics the Solution?" *Pharmacognosy Reviews* 11, no. 22 (2017): 57–72.

Chrzanowska, M., A. Grajewska, and M. D. Rozwadowska. "Asymmetric Synthesis of Isoquinoline Alkaloids: 2004–2015." *Chemical Reviews* 116, no. 19 (2016): 12369–465.

Cowan, M. M. "Plant Products as Antimicrobial Agents." *Clinical Microbiology Reviews* 12, no. 4 (1999): 564–82.

Dah-Nouvlessounon, D., M. Chokki, A. D. P. Noumavo, G. Cârâc, B. Furdui, H. Sina, C. Zongo, A. Savadogo, L. Baba-Moussa, R. M. Dinica, and F. Baba-Moussa. "Ethnopharmacological Value and Biological Activities via Antioxidant and Anti-Protein Denaturation Activity of Morinda lucida Benth and Momordica charantia L. Leaves Extracts from Benin." *Plants* 12, no. 6 (2023): 1228.

Dickson, R. A., L. Amponsah, A. N. Ankrah, and K. M. Mensah. "Antibacterial and Antioxidant Cassane Diterpenoids from Caesalpinia benthamiana." *Journal of Natural Products* 70, no. 12 (2007): 1904–8.

Eldeen, I. M., E. E. Elgorashi, and J. van Staden. "Antibacterial, Anti-inflammatory, Anti-cholinesterase and Mutagenic Effects of Extracts Obtained from Some Trees Used in South African Traditional Medicine." *Journal of Ethnopharmacology* 102, no. 3 (2005): 457–64.

Farnsworth, N. R. "The Role of Ethnopharmacology in Drug Development." *Ciba Foundation Symposium* 154 (1990): 2–11.

Ferrari, P. A., S. Zank, and N. Hanazaki. "Unraveling Sustainability in Brazilian Ethnobotany: An Analysis of the Sustainable Development Goals (SDGs)." *Economic Botany* 78, no. 2 (2024): 197–216.

Ferrazzano, G. F., T. Cantile, L. Roberto, A. Ingenito, M. R. Catania, E. Roscetto, G. Palumbo, A. Zarrelli, and A. Pollio. "Determination of the In Vitro and In Vivo Antimicrobial Activity on Salivary Streptococci and Lactobacilli and Chemical Characterisation of the Phenolic Content of a Plantago lanceolata Infusion." *BioMed Research International* 2015, no. 1 (2015): 286817.

Fitzgerald, M., M. Heinrich, and A. Booker. "Medicinal Plant Analysis: A Historical and Regional Discussion of Emergent Complex Techniques." *Frontiers in Pharmacology* 10 (2019): 423244.

Fuster, F., C. N. Kaiser-Bunbury, and J. M Olesen. "Pollination Effectiveness of Specialist and Opportunistic Nectar Feeders Influenced by Invasive Alien Ants in the Seychelles." *American Journal of Botany* 107, no. 7 (2020): 957–69.

Gao, Y., Y. Dong, Q. Guo, H. Wang, M. Feng, Z. Yan, and D. Bai. "Study on Supramolecules in Traditional Chinese Medicine Decoction." *Molecules* 27, no. 10 (2022): 3268.

Gleadow, R. M., and I. E. Woodrow. "Constraints on Effectiveness of Cyanogenic Glycosides in Herbivore Defense." *Journal of Chemical Ecology* 28, no. 7 (2002): 1301–13.

Goyal, M., D. Sasmal, and B. P. Nagori. "Review on Medicinal Plants Used by Local Community of Jodhpur District of Thar Desert." *International Journal of Pharmacology* 7, no. 3 (2011): 333–9.

Grange, J. M., and N. J. Snell. "Activity of Amorolfine against Mycobacterium Tuberculosis, Mycobacterium avium and Mycobacterium microti." *Journal of Antimicrobial Chemotherapy* 38, no. 1 (1996): 105–7.

Griffin, W. J., and G. D. Lin. "Chemotaxonomy and Geographical Distribution of Tropane Alkaloids." *Phytochemistry* 53, no. 6 (2000): 623–37.

Gupta, M., U. K. Mazumder, U. Rath, and D. Kumar. "Antibacterial Activity of Acacia catechu Wild. Bark Extract." *International Journal of Pharmacognosy* 42, no. 3 (2004): 248–50.

Haq, S. M., and B. Singh. "Ethnobotany as a Science of Preserving Traditional Knowledge: Traditional Uses of Wild Medicinal Plants from District Reasi, J & K (Northwestern Himalaya), India." In *Botanical Leads for Drug Discovery*, edited by B. Singh, 277–93, Springer: Singapore, 2020.

Humphries, R. M., J. Ambler, S. L. Mitchell, M. Castanheira, T. Dingle, J. A. Hindler, L. Koeth, and K. Sei. "CLSI Methods Development and Standardization Working Group Best Practices for Evaluation of Antimicrobial Susceptibility Tests." *Journal of Clinical Microbiology* 56, no. 4 (2018): 1–10.

Hossan, M. S., P. Roy, S. Seraj, S. M. Mou, M. N. Monalisa, S. Jahan, T. Khan, A. Swarna, R. Jahan, and M. Rahmatullah. "Ethnomedicinal Knowledge among the Tonchongya Tribal Community of Roangchaari Upazila of Bandarban District, Bangladesh." *American-Eurasian Journal of Sustainable Agriculture* 6, no. 4 (2012): 349–59.

Howes, M. J. R., C. L. Quave, J. Collemare, E. C. Tatsis, D. Twilley, E. Lulekal, A. Farlow, L. Li, M. E. Cazar, D. J. Leaman, T. A. K. Prescott, W. Milliken, C. Martin, M. N. De Canha, N. Lall, H. Qin, B. E. Walker, C. Vásquez-Londoño, B. Allkin, and E. Nic Lughadha. "Molecules from Nature: Reconciling Biodiversity Conservation and Global Healthcare Imperatives for Sustainable Use of Medicinal Plants and Fungi." *Plants, People, Planet* 2, no. 5 (2020): 463–81.

Izah, S. C., O. I.Ogidi, M. C. Ogwu, S. S. Salimon, Z. M. Yusuf, M. Akram, M. O. Raimi, and A. A. Iyingiala. "Historical Perspectives and Overview of the Value of Herbal Medicine." In *Reference Series in Phytochemistry*, Vol. Part F3164, 3–35, Cham: Springer, 2024.

Jain, S. K. "Ethnobotany and Research on Medicinal Plants in India." *Ciba Foundation Symposium* 185 (1994): 153–64.

Jamshidi-Kia, F., Z. Lorigooini, and H. Amini-Khoei. "Medicinal Plants: Past History and Future Perspective." *Journal of Herbmed Pharmacology* 7, no. 1 (2017): 1–7.

Khongsai, L., R. K. Yadav, and M. Singh. "Ethnomedicinal Plants Used by Tribal Communities of Arunachal Pradesh for Treating Microbial Infections." *Indian Journal of Traditional Knowledge* 10, no. 3 (2011): 528–30.

Kosalge, S. B., and R. A. Fursule. "Investigation of Ethnomedicinal Claims of Some Plants Used by Tribals of Satpuda Hills in India." *Journal of Ethnopharmacology* 121, no. 3 (2009): 456–61.

Kumar, A. "Evidenced Based Antimicrobial Potential of Medicinal Plants and Herbs Countering Bacterial Pathogens." *International Journal of Pharmacology* 10, no. 1 (2017): 1–43.

Kumar, A., S. Kumar, Komal, N. Ramchiary, and P. Singh. "Role of Traditional Ethnobotanical Knowledge and Indigenous Communities in Achieving Sustainable Development Goals." *Sustainability* 13, no. 6 (2021a): 3062.

Kumar, M., S. Rawat, B. Nagar, A. Kumar, N. A. Pala, J. A. Bhat, R. W. Bussmann, M. Cabral-Pinto, and R. Kunwar. "Implementation of the Use of Ethnomedicinal Plants for Curing Diseases in the Indian Himalayas and Its Role in Sustainability of

Livelihoods and Socioeconomic Development." *International Journal of Environmental Research and Public Health* 18, no. 4 (2021b): 1–26.

Lewis, Kim, and F. M. Ausubel. "Prospects for Plant-Derived Antibacterials." *Nature Biotechnology* 24, no. 12 (2006): 1504–7.

Li, H., L. Li, and D. Lockington. "Aeration for Plant Root Respiration in a Tidal Marsh." *Water Resources Research* 41, no. 9 (2005): 1–11.

Li, Y., D. Kong, Y. Fu, M. R. Sussman, and H. Wu. "The Effect of Developmental and Environmental Factors on Secondary Metabolites in Medicinal Plants." *Plant Physiology and Biochemistry* 148 (2020): 80–9.

Maikhuri, R. K., and K. S. Rao. "Plants and Wild Edibles Among Three." *Indigenous Knowledge and Development Monitor* 8 no. 2 (2000): 7–13.

Majekodunmi, S. O. "Review of Extraction of Medicinal Plants for Pharmaceutical Research." *Merit Research Journal of Medicine and Medical Sciences* 3, no. 11 (2015): 521–7.

Martínez, M. Carmen, et al. "Arabidopsis Formaldehyde Dehydrogenase. Molecular Properties of Plant Class III Alcohol Dehydrogenase Provide Further Insights into the Origins, Structure and Function of Plant Class P and Liver Class I Alcohol Dehydrogenases." *European Journal of Biochemistry* 241, no. 1 (1996): 75–82.

Masango, P. "Cleaner Production of Essential Oils by Steam Distillation." *Journal of Cleaner Production* 13, no. 8 (2005): 833–9.

Mejri, J., M. Abderrabba, and M. Mejri. "Chemical Composition of the Essential Oil of Ruta Chalepensis L: Influence of Drying, Hydro-distillation Duration and Plant Parts." *Industrial Crops and Products* 32, no. 3 (2010): 671–3.

Merkl, R., I. Hrádková, V. Filip, and J. Šmidrka. "Antimicrobial and Antioxidant Properties of Phenolic Acids Alkyl Esters." *Czech Journal of Food Sciences* 28, no. 4 (2010): 275–9.

Mogosanu, G. D., M. Semeniuc, P. Oana, and A. M. Grumezescu. "Prevention of Microbial Communities: Novel Approaches Based on Natural Products." In *Nanotechnology in Antimicrobial Sensing and Microbiological Analysis*, edited by A. M. Grumezescu, 433–52. Academic Press/Elsevier, 2015.

Mohagheghzadeh, A., P. Faridi, M. Shams-Ardakani, and Y. Ghasemi,. "Medicinal Plants Used in Traditional Medicine in Shiraz, Iran." *Iranian Journal of Pharmaceutical Research* 6, no. 2 (2007): 161–4.

Mohammadi, M., V. Zambare, L. Malek, C. Gottardo, Z. Suntres, and L. Christopher. "Lichenochemicals: Extraction, Purification, Characterization, and Application as Potential Anticancer Agents." *Expert Opinion on Drug Discovery* 15, no. 5 (2020): 575–601.

Moloney, M. G. "Natural Products as a Foundation for Drug Discovery." *Royal Society of Chemistry* (2016): 1–25.

Moraes, R. M., B. Klumpp, G. Klumpp, and G. M. F. Lima. "Air Pollutants and Leaf Anatomy of Tibouchina pulchra (Cham.) Cogn." *Journal of Applied Botany – Angewandte Botanik* 76 (2002): 104–9.

Morris, M. E., and S. Zhang. "Flavonoid–drug Interactions: Effects of Flavonoids on ABC Transporters." *Life Sciences* 78, no. 18 (2006): 2116–30.

Mustafa, A., and C. Turner. "Pressurized Liquid Extraction as a Green Approach in Food and Herbal Plants Extraction: A Review." *Analytica Chimica Acta* 703, no. 1 (2011): 8–18.

Nautiyal, B. P., M. C. Nautiyal, and V. Prakash. "Medicinal Plants of India: Conservation and Sustainable Utilization." *Botanical Survey of India (BSI), Ministry of Environment, Forest and Climate Change*, Government of India, 2015.

Negi, V. S., R. K. Maikhuri, and L. S. Rawat. "Non-timber Forest Products (NTFPs): A Viable Option for Biodiversity Conservation and Livelihood Enhancement in Central Himalaya." *Biodiversity and Conservation* 20, no. 3 (2011): 545–59.

Nishimura, H., and A. Satoh. "Antimicrobial and Nematicidal Substances from the Root of Chicory (Cichorium intybus)." In *Allelochemicals: Biological Control of Plant Pathogens and Diseases*, edited by Inderjit and K. G. Mukerji, 153–62. Dordrecht: Springer, 2006.

Nishteswar, K. "Pharmacological and Pharmaceutical Principles of Ayurvedic Drugs: A Concurrent Appraisal." In *Translational Ayurveda*, edited by S. Rastogi, 53–75. Singapore: Springer, 2019.

Oakenfull, D. "Saponins in Food—A Review." *Food Chemistry* 7, no. 1 (1981): 19–40.

Oliveira, A. C., A. R. Araçari, C. C. Teixeira, R. C. R. C. Pinto, and F. Fuchs. "Antimicrobial Activity of Syzygium cumini (Myrtaceae) Leaves Extract." *Revista Brasileira de Farmacognosia* 17, no. 2 (2007): 236–40.

Palit, D., and S. Gurung. "Some Phytoremedies Used Traditionally by Gurungs in Darjeeling, West Bengal, India." *Pleione* 2, no. 2 (2008): 171–4.

Pammi, S. S. S., B. Suresh, and A. Giri. "Antioxidant Potential of Medicinal Plants." *Journal of Crop Science and Biotechnology* 26, no. 1 (2023): 13–26.

Pandey, M. M., S. Rastogi, and A. K. S. Rawat. "Indian Traditional Ayurvedic System of Medicine and Nutritional Supplementation." *Evidence-Based Complementary and Alternative Medicine* 2013 (2013): 1–12.

Pant, P., S. Pandey, and S. Dall'Acqua. "The Influence of Environmental Conditions on Secondary Metabolites in Medicinal Plants: A Literature Review." *Chemistry & Biodiversity* 18, no. 11 (2021): e2100345.

Parekh, J., and S. V. Chanda. "In vitro Antimicrobial Activity and Phytochemical Analysis of Some Indian Medicinal Plants." *Turkish Journal of Biology* 31, no. 1 (2007): 53–8.

Park, K. M., J. S. You, H. Y. Lee, N. I. Baek, and J. K. Hwang. "Kuwanon G: An Antibacterial Agent from the Root Bark of Morus alba against Oral Pathogens." *Journal of Ethnopharmacology* 84, no. 2–3 (2003): 181–5.

Pizzi, A. "Tannins Medical / Pharmacological and Related Applications: A Critical Review." *Sustainable Chemistry and Pharmacy* 22 (2021): 100481.

Prakash, R. "Medicinal Plants Used By Tribal Communities : A Study of Uttarakhand Himalayan Region." *International Journal of Humanities and Social Science Invention* 4, no. 2 (2015): 55–61.

Prance, G. T. "What Is Ethnobotany Today?" *Journal of Ethnopharmacology* 32 (1991): 209–16.

Prassas, I., and E. P. Diamandis. "Novel Therapeutic Applications of Cardiac Glycosides." *Nature Reviews Drug Discovery* 7, no. 11 (2008): 926–35.

Quave, C. L., M. S. Lipsky, J. M. Kelley, Y. Jiang, J. T. Curé, and T. K. Wood. "Evaluation of the Antibacterial Potency of Medicinal Plants Used in Georgian Traditional Medicine against Clinical Strains of Pathogenic Bacteria." *Journal of Ethnopharmacology* 139, no. 2 (2012): 514–20.

Radulovic, N. S., P. D. Blagojevic, N. M. Stojanovic, and S. S. Sobcanić. "Antimicrobial Plant Metabolites: Structural Diversity and Mechanism of Action." *Current Pharmaceutical Design* 19, no. 11 (2013): 1871–98.

Raj, A. J., S. Biswakarma, N. A. Pala, G. Shukla, M. Kumar, S. Chakravarty, and R. W. Bussmann. "Indigenous Uses of Ethnomedicinal Plants among Forest-dependent Communities of Northern Bengal, India." *Journal of Ethnobiology and Ethnomedicine* 14, no. 1 (2018): 1–28.

Ralte, L., H. Sailo, and Y. T. Singh. "Ethnobotanical Study of Medicinal Plants Used by the Indigenous Community of the Western Region of Mizoram, India." *Journal of Ethnobiology and Ethnomedicine* 20, no. 1 (2024): 1–24.

Rani, P., and N. Khullar. "Antimicrobial Evaluation of Some Medicinal Plants for Their Anti-Infective Potential." *Phytotherapy Research* 18, no. 8 (2004): 670–3.

Rasingam, L. "Ethnobotanical Studies on the Wild Edible Plants of Irula Tribes of Pillur Valley, Coimbatore district, Tamil Nadu, India." *Asian Pacific Journal of Tropical Biomedicine* 2, no. 3 (2012): 1493–7.

Reyes-García, V. "The Relevance of Traditional Knowledge Systems for Ethnopharmacological Research: Theoretical and Methodological Contributions." *Journal of Ethnobiology and Ethnomedicine* 6, no. 1 (2010): 1–12.

Rizvi, M. M. A., M. Irshad, G. El Hassadi, and S. Ben Younis. "Bioefficacies of Cassia fistula: An Indian labrum." *African Journal of Pharmacy and Pharmacology* 3, no. 6 (2009): 287–92.

Rout, S. D., T. Panda, and N. Mishra. "Ethno-medicinal Plants Used to Cure Different Diseases by Tribals of Mayurbhanj District of North Orissa." *Ethno-Med* 3, no. 1 (2009): 27–32.

Sajem, A. L., and K. Gosai. "Traditional Use of Medicinal Plants by the Jaintia Tribes in North Cachar Hills District of Assam, Northeast India." *Journal of Ethnobiology and Ethnomedicine* 2 (2006): 1–7.

Saleem, M., M. T. Saeed, and S. I. Ahmad. "Antimicrobial Potential of Plant Extracts against Food-borne Pathogens." *World Applied Sciences Journal* 10, no. 11 (2010): 1274–8.

Sakulpanich, A., and W. Gritsanapan. "Determination of Anthraquinone Contents in Cassia Fistula Leaves for Alternative Source of Laxative Drugs." *Planta Medica* 75 (2009): 28–31.

Sanhueza, L., M. Faundez, and M. P. Paz. "Synergistic Interactions between Phenolic Compounds Identified in Grape pomace Extract with Antibiotics of Different Classes against Escherichia coli and Staphylococcus aureus Resistant Strains." *Journal of Applied Microbiology* 123, no. 1 (2017): 121–9.

Sarkar,J., M. C. Biswas, A. Naskar, and M. Kozarski. "Ganoderma: Antibacterial Effectiveness and Future Scope." *Ganoderma*, CRC Press, 2024, pp.20–48.

Savoia, D. "Plant-derived Antimicrobial Compounds: Alternatives to Antibiotics." *Future Microbiology* 7, no. 8 (2012): 979–90.

Semwal, D. K., A. Chauhan, A. Kumar, S. Aswal, R. B. Semwal, and A. Kumar. "Status of Indian Medicinal Plants in the International Union for Conservation of Nature and the Future of Ayurvedic Drugs: Shouldn't Think about Ayurvedic Fundamentals?" *Journal of Integrative Medicine* 17, no. 4 (2019): 238–43.

Schelz, Z., J. Molnar, and J. Hohmann. "Antimicrobial and Antiplasmid Activities of Essential Oils." *Fitoterapia* 77, no. 4 (2006): 279–85.

Serda, M., et al. "Synthesis and Characterization of Quinoline-Based Thiosemicarbazones and Correlation of Cellular Iron-Binding Efficacy to Anti-Tumor Efficacy." *Bioorganic & Medicinal Chemistry Letters* 22,no. 17 (2012): 5527–31.

Shahrajabian, M. H., Y. Kuang, H. Cui, L. Fu, and W. Sun. "Metabolic Changes of Active Components of Important Medicinal Plants on the Basis of Traditional Chinese Medicine under Different Environmental Stresses." *Current Organic Chemistry* 27, no. 9 (2023): 782–806.

Sharma, A., S. Khanna, G. Kaur, and I. Singh. "Medicinal Plants and Their Components for Wound Healing Applications." *Future Journal of Pharmaceutical Sciences* 7, no. 1 (2021): 1–13.

Sharma, J., S. Gairola, R. D. Gaur, and R. M. Painuli. "The Treatment of Jaundice with Medicinal Plants in Indigenous Communities of the Sub-Himalayan Region of Uttarakhand, India." *Journal of Ethnopharmacology* 143, no. 1 (2012): 262–91.

Sharma, N. K., P. K. Singh, V. Pramanik, B. Maji, and V. K. Mishra. "Traditional Ethnomedicinal Knowledge of Indian Tribes." *Current Science* 110, no. 4 (2016): 486–7.

Shen, L., S. Pang, M. Zhong, Y. Sun, A. Qayum, Y. Liu, A. Rashid, B. Xu, Q. Liang, H. Ma, and X. Ren. "A Comprehensive Review of Ultrasonic Assisted Extraction (UAE) for Bioactive Components: Principles, Advantages, Equipment, and Combined Technologies." *Ultrasonics Sonochemistry* 101 (2023): 106646.

Shewamene, Z., T. Dune, and C. A. Smith. "Use of Traditional and Complementary Medicine for Maternal Health and Wellbeing by African Migrant Women in Australia: A Mixed Method Study." *BMC Complementary Medicine and Therapies* 20, no. 1 (2020): 60.

Shil, S., M. D. Choudhury, and S. Das. "Indigenous Knowledge of Medicinal Plants Used by the Reang Tribe of Tripura State of India." *Journal of Ethnopharmacology* 152, no. 1 (2014): 135–41.

Signorini, M. A., M. Piredda, and P. Bruschi. "Plants and Traditional Knowledge: An Ethnobotanical Investigation on Monte Ortobene (Nuoro, Sardinia)." *Journal of Ethnobiology and Ethnomedicine* 5, no. 1 (2009): 1–14.

Silva, A.C.O., E.F. Santana, A. M. Saraiva, et al. "Which Approach Is More Effective in the Selection of Plants with Antimicrobial Activity?" *Evidence-Based Complementary and Alternative Medicine* 2013 (2013): 1–9.

Sparr Eskilsson, C., and E. Björklund. "Analytical-scale Microwave-assisted Extraction." *Journal of Chromatography A* 902, no. 1 (2000): 227–50.

Sreedevi, P., T. P. Ijinu, S. Anzar, A. J. Bincy, V. George, S. Rajasekharan, and P. Pushpangadan. "Ethnobiology, Ethnobotany, Ethnomedicine and Traditional Knowledge with Special Reference to India." *Annals of Phytomedicine* 2, no. 2 (2013): 4–12.

Stange, R. R., S. L. Midland, J. W. Eckert, and J. J. Sims. "An Antifungal Compound Produced by Grapefruit and Valencia Orange after Wounding of the Peel." *Journal of Natural Products* 56, no. 9 (1993): 1627–9.

Stickel, F., and D. Schuppan. "Herbal Medicine in the Treatment of Liver Diseases." *Digestive and Liver Disease* 39, no. 4 (2007): 293–304.

Syed, W., M. Gillani, M. Ahmad, M. Zafar, M. Haq, H. Manzoor, M. Shaheen, S. Waheed, F. Sultana, R. Ur, T. Makhkamov, C. Syed, W. Gillani, M. Ahmad, M. Zafar, M. Manzoor, H. Shaheen, M. Waheed, S. Sultana, and F. U. Rehman. "An Insight into Indigenous Ethnobotanical Knowledge of Medicinal and Aromatic Plants from Kashmir Himalayan Region." *Ethnobotany Research and Applications* 28 (2024): 1–21.

Takahashi, T., R. Kokubo, and M. Sakaino. "Antimicrobial Activities of Eucalyptus Leaf Extracts and Flavonoids from Eucalyptus maculata." *Letters in Applied Microbiology* 39, no. 1 (2004): 60–4.

Talekar, S., D. Choudhury, and M. Choudhury. "Inhibition of Bacterial Biofilm Formation by Bacteriophage." *Asian Pacific Journal of Tropical Biomedicine* 4, suppl. 1 (2014): S47–52.

Theodoridis, S., E. G. Drakou, T. Hickler, M. Thines, and D. Nogues-Bravo. "Evaluating Natural Medicinal Resources and Their Exposure to Global Change." *The Lancet Planetary Health* 7, no. 2 (2023): 155–63.

Tiwari, D. K., and A. Yadav. "Ethnobotanical Investigation of Some Medicinal Plants Availed by Gond Tribe of Naoradehi Wild Life Sanctuary, Madhya Pradesh." *The Anthropologist* 5, no. 3 (2003): 201–2.

Tokusoglu, O. "Food and Beverage Methylxanthines, Glycoalkaloids, Pyrolizidines and Phenolic Alkaloids: Processing Effects." *Journal of Food Health and Technology Innovations* 2, no. 5 (2019): 130–3.

Tripathi, M. K., and A. S. Mishra. "Glucosinolates in Animal Nutrition: A Review." *Animal Feed Science and Technology* 132, no. 1–2 (2007): 1–27.

Uniyal, B. "Utilization of Medicinal Plants by the Rural Women of Kullu, Himachal Pradesh." *Indian Journal of Traditional Knowledge* 2, no. 4 (2003): 366–70.

Upasana, S. "Ethnobotanical Study of Plants of Raigarh Area, Chattisgarh, India." *International Research Journal of Biological Sciences* 4, no. 6 (2015): 36–43.

Vaou, N., E. Stavropoulou, C. Voidarou, C. Tsigalou, and E. Bezirtzoglou. "Towards Advances in Medicinal Plant Antimicrobial Activity: A Review Study on Challenges and Future Perspectives." *Microorganisms* 9, no. 10 (2021): 2041.

Verpoorte, R. "Exploitation of Plant Biodiversity: Problems and Opportunities." In *Medicinal and Aromatic Plants – Industrial Profiles*, edited by G. Della Porta et al., vol. 3, Harwood Academic Publishers, 1998.

Vineeta, G. Shukla, J. A. Bhat, and S. Chakravarty. "Species Richness and Folk Therapeutic Uses of Ethnomedicinal Plants in West Bengal, India – A Meta-analysis." *Phytomedicine Plus* 2, no. 1 (2022): 100158.

Vitalini, S., M. Iriti, C. Puricelli, D. Ciuchi, A. Segale, and G. Fico. "Traditional Knowledge on Medicinal and food plants used in Val San Giacomo (Sondrio, Italy)—an Alpine Ethnobotanical Study." *Journal of Ethnopharmacology* 145, no. 2 (2013): 517–29.

Wang, J. X., X. H. Li, F. Gao, and X. L. Zhou. "An Unexpected Lewis Acid-mediated Structural Conversion of a Euphorbia Diterpene: From a Lathyrane Skeleton to Diterpene Pseudo-alkaloids." *Fitoterapia* 146 (2020): 104710.

Wang, W., F. Ding, H. Qu, and X. Gong. "Mechanism Modeling and Application of Salvia Miltiorrhiza Percolation Process." *Scientific Reports* 13, no. 1 (2023): 1–19.

Wright, P. "Plant-Derived Antimicrobials to Fight Against Multi-Drug-Resistant Bacteria." *BMC Complementary and Alternative Medicine* 17 (2017): 322.

Yunusova, H. M., Z. V. Turdieva, and N. B. Ilkhamova. "Development of Modern Technology for Obtaining Tinctures with Sedative Effect." *Cardiometry* 21 (2022): 90–4.

Zahin, M., F. Aqil, M. S. A. Khan, and I. Ahmad. "Ethnomedicinal Plants Derived Antibacterials and Their Prospects." *Helicobacter* 661, no. 2 (2010): 49–178.

Zhang, Q. W., L. G. Lin, and W. C. Ye. "Techniques for Extraction and Isolation of Natural Products: A Comprehensive Review." *Chinese Medicine (United Kingdom)* 13, no. 1 (2018): 1–26.

Zhou, J., Y. Chang, H. Tian, J. H. Qu, Q. Wang, J. Wang, and Z. Jiang. "Recent Advances in Accelerating Solid-phase Extraction." *Journal of Chromatography Open* 6 (2024): 100156.

12

Bioactive Compounds from Ethnomedicinal Plants with Antimicrobial Properties

Atreyi Ghosh[11*], Laiba Usmani[2], and Tanzila Alvi[1]

[1]Department of Microbiology, Sister Nivedita University, Kolkata, West Bengal, India

[2]Department of Biotechnology, Sister Nivedita University, Kolkata, West Bengal, India

*Corresponding Author's Email: atreyi.g@snuniv.ac.in

Introduction

The intimate connection between humans and plants is the primary emphasis of the scientific field of ethnobotany. US botanist John William Harsh Berger first introduced the word ethnobotany in 1895 to describe the study of plants used by Australia's indigenous people. It was continuously enhanced by different individuals. Martin claims that the term "ethnobiology" denotes an explanation of the local population's views on scientific and cultural knowledge. It explores each element, starting with the way human groups interact and relate to plant communities (Rishi et al. 2016). Man relied on the curative effects of medicinal plants before the thought of chemical-based treatments. Some people value these plants because of a centuries-old theory that claims plants were made to provide man with food, medicine, and other benefits. Since medicinal plants are regarded as the "backbone" of traditional medicine, over 3.3 billion people frequently consume them in less developed nations (Ahvazi et al. 2012).

India possesses a long history of practicing traditional medicine, and its citizens are generally conscious that they are notably more acquainted with medicinal plants than those living in any other nation on the planet. A wealth of information concerning traditions and folklore surrounding essential natural ingredients with medicinal value may be found in the Indian Materia Medica. Indian materia medica includes knowledge of plants, where they grow in all seasons, methods for storage, and shelf life of harvested materials. On the other hand, Indian traditional medicine is derived from several systems such as Siddha, Unani, and Ayurveda. These Ayurveda, Siddha, and Unani are all traditional medical systems that use a holistic approach to health and illness. They have been practiced for thousands of years and are used around the world. Acharya Charaka, Acharya Sushruta, and Dhanvantari Nighantu underlined that the individuals who are closest to forests, cowherds, shepherds, hermits, and members of ethnic communities are the ones who are most knowledgeable about identifying and using plants (Rishi et al. 2016).

Study Region

The study was conducted in the Chilapata Reserve Forest, which is part of the Cooch Behar Wildlife Division located in the Alipurduar district of West Bengal, India, spanning an area of 41 km^2. This reserve is situated 30 km from both Cooch Behar and Alipurduar and is intersected by National Highway 31C. The GPS coordinates for the location are latitude 26° 32.85′ N and longitude 89° 22.99′ E, with an elevation of 47 meters above sea level. The region experiences a subtropical climate, receiving 250–300 cm of rainfall annually, primarily between June and August, while temperatures can range from 34°C in May to 7.5°C in January. Surrounding the forest are villages such as Uttar Simlabari and Chaukakheti, which are home to around 1,000 families from various Indo-Mongoloid groups (including Raj-Bangshis, Mech, Ravas, Totos, Lepchas, Nageshias, Uraons, and Mundas) who depend on the forest and subsistence farming for their livelihoods (Raj et al. 2018).

Chilapata Reserve Forest under the jurisdiction of Cooch Behar wildlife division in West Bengal is home to a variety of flora including trees, orchids, and also medicinal plants. Here, the plant resources are used by different communities (Raj-Bangshis, Mech, Ravas, Totos, Lepchas, Nageshias, Uraons, and Mundas) for many purposes such as medicine, fuel, food, fodder, timber for house construction, agricultural equipment, religious, and other purposes. In general, communities living in the near vicinity of a forest closely interact with the forest and obtain their economic livelihood as well as their cultural spiritual identity. Due to the lack of availability of resources and poor socioeconomic conditions, the forest-originated products as well as medicinal plants like Neem, Haldi, Tulsi, Amla, and so on are mostly used by these communities for their survival.

In such a way, the plant *Azadirachta indica*, commonly known as Neem from the Miliaceae family, is used for treating stomach issues with its leaves. On the other hand, the plant *Asparagus racemosus*, or Shatavari from the Asparagaceae family, utilizes its roots to help with gastric ulcers. Again, the plant *Bacopa monnieri*, also called Brahmi from the Apiaceae family, is a herb whose leaves and seeds are consumed with milk to relieve suffocation, restlessness, and jaundice while also boosting memory. The powdered rhizome of *Curcuma domestica*, known as Haldi, Basaar, or Rahre from the Zingiberaceae family, is taken orally to heal cuts, wounds, internal bleeding, and fractures; it can also be applied externally to stop bleeding. Again, the plant *Ocimum tenuiflorum*, or Tulsi from the Lamiaceae family, uses its leaves to alleviate coughs and colds.

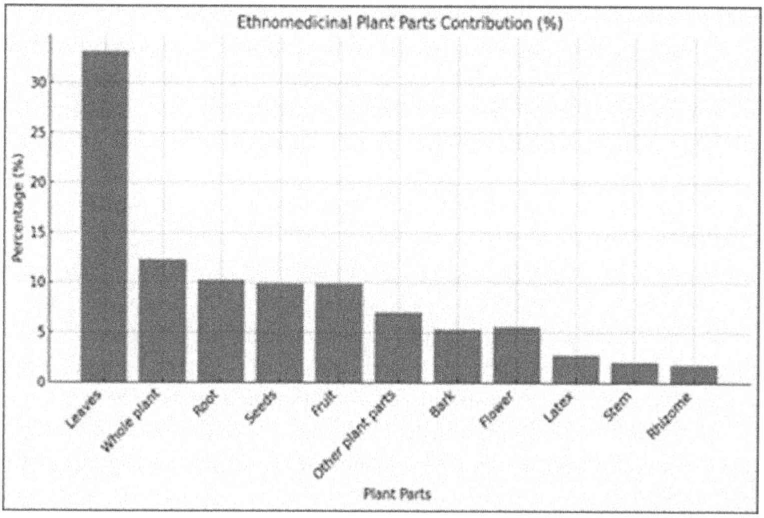

Figure 12.1. Ethnomedicinal plant parts contribution (%). Source: Bhatia, Sharma, and Singh 2014.

Yet again the plant *Phyllanthus emblica*, known as Amla and part of the Euphorbiaceae family provides health benefits through its fruit and acts as a blood purifier, appetizer, and helps to maintain blood pressure, while also promoting good eyesight and preventing acne and anorexia. Furthermore, the plant *Tinospora cordifolia*, referred to as Giloy from the Menispermaceae family, has its stem, roots, and leaves used in diabetes management by regulating blood glucose levels. Finally, *Withania somnifera*, called as Asgandh from the Solanaceae family, has fresh leaves that are chewed on an empty stomach to improve memory and aid in weight loss (Rao et al. 2015) (Figure 12.1).

Bioactive Compounds in Ethnomedicinal Plants

Ethnomedicinal plants are renowned for their rich content of bioactive compounds, which are responsible for their therapeutic properties. These compounds include phenolic compounds, tannins, terpenoids, alkaloids, and flavonoids, each of which contributes to the plant's ability to combat infections (Rasooli 2012).

(i) **Phenolic Compounds:** Phenolic compounds are a diverse group of chemical substances found in plants, characterized by one or more hydroxyl groups attached to an aromatic ring. They are known for their antioxidant, anti-inflammatory, and antimicrobial properties (Singh et al. 2016).

(ii) **Tannins and Flavonoids:** Tannins are a class of polyphenolic compounds that bind to proteins and other organic compounds, inhibiting the growth of bacteria and fungi. They work by precipitating microbial proteins, effectively inactivating them and preventing infections (Zahin et al. 2010). Flavonoids are a group of plant metabolites known for their antioxidant and anti-inflammatory effects. These compounds are widely distributed in the plant kingdom and are responsible for the vivid colors of many fruits and flowers (de Sousa Araújo et al. 2008).

(iii) **Terpenoids:** Terpenoids, also known as isoprenoids, are a large class of organic chemicals derived from five-carbon isoprene units. These compounds are responsible for the aromatic qualities of many plants and play a crucial role in plant defense against pathogens. Medicinal plants carrying terpenoids are *Azadirachta indica*, *Acacia catechu*, and *Salmalia malabarica*. *Azadirachta indica* (commonly known as neem) belongs to the family Meliaceae and is rich in terpenes like azadirachtin, which have been shown to have strong antibacterial, antifungal properties as well as immunosuppressive, anti-inflammatory, antiviral, antiulcer, antimalarial, and antioxidant properties. *Acacia catechu* (also called khair) of the family Fabaceae contains various immunopharmacological effects like anti-mycotic, hepatoprotective, antioxidant activities, and so on. *Salmalia malabarica* (commonly known as Saavar) of the family Bombacaceae is popular for its medicinal properties; for example, gum is useful for pulmonary tuberculosis (TB), flu, dysentery, and so on, and the flowers of this plant are used for eye complaints (Gupta and Chaphalkar 2016).

(iv) **Alkaloids:** Alkaloids are nitrogen-containing compounds that are often bitter-tasting and can be toxic to microorganisms. *Cleistanthus* and *Tiliacora* are rich in alkaloids and inhibit the growth of bacteria and viruses.

Phytochemical analysis of *Catharanthus roseus* detects different groups of compounds in the different parts of the plant by using various solvents. Saponins were present in methanolic extracts of leaves, stems, and roots, while also present in aqueous extracts. Tannins were detected in the leaves and roots in the methanolic and chloroform extracts. Terpenoids were found in the methanol, petroleum ether, and benzene extracts of leaves and roots, but higher amounts were found in the chloroform and aqueous extracts. Flavonoids were also found in the methanol extract of leaves and roots apart from their presence in the chloroform extract of leaves. Cardiac glycosides were present in leaves and root extracts using petroleum ether; they were also present in an aqueous leaf and stem extract. Alkaloids were soluble in methanol, petroleum ether, as well as in an aqueous extract for the various plant parts. Steroids appeared in both methanol and petroleum ether extracts of leaves and roots. Quinones have been detected in methanol and petroleum ether extracts from all parts of the plant; they were also detected in chloroform extract of leaves and stems. Phenols have been identified as being present in methanol and petroleum ether extracts from leaves and roots. This analysis reflects a good deal of bioactivity in diverse plant parts (Lahare et al. 2021) (Table 12.1).

Table 12.1. Comprehensive Overview of Medicinal Plants, Plant Parts, and Biological Activities of Key Phytochemicals

Plants Name	Plants Part	Activity
Acorus calamus	Rhizome	Phenolic compounds (α-asarone, β-asarone): Anti-inflammatory, neuroprotective, antimicrobial.
Achyranthes aspera	Whole plant	Phenolic acids (Gallic acid, Quercetin, Kaempferol): Antioxidant, anti-inflammatory, antimicrobial. Tannins: Astringent, antimicrobial.
Aloe vera	Fleshy leaves	Phenolic acids (Quercetin, Kaempferol): Antioxidant, UV protective. Tannins: Wound healing. Flavonoids (Apigenin): Antioxidant, anti-inflammatory.
Andrographis paniculata	Whole plant	Flavonoids (Apigenin, Luteolin): Anticancer, anti-inflammatory. Terpenoids (Andrographidine C): Antiviral, hepatoprotective.
Bacopa monnieri	Whole plant	Phenolic acids (Chlorogenic acid, Caffeic acid): Neuroprotective, antioxidant. Flavonoids (Luteolin): Cognitive enhancer, anti-inflammatory.
Berberis aristata	Root	Alkaloids (Berberine): Antimicrobial, antidiabetic, anti-inflammatory. Flavonoids (Rutin): Antioxidant, vascular health.
Biophytum sensitivum	Whole plant	Phenolic acids (Caffeic acid, Ferulic acid): Antioxidant, anti-inflammatory. Flavonoids (Rutin): Cardioprotective, antioxidant.
Centella asiatica	Whole plant	Flavonoids (Rutin, Quercetin, Kaempferol): Antioxidant, wound healing, neuroprotective. Tannins: Antimicrobial, astringent.
Costus speciosus	Rhizome	Phenolic acids (Ferulic acid, Quercetin): Antioxidant, antimicrobial. Terpenoids (Coumarin): Anticoagulant, anti-inflammatory.
Curcuma longa	Rhizome	Phenolic compounds (Curcumin, Caffeic acid): Anti-inflammatory, anticancer, antioxidant. Terpenoids: Antimicrobial, anti-inflammatory.
Datura metel	Fruits	Phenolic acids (Gallic acid, Quercetin): Antioxidant, antimicrobial. Terpenoids: Antimicrobial, anti-inflammatory.
Emblica officinalis	Fruits	Phenolic acids (Gallic acid, Quercetin): Antioxidant, anti-inflammatory. Tannins: Antimicrobial, astringent. Flavonoids: Antioxidant, cardiovascular health.
Gymnema sylvestre	Leaves	Flavonoids (Quercetin, Rutin): Antioxidant, antidiabetic. Tannins: Anti-inflammatory, antimicrobial.
Hymenaea courbaril	Bark	Flavonoids and Tannins: Antioxidant, antimicrobial, anti-inflammatory. Terpenoids: Antibacterial, antifungal.
Hyptis suaveolens	Leaves	Phenolic acids (Chlorogenic acid): Antioxidant, anti-inflammatory. Flavonoids: Antimicrobial, antioxidant.
Jatropha mollissima	Latex	Alkaloids: Antimicrobial, anti-inflammatory. Tannins: Antioxidant, antimicrobial.

(*Continued*)

Table 12.1 (Continued)

Plants Name	Plants Part	Activity
Mimosa tenuiflora	Bark	Alkaloids and Tannins: Antioxidant, wound healing, antimicrobial. Phenolic compounds: Anti-inflammatory, tissue regeneration.
Ocimum campechianum	Aerial portion	Phenolic acids (Chlorogenic acid): Antioxidant, neuroprotective. Flavonoids: Antioxidant, anti-inflammatory. Terpenoids: Antiviral, antimicrobial.
Spondias tuberosa	Bark	Flavonoids and Tannins: Antioxidant, anti-inflammatory, antimicrobial. Terpenoids: Hepatoprotective, immune modulating.
Tabebuia impetiginosa	Bark	Phenolic compounds (Quercetin, Gallic acid): Antioxidant, antimicrobial. Tannins: Anti-inflammatory, antimicrobial. Terpenoids: Antimicrobial, anti-inflammatory.
Anacardium occidentale	Bark	Phenolic compounds (Gallic acid): Antioxidant, antimicrobial. Flavonoids: Anti-inflammatory, anticancer. Tannins: Astringent, wound healing.
Anadenanthera colubrina	Bark	Phenolic acids and Tannins: Antioxidant, antimicrobial. Alkaloids: Anti-inflammatory, analgesic.
Caesalpinia ferrea	Bark	Tannins: Astringent, antimicrobial. Phenolic compounds: Antioxidant, wound healing. Alkaloids: Antimicrobial, anti-inflammatory.
Cereus jamacaru	Cladode	Phenolic acids (Ferulic acid): Antioxidant, anti-inflammatory. Flavonoids: Antidiabetic, anti-inflammatory.
Commiphora leptophloeos	Bark	Phenolic compounds and Tannins: Antioxidant, antimicrobial. Terpenoids: Anti-inflammatory, antimicrobial.
Erythrina velutina	Bark	Alkaloids: Antidepressant, sedative, anticonvulsant. Flavonoids (Quercetin): Antioxidant, anti-inflammatory.
Secondatia densiflora	Roots	Alkaloids: Antimicrobial, anticancer. Phenolic acids: Antioxidant, anti-inflammatory.
Senna occidentalis	Whole plant	Phenolic acids (Caffeic acid, Quercetin): Antioxidant, antimicrobial. Alkaloids: Antibacterial, antimalarial.
Schinopsis brasiliensis	Bark	Phenolic acids and Tannins: Antimicrobial, astringent. Flavonoids: Antioxidant, anti-inflammatory. Terpenoids: Anti-inflammatory, antimicrobial.
Maytenus rigida	Bark	Tannins: Antioxidant, wound healing. Phenolic compounds: Antimicrobial, anti-inflammatory. Terpenoids: Antifungal, antibacterial.
Passiflora foetida	Aerial portion	Flavonoids (Quercetin, Kaempferol): Antioxidant, sedative, neuroprotective. Alkaloids: Antimicrobial, analgesic.
Operculina macrocarpa	Roots	Phenolic acids and Tannins: Antioxidant, antimicrobial. Terpenoids: Anti-inflammatory, digestive stimulant.

(*Continued*)

Table 12.1 (Continued)

Plants Name	Plants Part	Activity
Vitex negundo	Leaves	Flavonoids (Luteolin, Kaempferol): Antioxidant, anti-inflammatory. Terpenoids: Antimicrobial, antifungal.
Tinospora cordifolia	Stem	Alkaloids: Immunomodulatory, anti-inflammatory. Phenolic acids (Chlorogenic acid): Antioxidant, antimicrobial.
Withania somnifera	Roots	Alkaloids: Adaptogenic, anti-inflammatory. Phenolic compounds: Antioxidant, neuroprotective.
Cassia fistula	Fruit	Flavonoids (Quercetin, Kaempferol): Antioxidant, antimicrobial. Tannins: Astringent, antimicrobial.
Solanum nigrum	Whole plant	Alkaloids: Anticancer, antimicrobial. Phenolic compounds (Gallic acid): Antioxidant, anti-inflammatory.
Azadirachta indica	Leaves	Terpenoids (Azadirachtin): Antifungal, antiviral. Flavonoids (Quercetin): Antioxidant, anti-inflammatory.
Tamarindus indica	Fruit pulp	Phenolic acids (Caffeic acid, Gallic acid): Antioxidant, anti-inflammatory. Tannins: Antimicrobial, antioxidant.
Trigonella foenum-graecum	Seeds	Alkaloids (Trigonelline): Antidiabetic, antimicrobial. Phenolic acids (Caffeic acid): Antioxidant, antimicrobial.
Zingiber officinale	Rhizome	Phenolic compounds (Gingerol): Anti-inflammatory, anticancer. Terpenoids: Antimicrobial, anti-inflammatory.

Source: de Sousa Araújo et al. 2008; Kumar et al. 2021; Lahare et al. 2021.

Growing Concern about Antimicrobial Resistance

An increasing concern is antimicrobial resistance. Antimicrobial resistance refers to the growing worry that bacteria, viruses, fungi, and parasites are becoming increasingly resistant to the medications used to treat them, making infections harder to cure and potentially leading to more severe illnesses and deaths due to the ineffectiveness of current antibiotics and other antimicrobial drugs; this is considered a major global health threat. Thus, microorganisms naturally develop resistance through genetic mutations, but human activities like overuse and misuse of antibiotics accelerate this process. Resistant infections can be harder to treat, leading to longer illnesses, increased healthcare costs, and potential complications from untreated infections. Accordingly, antimicrobial resistance threatens the effective prevention and treatment of an ever-increasing range of infections caused by bacteria, parasites, viruses, and fungi. Antimicrobial resistance is one of the top global public health threats in the twenty-first century, which requires action across all government sectors and society.

Throughout ancient scriptures like the Ayurveda and the Rig Veda (4500–1600 BC), emphasize natural cures in healthcare. The Rig Veda is an ancient Indian scripture that lists medicinal plants and their uses, and Ayurveda is a traditional medical system that uses these plants and other natural remedies. Thus, India has used medicinal plants since ancient time. Due to their varied chemical compositions and extensive history of therapeutic usage, medicinal plants offer promise in the face of the rising global rate of antimicrobial resistance (AMR), which includes India. The need for novel agents has increased because of the serious resistance problems and adverse consequences, including immunological suppression and hypersensitivity, brought on by the overuse of commercial antimicrobial medications. Rich in secondary metabolites such as tannins, flavonoids, and alkaloids, plant-based antimicrobials have the potential to treat a variety of illnesses with fewer side effects than synthetic counterparts (Newman and Cragg 2020). This is the reason this research has described a number of medicinal plants which have the potential to treat a variety of infections like Neem, Turmeric, Ashwagandha, Tulsi, Amla, Giloy, Brahmi, Shatavari, Echinacea, Ginger, and Garlic. The antimicrobial properties and bioactive compounds of these medicinal plants are given here.

(a) **Neem (*Azadirachta indica*):** More than 135 compounds have been isolated from various parts of Neem since Siddiqui's early report on the isolation of nimbin, the first bitter compound isolated from Neem oil. Several reviews have also been published on the chemistry and structural diversity of these compounds. A novel vaginal contraceptive made from Neem oil had an inhibitory effect on the growth of several pathogens, including bacteria, fungi, and viruses. The antimicrobial properties of Neem extract have been established against *Streptococcus mutans, S. faecalis*. A broad range of antibacterial activity is exhibited by the oil extracted from the leaves, seeds, and bark against both gram-positive and gram-negative bacteria, including strains of *M. tuberculosis* that are resistant to streptomycin (Siddiqui and Ali 1997).

(b) **Turmeric (*Curcuma longa*):** A member of the Zingiberaceae (ginger) family, turmeric is an herbaceous evergreen plant. Everywhere throughout India, the plant is grown. According to an in-depth examination of the literature, curcuma turmeric, a herbal remedy with a broad range of pharmacological activities, is generally recognized as a universal cure (Rafieian-Kopaei et al. 2014). Numerous studies have demonstrated the potential benefits of curcumin when employing herbs to treat cancer. On a molecular level, it can affect how cancer cells proliferate, divide, and spread. One powerful anticarcinogenic compound is cumin (Gautam et al. 1998). Turmeric's antioxidant properties help combat free radicals, reducing skin damage and offering therapeutic benefits. Key metabolites like curcuminoids, oils, flavonoids, phenolics, amino acids, proteins, and alkaloids contribute to its health advantages, including preventing cardiovascular diseases. Curcumin may stimulate bile production for better digestion and has shown antiviral effects in animal studies, including suppressing UV-stimulated HIV gene expression. Curcumin and its analogues hold potential for developing HIV treatments (Kumari et al. 2015). Moreover, turmeric has antifungal properties. Additionally effective against *Penicillium digitatum, Fusarium* *moniliforme*, *Aspergillus flavus*, and *A. parasiticus* is turmeric oil (Jayaprakasha et al. 2001; Verma et al. 2018).

(c) **Ashwagandha (*Withania somnifera*):** From the root tubers of *Withania somnifera*, a monomeric glycoprotein with a molecular mass of 28 kDa has been identified using SDS-PAGE. The protein known as WSG, or *Withania somnifera* glycoprotein, exhibited strong antibacterial action against the studied bacteria and phytopathogenic fungi. It has been shown that WSG has an antifungal impact by preventing spore germination and hyphal development in the fungi that are examined. Strong antibacterial activity against *Clavibacter michiganensis* subsp. michiganensis and strong antifungal activity against *Aspergillus flavus*, *Fusarium oxysporum*, and *F. verticilloides* were demonstrated by WSG. WSG is a nontoxic, acidic protease inhibitor that inhibits trypsin-chymotrypsin (Girish et al. 2006). Ashwagandha (*Withania somnifera*) has shown promise in treating burns, wounds, and skin conditions, as well as gastrointestinal, respiratory, and geriatric issues, including asthma, bronchitis, and cancer. Widely used in Ayurveda, it is included in formulas for musculoskeletal disorders like rheumatism and arthritis due to its anti-inflammatory properties. Additionally, it serves as a general tonic to enhance vitality, promote health and longevity, and prevent illness in pregnant women, the elderly, and athletes (Velu and Baskaran 2012).

(d) **Tulsi (*Ocimum sanctum*):** Tulsi, or Ocimum sanctum Linn., is the cornerstone of India's Ayurvedic holistic health system (Eswar, Devaraj, and Agarwal 2016). Tulsi contains rosmarinic acid, an antioxidant that protects against free radicals and excessive oxidation. It also has antibacterial compounds like carvacrol, terpene, and B-caryophyllene, which shield the body from bacteria causing illnesses (Kaur et al. 2020). Tulsi's adaptogenic and Rasayana properties, primarily from eugenol and caryophyllene, promote mental calmness and enhance immunity. Its essential oil has antiviral, antibacterial, and antiseptic qualities, inhibiting bacteria like B. anthracis, M. tuberculosis, and E. coli. Tulsi also shows antidiabetic effects and has been studied for its antifertility properties, linked to its anti-estrogenic activity (Kohli et al. 2020).

(e) **Amla (*Emblica officinalis*):** Amla extracts, with their antifungal, antiviral, and antibacterial properties, are being studied for new therapeutic alternatives. They show a strong zone of inhibition (ZOI) against pathogens like E. coli, K. pneumoniae, S. aureus, B. cereus, V. cholerae, and C. albicans. Extracts using ethanolic and aqueous solvents were effective against bacteria such as Salmonella and P. aeruginosa. Amla also demonstrated antibacterial activity against several gram-negative bacteria, although it was less effective against urinary infections. Additionally, methanol extracts of amla have shown potent antifungal effects and antiviral potential, especially in disrupting extracellular viral particles and inhibiting HPV transcriptional activity (Hassan et al. 2020).

(f) **Giloy (*Tinospora cordifolia*):** *Tinospora* has various therapeutic uses, including immune system strengthening and antidiabetic, anticancer, liver-protective, and immune-stimulating properties. Different parts of the plant offer specific benefits: the stem acts as a tonic, bile stimulant, fever reducer, and treats conditions like jaundice, skin diseases, diabetes, and more. The powdered root and stem are used in cancer treatments, as an aphrodisiac, and to treat snake bites and scorpion stings. The bark has antispasmodic, antiallergic, and antimicrobial properties, effective against bacteria like *Salmonella*, *E. coli*, and *Staphylococcus aureus* (Solanki and Goyal 2022). *Tinospora cordifolia* extracts in aqueous, ethanolic, and acetone forms demonstrate strong antibacterial efficacy, particularly against *Pseudomonas aeruginosa* and *Klebsiella pneumoniae*, which are linked to urinary infections. Silver nanoparticles synthesized from Tinospora stems also show effective antibacterial activity against drug-resistant *Pseudomonas aeruginosa* from burn patients. Tinospora exhibits broad-spectrum antibacterial activity against various microorganisms, including *Salmonella* species, *Proteus vulgaris*, *Staphylococcus aureus*, *Escherichia coli*, and *Enterobacter aeruginosa* (Solanki and Goyal 2022).

(g) **Brahmi (*Bacopa monnieri*):** *Bacopa monnieri* exhibits anti-infective properties against various bacteria and fungi and is also used medicinally for inflammatory conditions. Key compounds like flavonoids, tannins, and phenolic acids contribute to its antimicrobial effects. While all extracts, except aqueous ones, demonstrated antibacterial qualities, ethanolic extracts were particularly effective against fungi. The antibacterial activity of *Bacopa monnieri* extracts was evaluated against several microorganisms and compared to conventional medicines, such as ciprofloxacin and clotrimazole (Fazlul et al. 2019). The effectiveness of the brahmi extract as an antibacterial was evaluated against a range of gram-positive and gram-negative microorganisms. Inhibition zone (IZ) values for *P. vulgaris* and *P. aeruginosa* were highest and minimum, respectively (Vats and Tiwari 2014). The high phenolic and flavonoid content of the extract is primarily responsible for its antioxidant effect. Due to their demonstrated antioxidant activity, these phytochemicals are used to treat a wide range of illnesses (Fazlul et al. 2019).

(h) **Shatavari (*Asparagus racemosus*):** *Asparagus racemosus* aqueous extract demonstrated a modest level of antibacterial activity against the test pathogens, *Pseudomonas aeruginosa*, and Vibrio parahaemolyticus. With the exception of Pseudomonas aeruginosa, *Asparagus racemosus* methanol extract demonstrated efficacy against all test species. However, it was discovered that *Asparagus racemosus*'s methanol extract had strong anti-*Escherichia coli* and anti-Vibrio parahaemolyticus properties (Kumaran and Citarasu 2015).

(i) **Echinacea (*Echinacea purpurea*):** *Echinacea purpurea* extracts' antibacterial qualities were evaluated using both traditional and ultrasonic extraction methods, and they showed notable efficacy against a variety of bacteria and fungi. These extracts were very effective against bacterial strains such as *Escherichia coli*, *Pseudomonas aeruginosa*, *Bacillus subtilis*, and *Staphylococcus aureus*, as well as fungi like *Candida albicans* and *Saccharomyces cerevisiae.* Although neither technique proved successful against the mold *Aspergillus niger*, the traditional extraction method had somewhat stronger antibacterial effects than acoustic extraction. Additionally, the ethyl acetate fraction demonstrated the strongest antimicrobial activity when extracts made with different solvents (hexane, chloroform, and ethyl acetate) were tested. This was particularly true against bacteria such as *Bacillus cereus, Bacillus amyloliquefaciens, Staphylococcus aureus, Listeria monocytogenes, Escherichia coli, Pseudomonas aeruginosa*, and *Candida albicans* (Stanisavljević et al. 2009). Bioactive substances like medium-chain fatty acids and organic acids were shown to be responsible for the ethyl acetate extracts' increased activity. In contrast, the hexane extract exhibited moderate effects, which were attributed to its triterpene concentration, while the chloroform extract showed decreased antimicrobial activity, probably because it lacked alcohols, organic acids, and triterpenes. Although some action was seen against *Penicillium sp.* and yeasts like *Saccharomyces cerevisiae* and *Candida albicans*, all extracts were largely ineffective against fungi like *Aspergillus niger* and *Aspergillus flavus*, despite these encouraging results. These results demonstrate the potential of *Echinacea purpurea* as a natural source of antimicrobial compounds, especially in the fight against bacterial infections (Petkova et al. 2023).

(j) **Ginger (*Zingiber officinale*):** The antibacterial qualities of ginger (*Zingiber officinale*) have been acknowledged, especially regarding foodborne pathogens. *Escherichia coli, Pseudomonas aeruginosa, Staphylococcus aureus, Vibrio cholerae, Klebsiella* spp., *Salmonella* spp., and other bacteria have all been found to be significantly inhibited by ginger extracts made with soybean oil and heated for extraction. *Escherichia coli* showed the lowest sensitivity to ginger's antimicrobial action, whereas Salmonella spp. exhibited the maximum zone of inhibition. This demonstrates ginger's broad-spectrum antibacterial properties. It is thought that extracting ginger in oils, like soybean oil, increases its antibacterial activity and helps maintain its active ingredients even at high temperatures. This makes it a valuable component in cooking, particularly in Bangladesh and other countries where ginger is widely utilized. Additionally, it is believed that the antibacterial activity of ginger stems from bioactive molecules that are persistent under hot conditions and work in concert with soybean oil (Islam et al. 2014).

(k) **Garlic (Allium sativum):** Known for its broad range of antibacterial qualities, garlic can combat a variety of diseases, such as bacteria, fungi, viruses, and protozoa. Allicin, a sulfur-based molecule that is produced when garlic is chopped or crushed, is primarily responsible for this efficacy. By rupturing the integrity of cell membranes and interfering with vital enzymes that contain sulfhydryl groups, which are necessary for bacterial survival, allicin produces its antibiotic actions. Garlic is a powerful natural remedy against common bacterial pathogens because of this disruption, which has a broad-spectrum effect against bacteria like *Helicobacter pylori, Escherichia coli*, and *Staphylococcus aureus* (Harris et al. 2001). Garlic has strong antifungal activity in addition to its antibacterial properties, particularly against *Candida albicans*. It effectively stops fungal cells from growing by preventing them from synthesizing proteins and lipids. Garlic may also be effective against some viruses, such as HIV and influenza strains, according to some data, albeit it is less comprehensive. Garlic has long been used in both traditional and modern medicine and these antiviral properties support its historic usage in treating illnesses and preserving food. Garlic's potential as a natural medicinal agent is demonstrated by the combination of these antibacterial effects. In addition to supporting its traditional usage, garlic's capacity to target various microbial pathways makes it an intriguing topic for pharmacological and microbiological research (Wilson and Demmig-Adams 2007).

Health Benefits, Cultural Practices, and Conservation of Indian Ethnomedicinal Plants

Plants are essential to the lives of many indigenous tribes, offering food, fuel, animal feed, and herbal remedies for various health issues. India, often referred to as the world's botanical garden, boasts a rich variety of medicinal plants and stands as the largest producer globally. This abundance of resources underpins traditional medical systems such as Ayurveda, Unani, and Siddha. Historical texts like the Charaka Samhita (700 BC) and Sushruta Samhita (200 BC), along with the Vedas, provide early references to medicinal plants, underscoring their importance in ancient healing practices (Bhatia, Sharma, and Singh 2014). This particular research looks at traditional medical techniques used by different cultures, with an emphasis on using local plants and herbs as remedies (Bopana and Saxena 2007). These methods make use of medicinal herbs that have a number of health advantages, such as strengthened immunity, better digestion, and relief from long-term ailments.

The study highlights the role of cultural practices in the preservation and application of these medicinal plants. Traditional knowledge is often passed down through generations, maintaining cultural heritage. The significance of protecting these healing plants and the knowledge that goes along with them is emphasized. Documenting and preserving this knowledge is essential to preserving the effectiveness of ethnomedical techniques and guaranteeing their continuous application and benefits. The noteworthy health benefits, cultural practices, and conservation of a number of Indian plants that demonstrate the medicinal potential of ethnomedical herbs are as follows:

(1) **Neem (*Azadirachta indica*):** Native tribes in northern West Bengal use neem extensively to cure a wide range of conditions, such as microbial infections, diabetes, ulcers, and skin problems. Because these people have little access to modern healthcare facilities and a wealth of traditional knowledge, neem is important to them (Samanta, Ojha, and Ghosh 2023). Regarding health benefits, neem is utilized for its antibacterial, antioxidant, antidiabetic, anticancer, and anti-inflammatory properties. The report explains how tribal groups use various neem extracts to treat and prevent different kinds of illnesses. On the other hand, regarding cultural practices, neem in many communities is also used in

food, customs, and traditional healing practices. Neem sticks are used for dental hygiene, while neem leaves are ingested in various forms as a disease-prevention measure. Moreover, regarding conservation and knowledge transfer, there is still a lot of traditional knowledge about using Neem, it is gradually changing as a result of industrialization, globalization, and these communities' growing awareness and education.

(2) **Turmeric (*Curcuma longa*):** The Mullu Kuruma tribe uses 136 different plant species for traditional medicinal uses. These consist of therapies for inflammatory conditions of the skin, bronchial illnesses, asthma, urinary problems, anemia, and more. Generation after generation of people have inherited this knowledge of these plants and their uses, which reflects the tribe's extensive knowledge of the regional flora and its applications (Silja, Varma, and Mohanan 2008). Regarding health benefits, these plants have a wide range of health advantages. They cover remedies for common conditions like anemia, piles, asthma, and skin disorders. *Adhatoda zeylanica*, for example, works well for respiratory conditions including cough and asthma, whereas *Abrus precatorius* is utilized as an anti-inflammatory and abortifacient. The tribe, whose medical requirements are met primarily by natural resources, benefits greatly from these treatments. Conversely, regarding cultural practices, the Mullu Kuruma tribe's traditional customs are intricately entwined with the usage of medicinal plants. Elders are crucial in preserving and transmitting the traditional wisdom that is passed down over the years. The tribe's cultural identity and customs, including ceremonies and rituals, are closely associated with their dependence on medicinal plants. Finally, regarding conservation and knowledge transfer, the survival of the tribe depends on the preservation of medicinal plants and the dissemination of ethnomedical knowledge. The tribe harvests plants from their environment, making sure that resource depletion is avoided through sustainable collecting methods. Oral knowledge transfer takes place, with younger generations picking up knowledge from older ones through involvement in medical procedures and observation. The tribe's ethnobotanical legacy is preserved through this kind of information transfer.

(3) **Ashwagandha (*Withania somnifera*):** In drier regions of India, like Madhya Pradesh, Rajasthan, and Gujarat, ashwagandha is mostly grown. It plays a crucial role in these regions' traditional medical procedures (Verma 2010). For thousands of years, Ayurvedic medicine in India has made considerable use of *Withania somnifera*, also known as ashwagandha. It is used as a general health tonic and to cure a variety of illnesses, such as stress, arthritis, and skin disorders. The herb is especially prized for its revitalizing qualities, which increase life and longevity (Umadevi et al. 2012). Regarding health benefits, the adaptogenic qualities of ashwagandha are widely known for their ability to lower stress and enhance both mental and physical well-being. It has been demonstrated to decrease cortisol levels, which lessen stress and increase resilience. Ashwagandha has demonstrated promise in improving memory, cognitive function, and offering neuroprotection, especially for diseases like

Parkinson's and Alzheimer's (Verma 2010). Significant anticancer capabilities have been revealed by research conducted in India on Withaferin A, a major component found in ashwagandha. It has been demonstrated to stop cancer cells from growing and improve chemotherapy's efficacy (Umadevi et al. 2012). On the other hand, regarding cultural practices, ashwagandha in Indian tradition is a key component of Ayurvedic therapy. Since it is regarded as a Rasayana, it prolongs life and rejuvenates. The plant is used to treat a number of ailments, such as nervous tiredness, debility, and weariness (Verma 2010). Finally, regarding conservation and knowledge transfer, overharvesting of ashwagandha is causing worry for its conservation in India. Sustainable production methods must be followed to protect this priceless medicinal plant. In India, the traditional knowledge of ashwagandha's medicinal applications is being recorded and researched more and more in order to preserve it and confirm its potential for use in treatment through science (Umadevi et al. 2012).

(4) **Tulsi (Ocimum sanctum):** For decades, *Ocimum sanctum*, often known as tulsi, has been an essential part of traditional medicine among Bangladesh's rural and ethnic communities. For example, Tulsi leaves are frequently used by traditional healers to treat respiratory conditions like bronchitis and persistent coughs. In another instance, Tulsi is used to treat stomach problems such as dysentery and ulcers through the chewing of fresh leaves or the consumption of extract. The plant's importance in regional health care systems is highlighted by this common habit that is passed down through the generations (Mamun-or-rashid et al. 2013). Regarding health benefits, several ailments have been shown to benefit from Tulsi's benefits, as demonstrated by case studies. For instance, Tulsi may play a part in the management of diabetes as scientific research has demonstrated its potential to lower blood glucose levels in diabetic patients. Tulsi extract's radioprotective qualities were demonstrated in another instance when it was used to lessen the negative effects of radiation treatment on cancer patients. These illustrations highlight the potential of tulsi as a multipurpose medicinal herb. On the other hand, regarding cultural practices, Tulsi in many South Asian traditions, is not just a medical herb but also a plant with cultural significance. For instance, Tulsi is frequently shown in the courtyard and is regularly worshipped in Hindu homes. The concept that Tulsi is a sacred plant with divine characteristics is the source of this tradition. A particular instance from Varanasi, India, shows how a family has been using Tulsi in religious rites for generations, thinking it will protect the home from harm. These customs highlight the profound cultural respect that Tulsi possesses, elevating it above the status of a mere therapeutic herb. Lastly, regarding conservation and knowledge transfer, modernization and overexploitation of natural resources pose a threat to the traditional knowledge related with Tulsi. In a case study from Uttarakhand, India, it was discovered that the introduction of modern medicine had caused the local community to lose memory of the traditional usage of Tulsi. This emphasizes how vital it is to carry out conservation initiatives, including documenting and passing along ethnomedical knowledge to future generations.

To ensure that this important information is maintained, community-led projects to cultivate Tulsi and other medicinal plants have started in several places.

(5) **Amla (*Emblica officinalis*):** *Emblica officinalis*, or Amla, is a highly esteemed herb in Ayurvedic medicine and traditional Indian medicine. It is utilized to treat a variety of illnesses, including diarrhea, jaundice, and inflammation. It is regarded as a potent "Rasayana," or rejuvenating agent. Treatments for fever, common colds, and more serious ailments like liver and heart disorders are all made with the fruit and other parts of the tree (Pandey, Karmakar, and Raja 2023). Regarding health benefits, Amla has numerous, well-researched health advantages. It has been demonstrated to enhance cardiovascular health by raising High-density Lipoprotein (HDL) and lowering Low-density Lipoprotein (LDL) cholesterol. In addition to its antibacterial and anticancer capabilities, it also demonstrates antidiabetic qualities that help to manage blood sugar levels. Amla also strengthens the skin, strengthens the immune system, and guards against a number of age-related illnesses. On the other hand, in the context of cultural practices, Indian customs are strongly rooted in the use of Amla, a plant known for both its therapeutic benefits and its lifespan as a symbol of health. It is frequently incorporated into daily eating routines and rituals to enhance well-being. In various Indian cultures, the tree itself is revered, underscoring its significance for reasons other than health. Finally, in the context of conservation and knowledge transfer, with the increasing recognition of Amla's medicinal potential, there is a growing need to conserve this plant and ensure the transfer of traditional knowledge to future generations. This involves sustainable harvesting practices and integrating modern scientific research with traditional wisdom to maximize its benefits while preserving its natural habitat. The document underscores the need for continued research to explore Amla's molecular mechanisms and its potential in modern medicine.

(6) **Giloy (*Tinospora cordifolia*):** One important medicinal plant that is frequently utilized in Ayurvedic medicine and other ancient Indian medical systems is giloy (*Tinospora cordifolia*). It goes by several names, including Heart-leaved Moonseed, Guduchi, and Amrita. It has historically been used to treat a variety of conditions, such as diabetes, asthma, persistent fever, and skin problems. Its function in enhancing immunity has come to light recently, especially during the Covid-19 pandemic. For increased therapeutic benefits, the plant is frequently used with other herbs including neem, tulsi, and ashwagandha (Jayswal Ali and Jayswal 2021). Regarding health benefits, Giloy is a versatile medicinal herb that provides a multitude of health benefits. It has antidiabetic, anticancer, antimicrobial, immunomodulatory, and cardioprotective qualities. The plant has been used to lower oxidative stress, boost immunity, guard against infections, and manage diabetes. Furthermore, studies on its extracts have indicated promise in the treatment of HIV and even rheumatoid arthritis and asthma. On the other hand, regarding cultural practices, Indian traditional medicine has a long history of using Giloy. Because of its many health benefits, Ayurvedic

practitioners frequently suggest it. To increase the plant's therapeutic qualities, neem trees are typically used for cultivation. Its usage as an immune booster during the Covid-19 pandemic is another indication of its cultural relevance. Lastly, regarding conservation and knowledge transfer, Giloy's flexibility is demonstrated by the fact that it can be grown in a range of soil types and climates. Sustainable farming methods, such as rain-fed agriculture and the use of organic fertilizers, are the main focus of conservation initiatives. Generations have passed down knowledge of its medical qualities, and contemporary study keeps confirming and developing long-standing applications. To protect this information and guarantee Giloy's sustainable use going forward, more public awareness and documentation are necessary.

(7) **Brahmi (*Bacopa monnieri*):** *Bacopa monnieri*, commonly known as Brahmi, is a significant herb in Ayurvedic medicine and is used for its memory-boosting, anti-anxiety, and cognitive-boosting qualities. Brahmi has been prescribed for mental disorders, improving intellect, and relieving anxiety in ancient texts such as the Charaka Samhita and Sushruta Samhita. The entire plant is used in medicine in different forms, such as extracts and powders (Bopana and Saxena 2007). Regarding health benefits, Brahmi is well-known for its capacity to boost memory, lessen anxiety, and improve cognitive performance. It is used to treat a number of neurological conditions, such as ADHD, epilepsy, and Alzheimer's disease. Brahmi is good for general health and well-being because it also has hepatoprotective, antioxidant, and anti-inflammatory qualities. Brahmi is supposed to support emotional balance, lessen stress, and improve mental clarity when taken regularly. On the other hand, regarding cultural practices, Brahmi in Indian tradition is highly esteemed, especially in Ayurvedic treatment, where it is referred to as a "Medhya Rasayana" (a mental rejuvenator). Because the plant is linked to brain health and creativity, the term "Brahmi" is taken from "Brahma," the Hindu god of creation. Its significance in preserving mental and spiritual well-being has been emphasized by its centuries-long use in a variety of cultural ceremonies and traditional healing techniques. Lastly, in the context of conservation and knowledge transfer, Brahmi must be conserved for future generations to have access to it because of its important therapeutic qualities. Sustainable cultivation of Brahmi is being attempted to prevent depletion of wild populations. Another important component is information transfer, with contemporary scientists and traditional practitioners collaborating to conserve and disseminate Brahmi-related ethnomedical knowledge. This guarantees that the advantages of this age-old plant will always be acknowledged and applied in modern medicine.

(8) **Shatavari (*Asparagus racemosus*):** *Asparagus racemosus* has antioxidant and antibacterial effects. It also stimulate the immune system. People use *Asparagus racemosus* for athletic performance, diabetes, HIV/AIDS, lactation, and many other purposes. Shatavari is used in Indian traditional medicine. Despite its long history of use in Ayurveda, no high-quality clinical evidence exists to support using shatavari as a therapy for any disease. Studies of its effects on lactation have

shown mixed results. Being a powerful adaptogenic herb, it not only relieves one from physical and emotional stress but also manages diabetes mellitus, prevents high cholesterol and triglyceride levels, and helps in the treatment of bacterial and fungal infections, edema, infertility, depression, and cancer. *Asparagus racemosus* is an endangered medicinal plant that requires conservation efforts. Conservation efforts include protecting its habitat, genetic improvement, tissue culture, agro-techniques, and marketing.

(9) **Echinacea (*Echinacea purpurea*):** Echinacea purpurea: This traditional medicinal herb is said to provide immunoenhancement and antiviral properties. This medicinal herb is getting attention in India with respect to health care (Ghatas and Abdallah 2016). India is researching the possibility of its sustainable cultivation to improve growth and increase the medicinal value of the crop (Anandan et al. 2020). Regarding health benefits, *Echinacea purpurea*, commonly known as the medicinal herb purple coneflower, is an immunostimulant that has been used for a long time. The plant fights off several infections in the respiratory tract, viruses, and the common cold/flu; it also possesses antiviral activity against coronaviruses, according to various studies (Anandan et al. 2020). Caffeic acid derivatives, alkamides, and polysaccharides are some of the bioactive constituents responsible for their antioxidant, anti-inflammatory, and immuno-enhancing properties (Ghatas and Abdallah 2016). Conversely, regarding cultural practices, Echinacea is an exotic species in India, with natural medicinal properties, and hence has been introduced and cultivated in some regions (Anandan et al. 2020). The crop is mainly produced in herbal gardens and farms that specialize in medicinal and aromatic plants. It is cultivated to prepare herbal teas, tinctures, and extracts. This crop involves organic farming where compost, bio-fertilizers, and so on, are used for better health of the soil (Ghatas and Abdallah 2016). Finally, with the increasing global demand, conservation of Echinacea should also be highlighted. This can include employing the best practices and sustainable cultivation practices as well as conserving the genetic resource with seed banks. Knowledge transfer in India is done through agricultural universities and research centers focused on medicinal plants. Workshops and training programs help farmers increase awareness of organic farming techniques so that Echinacea could be produced without draining the natural resources of earth (Ghatas and Abdallah 2016).

(10) **Ginger (*Zingiber officinale*):** India stands as the largest producer of ginger globally, playing a crucial role in both the medicinal and economic fields (Bhutia and Mula 2022). Key regions for ginger cultivation, including Assam, Kerala, and Meghalaya, contribute more than 60 percent of the country's total ginger output, highlighting its significance in the agricultural sector (Gohain, Atibudhi, and Kumar 2020). Regarding health benefits, *Zingiber officinale* is well-known for its medicinal qualities and is widely utilized in Ayurvedic, Chinese, and Unani medicine. It is celebrated for its anti-inflammatory, antioxidant, and digestive properties, helping to relieve nausea, digestive

problems, and joint pain (Bhutia and Mula 2022). Additionally, ginger is effective against common issues such as colds, headaches, and asthma, with regular intake boosting immunity and circulation, thereby lowering the risk of chronic illnesses (Gohain, Atibudhi, and Kumar 2020). Regarding cultural practices, ginger in India is cultivated extensively in states like Assam, Kerala, and Meghalaya, where there is a strong focus on organic farming, particularly in hilly areas (Bhutia and Mula 2022). Traditional methods include intercropping ginger with legumes, using organic fertilizers, and manual weeding (Gohain, Atibudhi, and Kumar 2020). The production is primarily managed by smallholder farmers, and organic ginger is mainly sold through local trading networks, with minimal reliance on advanced technology (Bhutia and Mula 2022). Finally, the conservation efforts for ginger focus on growing native seed varieties and implementing organic practices to enhance soil health (Bhutia Bidhan Chandra Krishi Viswavidyalaya and Mula Uttar Banga Krishi Vishwavidyalaya 2022). Knowledge sharing primarily happens through farmer networks and occasional training sessions, but access to better seeds and modern processing facilities is still limited. This highlights the need for greater institutional support to safeguard traditional methods while encouraging sustainable development in ginger farming (Gohain, Atibudhi, and Kumar 2020).

(11) **Garlic (*Allium sativum*):** Garlic is a highly valued horticultural crop around the world, widely grown for its culinary, medicinal, and antimicrobial benefits. However, in India, garlic production is not reaching its full potential due to a range of internal and external challenges, highlighting the need for focused improvement and cultivation strategies (Malik et al. 2017). Regarding health benefits, garlic is celebrated for its many health benefits, largely thanks to allicin, a sulfur-containing compound known for its strong antimicrobial and anti-inflammatory effects (Malik et al. 2017). Incorporating garlic into your diet can help lower cholesterol levels, boost heart health, and manage blood pressure. Furthermore, garlic is known to strengthen the immune system, offering defense against common colds and infections. Its antioxidant properties also play a role in minimizing oxidative stress in the body, which may help reduce the risk of chronic illnesses (Malik et al. 2017). In the context of cultural practices, garlic in India is grown in well-drained soils rich in organic matter, mainly in states like Madhya Pradesh, Rajasthan, and Uttar Pradesh. The planting season typically falls in September–October for long-day varieties, which thrive under longer daylight hours and specific temperature conditions to develop optimal bulbs (Malik et al. 2017). Traditional farming methods often involve using organic fertilizers, such as farmyard manure and compost, to sustain soil fertility and encourage robust crop growth (Sharma et al. 2018). Additionally, farmers practice crop rotation with legumes to boost soil nutrients and minimize pest problems (Rajendran et al. 2009). Finally, the efforts to conserve garlic genetic resources in India include both in-situ and ex-situ methods, such as creating germplasm banks and developing disease-

resistant varieties (Malik et al. 2017). Agricultural research institutes and universities are essential in sharing knowledge with farmers through training programs focused on advanced cultivation techniques, pest management, and postharvest handling (Rajendran et al. 2009). Additionally, extension services and agricultural cooperatives assist farmers by spreading innovative practices and offering access to improved seed varieties, which helps ensure sustainable cultivation and increased productivity of garlic in India (Sharma et al. 2018; Malik et al. 2017).

Mechanisms of Action

The mechanisms of action of anti-inflammatory and analgesic plants involve inhibiting various pathways associated with pain and inflammation. For instance, plants like *Boswellia serrata* inhibit 5-lipoxygenase and reduce the synthesis of leukotrienes, which play a role in inflammation. Similarly, *Curcuma longa* (turmeric) and its active compound, curcumin, inhibit multiple enzymes such as cyclooxygenase (COX) and lipoxygenase (LOX), which are involved in the production of inflammatory mediators like prostaglandins and leukotrienes. These actions typically reduce the production of proinflammatory compounds, leading to a reduction in inflammation and pain. Many of these compounds also have antioxidant properties, further aiding in the reduction of oxidative stress in tissues, which is another contributor to inflammatory responses (Kumar et al. 2021).

Many plant-derived compounds inhibit the replication of viruses by interacting with viral enzymes such as reverse transcriptase (RTase) or integrase, essential for viral genome synthesis. For example, phenolic acids like caffeic and chlorogenic acids prevent the adsorption of viruses to host cells and inhibit enzymes crucial for RNA and DNA synthesis (Chattopadhyay and Naik 2007). On the other hand, some flavonoids and coumarins interfere with virus entry into host cells. For instance, flavonoids such as quercetin block viral proteins necessary for cell attachment and entry, preventing the virus from invading host cells (Chattopadhyay and Naik 2007). Furthermore, terpenes and polyphenols can bind and inactivate viral proteins, disrupting key processes like protease function that viruses need for their replication cycles. This reduces the virus's ability to infect new cells and sustain an infection (Chattopadhyay and Naik 2007).

Challenges in Utilizing Ethnomedicinal Plants

It is difficult to use ethnomedical herbs in India for a variety of reasons. The lack of uniform data about safety, effectiveness, and dosage causes irregularities and possible hazards while using them. The preservation of traditional knowledge, which is essential for efficient utilization, is threatened by cultural erosion brought on by modernity and the extinction of indigenous languages. Furthermore, as big businesses take advantage of indigenous knowledge without paying fair compensation, biopiracy and intellectual property issues surface. These communities also lack effective legal protection, which makes it more difficult to defend their rights and advance sustainable development in ethnomedicine (Gupta and Wagh 2024). Numerous obstacles impact the application of ethnomedicinal herbs in India. Degradation of the environment, such as habitat destruction and deforestation brought on by urbanization and industry, disturbs biodiversity and has an impact on the sustainability and availability of these plants.

The dissemination of ethnomedical knowledge is restricted by oral tradition; most of it is held by few people and is in danger of vanishing as interest in it wanes in younger generations. Furthermore, tribal societies' reluctance to combine traditional medical methods with modern ones may prevent these important resources from being widely accepted and used in healthcare today (Tripathi 2019). The usage of ethnomedical herbs is beset with difficulties in India. A growing number of high-value species are in danger of going extinct due to overharvesting brought on by increased demand. Lack of technology and understanding about cultivation hinders large-scale production, which affects availability and pricing. Furthermore, obstacles to equitable pricing and commercialization include the unregulated market, middlemen's exploitation, intricate legal systems, and challenging permit acquisition (Kala, Dhyani, and Sajwan 2006).

Synergy of Tradition and Science

The combination of contemporary scientific study and traditional knowledge is evident in the Indian usage of ethnomedicinal plants to heal skin conditions. Medicinal plants have long been used for their therapeutic qualities in traditional ethno-dermatological methods, which have their roots in Ayurveda and Unani medicine. Contemporary research is now verifying these traditions by examining the pharmacological effects of these herbs, such as their antibacterial, anti-inflammatory, and wound-healing qualities. This combination of modern science and traditional wisdom validates existing knowledge and helps search for brand-new, all-natural skin care solutions (Anand, Subbaiya, and Perumal 2022).

This research examines how contemporary science and age-old Vedic traditions can work together to better understand ethnomedicinal plants. Ayurveda is a comprehensive approach to health that incorporates mental, physical, and spiritual well-being. It has its roots in books such as the Rigveda, Atharvaveda, Charaka Samhita, and Sushruta Samhita. The medicinal benefits of these plants, as reported by ancient sages and healers, are being further explored and validated by contemporary scientific research. Through this integration, ancient information has been preserved and our comprehension of these therapies has improved. The result has been the development of nutritional supplements and herbal compositions that combine traditional wisdom with contemporary scientific methodologies. This combination guarantees that the ageless precepts of Vedic medicine will continue to inform and direct modern medical procedures (Acharya 2024).

The use of ethnomedicinal plants in Solan, Himachal Pradesh, highlights the importance of traditional knowledge in rural healthcare that has been passed down through the centuries but is currently in jeopardy due to modernity and a decline in youth interest. The urgency of recording and preserving this knowledge before it is gone is emphasized throughout the text. The medicinal benefits of these herbs for conditions like diabetes, respiratory disorders, and skin diseases must be validated by science. These natural resources can be preserved, and new herbal remedies can be developed by combining traditional knowledge with contemporary research (Kumar et al. 2021).

Conclusion and Future Prospects

With growing commercial production and potential for expansion in the pharmaceutical business, India's future for ethnomedicinal plants is bright. Ongoing research into plant-based medications and the growing interest in herbal medicine worldwide highlights the necessity for sustainable methods and conservation. Preserving traditional knowledge and resources is vital because of worries about biopiracy and overexploitation. The trend in contemporary medicine toward the use of synergistic plant extracts contributes to the growing importance of ethnomedicinal plants in both local and international markets (Rishi et al. 2016). This research highlights the increased commercial demand for pharmacopoeia pharmaceuticals, which has led to the localized cultivation of various medicinal plants like poppy, isabgol, and senna. This highlights the prospects of ethnomedicinal plants in India. India's pharmaceutical sector has a lot of room to grow because of the continuous research being done on plant-based medications. To guarantee that these plants will still be around for future generations, sustainable practices and conservation initiatives are essential as there is worry about overexploitation of these species.

Furthermore, the trend in contemporary medicine is moving toward the use of plant extracts that have synergistic effects, which strengthens the position of ethnomedicinal plants in both domestic and international markets (Kundu et al. 2020). Because of the great biodiversity and ideal agro-climatic conditions in Tripura, ethnomedicinal plants have a bright future in India. Commercial cultivation could be possible, utilizing traditional expertise to support local healthcare and economic development. But problems like overuse, habitat degradation, and illicit commerce still exist. For these plants to be safely and effectively incorporated into contemporary healthcare, conservation initiatives, sustainable practices, and scientific verification of traditional applications are essential.

In a nutshell, ethnomedicine practices have an extensive reservoir of unregulated medical plants that have centuries of traditions married with modern scientific practices. These plants comprise active components like phenolics, tannins, flavonoids, terpenes, and alkaloids, making them natural and environmentally friendly solutions with negligible or no side effects compared to synthetic drugs. The compounds have therapeutic value because they possess antimicrobial properties that fight infections, are antioxidants that counter cell damage and inflammation, and have immunomodulatory activity that can be used in cancers, diabetes, and other inflammatory conditions. The need to document and protect ethnic medicine practices can be explained with examples of the rapid increase in behavioral changes of microbes, which has led to the development of antimicrobial resistance—a critical concern for healthcare worldwide. Plants with medicinal values and used ethnically well include Neem, Ashwagandha, Turmeric, and Brahmi that have shown antibacterial, antiviral, and anticancer actions. With the research proving these beliefs and practices right, there is little doubt that the incorporation of ethnomedicinal plants into modern-day practices serves to improve health outcomes in a better and more enduring way.

Moreover, ethnomedicine is very much dependent on the conservation of biodiversity and traditional knowledge. Globalization has led to a decline of these plants as well as the cultures that sustain them through overexploitation, habitat degradation, and encroachment of Western culture. Both sustainable use through cultivation and strict monitoring and scientific research of these practices will be important for the availability of these plants to the next generations. Ethnomedicinal plants have a promising future, not just because their customary uses must be safeguarded but also because their full potential must be realized with the aid of modern technology. With the evolution of research, it is anticipated that the formulation of phytopharmaceuticals will intensify as new diseases resistant to present treatment modalities emerge. Since there is a growing tendency for people to prefer plant-derived cures over synthetic ones in response to side effects of chemical drugs, ethnomedicine is bound to play a central role in healthcare developments of the future.

References

Acharya, S. K. "Ethnomedicinal Plants Used in Vedic Medicine." *International Journal of Multidisciplinary Research in Science, Engineering, and Technology (IJMRSET)* 7, no. 3 (2024): 4719–25.

Ahvazi, M., F. Khalighi-Sigaroodi, M. M. Charkhchiyan, F. Mojab, V. A. Mozaffarian, and H. Zakeri. "Introduction of Medicinal Plants Species with the Most Traditional Usage in Alamut Region." *Iranian Journal of Pharmaceutical Research* 11, no. 1 (2012): 185–94.

Anand, U., R. Subbaiya, and K. Perumal. "Natural Bioactive Products as Promising Therapeutics: A Review of Chemical Profiling, Preclinical Assessment, and Commercialization." *Environmental Research* 215, no. 2 (2022): 1234–45.

Anandan, R., G. Suseendran, N. Zaman, S. Nawaz Brohi, and D. B. S. "Echinacea purpurea to Treat Novel Coronavirus (2019-nCoV)." *CC-BY-SA* 4 (2020). https://doi.org/10.36227/techrxiv.12241223.v1

Bhatia, H., S. Sharma, and R. Singh. "A Short History of Evolution of Indigenous Plants and Medicine System." *Journal of Pharmacognosy and Phytochemistry* 3, no. 5 (2014): 1–4.

Bhutia , D. and Mula G. . "Marketing Strategies and Constraints Perceived by Farmers in Adoption of Organic Ginger Cultivation—A Case Study in Hill Zone of West Bengal." *International Journal of Agricultural Sciences* 14, no. 6 (2022): 11419–23.

Bopana, N., and S. Saxena. "Asparagus Racemosus—Ethnopharmacological Evaluation and Conservation Needs." *Journal of Ethnopharmacology* 110, no. 1 (2007): 1–15.

Chattopadhyay, D., and T. N. Naik. "Mini-Reviews in Medicinal Chemistry." *Mini-Reviews in Medicinal Chemistry* 7 (2007).

de Sousa Araújo, T. A., N. L. Alencar, E. L. C. de Amorim, and U. P. de Albuquerque. "A New Approach to Study Medicinal Plants with Tannins and Flavonoids Contents from the Local Knowledge." *Journal of Ethnopharmacology* 120, no. 1 (2008): 72–80.

Eswar, P., C. G. Devaraj, and P. Agarwal. "Anti-Microbial Activity of Tulsi (Ocimum sanctum Linn.) Extract on a Periodontal Pathogen in Human Dental Plaque: An In Vitro Study." *Journal of Clinical and Diagnostic Research: JCDR* 10, no. 3 (2016): ZC53.

Fazlul, M. K. K., S. P. Deepthi, I. Mohammed, Y. Farzana, B. Munira, and M. H. M. Nazmul. "Antibacterial and Antifungal Activity of Various Extracts of *Bacopa monnieri*." *International Journal of Pharmaceutical Research* 11, no. 1 (2019): 1698–702.

Gautam, S. C., Y. K. Xu, K. R. Pindolia, N. Janakiraman, and R. A. Chapman. "Nonselective Inhibition of Proliferation of Transformed and Non-transformed Cells by the Anticancer Agent Curcumin (Diferuloylmethane)." *Biochemical Pharmacology* 55 (1998): 1333–7.

Girish, K. S., K. D. Machiah, S. Ushanandini, K. H. Kumar, S. Nagaraju, M. Govindappa, M. Vedavathi, and K. Kemparaju. "Antimicrobial Properties of a Non-toxic Glycoprotein (WSG) from Withania somnifera (Ashwagandha)." *Journal of Basic Microbiology* 46, no. 5 (2006): 365–74.

Ghatas, Y. A. A., and W. H. Abdallah. "Effect of Some Fertilization and Micro-nutrients Treatments on Growth and Chemical Constituents of Echinacea purpurea Plant." *Journal of Plant Production* 7, no. 7 (2016): 709–19.

Gohain, N., H. N. Atibudhi, and A. Kumar. "A Study on Economics of Ginger Cultivation in Assam—A Case Study of Tinsukia District." *Plant Archives* 20, no. 2 (2020): 2522–6.

Gupta, A., and S. R. Chaphalkar. "Terpenoids from Three Medicinal Plants and Their Potential Anti-Inflammatory and Immunosuppressive Activity on Human Whole Blood and Peripheral Blood Mononuclear Cells." *Asian Journal of Ethnopharmacology and Medicinal Foods* 2, no. 1 (2016): 13–17.

Gupta, V., and V. V. Wagh. "Traditional Plant Knowledge and Medicinal Practices in Yavatmal District, Maharashtra, India: An Ethnobotanical Review." Plant Biosystems 158, no. 4 (2024): 704–45.

Harris, J. C., S. L. Cottrell, S. Plummer, and D. Lloyd. "Antimicrobial Properties of Allium sativum (Garlic)." *Applied Microbiology and Biotechnology* 57, no. 3 (2001): 282–6.

Hassan, M. S., S. S. Mughal, A. Aslam, M. Mushtaq, M. Munir, S. Pervez, N. Shabbir, A. Raza Ayub, and M. Farman. "*Emblica Officinalis* (Amla): A Prospective Review on Distinctive Properties and Therapeutic Applications of Amla." *Innovare Journal of Ayurvedic Sciences* 8, no. 3 (2020): 1–6.

Islam, K., A. A. Rowsni, M. M. Khan, and M. S. Kabir. "Antimicrobial Activity of Ginger (*Zingiber officinale*) Extracts Against Food-borne Pathogenic Bacteria." *International Journal of Science, Environment and Technology* 3, no. 3 (2014): 867–71.

Jayaprakasha, G. K., P. S. Negi, C. Anandharamakrishnan, and K. K. Sakariah. "Chemical Composition of Turmeric Oil – A Byproduct from Turmeric Oleoresin Industry and Its Inhibitory Activity against Different Fungi." *Z. Naturforsch* C 56 (2001): 40–4.

Jayswal, M. G., and A. Jayswal. "A Comprehensive Review on *Tinospora cordifolia* (Giloy): The Medicinal Plant." *International Journal of Multidisciplinary Research and Development* 8, no. 6 (2021): 80–5.

Kala, C. P., P. P. Dhyani, and B. S. Sajwan. "Developing the Medicinal Plants Sector in Northern India: Challenges and Opportunities." *Journal of Ethnobiology and Ethnomedicine* 2 (2006): 1–15.

Kaur, S., S. Sabharwal, N. Anand, S. Singh, D. Singh Baghel, and A. Mittal. "An Overview of Tulsi (Holy Basil)." *European Journal of Molecular & Clinical Medicine* 7, no. 7 (2020): 2833–9.

Kohli, K., A. Chaudhary, R. Singh, and M. Sharma. "Pharmacological Actions of Tulsi." In *Tulsi: Sacred Plant of India*, edited by A. Kak, 45–62. Springer, 2020.

Kumar Acharya, S. "Ethnomedicinal Plants Used in Vedic Medicine." *International Journal of Multidisciplinary Research in Science, Engineering and Technology (IJMRSET)* 7, no. 3 (2024): 4719.

Kumar, M., S. Rawat, B. Nagar, A. Kumar, N. A. Pala, J. A. Bhat, and R. W. Bussmann. "Implementation of the Use of Ethnomedicinal Plants for Curing Diseases in the Indian Himalayas and Its Role in Sustainability of Livelihoods and Socioeconomic Development." *Sustainability* 13 (2021): 1785.

Kumaran, T., and T. Citarasu. "Phytochemical Screening, Bioautography and Antibacterial Evaluation of the Methanolic Extract of Glycine Max (Soybean)." *Screening* 9 (2015): 10–16.

Kumari, N., A. A. Kulkarni, X. Lin, C. McLean, T. Ammosova, A. Ivanov, M. Hipolito, S. Nekhai, and E. Nwulia. "Inhibition of HIV-1 by Curcumin A, a Novel Curcumin Analog." *Drug Design, Development and Therapy* 9, no. 3 (2015): 5051–60.

Kundu, P., P. Sharma, R. Mahato, M. Saha, S. Das, and P. Ghosh. "A Brief Review for the Development of Bio-nanoparticles Using Some Important Indian Ethnomedicinal Plants." *Journal of Medicinal Plant Studies* 8, no. 6 (2020): 26–33.

Lahare, R. P., H. S. Yadav, Y. K.Bisen, and A. K. Dashahre. "Estimation of Total Phenol, Flavonoid, Tannin and Alkaloid Content in Different Extracts of *Catharanthus roseus* from Durg District, Chhattisgarh, India." *Scholars Bulletin* 7, no. 1 (2021): 1–6.

Malik, G., V. Mahajan, A. Sharma, J. I. Mir, S. Yousuf, A. Shabir, A. A. Malik, A. S. Dhatt, D. B. Singh, and S. H. Wani. "Present Status and Future Prospects of Garlic (Allium sativum L.) Improvement in India with Special Reference to Long Day Type." *Journal of Pharmacognosy and Phytochemistry* 6, no. 5 (2017).

Mamun-Or-Rashid, A. N. M., M. M. Azam, B. K. Dash, F. B. Hafiz, and M. K. Sen. "Ethnomedicobotanical Study on Ocimum sanctum L. (Tulsi)—A Review." *Mintage Journal of Pharmaceutical and Medical Sciences* 2, no. 2 (2013): 37–42.

Newman, D. J., and G. M. Cragg. "Natural Products as Sources of New Drugs Over the Nearly Four Decades from 1981 to 2019." *Journal of Natural Products* 83, no. 3 (2020): 770–803.

Pandey, A. S. P., S. Karmakar, and W. Raja. "Emblica Officinalis (Amla): A Review for Its Phytochemistry, Ethnomedicinal Uses, and Medicinal Potentials." *Journal of Advancement in Pharmacognosy* 4, no. 1 (2023).

Petkova, N., A. Petrova, I. Ivanov, I. Hambarlyiska, Y. Tumbarski, I. Dincheva, M. Ognyanov, and P. Denev. "Chemical Composition of Different Extracts from Echinacea Purpurea (L.) Moench Roots and Evaluation of Their Antimicrobial Activity." *ChemEngineering* 7, no. 5 (2023): 94.

Rafieian-Kopaei, M., H. Nasri, N. Sahinfard, M. Rafieian, S. Rafieian, and M. Shirzad. "Turmeric: A Spice with Multifunctional Medicinal Properties." *Journal of Herbmed Pharmacology* 3, no. 1 (2014): 5–8.

Raj, A. J., S. Biswakarma, A. N. Pala, G. Shukla, Vineeta, M. Kumar, and R. W. Bussmann. "Indigenous Uses of Ethnomedicinal Plants Among Forest-Dependent Communities of Northern Bengal, India." *Journal of Ethnobiology and Ethnomedicine* 14 (2018): 1–28.

Rajendran, S., M. Kalpana Devi, A. Peter Pascal Regis, A. J. Amalraj, J. Jeyasundari, and M. Manivannan. "Electroplating Using Environmentally Friendly Garlic Extract: A Case Study." *Zaštita materijala* 50, no. 3 (2009): 131–40.

Rao, P. K., S. S. Hasan, B. L. Bhellum, and R. K. Manhas. "Ethnomedicinal Plants of Kathua District, J&K, India." *Journal of Ethnopharmacology* 171 (2015): 12–27.

Rasooli, I. *Bioactive Compounds in Phytomedicine*. London: IntechOpen, 2012.

Rishi, A., D. C. Singh, R. C. Tiwari, and B. M. Tripathi. "An Overview of Ethnomedicine and Future Aspects of Ethnomedicinal Plants." *International Journal of Ayurveda and Pharma Research* 4, no. 5 (2016): 29–33.

Samanta, S. K., A. K. Ojha, and K. Ghosh. "Biochemical Properties of Neem (Azadirachta Indica) and Its Use by the Tribals of Northern West Bengal: A Brief Review." *European Chemical Bulletin* 12, no. 1 (2023): 5434–49.

Sharma, L., M. K. Vaidya, P. Singh, and K. Dev. "Economic Analysis of Input Use Efficiency of Garlic in Himachal Pradesh: A Case Study of Sirmaur District." *Journal of Agricultural Development and Policy* 28, no. 2 (2018): 141–8.

Siddiqui, A. A., and M. Ali. *Practical Pharmaceutical Chemistry*. New Delhi: CBS Publishers and Distributors, 1997.

Silja, V. P., K. S. Varma, and K. V. Mohanan. "Ethnomedicinal Plant Knowledge of the Mullu Kuruma Tribe of Wayanad District, Kerala." *Indian Journal of Traditional Knowledge* 7, no. 4 (2008): 604–12.

Singh, G., A. K. Passsari, V. V. Leo, V. K. Mishra, S. Subbarayan, B. P. Singh, B. Kumar, S. Kumar, V. K. Gupta, H. Lalhlenmawia, and S. K. Nachimuthu. "Evaluation of Phenolic Content Variability Along with Antioxidant, Antimicrobial, and Cytotoxic Potential of Selected Traditional Medicinal Plants from India." *Frontiers in Plant Science* 7 (2016): 407.

Solanki, P., and S. Goyal. "Evaluation of the Antibacterial Properties and Phytochemicals of Giloy (*Tinospora cordifolia*)." *World Journal of Pharmaceutical Research* 11, no. 5 (2022): 2450–61.

Stanisavljević, I., S. Stojičević, D. Veličković, V. Veljković, and M. Lazić. "Antioxidant and Antimicrobial Activities of Echinacea (Echinacea Purpurea L.) Extracts Obtained by Classical and Ultrasound Extraction." *Biotechnology and Bioengineering* 17, no. 3 (2009).

Tripathi, S. "Ethnomedicine and Future Challenges." *Global Journal of Archaeology & Anthropology* 10, no. 5 (2019): 87–90.

Umadevi, M., R. Rajeswari, C. S. Rahale, S. Selvavenkadesh, R. Pushpa, K. P. S. Kumar, and D. Bhowmik. "Traditional and Medicinal Uses of *Withania somnifera*." *The Pharma Innovation* 1, no. 9 (2012): 102–10.

Vats, S., and R. Tiwari. "Evaluation of Antioxidant and Antimicrobial Potential of *Bacopa monnieri* L." *Researcher* 6, no. 9 (2014): 20–3.

Velu, S., and C. Baskaran. "Phytochemical Analysis and In-Vitro Antimicrobial Activity of Withania somnifera (Ashwagandha)." *Journal of Natural Products and Plant Resources* 2, no. 6 (2012): 711–16.

Verma, K. C. "Ashwagandha (Withania Somnifera Dunal): Wonder Medicinal Plant." *Agricultural Reviews* 31, no. 4 (2010): 292–7.

Verma, R. K., P. Kumari, R. K. Maurya, V. Kumar, R. B. Verma, and R. K. Singh. "Medicinal Properties of Turmeric (Curcuma Longa L.): A Review." *International Journal of Chemical Studies* 6, no. 4 (2018): 1354–7.

Wilson, E. A., and B. Demmig-Adams. "Antioxidant, Anti-Inflammatory, and Antimicrobial Properties of Garlic and Onions." *Nutrition and Food Science* 37, no. 3 (2007): 178–83.

Zahin, M., F. Aqil, M. S. A. Khan, and I. Ahmad. "Ethnomedicinal Plants Derived Antibacterials and Their Prospects." In *Ethnomedicine: A Source of Complementary Therapeutics*, edited by D. Chattopadhyay, 149–78. Kerala: Research Signpost, 2010.

13

Nutraceutical, Phytochemical, and Pharmacological Value of Lactuca

A Review

Saroj Kumar Pradhan[11*], Raspinder Kaur[2], Pooja Mawal[3], Jyoti Rani[4], and Rohita Singla[5]

[1]Department of Botany and Environmental Sciences, Sri Guru Granth Sahib World University, Fatehgarh Sahib, Punjab, India

[2]Post Graduate Department of Botany, Dev Samaj College for Women, Ferozepur, Punjab, India

[3]Department of Botany, Central University of Jammu, J & K, India

[4]Department of Botany, Chaudhary Devi Lal University, Sirsa, Haryana, India

[5]Department of Botany, Eternal University, Baru Sahib, Himachal Pradesh, India

*Corresponding Author's Email: pradhan_sarojkumar@yahoo.com

Introduction

Lactuca genus belongs to tribe Cichorieae of the family Asteraceae, composed of *ca.* 100 species spread across Europe, North America, Africa, Australia, and Asia. Twenty-four species from the Himalayan regions of Himachal Pradesh, Jammu and Kashmir, Uttarakhand, and Arunachal Pradesh have been documented in India (Bhellum and Singh 2015). The identifying characters of the genus are herbs with abundant latex, underground stolons, erect stems, spirally arranged leaves with a rosette basal condition. The inflorescence is spike-like, pyramidal, or corymbose. The involucre is cylindrical, with short bracts with or without anthocyanin; ligules are blue, yellow, and rarely white. The achenes are beaked, pale brown, black, or olive colored, and the pappus may be brown, yellow, or white in color. The genus falls into seven sections, namely, *Lactuca* subsect *Cyanicae* DC. *Phoenix opus* (Cass.) Benth., *Mulgedium* (Cass.) C.B. Clarke, *Lactucopsis* (Schultz Bip. ex Vis. et Pančič) Rony, *Tuberose* Boiss., *Micranthae* Boiss., and *Sororiae* Franchet. Asia has fifty-one species of *Lactuca*, Africa has forty-three species, Europe has seventeen species, North America has twelve species, and Australia has three species as centers of wild germplasm (Lebeda et al. 2004).

Most of the researchers used morphological data along with molecular markers for the germplasm evaluation of worldwide accessions (Koopman 2002; Doležalova et al. 2002, 2004; Rajičić et al. 2008; Křístková et al. 2008; Lebeda et al. 2009; Jemelková et al. 2015). On the basis of morphology, chromosome number, and biogeography, Wei et al. (2017) splitted *Lactuca* into two major clades (Pterocypsela and crop clade), while other species from North America and Asia form smaller clades with the Melanoseris species. The Mediterranean region, Southwestern Asia, and Middle East are the hotspots of biodiversity of *Lactuca* and the possible center of domesticated lettuce (Lebeda et al. 2009). The most common vegetable species of the *Lactuca* genus is L. *sativa*, having all essential minerals, trace elements, pigments, amino acids, and other beneficial secondary metabolites for human nutrition (Pinto et al. 2014). So far seven wild species of *Lactuca* (*L. scarioloides, L. aculeata, L. dregeana, L. altaica, L. georgica, L. serriola, L. azerbaijanica*) have been reported as close wild relatives of *L. sativa* on the basis of morphological data and also have genetic affinities (Zohary 1991). The breeding and domestication of wild species have been mainly focused on enhancing the nutritional quality, disease resistance, reduced bitterness, different forms of heads and leaf color, and so on (Lebeda et al. 2019).

Traditional Uses of Lactuca

In addition to the nutritional value, different species have been utilized to treat a variety of illnesses in traditional medical systems. The fresh leaves of *L. canadensis, L. ludoviciana, L. tatarica* subsp. *pulchella* (North America), *L.* sativa (North America, Italy, Jammu and Kashmir), *L. serriola* (Italy, Croatia), and *L. lessertiana* (Jammu and Kashmir) were used as salads or in preparations of boiled vegetables (Geraci, Polizzano, and Schicchi 2018; Lebeda et al. 2019; Singh et al. 2016; Varga et al. 2019). Native Americans from Florida, North America, including the Cherokee, Iroquois, Meskwakis, and Ojibwa, employed *L. canadensis* in the past as a nerve tonic, sedative pain reliever, diuretic, to promote lactation, medication for warts, pimples, skin disorders, and to stop bleeding (Austin 2004). North Americans used *L. virosa* for the treatment of gastroenteritis and also as sedative for nervous and vision disorders, *L. biennis* to ease lactation, and roots of *L. tatarica* subsp. *pulchella* as chewing gum and to treat diarrhea (Lebeda et al. 2019). There are also reports on traditional uses of *L. intybacea* and *L. capensis* for the treatment of gout disorders, ulcers, skin disorders, arthritis, and hepatitis (Johnson 1998).

The decoction or infusions of leaves and flowers of *L. serriola* (ver. *Agriomarulo*) were used to treat hypercholesterolemia, insomnia, and otitis by the local peoples of Edessa and Naoussa (Central Macedonia region, Northern Greece). Leaves were used as neutralizer for scorpion venom in the traditional medicine system of El Kelaa of Seraghna region (Morocco), and powdered seeds for the management of chronic cough and insomnia disease in Jammu and Kashmir, India (Tsioutsiou et al. 2019; Kpodar et al. 2016; Bhellum and Singh 2015). Various folk medicine systems have reported the sedative and aphrodisiac effects of milky latex "lactucarium" of *L. virosa*. The compound responsible for the sedative-hypnotic effect is Lactucin and its esters (Rätsch 2005; Lebeda et al. 2019; Ilgün et al. 2020). The Persian and Indian folks used the seeds of *L. sativa* (ver. *Khas*) for the treatment of sleeping disorders in pregnant women and also to relieve pain (Pour et al. 2018).

In some areas of Southern and Central Italy (Campania, Calabria, Marche, Abruzzo, Latium) leaves of *L. sativa* were used as antiodontalgic and for the treatment of dental abscesses or spots (Motti and Motti 2017). The leaves of *L. taraxacifolia* in the form of decoction were used for curing liver diseases in the Maritime region of Togo (Touloun 2012). The decoction of *L. sativa* (ver. *Alface*) roots is used as a tranquilizer to treat mental and behavioral disorders in the North Araguaia microregion of Mato Grosso, Brazil (Ribeiro et al. 2017). Additionally, several researchers documented the ethno-veterinary usage of *L. muralis* to cure rheumatoid arthritis, joint discomfort, and acute stress in pet animals, and *L. tatarica* for fodder (Bhellum and Singh 2015; Lans 2019).

Nutraceutical Value of Lactuca

Lactuca species were consumed worldwide as they provide vitamins, minerals, and fiber for the diet, are low in calories, and are a source of many other bioactive compounds. Most of them are consumed fresh as salads and are also available in packed forms. Various cultivars are available with different forms and colors, contributing to a variety of salads. The different types of lettuce used in the diet are crisphead (iceberg), butterhead, romaine (cos), and leaf lettuce (Kim et al. 2016). Mou (2012) described that horticultural types, genotypes, environmental influence, head structure, and moisture content greatly influence the nutritional quality of lettuce. Compared to leaf and romaine lettuce, crisphead lettuce is the least nutritious of the three commonly grown kinds. The quality of species for edibility and consumption depends on the taste, shelf life, postharvest, and growing conditions (Shalaby et al. 2017). There were many factors during growing conditions that affected the nutrient composition of lettuce (McKeehen et al. 1996; Varoquaux, Mazollier, and Albagnac 1996; Wießner et al. 2009; Konstantopoulou et al. 2010; Serna et al. 2012).

Increased levels of salinity during growing reduced oxidase activities during storage as proposed by Chisari et al. (2010). However, low salinity stress could enhance the levels of ascorbic acid, phenolic, and flavonoid content in baby lettuce, also with the altered levels of mineral composition (Neocleous et al. 2014). Long-term deficit or low irrigation also decreased the browning of cut pieces and enhanced the level of phenolics (128–213 μg/g) in iceberg lettuce (*L. sativa*) (Luna et al. 2012). Chicoric acid and chlorogenic acid, two derivatives of caffeic acid, were more prevalent, while flavonoids remained moderately stable. Bonasia et al. (2013) found that application of nitrogen fertilizer and strobilurin improved the visual indices, physiological factors, nutritional value, and quality of raw material in lettuce. Złotek, Świeca, and Jakubczyk (2014) enhanced the phytochemical levels and quality of *L. sativa* by using various chemical elicitors, such as abscisic acid, jasmonic acid, and arachidonic acid. Among them, jasmonic acid and abscisic acid increased the amount of phenolic acids, flavonoids, chlorophyll, carotenoids, and vitamins. Luteolin, *o*-coumaric acid, caffeic acid, ferulic acid, chlorogenic acid, quercetin, and kaempferol were among the members of the polyphenols group that rose.

Similarly, Viacava and Roura (2015) increased the phytochemical content and antioxidant activity of lettuce sprouts by using natural elicitors (tea tree and chitosan). Since the overall phenol and flavonoid content of lettuce increased by 13 percent and 19 percent, respectively, these elicitors enhance the plant's nutritional value. However, Zhao et al. (2016) discovered that the nutritional value of lettuce is generally negatively impacted by the foliar application of copper-based nanopesticides. The growth and quality of lettuce are negatively impacted by high metal contamination areas; however, this can be corrected by using altered biochar (Quartacci, Sgherri, and Frisenda 2017). Application of microorganisms was also studied to enhance the nutritional quality of lettuce. Radhakrishnan and Lee (2016) used *Bacillus methylotrophicus KE2* as a bacterial treatment for the growth of L. sativa. The treated plants show significantly better morphological characters and have a high content of fructose, micro minerals, protein, amino acids, and gamma-aminobutyric acid as compared to the untreated group.

The browning of cut lettuce is the main issue with minimally processed lettuce, and different methods and treatments have been suggested to combat the enzymatic processes (López-Gálvez, Saltveit, and Cantwell 1996; Martınez and Artés 1999). Techniques that retard browning and enhance shelf life include low storage temperatures, UV treatments, vacuum cooling, green tea extract, hypobaric packaging, aqueous chlorine dioxide, and so on (Allende et al. 2006; Martín-Diana, Rico, and Barry-Ryan 2008; An, Park, and Lee 2009; López-Gálvez et al. 2010; Ordidge et al. 2010). The combined effects of high light and enhanced CO_2 on the nutritional quality of two cultivars of *L. sativa* (red-leaf Clemente Viven and green-leaf Blonde) were investigated by Pérez-López et al. (2013). While the concentrations of practically all minerals stayed constant, high light intensity alone raised the concentrations of soluble proteins, carbohydrates, carotenoids, glutathione, total phenols, and anthocyanins. Along with higher CO_2 levels, total biomass boosted while levels of anthocyanins, carotenoids, total phenols, and chlorophyll a were lowered. By sustaining high net photosynthetic rates, blue and red light supplemented with green light also enhance the nutritional qualities of *L. sativa* cv. Butterhead.

After postharvest, Lee and Chandra (2018) discovered that packing *L. sativa* cv. Tojong-mats with non-perforated polypropylene that has anti-fogging qualities prolongs the pigmentation and shelf life for up to two weeks. After seventeen days of storage at 12°C, Witkowska and Woltering (2014) observed that even though undamaged lettuce heads remain fresh, their sugar and chlorophyll contents decreased. Using pepper essential oils rich in β-caryophyllene can help prevent microorganisms from destroying fresh cut lettuce while it's being stored (Myszka et al. 2017). As before, Chen et al. (2017) employed eugenol solutions and clove essential oil to prevent lettuce from browning and losing its texture. Eugenol, carvacrol, and trans-anethole are found in bio-based emitting sachets that can be used to boost phenolic production and give organic, ready-to-eat iceberg lettuce significant antioxidant properties (Wieczyńska and Cavoski 2018).

Mou (2005) investigated the differences in lutein and β-carotene levels among fifty-two lettuce genotypes. The wild species have the highest concentration as compared to the cultivated ones and among the latter type, green leaf or romaine have the highest content. Koudela and Petříková (2008) compared the nutritional quality of five cultivars of *L. sativa* var. *crispa*, that is, Bergamo, Dubáček, Frisby, Lollo Rossa, and Redin. Lollo Rossa had the highest levels of calcium, fiber, nitrates, potassium, sodium, dry weight, and leaf rosette weight in Redin, whereas Frisby had the highest levels of magnesium and vitamin C. The content of all these nutrients also varies among the cultivars, depending upon the time of plantation. Belitz et al. (2009) found that romaine lettuce is the richest source of dietary fiber, potassium, manganese, iron, vitamins, and omega-3 fatty acids.

Linolenic acid, linoleic acid, and palmitic acid were the principal fatty acids found in lettuce. The overall amount of polyunsaturated fatty acids in various cultivars varied from 14 to 32 mg/g DW, with the cultivar romaine having the highest amount (Le Guedard et al. 2008). Further, the dietary fiber content ranged from 180 to 420 mg/g DW with the peak content in the romaine lettuce (USDA 2015). The content of minerals in the different lettuce types as per USDA (2015) are 1.0–6.0 mg/g DW for Na, K (28–50 mg/g DW), Ca (4–8 mg/g DW), Mg (1.4–2.8 mg/g DW), P (4–6 mg/g DW), Fe (172–248 μg/g DW), and Zn (35.7–50.5 μg/g DW). The nutritional value of the inner and outer leaves of lettuces with green and red pigments (*L. sativa* var. *capitata*) was compared by Baslam et al. (2013). The level of ß-carotene was high in outer leaves (0.39–0.48 mg/g DM) in all the cultivars as compared to inner leaves (0.18–0.46 mg/g DM). The amounts of elemental nutrients were also high in the outer leaves as Mg (7.6–9.5 g/kg), S (1.3–3.6 g/kg), Ca (15.3–20.6 g/kg), Fe (75.71–112.37

mg/kg), Na (2946.20–4125.98 mg/kg), Cu (1.22–3.13 mg/kg), Mn (149.16–202.96 mg/kg), and Zn (35.07–50.51 mg/kg). In contrast to this, the phenolic content was high in the inner leaves as compared to the former one in all the three cultivars studied (Batavia Rubia Munguía, Cogollos de Tudela, and Maravilla de Verano).

Previously, Mou and Ryder (2004) stated that, there is a definite variation in the dietary value according to the head arrangement of lettuce. They found that the content of Fe, Ca, and β-carotene was higher in outer leaves, while artificially opened leaves have greater nutrient content compared to normal romaine lettuce. Therefore, the closed outer leaves in the head structure of crisphead lettuce are the cause of its low nutritional content. Cruz et al. (2012) found that supplementation of 10 percent coffee residues can also increase the level of β-carotene (90 percent) and lutein (72 percent) in *L. sativa* var. *capitata*. Additionally, López et al. (2014) discovered that regular-sized and baby-sized lettuces differ in terms of their concentration of nitrate, organic acids, sugars, and antioxidant chemicals. The content of sugars, carotenoids, and organic acids was found to be greater in Mini Romaine type, while folates, vitamin C, and phenolic compounds were more in the case of regular-sized romaine type. The third variety studied, Little Gem, has the highest content of nitrates, which is a negative factor for the lettuce. Size and head structure, which control sunlight penetration and the synthesis of light-dependent metabolites, were the primary causes of these content variations.

Chadwick et al. (2016) compared the bitterness, sweetness, and liking of recombinant inbred lines and parental (*L. serriola* and *L. sativa* cv. salinas) lettuce. According to their hypothesis, the proportions of sugars and sesquiterpene lactones play a significant role in how taste is perceived, with the bitter and sweet ingredients acting to balance each other out more so than the amounts of individual metabolites. The primary factor for sweetness was glucose, and the only sesquiterpene lactone that counteracts the perceptible change in bitterness was 15-p-hydroxyl phenylacetyl lactucin-8-sulfate. Santos et al. (2014) investigated the amount of nine macro and micro minerals in seven baby leaf vegetables, including green lettuce (*L. sativa* var. crispa). The amount of manganese (0.79–0.84 mg/100g FW) was found to be highest in the species alone, while the rest of the minerals were found to be high in other baby leaf vegetables. The nutritional value of lettuce is low among the other leafy vegetables, but still, it can provide specific nutrients, such as carotenoids, folates, and phenolic compounds. Recently, Kim et al. (2016) reviewed the nutritional quality of different cultivars of *L. sativa* and recommended different types for each type of specific nutrients. They found that the romaine type was rich in dietary fibers, while butterhead, red leaf, and baby green leaf were high in iron content. The butterhead and romaine types are the richest sources of folate, β-carotene, and lutein. The red romaine and red leaf types have maximum phenolic compounds, while green leaf and baby green romaine have vitamin C.

Phytochemicals of Lactuca

In Tables 13.1 to 13.3, 253 compounds have been isolated and characterized from different plant organs of the genus *Lactuca*. The plants of the genus contain sesquiterpenoids, phenols, and flavonoids. Initially, the latex of *L. virosa* and *L. sativa* has been examined by many researchers and led them to the isolation of crystalline mixtures of α-Lactucerol and β-Lactucerol (Bauer and Schub 1929; Kassner 1887; Hesse 1886; Pomeranz and Sperling 1904). Later on Simpson (1944) isolated taraxasterol (pure form of *α-Lactucerol*), β-amyrin, and germanicol from non-saponifiable matter of dried latex of *L. virosa*. Hui and Lee (1971) isolated β-amyrenyl, germanicol, taraxasterol acetate, and taraxasterol from petroleum extract of *L. denticulata* and *L. indica*.

(a) **Terpenoids:** The sesquiterpene lactones are the major compounds found in the aerial parts and roots of the genus *Lactuca*. Cichorioside B, Lactucin, 11β,13-dihydrolactucin, 8-Deoxylactucin, Lactucopicrin, Jacquinelin, and 9α-hydroxyzaluzanin C are the guaianolides reported from the leaves, roots, aerial parts, and whole plant of the genus *Lactuca*. The major guaianolide glycosides, namely: crepidiaside B, picriside A, macrocliniside A, ixerin F, and scorzoside are widely distributed in the genus. Most triterpenoids exist in various forms including germacrolide, melampolide, eudesmanolide, guanine. lupane type, diterpene alcohol, and norsesquiterpene along with their glycosides (see Table 13.1).

(b) **Phenolic compounds and Flavonoids:** Phenolics are among the dominant compounds of this plant. Hydroxycinnamic acid and its derivatives including caffeoylquinic acids, dicaffeoylquinic acids, p-coumaroylquinic acids, caffeoyltartaric acid, dicaffeoyltartaric acids, p-coumaroyltartaric acid, caffeoylmalic acid, p-coumaroylcaffeoylquinic acids along with hydroxybenzoic acid and hydroxyphenyl acid derivatives were isolated from various species as shown in Table 13.2. Flavonoids from the genus *Lactuca* were mainly flavonols and mostly isolated from the whole plant and aerial parts of the members. Quercetin, kaempferol, luteolin, apigenin, and their derivatives are the most common compounds isolated from the leaves and whole plant of *L. sativa*, *L. serriola*, *L. tatarica*, *L. indica*, and *L. virosa* (see Table 13.2).

(c) **Lignans and Coumarins:** To date, some of the lignans and coumarins are also isolated from various plant parts (aerial parts, roots, and whole plant) and callus tissue of *L. aculeata*, *L. indica*, *L. sibirica*, *L. orientalis*, and *L. sativa*. To mention, some of the compounds are loliolide, lactucaside, esculetin–6–*O*–glucoside, dihydroxycoumarin, syringaresinol, and its derivatives (see Table 13.3).

Table 13.1. Terpenoids Isolated from Members of the Genus *Lactuca*

Terpenoid Compounds	Species	Plant Part	References
		Guaianolide	
Cichorioside B	*L. tatarica*	Roots	Kisiel, Barszcz, and Szneler 1997;
		Whole Plant	Wang, Gao, and Jia 2010;
	L. indica		Hou et al. 2003;
		Aerial parts	Kim et al. 2008;
	L. sativa var. *anagustata*		Han et al. 2010; Beharav et al. 2015;
	L. georgica	Leaves and Roots	Michalska, Beharav, and Kisiel 2014;
			Nishimura et al. 1986;
	L. lacinata		Michalska, Żylewski, and Kisiel 2008;
	L. triangulata		Michalska, Szneler and Kisiel 2010;
	L. altaica		Michalska, Kisiel, and Stojakowska 2015;
	L. dregeana		Michalska, Michalski, and Stojakowska 2017
	L. sativa var. *anagustata*		
Lactucin	*L. virosa*	Aerial parts Roots	Gromek 1989, 1991;
		Aerial parts	Kisiel et al. 1995;
	L. saligna		Kisiel and Gromek 1993;
		Leaves and Roots	Khalil, Abd El-fattah, and Mansour 1991;
		Whole plant	Michalska et al. 2009;
	L. tatarica	Stem	Kisiel, Barszcz, and Szneler 1997;
		Leaves and Roots	Wang, Gao, and Jia 2010;
	L. sativa cv. Diana		Sessa et al. 2000;
	L. dregeana		Michalska et al. 2009;
	L. perennis		
	L. sativa cv. British Hilde		
	L. serriola		
	L. tatarica		
	L. virosa	Roots	
	L. altaica		Michalska, Szneler and Kisiel 2010; Michalska, Michalski, and Stojakowska 2017;
	L. sativa var. *anagustata*		
	L. georgica		Beharav et al. 2015

Lactucin-15-oxalate	*L. sativa* cv. Diana	Aerial parts	Sessa et al. 2000
Lactucopicrin-15-oxalate	*L. serriola*		
8-deoxy lactucin-15-oxalate	*L. virosa*		
15-deoxy lactucin-8-sulfate			
15-p-hydroxyphenylacetic-lactucin-8-sulfate			
Lactucin-8-*O*-acetate	*L. floridana*	Roots	Song et al. 1995;
	L. georgica		Michalska, Beharav, and Kisiel 2014
Lactucin methacrylate	*L. georgica*	Roots	Michalska, Beharav, and Kisiel 2014
11β H, 13-dihydro lactucin-8-P-methoxyphenyl acetate	*L. tatarica*	Roots	Kisiel, Barszcz, and Szneler 1997
11β,13-dihydrolactucin	*L. indica*	Whole plant	Nishimura et al. (1986); Hou et al. (2003);
			Michalska, Żylewski, and Kisiel (2008); Kisiel and Michalska (2008);
	L. triangulata	Roots	Michalska and Kisiel (2009);
	L. sibirica	Aerial parts	Michalska et al. (2009)
	L. saligna		
	L. sativa cv. British Hilde		Wang, Gao, and Jia 2010;
	L. serriola		Michalska, Szneler and Kisiel 2010;
	L. virosa		Michalska, Kisiel, and Stojakowska 2015;
	L. tatarica		Han et al. 2010;
		Whole plant	Beharav et al. 2015;
	L. altaica		Michalska, Beharav, and Kisiel 2014
	L. dregeana	Aerial parts	
	L. sativa var. *anagustata*		
	L. georgica	Roots	
11β,13-dihydrolactucin-8-*O*-acetate	*L. floridana*	Roots	Song et al. 1995;
	L. georgica		Michalska, Beharav, and Kisiel 2014;
			Beharav et al. 2015

(*Continued*)

Table 13.1 (Continued)

Terpenoid Compounds	Species	Plant Part	References
8-Deoxy Lactucin	*L. virosa*	Leaves	Gromek 1989;
		Roots,Leaves	Michalska et al. 2009;
	L. saligna	Roots Roots,Leaves	Kisiel and Gromek 1993;
		Roots	Michalska et al. 2009;
	L. sibirica		Kisiel and Michalska 2008;
			Michalska and Kisiel 2009;
			Song et al. 1995;
	L. floridana	Roots	Michalska, Żylewski, and Kisiel 2008;
	L. triangulata		
	L. aculeata		Michalska et al. 2009;
		Roots	Michalska and Kisiel 2010; Michalska et al. 2009
	L. dregeana	Whole plant	
	L. indica		
	L. sativa cv. British Hilde	Roots	
	L. serriola		Michalska and Kisiel 2013
	L. tatarica		
	L. viminea		
Intybulide	*L. altaica*	Whole plant	Michalska, Szneler and Kisiel 2010
Lactucopicrin	*L. virosa*	Aerial parts Roots	Gromek 1989, 1991;
		Roots,Leaves	Kisiel et al. 1995;
		Aerial parts	Michalska et al. 2009;
	L. saligna	Roots	Khalil, Abd El-fattah, and Mansour 1991;
		Roots,Leaves	Kisiel and Gromek 1993;
		Whole plant	Michalska et al. 2009;
	L. tatarica	Roots,Leaves	Kisiel, Barszcz, and Szneler 1997;
		Whole plant	Michalska et al. 2009;
			Wang, Gao, and Jia 2010;
	L. sativa cv. Diana		Sessa et al. 2000;
	L. dregeana		Michalska et al. 2009;
	L. indica		
	L. sativa cv. British Hilde		
	L. serriola		
	L. altaica	Roots	Michalska, Szneler and Kisiel 2010;
	L. georgica		Michalska, Beharav, and Kisiel 2014

11β, 13-dihydro lactucopicrin	*L. virosa*	Aerial parts	Gromek 1989, 1991;
	L. sativa var. *anagustata*	Roots	Han et al. 2010;
	L. georgica		Michalska, Beharav, and Kisiel 2014;
			Beharav et al. 2015;
	L. dregeana		Michalska, Kisiel, and Stojakowska 2015
Lettucenin A	*L. sativa*	Seedlings	Bestwick et al. 1995
	L. sativa var. *capitata*	Leaves	Takasugi et al. 1985
Lettucenin B	*L. sativa*	Aerial parts	Mai and Glomb 2014
Leucodin	*L. sativa* var. *anagustata*	Whole plant	Michalska, Michalski, and Stojakowska 2017 Stojakowska et al. 2018 Michalska and Kisiel 2013
	L. orientalis		
	L. viminea		
Jacquinelin	*L. virosa*	Aerial parts Roots	Gromek 1989, 1991;
		Roots,Leaves	Kisiel et al. 1995;
		Aerial parts	Michalska et al. 2009;
	L. saligna	Roots	Khalil, Abd El-fattah, and Mansour 1991;
		Roots,Leaves	Kisiel and Gromek 1993;
		Aerial parts	Michalska et al. 2009;
	L. tatarica	Roots,Leaves	Kisiel, Barszcz, and Szneler 1997;
		Aerial parts	Michalska et al. 2009;
	L. sibirica		Kisiel and Michalska 2008;
		Roots	Michalska and Kisiel 2009;
			Michalska and Kisiel 2010;
			Michalska and Kisiel 2013;
	L. aculeata		Michalska et al. 2009
	L. viminea		
	L. dregeana		
	L. indica		
	L. perennis		
	L. sativa cv. British Hilde		
	L. serriola		
11β,13-dihydrolactucin-8-*O*-methacrylate	*L. virosa*	Roots	Kisiel and Barszcz 1997;
	L. georgica		Michalska, Beharav, and Kisiel 2014;
			Beharav et al. 2015

(*Continued*)

Table 13.1 (Continued)

Terpenoid Compounds	Species	Plant Part	References
11,13-dehydrolactuside	*L. canadensis*	Roots	Michalska, Szneler and Kisiel 2013
Zaluzanin C			
3-epizaluzanin C			
11β,13-dihydro-3-epizaluzanin C			
11β,13- dihydrozaluzanin C	*L. aculeata*	Whole plant	Michalska and Kisiel 2010;
		Roots	Michalska, Szneler and Kisiel 2010;
	L. altaica		Michalska, Szneler and Kisiel 2010
	L. canadensis		
11β-hydroxy-11, 13-dihydrolactucin	*L. tatarica*	Whole plant	Kisiel, Barszcz, and Szneler 1997;
			Wang, Gao, and Jia 2010
9α-hydroxyzaluzanin C	*L. indica*	Whole plant	Nishimura et al. 1986;
	L. aculeata		Michalska and Kisiel 2010;
	L. altaica		Michalska, Szneler and Kisiel 2010;
	L. viminea	Roots	Michalska and Kisiel 2013;
			Michalska and Kisiel 2014
	L. inermis		
9α-hydroxy-11,13α-dihydrozaluzanin C	*L. indica*	Aerial parts	Nishimura et al. 1986;
		Roots	Hou et al. 2003;
			Kim et al. 2008;
	L. viminea		Michalska and Kisiel 2013;
			Michalska and Kisiel 2014
	L. inermis		
9α-hydroxy-4β, 15, 11β,13-tetrahydro dehydrozaluzanin C	*L. indica*	Whole plant	Nishimura et al. 1986; Michalska and Kisiel 2010
	L. aculeata		
9β-hydroxyl-4β, 11β, 13, 15-tetrahydrozaluzanin C	*L. sativa* var. *anagustata*	Aerial parts	Han et al. 2010
10β, 14-dihydroxyl-11βH-guaiane-4(15)-ene-12, 6α-olide			
9α-hydroxy-11,13-dehydroleucodin-9-O-β-xyl opyranoside	*L. triangulata*	Roots	Michalska, Żylewski, and Kisiel 2008
9α-hydroxyleucodin-9-O-β-xylopyranoside			
Hieracin I	*L. aculeata*	Whole plant	Michalska and Kisiel 2010
Hieracin II			

Deacetylmatricarin	*L. tatarica*	Whole plant	Wang, Gao, and Jia 2010
8-deacetyl matricarin-8-O-sulfate	*L. dregeana*	Whole plant	Michalska, Kisiel, and Stojakowska 2015;
	L. sativa var. *anagustata*		Michalska, Michalski, and Stojakowska 2017
Guaianolide glycosides			
Crepidiaside B	*L. virosa*	Aerial parts	Gromek 1989, 1991;
		Roots	Kisiel et al. 1995;
		Roots,Leaves	Michalska et al. 2009;
	L. tatarica	Aerial parts	Kisiel, Barszcz, and Szneler 1997;
		Roots,Leaves	Michalska et al. 2009;
	L. saligna	Roots	Khalil, Abd El-fattah, and Mansour 1991;
		Aerial parts and Roots	Kisiel and Gromek 1993;
		Aerial parts	Michalska et al. 2009;
	L. perennis		Kisiel and Zielińska 2000;
		Roots,Leaves	Michalska et al. 2009;
		Roots	Kisiel and Michalska 2008;
	L. sibirica		Michalska and Kisiel 2009;
			Michalska, Żylewski, and Kisiel 2008;
			Michalska et al. 2009
	L. triangulata		
	L. capensis		
	L. dregeana		
	L. indica		Michalska, Szneler and Kisiel 2010;
	L. sativa cv. British Hilde		Michalska, Beharav, and Kisiel 2014;
	L. serriola		Michalska, Michalski, and Stojakowska 2017;
	L. altaica		Michalska and Kisiel 2010;
	L. georgica		Michalska and Kisiel 2013
	L. sativa var. *anagustata*		
	L. aculeata		
	L. viminea		
Ixerin H	*L. viminea*	Roots	Michalska and Kisiel 2013

(*Continued*)

Table 13.1 (Continued)

Terpenoid Compounds	Species	Plant Part	References
Ixerin F	*L. virosa*	Aerial parts Roots	Gromek 1989, 1991;
			Kisiel et al. 1995;
	L. saligna	Aerial parts	Khalil, Abd El-fattah, and Mansour 1991;
			Kisiel and Gromek 1993 ;Kisiel, Barszcz, and Szneler 1997;
	L. tatarica	Roots	Michalska and Kisiel 2009;
	L. sibirica		Michalska and Kisiel 2010
	L. aculeata		Michalska, Szneler and Kisiel 2010;
			Michalska, Szneler and Kisiel 2013;
			Michalska, Michalski, and Stojakowska 2017;
	L. altaica		Michalska and Kisiel 2013;
	L. canadensis		Michalska and Kisiel 2014
	L. sativa var. *anagustata*		
	L. viminea		
	L. inermis		
Macrocliniside A	*L. indica*	Whole plant	Nishimura et al. 1986
	L. sativa	Roots	Ishihara, Miyase, and Ueno 1987
	L. virosa		Kisiel et al. 1995
	L. tatarica	Aerial parts	Kisiel, Barszcz, and Szneler 1997
	L. sibirica	Roots	Michalska and Kisiel 2009
			Michalska and Kisiel 2010
	L. aculeata		Han et al. 2010
			Michalska, Michalski, and Stojakowska 2017
	L. sativa var. *anagustata*	Aerial parts	Michalska, Szneler and Kisiel 2010
		Roots	Michalska, Szneler and Kisiel 2013
	L. altaica		Michalska, Beharav, and Kisiel 2014
	L. canadensis		
	L. georgica		
Salignoside	*L. saligna*	Roots	Kisiel and Gromek 1993
	L. viminea		Michalska and Kisiel 2013
Scorzoside	*L. virosa*	Roots	Kisiel et al. 1995
	L. perennis		Kisiel and Zielińska 2000
			Michalska, Michalski, and Stojakowska 2017 Michalska and Kisiel 2013
	L. sativa var. *anagustata*		

Vernoflexuoside	*L. indica*	Whole plant	Nishimura et al. 1986
		Roots	Michalska et al. 2009
	L. dregeana		
	L. perennis		
	L. saligna		
	L. serriola		
	L. tatarica		
	L. virosa		
	L. altaica		Michalska, Szneler and Kisiel 2010
	L. canadensis		Michalska, Szneler and Kisiel 2013
	L. sibirica		Michalska and Kisiel 2009
11β,13-dihydrovernoflexuoside	*L. aculeata*	Whole plant	Michalska and Kisiel 2010 Michalska, Michalski, and Stojakowska 2017 Michalska, Szneler and Kisiel 2013
	L. sativa var. *anagustata*	Roots	
	L. canadensis	Whole plant	Michalska, Szneler and Kisiel 2010
	L. altaica		
11β ,13-dihydroglucozaluzanin C	*L. indica*	Whole plant	Nishimura et al. 1986
	L. tatarica	Aerial parts	Kisiel, Barszcz, and Szneler 1997
	L. perennis		Kisiel and Zielińska 2000
			Michalska and Kisiel 2009
	L. sibirica	Roots	Michalska, Szneler and Kisiel 2013
			Michalska and Kisiel 2013
	L. canadensis		Michalska, Beharav, and Kisiel 2014
	L. viminea		Michalska and Kisiel 2014
	L. georgica		
	L. inermis		
3-epizaluzanin C-3-*O*-β-glucopyranoside	*L. canadensis*	Roots	Michalska et al. 2013
11,13 dihydro-8-deoxylactucin 15-glycoside (jacquinellin glycoside)	*L. sativa*	Aerial parts	Sessa et al. 2000
	L. serriola		
	L. virosa		

(*Continued*)

Table 13.1 (Continued)

Terpenoid Compounds	Species	Plant Part	References
4α-*O*-β-D-glucopyranosyl-15-hydroxyl-5α, 6βH-guaiane-10(14), 11(13)-dien-12, 6α-olide	*L. sativa* var. *anagustata*	Aerial parts	Han et al. 2010
11β(13)-tetrahydro-8, 9-didehydro-3-deoxyzaluzanin C-10-*O*-β-glucopyranoside			
10β, 14-dihydroxy-10(14), 11 β(13)-tetrahydro-8,9-didehydro-3-deoxyzaluzanin C-10-*O*-β-glucopyranoside	*L. altaica* *L. sativa* var. *anagustata*	Whole plant	Michalska, Szneler and Kisiel 2010, Michalska, Michalski, and Stojakowska 2017
3-deoxyzaluzanin C derivative	*L. viminea*	Roots	Michalska and Kisiel 2013
Germacranolide			
3β,14-dihydroxy-11β,13-dihydrocostunolide	*L. sativa* var. *anagustata*	Roots	Michalska, Michalski, and Stojakowska 2017
Germacranolide glucoside			
Tataroside (3β,1 l β,14-trihydroxy-11,13-dihydrocostunolide-3-β-glucopyranoside)	*L. tatarica*	Whole plant	Kisiel and Barszcz 1998
Sonchuside A	*L. tatarica* *L. sativa* var. *anagustata* *L. viminea* *L. georgica*	Roots	Kisiel, Barszcz, and Szneler 1997 Michalska, Michalski, and Stojakowska 2017 Michalska and Kisiel 2013 Michalska, Beharav, and Kisiel 2014
3β,14-dihydroxy-11β,13-dihydrocostunolide-3-*O*-β-glucopyranoside	*L. virosa* *L. triangulata* *L. altaica* *L. sibirica* *L. aculeata* *L. georgica*	Roots	Kisiel and Barszcz 1997 Michalska, Żylewski, and Kisiel 2008 Michalska, Szneler and Kisiel 2010 Michalska and Kisiel 2009 Michalska and Kisiel 2010 Michalska, Beharav, and Kisiel 2014
Hypochoeroside B	*L. georgica*	Roots	Michalska, Beharav, and Kisiel 2014
Picriside A	*L. virosa* *L. tatarica* *L. saligna*	Aerial parts Roots Aerial parts Roots	Gromek 1989, 1991 Kisiel et al. 1995 Khalil, Abd El-fattah, and Mansour 1991 Kisiel and Gromek 1993

Picriside B	*L. tatarica*	Roots	Kisiel, Barszcz, and Szneler 1997
	L. aculeata		Michalska and Kisiel 2010
			Michalska, Szneler and Kisiel 2013
	L. canadensis		Michalska, Michalski, and Stojakowska 2017
	L. sativa var. *anagustata*		Michalska and Kisiel 2013
	L. viminea		
Picriside C	*L. tatarica*	Whole plant	Kisiel, Barszcz, and Szneler 1997
Lactucopicriside	*L. indica*	Aerial parts	Nishimura et al. 1986
Melampolide			
Lactulide A	*L. indica*	Whole plant	Nishimura et al. 1986
	L. aculeata		Michalska and Kisiel 2010
Lactulide B	*L. sativa* var. *anagustata*	Roots	Michalska, Michalski, and Stojakowska 2017
Melampolide glucoside			

(*Continued*)

Table 13.1 (Continued)

Terpenoid Compounds	Species	Plant Part	References
Lactuside A	*L. indica*	Aerial parts	Nishimura et al. 1986
		Roots	Michalska et al. 2009
	L. sativa		Ishihara, Miyase, and Ueno 1987
	L. virosa	Aerial parts	Gromek 1989, 1991
		Roots	Michalska et al. 2009
	L. tatarica		Kisiel et al. 1995
			Michalska et al. 2009
			Kisiel, Barszcz, and Szneler 1997
	L. saligna	Aerial parts	Khalil, Abd El-fattah, and Mansour 1991
		Roots	Michalska et al. 2009
			Kisiel and Gromek 1993 Kisiel and Zielińska 2000
	L. perennis		Michalska et al. 2009
			Michalska and Kisiel 2010
			Michalska et al. 2009
	L. aculeata		
	L. dregeana		
	L. perennis		Michalska, Szneler and Kisiel 2010
	L. sativa cv. British Hilde		Michalska, Beharav, and Kisiel 2014
	L. serriola		Beharav et al. 2015
	L. altaica		
	L. georgica		Michalska and Kisiel 2013
	L. canadensis		
Lactuside B	*L. indica*	Aerial parts	Nishimura et al. 1986
			Hou et al. 2003
			Kim et al. 2008
Lactuside C (9α-hydroxyleucodin-9-O-β-glucopyranoside)	*L. sativa*	Roots	Ishihara, Miyase, and Ueno 1987
	L. triangulata		Michalska, Żylewski, and Kisiel 2008
	L. canadensis		Michalska, Szneler and Kisiel 2013
	L. dregeana		Michalska, Kisiel, and Stojakowska 2015 Michalska, Michalski, and Stojakowska 2017
	L. sativa var. *anagustata*		
11β-hydroxyleucodin-11-O-β-glucopyranoside	*L. sativa* var. *anagustata*	Roots	Michalska, Michalski, and Stojakowska 2017

		Eudesmanolide	
1β-hydroxyl-15-O-(*p*-methoxyphenylacetyl)-5α, 6β, 11βH-eudesma-3-en-12, 6α-olide	*L. sativa* var. *anagustata*	Aerial parts	Han et al. 2010
Reynosin	*L. floridana*	Roots	Song et al. 1995
Santamarin	*L. floridana*	Roots	Song et al. 1995
	L. canadensis		Michalska, Szneler and Kisiel 2013
	L. viminea		Michalska and Kisiel 2013
Tauremisin (=vulgarin)	*L. viminea*	Roots	Michalska and Kisiel 2013
11β,13-dihydrosantamarin	*L. indica*	Whole plant	Nishimura et al. 1986
	L. tatarica	Roots	Wang, Gao, and Jia 2010
	L. canadensis		Michalska, Szneler and Kisiel 2013
	L. viminea		Michalska and Kisiel 2013
2-oxo-11β, 13-dihydrosantamarin	*L. tatarica*	Roots	Kisiel, Barszcz, and Szneler 1997
			Wang, Gao, and Jia 2010
	L. viminea		Michalska and Kisiel 2013
1-epiisoerivanin	*L. canadensis*	Roots	Michalska, Szneler and Kisiel 2013
1-epierivanin	*L. viminea*		Michalska and Kisiel 2013
1-epidehydroisoerivanin			
Armexifolin	*L. canadensis*	Roots	Michalska, Szneler and Kisiel 2013
Armefolin			
3α-hydroxyreynosin			
2β-hydroxy-11β, 13-dihydrodouglanin	*L. tatarica*	Whole plant	Wang, Gao, and Jia 2010
1β-O-β-D-glucopyranosyl-4α hydroxyl-5α, 6β, 11βH-eudesma-12, 6 α -olide	*L. sativa* var. *anagustata*	Aerial parts	Han et al. 2010
1β-hydroxyl-5α, 6βH-eudesman-3-ene-12, 6α-olide			
methyl 3β-(β-glucopyranosyloxy)-6α-hydroxy eudesma-1,4(15), 11(13)-trien-12-oate	*L. altaica*	Whole plant	Michalska, Szneler and Kisiel 2010
2β-hydroxy-11β, 13-dihydrodouglanin	*L. tatarica*	Whole plant	Wang, Gao, and Jia 2010
Guanine			
Lactucain A	*L. indica*	Aerial parts	Hou et al. 2003
Lactucain B			
Lactucain C			

(*Continued*)

Table 13.1 (Continued)

Terpenoid Compounds	Species	Plant Part	References
Lupane			
Lactucenyl acetate	*L. indica*	Roots	Shinozaki et al. 2011
Tarolupenyl acetate			
Bauerenyl acetate			
α-amyrin acetate	*L. denticulata*	Whole plant	Hui and Lee 1971
β-amyrin acetate	*L. denticulata*	Whole plant	Hui and Lee 1971
Germanicyl acetate	*L. indica*	Roots	Shinozaki et al. 2011
Taraxasteryl acetate			
Taraxasterol			
Lupenyl acetate			
3β-Hydroxyglutin-5-ene	*L. indica*	Aerial parts	Kim et al. 2008
Diterpene alcohol			
trans-Phytol	*L. indica*	Aerial parts	Kim et al. 2008
Norsesquiterpene glycoside			
(6*S*,9*S*)-Roseoside	*L. indica*	Aerial parts	Kim et al. 2008
5,6-Epoxy-3-hydroxy-7-megastigmen-9-one			
Monoterpene glycoside			
1-Hydroxy Linalool-6-O-β-D-glucopyranoside	*L. indica*	Aerial parts	Kim et al. 2008

Table 13.2. Phenolic Compounds and Flavonoids Isolated from Members of the Genus *Lactuca*

Phenolic Compounds	Species	Plant Parts	Reference
	Hydroxycinnamic acid		
Caffeic acid (3,4-dihydroxy-cinnamic acid)	*L. indica*	Whole head and Roots	Wang et al. 2003
	L. sativa var *capitata*		Mai and Glomb 2013
	L. tuberosa		Stojakowska et al. 2013, 2018
	L. orientalis		Llorach et al. 2008
	L. sativa	Leaves	Abu-Reidah et al. 2013
	L. sativa cv Baby		
	L. sativa cv Romaine		
	L. sativa cv Iceberg		
p-Coumaric acid	*L. sativa*	Whole plant	Llorach et al. (2008)
Hydroxycinnamic acid derivatives			
Caffeoylquinic acids			
1-**O**-caffeoylquinic acid	*L. sativa* cv Krysthine RZ	Leaves	Viacava et al. 2017, 2018
4-**O**-caffeoylquinic acid	*L. sativa* cv Versai RZ		
	L. sativa var Lores		
5-*O*-caffeoylquinic acid	*L. indica*	Aerial parts	Kim, Kim, and Lee 2007
3-*O*-caffeoylquinic acid	*L. sativa* cv Krysthine RZ	Leaves	Viacava et al. 2017, 2018
	L. sativa cv Versai RZ		
	L. sativa var Lores		Abu-Reidah et al. 2013
	L. sativa cv Baby		
	L. sativa cv Romaine		
	L. sativa cv Iceberg		

(*Continued*)

Table 13.2 (Continued)

Phenolic Compounds	Species	Plant Parts	Reference
Chlorogenic acid (5-*O*-caffeoylquinic acid)	*L. indica*	Whole plant	Hou et al. 2003
	L. sativa		Llorach et al. 2008
	L. sativa var. *capitata*		Li et al. 2010
			Ribas-Agustí et al. 2011
			Mai and Glomb 2014
			López et al. 2014
	L. aculeata		Stojakowska and Malarz 2017
			Stojakowska et al. 2018
	L. orientalis		Abu-Reidah et al. 2013
	L. sativa cv Baby		
	L. sativa cv Romaine		
	L. sativa cv Iceberg		
Caffeoylquinic acid–hexoside	*L. sativa* cv Krysthine RZ	Leaves	Viacava et al. 2017, 2018
	L. sativa cv Versai RZ		
	L. sativa var Lores		
Dicaffeoylquinic acids			
Isochlorogenic acid (3,5-Dicaffeoylquinic acid)	*L. indica*	Whole plant	Wang et al. 2003
	L. sativa	Aerial parts	Kim, Kim, and Lee 2007
			Li et al. 2010
		Whole plant	Ribas-Agustí et al. 2011
			Llorach et al. 2008
	L. sativa cv Audran	Leaves	Romani et al. 2002
	L. sativa var. *capitata*	Whole plant	Mai and Glomb 2014
	L. sativa cv Baby	Leaves	Abu-Reidah et al. 2013
	L. sativa cv Romaine		
	L. sativa cv Iceberg		
Dicaffeoylquinic acid	*L. sativa* cv Baby	Leaves	Abu-Reidah et al. 2013
	L. sativa cv Romaine		
	L. sativa cv Iceberg		
3,4-di-*O*-caffeoylquinic acid	*L. indica*	Aerial parts	Kim, Kim, and Lee 2007
3,5-di-*O*-caffeoyl-muco-quinic acid			
4,5-di-*O*-caffeoylquinic acid			

1,5-dicaffeoylquinic acid 4,5-dicaffeoylquinic acid	*L. aculeata*	Callus tissue	Stojakowska and Malarz 2017
1,5–di–*O*–Caffeoylquinic acid 3,5–di–*O*–Caffeoylquinic acid 4,5–di–*O*–Caffeoylquinic acid	*L. sativa* cv Krysthine RZ *L. sativa* cv Versai RZ L. sativa var Lores	Leaves	Viacava et al. 2017, 2018
p-Coumaroylquinic acids			
5-*p*-Coumaroylquinic acid	*L. sativa* *L. sativa* cv Krysthine RZ *L. sativa* cv Versai RZ *L. sativa* var Lores	Leaves	Ribas-Agustí et al. 2011 Viacava et al. 2017, 2018
p-coumaroylquinic acid	*L. sativa* cv Baby *L. sativa* cv Romaine *L. sativa* cv Iceberg	Leaves	Abu-Reidah et al. 2013
3–**p**–Coumaroylquinic acid	*L. sativa* cv Krysthine RZ *L. sativa* cv Versai RZ *L. sativa* var Lores	Leaves	Viacava et al. 2017, 2018
5-*O*-(E)-*p*-coumaroylquinic acid	*L. indica*	Aerial parts	Kim, Kim, and Lee 2007
Caffeoyltartaric acid			
Caftaric acid (Caffeoyltartaric acid)	*L. sativa* cv Krysthine RZ *L. sativa* cv Versai RZ	Leaves	Viacava et al. 2017, 2018
	L. sativa var Lores *L. sativa*	Whole plant Leaves	Llorach et al. 2008 Li et al. 2010 Ribas-Agustí et al. 2011 Abu-Reidah et al. 2013
	L. sativa cv Baby *L. sativa* cv Romaine *L. sativa* cv Iceberg *L. aculeata*		Stojakowska and Malarz 2017
	L. orientalis		Stojakowska et al. 2018
Dicaffeoyltartaric acids			
Chicoric acid (Dicaffeoyltartaric acid)	*L. sativa* *L. sativa* var. *capitata*	Leaves Whole plant	Li et al. 2010 Llorach et al. 2008 Ribas-Agustí et al. 2011

(*Continued*)

Table 13.2 (Continued)

Phenolic Compounds	Species	Plant Parts	Reference
			Mai and Glomb 2014
	L. aculeata	Callus tissue	Stojakowska and Malarz
	L. orientalis		Stojakowska et al. 2018
		Leaves	
	L. sativa cv Krysthine RZ		Viacava et al. 2017, 2018
	L. sativa cv Versai RZ		
	L. sativa var Lores		Abu-Reidah et al. 2013
	L. sativa cv Baby		
	L. sativa cv Romaine		
	L. sativa cv Iceberg		
messo–di–O–Caffeoyl Tartaric acid	*L. sativa*	Whole plant	Llorach et al. 2008
	L. sativa cv Krysthine RZ	Leaves	Viacava et al. 2017, 2018
	L. sativa cv Versai RZ		
	L. sativa var Lores		
p-Coumaroyltartaric acid			
Coutaric acid (p–Coumaroyltartaric acid)	*L. sativa*	Leaves	Ribas-Agustí et al. 2011
	L. sativa cv Krysthine RZ		Viacava et al. 2017, 2018
	L. sativa cv Versai RZ		
	L. sativa var Lores		Abu-Reidah et al. 2013
	L. sativa cv Baby		
	L. sativa cv Romaine		
	L. sativa cv Iceberg		
di-*p*-Coumaroyltartaric acid	*L. sativa*	Leaves	Ribas-Agustí et al. 2011
Caffeoylmalic acid			
Caffeoylmalic acid	*L. sativa*	Whole plant	Llorach et al. 2008
			Ribas-Agustí et al. 2011
	L. sativa cv Krysthine RZ	Leaves	Viacava et al. 2017, 2018
	L. sativa cv Versai RZ		
	L. sativa var Lores		Mai and Glomb 2014
	L. sativa var. *capitata*	Whole head	Abu-Reidah et al. 2013
	L. sativa cv Baby	Leaves	
	L. sativa cv Romaine		
	L. sativa cv Iceberg		

p-Coumaroylcaffeoylquinic acids			
4−Caffeoyl−5−*p*−coumaroylquinic acid	*L. sativa* cv Krysthine RZ	Leaves	Viacava et al. 2017, 2018
	L. sativa cv Versai RZ		
	L. sativa var Lores		
p-Coumaroylcaffeoylquinic acids	*L. sativa* cv Baby	Leaves	Abu-Reidah et al. 2013
	L. sativa cv Romaine		
	L. sativa cv Iceberg		
3−*p*−Coumaroyl−4−caffeoylquinic acid	*L. sativa* cv Krysthine RZ	Leaves	Viacava et al. 2017, 2018
	L. sativa cv Versai RZ		
	L. sativa var Lores	Whole head	
Other Hydroxycinnamic acid			
Methyl caffeate	*L. tuberosa*	Roots	Stojakowska et al. 2013
	L. aculeata	Callus tissue	Stojakowska and Malarz 2017
Ethyl caffeate	*L. tuberosa*	Roots	Stojakowska et al. 2013
p−Coumaric acid−hexoside	*L. sativa* cv Krysthine RZ	Leaves	Viacava et al. 2017, 2018
Sinapic acid−hexoside	*L. sativa* cv Versai RZ		
	L. sativa var Lores		
Dihydrocaffeic acid−hexoside	*L. sativa* cv Baby	Leaves	Abu-Reidah et al. 2013
Caffeoyl-hexose	*L. sativa* cv Romaine		
Ferulic acid methyl ester	*L. sativa* cv Iceberg		
	L. sativa cv Krysthine RZ		Viacava et al. 2017, 2018
	L. sativa cv Versai RZ		
	L. sativa var Lores		
Dihydrocaffeic acid sulfate	*L. sativa* cv Baby	Leaves	Abu-Reidah et al. 2013
Ferulic acid glucoside	*L. sativa* cv Romaine		
Sinapoyl glucoside	*L. sativa* cv Iceberg		
p-Coumaroyl glucoside			
Cinnamic acid-dihydrothymine			
p-coumaryl alcohol	*L. tuberosa*	Roots	Stojakowska et al. 2013
Ethyl 4'-hydroxy-*trans*-cinnamate	*L. perennis*	Aerial parts and Roots	Kisiel and Zielińska 2000
Ethyl 3'4'-dihydroxy-*trans*-cinnamate			
	Hydroxybenzoic acid and derivatives		
Protocatechuic acid (3,4-dihydroxybenzoic acid)	*L. indica*	Whole plant	Wang et al. 2003
	L. sativa		Llorach et al. 2008
	L. tuberosa		Stojakowska et al. 2013

(*Continued*)

Table 13.2 (Continued)

Phenolic Compounds	Species	Plant Parts	Reference
Methyl p-hydroxybenzoate	*L. indica*	Whole plant	Wang et al. 2003
Gallic acid (3,4,5-trihydroxybenzoic acid)	*L. aculeata*	Callus tissue	Stojakowska and Malarz 2017
Methyl 4-hydroxybenzoate	*L. orientalis*	Roots	Stojakowska et al. 2018
Hydroxybenzoic acid	*L. sativa* cv Krysthine RZ	Leaves	Viacava et al. 2017, 2018
Dihydroxybenzoic acid	*L. sativa* cv Versai RZ		
Hydroxybenzoyl gallic acid–hexoside	*L. sativa* var Lores		
Hydroxybenzoyl–*O*–dihydroxybenzoic acid–hexoside			
Syringaldehyde	*L. altaica*	Roots	Michalska, Szneler and Kisiel 2010
Syringic acid	*L. inermis*	Roots	Michalska and Kiesel 2014
Hydroxybenzoic acid–hexoside	*L. sativa* cv Baby	Leaves	Abu-Reidah et al. 2013
Dihydroxybenzoic acid–hexoside	*L. sativa* cv Romaine		
Galloyl hexose	*L. sativa* cv Iceberg		
Syringic acid–hexoside	*L. sativa* cv Krysthine RZ		Viacava et al. (2017, 2018)
	L. sativa cv Versai RZ		
	L. sativa var Lores		
Tachioside (3-Methoxy-4-hydroxyphenyl-1-O-β-D-glucoside)	*L. sativa* cv Baby	Leaves	Abu-Reidah et al. 2013
Vanillic acid glucoside	*L. sativa* cv Romaine		
2-*O*-*p*-hydroxybenzoyl-6-*O*-galloyl glucoside	*L. sativa* cv Iceberg		
Hydroxybenzoyl dihydroxybenzoyl hexose			
Hydroxyphenyl acid derivatives			
4-hydroxyphenylacetic acid	*L. sativa* cv Krysthine RZ	Leaves	Viacava et al. 2017, 2018
	L. sativa cv Versai RZ		
	L. sativa var Lores		
	L. sativa cv Baby		Abu-Reidah et al. 2013
	L. sativa cv Romaine		
	L. sativa cv Iceberg		Michalska and Kisiel 2014
	L. inermis	Roots	
4–hydroxyphenylacetic acid–hexoside	*L. sativa* var Lores	Whole head	Viacava et al. 2018
Methyl 4-hydroxyphenyl acetate	*L. altaica*	Roots	Michalska, Szneler and Kisiel 2010
Methyl *p*-hydroxyphenyl acetate	*L. tuberosa*	Roots	Stojakowska et al. 2013
4-hydroxyphenylacetyl glucoside	*L. sativa* cv Baby	Leaves	Abu-Reidah et al. 2013
Di(4-hydroxyphenylacetyl)-hexose	*L. sativa* cv Romaine		
	L. sativa cv Iceberg		
Ethyl 4’-hydroxyphenylacetates	*L. perennis*	Aerial parts and Roots	Kisiel and Zielińska 2000
Methyl 4’-hydroxyphenylacetates			

	Other Phenolics		
p-Coumaroylcaffeoyltartaric acid	*L. sativa*	Leaves	Ribas-Agustí et al. 2011
	L. sativa cv Baby		Abu-Reidah et al. 2013
	L. sativa cv Romaine		
	L. sativa cv Iceberg		
3-n-Pentadecyl-2,4-dinitrophenol	*L. runcinata*	Whole plant	Kanthal et al. 2014
Vanillaldehyde	*L. altaica*	Roots	Michalska, Szneler and Kisiel 2013
Coniferyl aldehyde			
2,6-dimethoxybenzoquinone			
Eugenyl-4-*O*-β-glucopyranoside			
Dihydrodehydrodiconiferyl alcohol 9-*O*-β-glucopyranoside			
Dihydroconiferin	*L. tenerrima*	Whole plant	Michalska, Szneler and Kisiel 2012
Dihydrosyringin			
Dihydrodehydrodiconiferyl alcohol 9-*O*-β-glucopyranoside			
Vanillin	*L. orientalis*	Roots	Stojakowska et al. 2018
Flavonoid compounds			
Flavonols			
Quercetin	*L. acanthifolia*	Whole plant	Rees and Harborne 1984
	L. altaica		
	L. graeca		
	L. saligna		
	L. serriola		
	L. tatarica		
	L. virosa		
	L. tetrantha		
	L. viminea		Terencio et al. 1992
	L. indica		Hou et al. 2003

(*Continued*)

Table 13.2 (Continued)

Phenolic Compounds	Species	Plant Parts	Reference
Isoquercetin (Quercetin-3-*O*-glucoside)	*L. tatarica*	Aerial parts	Kisiel (1998)
	L. quercina		
	L. indica		Kim, Kim, and Lee 2007
		Whole plant	Wang et al. 2003
	L. sativa var *capitata*	Whole heads	Mai and Glomb 2013
	L. sativa cv Baby	Leaves	Abu-Reidah et al. 2013
	L. sativa cv Romaine		
	L. sativa cv Iceberg	Whole plant	
	L. sativa	Leaves	Llorach et al. 2008
	L. tenerrima		Michalska et al. 2012
	L. viminea		Terencio et al. 1992
	L. sativum		DuPont et al. 2000
	L. indica		Hou et al. 2003
	L. sativa cv Audran		Romani et al. 2002
	L. muralis		Mańez et al. 1994
	L. virosa		
Quercetin 3-*O*-glucuronide	*L. sativum*	Whole plant	DuPont et al. 2000
	L. sativa cv Audran	Leaves	Romani et al. 2002
	L. sativa	Whole plant	Llorach et al. 2008
			Ribas-Agustí et al. 2011
	L. sativa var. *capitata*	Whole heads	Mai and Glomb 2013
	L. sativa cv Krysthine RZ	Leaves	Viacava et al. 2017
	L. sativa cv Versai RZ		
	L. sativa var Lores		Viacava et al. 2018
Quercetin-3-*O*-galactoside	*L. indica*	Whole heads	Kaneta et al. 1978
	L. sativa var. *capitata*		Mai and Glomb 2013
	L. sativum		DuPont et al. 2000
	L. sativa cv Krysthine RZ	Leaves	Viacava et al. 2017
	L. sativa cv Versai RZ		
	L. sativa var Lores		Viacava et al. 2018
Quercetin hexose glucuronide	*L. sativa* cv Baby	Leaves	Abu-Reidah et al. 2013
	L. sativa cv Romaine		
	L. sativa cv Iceberg		

Quercetin 3-*O*-(6-*O*-malonyl)glucoside	*L. sativa* cv Audran	Leaves	Romani et al. 2002
	L. sativa	Whole plant	Li et al. 2010
			Llorach et al. 2008
			Ribas-Agustí et al. 2011
	L. sativum	Leaves	DuPont et al. 2000
	L. sativa var. *capitata*	Whole plant Whole heads	Mai and Glomb 2013
	L. sativa cv Krysthine RZ		Viacava et al. 2017
	L. sativa cv Versai RZ		
	L. sativa var Lores		Viacava et al. 2018
Quercetin-7-*O*-glucuronide-3-O-(6”-*O*-malonyl)-glucoside	*L. sativa*	Whole plant	Llorach et al. 2008
	L. sativa cv Baby	Leaves	Abu-Reidah et al. 2013
	L. sativa cv Romaine		
	L. sativa cv Iceberg		
Quercetin 3-*O*-α-L-rhamnopyranosyl(1→6)-β-D-glucopyranoside	*L. indica*	Aerial parts	Kim, Kim, and Lee 2007
Quercetin 5-*O*-β-D-glucopyranoside			
Quercetin 3-*O*-rhamnoside	*L. sativum*	Whole head	DuPont et al. 2000
Quercetin 5-*O*-glucoside	*L. indica*	Aerial parts	Kim, Kim, and Lee 2007
Quercetin-*O*-hexoside	*L. sativa* cv Krysthine RZ	Leaves	Viacava et al. 2017
Quercetin hexose-glucuronide	*L. sativa* cv Versai RZ		
Quercetin-3-*O*-(6”-*O*-malonyl)-glucoside-7-*O*-glucuronide	*L. sativa* var Lores		Viacava et al. 2018
Quercetin-*O*-di-hexoside			
Quercetin-*O*-rhamnosyl-gluconide			
Rutin (Quercetin-3-*O*-rutinoside)	*L. sativa*	Whole plant	Llorach et al. 2008
			López et al. 2014
	L. indica	Aerial parts	Kim, Kim, and Lee 2007
		Whole plant	Hou et al. 2003
Kaempferol	*L. sativa*	Whole plant	Bilyk and Sapers 1985
			López et al. 2014
	L. sativa cv Krysthine RZ		Viacava et al. 2017
	L. sativa cv Versai RZ		
	L. sativa var Lores		Viacava et al. 2018

(*Continued*)

Table 13.2 (Continued)

Phenolic Compounds	Species	Plant Parts	Reference
Kaempferol 3-*O*-glucoside (Kaempferol 3-*O*-β-glucopyranoside)	*L. tatarica*	Whole plant	Kisiel 1998
	L. tenerrima		Michalska, Stojakowska, and Kisiel 2012
	L. sativa cv Krysthine RZ	Leaves	Viacava et al. 2017
	L. sativa cv Versai RZ		
	L. sativa var Lores		Viacava et al. 2018
Kaempferol-3-*O*-glucuronide	*L. sativa*	Whole plant	Llorach et al. 2008
Kaempferol-3-*O*-(6"-*O*-malonyl)-glucoside	*L. sativa* cv Krysthine RZ	Leaves	Viacava et al. 2017
	L. sativa cv Versai RZ		
	L. sativa var Lores		Viacava et al. 2018
Kaempferol-hexoside	*L. sativa* cv Krysthine RZ	Leaves	Viacava et al. 2017
	L. sativa cv Versai RZ		
	L. sativa var Lores		Viacava et al. 2018
Luteolin	*L. acanthifolia*	Whole plant	Rees and Harborne 1984
	L. altaica		
	L. graeca		
	L. saligna		
	L. serriola		
	L. virosa		
	L. tetrantha		
	L. viminea		Terencio et al. 1992
	L. quercina		Kisiel 1998
	L. tatarica		
	L. perennis	Aerial parts and Roots	Kisiel and Zielińska 2000
		Whole plant	Hou et al. 2003
	L. indica		López et al. 2014
	L. sativa		Viacava et al. 2017
	L. sativa cv Krysthine RZ		
	L. sativa cv Versai RZ		Viacava et al. 2018
	L. sativa var Lores		
Luteolin 7-*O*-glucoside (Luteolin 7-O-β-glucopyranoside)	*L. muralis*	Aerial Parts	Kaneta et al. 1978
	L. viminea		Terencio et al. 1992
	L. virosa		Mańez et al. 1994
	L. tenerrima		Michalska, Stojakowska, and Kisiel 2012
	L. quercina	Whole plant	Kisiel 1998
	L. indica		Wang et al. 2003
			Llorach et al. 2008

Luteolin 7-*O*-glucuronide	*L. sativum*	Whole plant	DuPont et al. 2000
	L. indica		Hou et al. 2003
	L. sativa var. *capitata*		Kim, Kim, and Lee 2007
			Mai and Glomb 2013
	L. sativa		Llorach et al. 2008
	L. sativa cv Krysthine RZ	Leaves	Viacava et al. 2017
	L. sativa cv Versai RZ		
	L. sativa var Lores		Viacava et al. 2018
	L. indica	Aerial Parts	Kim, Kim, and Lee 2007
Luteolin 7-*O*-glucuronide methyl ester	*L. viminea*	Aerial Parts	Terencio et al. 1992
	L. tenerrima		Mańez et al. 1994
	L. virosa		
Luteolin-7-*O*-rutinoside	*L. sativa*	Whole plant	Llorach et al. 2008
	L. sativa cv Krysthine RZ	Leaves	Viacava et al. 2017
	L. sativa cv Versai RZ		
	L. sativa var Lores		Viacava et al. 2018
Luteolin-7-*O*-rhie	*L. sativa* cv Krysthine RZ	Leaves	Viacava et al. 2017
	L. sativa cv Versai RZ		
	L. sativa var Lores		Viacava et al. 2018
Luteolin-hydroxymalonylhexoside	*L. sativa* cv Krysthine RZ	Leaves	Viacava et al. 2017
	L. sativa cv Versai RZ		
Apigenin	*L. saligna*	Whole plant	Rees and Harborne 1984
	L. aculeata		
	L. triquetra		
	L. serriola		
	L. tenerrima		
	L. virosa		
	L. perennis		Kisiel and Zielińska 2000
			López et al. 2014
	L. sativa		Hou et al. 2003
	L. indica		Terencio et al. 1992
	L. viminea		Kisiel 1998
	L. quercina		
	L. tatarica		

(*Continued*)

Table 13.2 (Continued)

Phenolic Compounds	Species	Plant Parts	Reference
Apigenin 7-*O*-glucoside (Apigenin-7-*O*-β-glucopyranoside)	*L. muralis*	Aerial Parts	Kaneta et al. 1978
	L. tenerrima		Mańez et al. 1994
	L. tatarica		Kisiel 1998
	L. indica		Hou et al. 2003
	L. perennis	Roots	Kisiel and Zielińska 2000
			López et al. 2014
	L. sativa	Leaves	Viacava et al. 2017
	L. sativa cv Krysthine RZ		
	L. sativa cv Versai RZ		Viacava et al. 2018
	L. sativa var Lores		
Apigenin-glucuronide	*L. sativa* cv Krysthine RZ	Leaves	Viacava et al. 2017
Apigenin-*O*-rhamnosyl-hexoside	*L. sativa* cv Versai RZ		
	L. sativa var Lores		Viacava et al. 2018
Apigenin-pentahydroxyhexanoide	*L. sativa* cv Krysthine RZ	Leaves	Viacava et al. 2017
	L. sativa cv Versai RZ		
5,2'-dihydroxy-7-*O*-β-D-glucuronylflavone	*L. indica*	Aerial parts	Kim, Kim, and Lee 2007
5,7,2'-trihydroxyflavone7-*O*-glucoside			
Rutin	*L. indica*	Whole plant	Hou et al. 2003
	L. sativa		López et al. 2014
Eriodictyol-*O*-glucuronide	*L. sativa* cv Krysthine RZ	Leaves	Viacava et al. 2017
	L. sativa cv Versai RZ		
	L. sativa var Lores		Viacava et al. 2018
Anthocyanidin			
Cyanidin-3-*O*-glucoside	*L. sativa*	Whole plant	Li et al. 2010
Cyanidin-3-*O*-(6"-O-malonyl)-glucoside	*L. sativa* cv Krysthine RZ	Leaves	Viacava et al. 2017
	L. sativa cv Versai RZ		
	L. sativum	Whole head	DuPont et al. 2000
Cyanidin-3-*O*-(6"-O-acetyl)-glucoside	*L. sativa* cv Krysthine RZ	Leaves	Viacava et al. 2017
	L. sativa cv Versai RZ		
Cyanidin-3-*O*-(3"-O-malonyl)-glucoside	*L. sativa*	Whole plant	Li et al. 2010
	L. sativa cv Krysthine RZ	Leaves	Viacava et al. 2017
	L. sativa cv Versai RZ		
Others			
Phloridzin	*L. sativa*	Whole plant	López et al. 2014

Table 13.3. Lignans and Coumarins Isolated from Members of the Genus *Lactuca*

Lignans and Others	Species	Plant Part	References
8α-hydroxypinoresinol-4α-*O*-β-(6-p-methoxyphenylacetyl)-glucopyranoside	*L. sibirica*	Aerial parts	Kisiel and Michalska 2008
8α-hydroxypinoresinol-4α-*O*-β-(6-p-hydroxyphenylacetyl)-glucopyranoside			
(+)-5-methoxybalanophonin (+)-buddlenol A	*L. aculeata*	Callus tissue	Stojakowska and Malarz 2017
(+)-balanophonin-9-*O*-β-glucopyranoside			
(-)-dihydrodehydrodiconiferyl alcohol-4-*O*-β-glucopyranoside			
(-)-dihydrodehydrodiconiferyl alcohol-9-*O*-β-glucopyranoside			
(±) 4-*O*-methyldihydrodehydrodiconiferyl alcohol (±) dihydrodehydrodiconiferyl alcohol	*L. orientalis*	Aerial parts and Roots	Stojakowska et al. 2018
dihydrodehydrodiconiferyl alcohol 9-O-β-glucopyranoside			
(−) dihydrodehydrodiconiferyl alcohol 9-O-β-glucopyranoside			
(+) 4-*O*methyldihydrodehydrodiconiferyl alcohol 9′-O-β-glucopyranoside			
(±) 4-*O*-methyldihydrodehydrodiconiferyl alcohol 9-*O*-			
β-glucopyranoside			
Dihydroconiferyl alcohol, 3-indolecarbaldehyde	*L. aculeata*	Whole plant	Michalska and Kisiel 2010
Loliolide	*L. aculeata* *L. orientalis*	Whole plant	Michalska and Kisiel 2010 Stojakowska et al. 2018
Lactucaside	*L. indica* *L. sibirica*	Aerial parts	Hou et al. 2003 Kisiel and Michalska 2008
Coumarins			

(*Continued*)

Table 13.3 (Continued)

Lignans and Others	Species	Plant Part	References
Esculetin–6–*O*–glucoside	*L. sativa* cv Krysthine RZ	Leaves	Viacava et al. 2017, 2018
Dihydroxycoumarin	*L. sativa* cv Versai RZ		
6,7–dihydroxycoumarin	*L. sativa* var Lores		
Maloyl–dihydroxycoumarin			
Tri–4–hydroxyphenylacetic acid–glucoside			
Syringaresinol	*L. sativa* var Lores	Whole heads	Viacava et al. (2018)
	L. aculeata	Callus tissue	Stojakowska and Malarz 2017
Syringaresinol–hexose	*L. sativa* cv Krysthine RZ	Whole heads	Viacava et al. 2017, 2018
Syringaresinol–acetylhexose	*L. sativa* cv Versai RZ		
Dimethoxy–hexosyl–lariciresinol	*L. sativa* var Lores		
Scopolin	*L. tenerrima*	Aerial parts and Roots	Michalska, Stojakowska and Kisiel 2012
	L. inermis		Michalska and Kisiel 2014
Fraxetin 7- O-b-glucopyranoside (isofraxoside)	*L. inermis*	Aerial parts and Roots	Michalska and Kisiel 2014
α-xylofuranosyluracil			

Bioactivities of Lactuca

Bioactivity is the ability of a substance to have an effect on a living organism or tissue. It can also refer to the ability of a material to elicit a biological response. Bioactive compounds have actions in the body that may promote good health. They are being studied in the prevention of cancer, heart disease, and other diseases. Examples of bioactive compounds include lycopene, resveratrol, lignan, tannins, and indoles. Bioactive compounds found in Lactuca species (commonly known as lettuce) include phenolic compounds like flavonoids, carotenoids, vitamins (particularly vitamin C and folate), phytosterols, antioxidants like lutein and zeaxanthin, and lactones (particularly lactucin and lactucopicrin), which contribute to potential health benefits like anti-inflammatory, antioxidant, and anticancer properties depending on the specific lettuce variety. The detailed health benefits of Lactuca species are given here.

(a) **Antimicrobial activity:** Despite the fact that *Lactuca* species have high nutritional value and biologically active compounds, there were also few reports of their antimicrobial activity. A new antibacterial triterpenoid saponin having potential against six bacteria strains was isolated from the stem and seeds of *L. serriola* (Yadava and Jharbade 2007, 2008). Zdravković and colleagues (2012) investigated the antibacterial properties of ethanol-based extracts of lettuce leaves against eight strains of bacteria and fungi that were cultivated in two different types of environments, namely glass and plastic houses. The leaf extract shows maximum antimicrobial activity against *Aspergillus niger*, *Bacillus subtilis*, *Proteus mirabilis*, and *Staphylococcus aureus*, in the range of 1953–78125 µg/mL. The decoction of *L. indica* decreased the colonization of *E. coli* strains in the epithelial cells of the bladder by lowering the activation of focal adhesion kinase (Lüthje, Dzung, and Brauner 2011). Aqueous and methanol extracts of *L. sativa* var *longifolia* were tested for their antibacterial properties against five gram-positive and six gram-negative bacteria by Edziri et al. (2011). In contrast to aqueous extracts, methanol extracts exhibit a higher phenolic content and radical-scavenging activity. When used against all types of bacteria, the extract worked best at a dose of 2.5 mg/mL. Furthermore, it demonstrated antiviral activity against coxsackie B virus type 3 and human cytomegalovirus (HCMV) strain AD-169, with an IC_{50} of 200 g/mL. Recently, Jaradat et al. (2018) demonstrated the antimicrobial potential of aqueous and organic extracts of *L. orientalis* against six bacterial strains. The minimum inhibitory concentration of organic extracts was found to be in the range of 1.5–6.25 mg/mL, which is very much lower compared to DMSO.

(b) **Antioxidant activity:** The presence of micronutrients, minerals, vitamins, phenolics, and triterpenes imparts the highest antioxidant activity in the lettuce. Through genetic engineering, the content of vitamins, total phenolics, and cellular antioxidant activities can be increased in the commonly used lettuce (Guo et al. 2013). Garg et al. (2004) evaluated antioxidant potential of methanolic extracts of *L. sativa* in both *in vitro* and *in vivo* conditions. The extracts show significant antioxidative potential against oxidative damage done by UV radiations. Liu et al. (2007) compared the total phenol content and radical-scavenging activity of twenty-five cultivars of lettuce grown in Colorado. The leafy red pigmented lettuce cultivar possesses the highest phenolic content and also antioxidant capacity. According to the study, harvesting time and environmental factors directly affect the amount of bioactive chemicals present. Altunkaya et al. (2009) found that combination of lettuce extract with either α-tocopherol, quercetin, or ascorbic acid caused increasing synergism against the lipid peroxidation of liposomes. Al Nomaani et al. (2013) discovered that the crude extracts of Omani lettuce's essential oils are promising contenders for their antioxidant qualities. The major chemical constituents were durenol, thymol, camphene, α-pinene, spathulenol, caryophyllene, γ-cymene, α-terpinene, limonene, and thymol acetate. The impact of various treatments and storage conditions on lettuce's antioxidant potential has also been investigated by a number of authors (Malejane et al. 2017). According to Serafini et al. (2002), eating fresh lettuce has a greater impact on a person's plasma total radical-trapping antioxidant capacities than eating preserved lettuce. According to Samuolienė et al. (2012), red, green, and light-green leaf baby lettuces with increased phenol content and strong antioxidant potential have higher levels of tocopherol and ascorbic acid when exposed to more light. The impact of high CO_2 and its combination with salinity or strong light on the antioxidant capacity of red and green leaf lettuce was also investigated by Pérez-López et al. (2013). These combinations or alone conditions have a positive effect on the antioxidant potential in both cultivars. In order to maximize the overall reducing and antioxidant capabilities for extracts of lettuce by-products, Gomes et al. (2013) optimized the extraction parameters with regard to solvents (acetone, water and methanol), extraction temperatures (30 to 60°C), and time (10 to 60 min). The best extraction parameters for maximum antioxidant capacity were 60°C, 60 minutes, and 30 percent methanol (v/v). Recently, Yang et al. (2017) have showed that exogenous application of glycine nitrogen to two cultivars of *L. sativa* (Shenxuan 1 and Lollo Rossa) enhances the accumulation of luteolin and quercetin derivatives and high antioxidant activity in hydroponically grown plants.

(c) **Anti-inflammatory activity:** In a carrageenan model of inflammation, Sayyah, Hadidi, and Kamalinejad (2004) discovered that the crude petroleum ether or methanol extract of *L. sativa* seeds exhibited dose-dependent anti-inflammatory action. Two anti-inflammatory substances, 3,14-Dihydroxy-11,13-dihydro costunolide and 8-Tigloyl-15-Deoxy-actucin, were extracted from *L. sativa* by Araruna and Carlos (2010). The presence of polyphenols in the lettuce has anti-inflammatory and antioxidant potential, as reported by Pepe et al. (2014). Nitric oxide release and reactive oxygen species were considerably reduced by the lettuce extract, but cyclooxygenase-2 and nitric oxide synthase expression were elevated. Similarly, polyphenolic extracts in the range of 250–2.5 μg mL^{-1} from *L.*

sativa demonstrated both oxidative and inflammatory activity in LPS-stimulated macrophage cells, according to Adesso et al. (2016). According to Ismail and Mirza (2015), the highest anti-inflammatory, antidepressant, and analgesic properties were found in an aqueous extract of *L. sativa* (cv. grand rapids) leaves at a dose of 1 g/Kg. These were followed by methanolic/chloroform extracts of the leaves, cell suspension exudates, and aqueous and methanolic/chloroform seed extracts. The polyphenolic profile of *L. sativa* (var. Maravilla de Verano) was higher in case of mineral-fertilized treatment. The main active content proposed for the anti-inflammatory activities were quercetin and chicoric acid, as the levels were found to increase by various treatments and positively correlated with the higher activity (Adesso et al. 2016; Złotek and Świeca 2016).

(d) **Analgesic activity:** Ahmad, Khan, and Rasheed (1992) found that extracts of *L. scariola* (300, 500 and 1000 mg/kg) showed potent analgesic activity, as compared to acetylsalicylic acid as a standard drug (300 mg/kg). When comparing the test extract to various doses of morphine sulfate, Morshedi, Dashti-Rahmatabadi, and Rafati (2006) investigated the analgesic effect of L. sativa seed extracts and discovered that there was no discernible increase in Tail-Flick latency. Similarly, Sayyah, Hadidi, and Kamalinejad (2004) found that lettuce seed extracts had no analgesic effect at the highest dosage of 6 g/kg. Recently, Ismail et al. (2016) investigated the effects of *Agrobacterium*-mediated transformed *rol ABC* genes in lettuce. High levels of phenols, flavonoids, and antioxidant capacity are present in the transformed plants, which also exhibit 80 percent inhibition in analgesic assay. However, additional research was required to evaluate lettuce's analgesic effects in various pain models.

(e) **Anxiolytic activity:** Harsha and Anilakumar (2012) explored the anxiolytic activity of leaves of *L. sativa* (100, 200, 400 mg/kg). The dried extract shows significant exploratory behavior, locomotor and anxiolytic activities. Later on, they analyzed the active content of extracts by HPLC method and found bioactive components as caffeic acid, chlorogenic acid, epicatechin, p-coumaric, rutin hydrate, sinapic acid, quercetin, quercetin-3-rhamnoside, and vanillin. The associated biochemical changes in the treated mice were increased levels of catalase and glutathione, and decreased malondialdehyde and nitrite levels (Harsha and Anilakumar 2013).

(f) **Anticancer activity:** The ethanol extracts of *L. indica* show antiproliferative activity on human leukemic HL-60 cell lines. The lettuce extract at a concentration of 313 μg/mL induced apoptosis in the cell lines by disturbing mitochondrial membrane potential and arresting the cell cycle. Majorly, phenolic compounds were responsible for the inhibition against cell viability (Chen et al. 2007). In addition to the MCF-7 breast cancer cells, Gridling et al. (2010) showed that the aqueous extract of *L. sativa* also suppresses the viability of the former cell lines. Additionally, 3 kg of lettuce was determined to be the lowest amount of human ingestion needed to achieve 50 percent suppression of HL-60 growth. The methanolic extracts of *L. serriola* showed maximum cytotoxic action counter to MCF-7 breast cancer cell lines and moderate activity against HCT116, A549, and HepG2. The triterpenoids and phytosterols in the aerial parts of the plant were found to be responsible for the cytotoxic activity (Elsharkawy and Alshathly 2013). Recently, Qin et al. (2018) found that the cultivar B-2 (*L. sativa*), possessing the highest antioxidant activity, also showed antitumor activity against the human cancer colorectal adenoma (HCT-8), lung adenocarcinoma (A549), colon cancer (HT-29), and hepatoma (Bel7402) cell lines. The metabolite profiling of the plant displays high levels of anthocyanin, flavones, and phenolic acids. Daily eating of lettuce and other vegetables rich in carotenoids, beta-carotene, and retinol can lower the likelihood of lung cancer by at least 25 percent or more among lifetime non-smokers, as proven in a case study done in Europe (Brennan 2005).

(g) **Hepatoprotective activity:** From the aerial portions of *L. indica*, Kim, Kim and Lee (2007) extracted five flavonoids and seven quinic acid derivatives that had hepatoprotective action in the human HBV-transfected liver cell line (HepG2.2.15). The ethanol extracts of leaves (200 mg/kg body weight) of *L. sativa* showed protective effect against CCl_4 induced injury by increasing the action of antioxidant enzymes, restoring cellular metabolism and hormone levels (Hefnawy and Ramadan 2013). Kanthal et al. (2017) recently showed that other species of lettuce, *L. runcinata*, has hepatoprotective properties. They studied the influence of methanolic extracts (50–100 mg/kg body weight) on serum biological parameters. There was moderate improvement in the hepatic lesions induced by the chemical treatment.

(h) **Other Bioactivities:** The regular feeding of a 20 percent lettuce diet for three weeks has been reported to have beneficial effects on tissue oxidation and lipid metabolism. There was a total decrease of 41 percent in the cholesterol LDL/HDL ratio and 37 percent in the absorption of dietary cholesterol, while there was a 44 percent increase in fecal total steroid excretion. As lutein, α-tocopherol, ascorbic acid, and vitamin E accumulated within two hours of ingestion, there was also decreased lipid peroxidation in the heart tissue and an increase in plasma antioxidant capacity (Nicolle et al. 2004). According to Lee et al. (2009), C57BL/6J mice's levels of cholesterol were considerably reduced when they were fed 8 percent freeze-dried green lettuce (red-pigmented). The content of antioxidant compounds and activity increased in blood or liver tissues, while there was lesser oxidative damage of DNA and lipid peroxidation in the heart, kidney, plasma, and liver of the mice. Han et al. (2018) used a particular line of mice to show that animals who consumed a lot of fat either by itself or in conjunction with 2.5–10 percent purple lettuce had reduced metabolic abnormalities in diet-induced obesity. Typically, due to the existence of high amounts of bioactive compounds (esculin and chlorogenic acid) in the purple lettuce, it reduced fat mass accumulation along with an increase in glucose homeostasis, insulin sensitivity, and energy expenditure. It also improved the lipid profile and affected the intestinal microbiota, predominantly decreasing the amount of firmicutes bacteria (*Lachnospiraceae*). Rutgers Scarlet lettuce's polyphenol-rich extract (100–300 mg/kg) has been shown to have antidiabetic effects in obese mice. The primary substances linked to the bioactivity in the extracts include quercetin malonyl-glucoside (35.7 mg/g DW), chlorogenic acid (27.6 mg/g DW), and cyanidin malonyl-glucoside (20.5 mg/g DW). The lettuce extract and chlorogenic acid demonstrated a dose-dependent suppression of glucose synthesis *in vitro*, but *in vivo* the extract enhanced insulin sensitivity, reduced the amount of total liver lipids, and improved glucose metabolism (Cheng et al. 2014). Janbaz et al. (2013) demonstrated that methanolic extracts of *L. serriola* (0.03–5.0 mg/mL) have a protective effect for various types of ailments like gastrointestinal, respiratory, and vascular ailments on isolated rabbit tissue preparations. Ghorbani, Rakhshandeh, and Sadeghni (2013) showed that a 400 mg/kg hydro-alcoholic extract can lengthen the time that mice sleep after being given pentobarbital, and the extract's n-butanol fraction can lengthen sleep for as long as diazepam. Ahangarpour, Oroojan, and Radan (2014) found the antispermatogenic effects of aqueous/alcoholic extracts of lettuce seed (50 mg/kg). The methanolic extract (100, 200 mg/kg) of leaves of *L. capensis* caused memory impairment in an Alzheimer's disease rat model. The plant extract reverses the effect by restoring oxidant–antioxidant balance, acetylcholinesterase activity, and brain-derived neurotrophic factor (BDNF) (Postu et al. 2017).

Conclusion

The genus Lactuca is widely used to treat sleeplessness, chronic cough, skin conditions, and neurological and visual abnormalities. According to in vitro research, the genus's members may have an impact on various microbial strains and cancer lines. Significant analgesic, anxiolytic, hepatoprotective, anti-inflammatory, and antioxidant properties were also demonstrated by them. Future advanced study will surely depend on combining phytochemical analysis with their well-known bioactive qualities, particularly the associated mechanism to promote the creation of pharmaceutical products. Furthermore, further research on the characterization of the less common species is also desperately needed. A number of techniques for quality improvement have been developed to guarantee the quality of *Lactuca* species for safe and effective use as a food diet.

References

Abu-Reidah, I. M., M. M. Contreras, D. Arráez-Román, A. Segura-Carretero, and A. Fernández-Gutiérrez. "Reversed-phase Ultra-high-performance Liquid Chromatography Coupled to Electrospray Ionization-quadrupole-time-of-flight Mass Spectrometry as a Powerful Tool for Metabolic Profiling of Vegetables: *Lactuca sativa* as an Example of Its Application." *Journal of Chromatography A* 1313 (2013): 212–27.

Adesso, S., G. Pepe, E. Sommella, M. Manfra, A. Scopa, A. Sofo, G. C. Tenore, et al. "Anti-inflammatory and Antioxidant Activity of Polyphenolic Extracts from Lactuca

Sativa(Var.Maravilla De Verano) Under Different Farming Methods." *Journal of the Science of Food and Agriculture* 96 (2016): 4194–206.

Ahangarpour, A., A. A. Oroojan, and M. Radan. "Effect of Aqueous and Hydro-alcoholic Extracts of Lettuce (*Lactuca sativa*) Seed on Testosterone Level and Spermatogenesis in NMRI Mice." *Iranian Journal of Reproductive Medicine* 12 (2014): 65.

Ahmad, F., R. A. Khan, and S. Rasheed. "Study of Analgesic and Anti-inflammatory Activity from Plant Extracts of *Lactuca scariola* and *Artemisia absinthium*." *Journal of Islamic Academy of Sciences* 5 (1992): 111–14.

Al Nomaani, R. S. Salim Al, M. A. Hossain, A. M. Weli, Q. Al-Riyami, and J. N. Al-Sabahi. "Chemical Composition of Essential Oils and in Vitro Antioxidant Activity of Fresh and Dry Leaves Crude Extracts of Medicinal Plant of *Lactuca sativa* L. Native to Sultanate of Oman." *Asian Pacific Journal of Tropical Biomedicine* 3 (2013): 353–7.

Allende, A., J. L. McEvoy, Y. Luo, F. Artes, and C. Y. Wang. "Effectiveness of Two-Sided UV-C Treatments in Inhibiting Natural Microflora and Extending the Shelf-Life of Minimally Processed 'Red Oak Leaf' Lettuce." *Food Microbiology* 23 (2006): 241–9.

Altunkaya, A., E. M. Becker, V. Gökmen, and L. H. Skibsted. "Antioxidant Activity of Lettuce Extract (*Lactuca sativa*) and Synergism with Added Phenolic Antioxidants." *Food Chemistry* 115 (2009): 163–8.

An, D. S., E. Park, and D. S. Lee. "Effect of Hypobaric Packaging on Respiration and Quality of Strawberry and Curled Lettuce." *Postharvest Biology and Technology* 52 (2009): 78–83.

Araruna, K., and B. Carlos. "Anti-inflammatory Activities of Triterpene Lactones from *Lactuca sativa*." *Phytopharmacology* 1 (2010): 1–6.

Austin, D. F. *Florida Ethnobotany*. Boca Raton: CRC Press, 2004.

Baslam, M., F. Morales, I. Garmendia, and N. Goicoechea. "Nutritional Quality of Outer and Inner Leaves of Green and Red Pigmented Lettuces (*Lactuca sativa* L.) Consumed as Salads." *Scientia Horticulturae* 151 (2013): 103–11.

Bauer, K. H., and H. Schub. "On the Knowledge of the Ingredients of the Latex of Lactuca virosa L. and Lactuca sativa L." *Archiv der Pharmazie und Berichte der Deutschen Pharmazeutischen Gesellschaft* 267, no. 6–7 (1929): 322–31.

Beharav, A., A. Stojakowska, R. Ben-David, J. Malarz, K. Michalska, and W. Kisiel. "Variation of Sesquiterpene Lactone Contents in *Lactuca georgica* Natural Populations from Armenia." *Genetic Resources and Crop Evolution* 62 (2015): 431–41.

Belitz, H.-D., W. Grosch, and P. Schieberle. "Food Additives." *Food Chemistry* (2009): 429–66.

Bestwick, C. S., I. R. Brown, J. W. Mansfield, and D. E. Mathews. "Accumulation of the Phytoalexin Lettucenin A and Changes in 3-hydroxy-3-methylglutaryl coenzyme A Reductase Activity in Lettuce Seedlings with the Red Spot Physiological Disorder." *Phytochemistry* 38, no. 4 (1995): 793–8.

Bhellum, B., and B. Singh. "Taxonomic Novelties of the Genus Lactuca L. in Jammu and Kashmir (India): Diversity, Phenology and Distribution." *Current Life Sciences* 1 (2015): 93–102.

Bonasia, A., G. Conversa, C. Lazzizera, and A. Elia. "Pre-Harvest Nitrogen and Azoxystrobin Application Enhances Postharvest Shelf-Life in Butterhead Lettuce." *Postharvest Biology and Technology* 85 (2013): 67–76.

Brennan, C. S. "Dietary Fibre, Glycaemic Response, and Diabetes." *Molecular Nutrition & Food Research* 49 (2005): 560–70.

Chadwick, M., F. Gawthrop, R. W. Michelmore, C. Wagstaff, and L. Methven. "Perception of Bitterness, Sweetness and Liking of Different Genotypes of Lettuce." *Food Chemistry* 197 (2016): 66–74.

Chen, X., L. Ren, M. Li, J. Qian, J. Fan, and B. Du. "Effects of Clove Essential Oil and Eugenol on Quality and Browning Control of Fresh-Cut Lettuce." *Food Chemistry* 214 (2017): 432–39.

Chen, Y.-H., H.-Y. Chen, C.-L. Hsu, and G.-C. Yen. "Induction of Apoptosis by the *Lactuca indica* L. in Human Leukemia Cell Line and Its Active Components." *Journal of Agricultural and Food Chemistry* 55 (2007): 1743–9.

Cheng, D. M., N. Pogrebnyak, P. Kuhn, A. Poulev, C. Waterman, P. Rojas-Silva, W. D. Johnson, and I. Raskin. "Polyphenol-rich Rutgers Scarlet Lettuce Improves Glucose Metabolism and Liver Lipid Accumulation in Diet-induced Obese C57BL/6 Mice." *Nutrition* 30 (2014): S52–8.

Chisari, M., A. Todaro, R. N. Barbagallo, and G. Spagna. "Salinity Effects on Enzymatic Browning and Antioxidant Capacity of Fresh-cut Baby Romaine Lettuce (*Lactuca sativa* L. cv. Duende)." *Food Chemistry* 119 (2010): 1502–6.

Cruz, R., P. Baptista, S. Cunha, J. A. Pereira, and S. Casal. "Carotenoids of Lettuce (*Lactuca sativa* L.) Grown on Soil Enriched with Spent Coffee Grounds." *Molecules* 17 (2012): 1535–47.

Dietary Guidelines Advisory Committee, HHS, Office of Disease Prevention, Health Promotion (US), USDA, and Center for Nutrition Policy Promotion (US). *Dietary Guidelines for Americans, 2015–2020*. Government Printing Office, 2015.

Dolezalová, I., A. Lebeda, I. Tiefenbachová, and E. Křistková. "Taxonomic Reconsideration of Some Lactuca spp. Germplasm Maintained in World Genebank Collections." *Acta Horticulturae* 634 (2004): 193–201.

Doležalová, I., E. Křístková, A. Lebeda, and V. Vinter. "Description of Morphological Characters of Wild Lactuca L. Spp. Genetic Resources (English-Czech Version)." *Horticultural Science* 29 (2002): 56–83.

DuPont, M. S., Z. Mondin, G. Williamson, and K. R. Price. "Effect of Variety, Processing, and Storage on the Flavonoid Glycoside Content and Composition of Lettuce and Endive." *Journal of Agricultural and Food Chemistry* 48 (2000): 3957–64.

Edziri, H. L., M. A. Smach, S. Ammar, M. A. Mahjoub, Z. Mighri, M. Aouni, and M. Mastouri. "Antioxidant, Antibacterial, and Antiviral Effects of *Lactuca sativa* Extracts." *Industrial Crops and Products* 34 (2011): 1182–5.

Elsharkawy, E., and M. Alshathly. "Anticancer Activity of Lactuca steriolla Growing under Dry Desert Condition of Northern Region in Saudi Arabia." *Journal of Natural Sciences Research* 3 (2013): 5–18.

Garg, M., C. Garg, P. K. Mukherjee, and B. Suresh. "Antioxidant Potential of *Lactuca sativa*." *Ancient Science of Life* 24 (2004): 6–10.

Geraci, A., V. Polizzano, and R. Schicchi. "Ethnobotanical Uses of Wild Taxa as Galactagogues in Sicily (Italy)." *Acta Societatis Botanicorum Poloniae* 87, no. 2 (2018): 1–18.

Ghorbani, A., H. Rakhshandeh, and H. R. Sadeghnia. "Potentiating Effects of Lactuca sativa on Pentobarbital-induced Sleep." *Iranian Journal of Pharmaceutical Research* 12 (2013): 401.

Gomes, T., T. Delgado, A. Ferreira, J. A. Pereira, P. Baptista, S. Casal, and E. Ramalhosa. "Application of Response Surface Methodology for Obtaining Lettuce (*Lactuca sativa*

L.) By-products Extracts with High Antioxidative Properties." *Industrial Crops and Products* 44 (2013): 622–9.
Gridling, M., R. Popescu, B. Kopp, K.-H. Wagner, L. Krenn, and G. Krupitza. "Anti-leukaemic Effects of Two Extract Types of *Lactuca sativa* Correlate with the Activation of Chk2, Induction of p21, Downregulation of Cyclin D1 and Acetylation of α-tubulin." *Oncology Reports* 23 (2010): 1145–51.
Gromek, D. "Lactuside A from *Lactuca virosa*." *Polish Journal of Chemistry* 65 (1991): 11–12.
Gromek, D. "Sesquiterpene Lactones from *Lactuca virosa* L." *Polish Journal of Chemistry* 63 (1989): 297–301.
Guedard, M. L., B. Schraauwers, I. Larrieu, and J.-J. Bessoule. "Development of a Biomarker for Metal Bioavailability: The Lettuce Fatty Acid Composition." *Environmental Toxicology and Chemistry: An International Journal* 27 (2008): 1147–51.
Guo, X., R. H. Liu, X. Fu, X. Sun, and K. Tang. "Over-expression of l-galactono-γ-lactone Dehydrogenase Increases Vitamin C, Total Phenolics and Antioxidant Activity in Lettuce through Bio-fortification." *Plant Cell, Tissue and Organ Culture* 114 (2013): 225–36.
Han, Y.-F., G.-X. Cao, X.-J. Gao, and M. Xia. "Isolation and Characterisation of the Sesquiterpene Lactones from *Lactuca sativa* L var. *anagustata*." *Food Chemistry* 120, no. 4 (2010): 1083–8.
Han, Y., C. Zhao, X. He, Y. Sheng, T. Ma, Z. Sun, X. L. et al. "Purple Lettuce (*Lactuca sativa* L.) Attenuates Metabolic Disorders in Diet Induced Obesity." *Journal of Functional Foods* 45 (2018): 462–70.
Harsha, S. N., and K. R. Anilakumar. "Anxiolytic Property of *Lactuca sativa*, Effect on Anxiety Behaviour Induced by Novel Food and Height." *Asian Pacific Journal of Tropical Medicine* 6 (2013): 532–6.
Harsha, S. Nagesh, and K. R. Anilakumar. "Effects of *Lactuca sativa* Extract on Exploratory Behavior Pattern, Locomotor Activity and Anxiety in Mice." *Asian Pacific Journal of Tropical Disease* 2 (2012): S475–S479.
Hefnawy, H. T. M., and M. F. Ramadan. "Protective Effects of Lactuca sativa Ethanolic Extract on Carbon Tetrachloride Induced Oxidative Damage in Rats." *Asian Pacific Journal of Tropical Disease* 3, no. 4 (2013): 277–85.
Hesse, O. "Über die Bestandteile des Milchsaftes von Lactuca virosa und Lactuca sativa." *Berichte der Deutschen Chemischen Gesellschaft* 19 (1886): 297–99.
Hou, C.-C., S.-J. Lin, J.-T. Cheng, and F.-L. Hsu. "Antidiabetic Dimeric Guianolides and a Lignan Glycoside from *Lactuca indica*." *Journal of Natural Products* 66 (2003): 625–9.
Hui, W. H., and W. K. Lee. "Triterpenoid and Steroid Constituents of Some Lactuca and Ageratum Species of Hong Kong." *Phytochemistry* 10, no. 4 (1971): 899–901.
Ilgün, S., E. K. Akkol, M. Ilhan, D. Ç. Polat, A. B. Kılıç, M. Coşkun, and E. Sobarzo-Sánchez. "Sedative Effects of Latexes Obtained from some Lactuca L. Species Growing in Turkey." *Molecules* 25, no. 7 (2020): 1587.
Ishihara, N., T. Miyase, and A. Ueno. "Sesquiterpene Glycosides from *Lactuca sativa* L." *Chemical and Pharmaceutical Bulletin* 35 (1987): 3905–8.
Ismail, H., and B. Mirza. "Evaluation of Analgesic, Anti-inflammatory, Anti-depressant and Anti-coagulant Properties of *Lactuca sativa* (CV. Grand Rapids) Plant Tissues and Cell Suspension in Rats." *BMC Complementary and Alternative Medicine* 15 (2015): 1–7.

Ismail, H., E. Dilshad, M. T. Waheed, and B. Mirza. "Transformation of Lettuce with Rol ABC Genes: Extracts Show Enhanced Antioxidant, Analgesic, Anti-Inflammatory, Antidepressant, and Anticoagulant Activities in Rats." *Applied Biochemistry and Biotechnology* 181 (2016): 1179–98.

Janbaz, K. Hussain, M. F. Latif, F. Saqib, I. Imran, M. Zia-Ul-Haq, and V. De Feo. "Pharmacological Effects of *Lactuca serriola* L. in Experimental Model of Gastrointestinal, Respiratory, and Vascular Ailments." *Evidence-Based Complementary and Alternative Medicine* 2013 (2013): 1–9.

Jaradat, N., M. AlMasri, A. N. Zaid, and D. G. Othman. "Pharmacological and Phytochemical Screening of Palestinian Traditional Medicinal Plants *Erodium laciniatum* and *Lactuca orientalis*." *Journal of Complementary and Integrative Medicine* 15 (2018): 20170059.

Jemelková, M., M. Kitner, E. Kristková, A. Beharav, and A. Lebeda. "Biodiversity of Lactuca aculeata Germplasm Assessed by SSR and AFLP Markers, and Resistance Variation to Bremia lactucae." *Biochemical Systematics and Ecology* 61 (2015): 344–56.

Johnson, Tim. *CRC Ethnobotany Desk Reference*. Boca Raton, FL: CRC Press, 2019. (First edition 1998)

Kaneta, M., H. Hikichi, S. Endo, and N. Sugiyama. "Identification of Flavones in Sixteen Compositae Species." *Agricultural and Biological Chemistry* 42 (1978): 475–77.

Kanthal, L. K., A. Dey, K. Satyavathi, and P. J. P. R. Bhojaraju. "GC-MS Analysis of Bio-active Compounds in Methanolic Extract of *Lactuca runcinata* DC." *Pharmacognosy Research* 6 (2014): 58.

Kanthal, L. K., K. Satyavathi, P. Bhojaraju, and M. P. Kumar. "Hepatoprotective Activity of Methanolic Extracts of *Lactuca runcinata* DC and *Gyrocarpus asiaticus* Willd." *Beni-Suef University Journal of Basic and Applied Sciences* 6 (2017): 321–5.

Kassner, A. "Ueber die unverseifbaren Bestandtheile des Lactucariums (On the Unsaponifiable Components of Lactucarium)." *Archiv der Pharmazie* 225, no. 9 (1887): 441–7.

Khalil, A. T., H. Abd El-fattah, and E. S. Mansour. "Guaianolides from *Lactuca saligna*." *Planta Medica* 57 (1991): 190–1.

Kim, K. H., K. H. Lee, S. U. Choi, Y. H. Kim, and K. R. Lee. "Terpene and Phenolic Constituents of *Lactuca indica* L." *Archives of Pharmacal Research* 31 (2008): 983–8.

Kim, K. H., Y. H. Kim, and K. R. Lee. "Isolation of Quinic Acid Derivatives and Flavonoids from the Aerial Parts of *Lactuca indica* L. and Their Hepatoprotective Activity in *vitro*." *Bioorganic & Medicinal Chemistry Letters* 17 (2007): 6739–43.

Kim, M. J., Y. Moon, J. C. Tou, B. Mou, and N. L. Waterland. "Nutritional Value, Bioactive Compounds and Health Benefits of Lettuce (*Lactuca sativa* L.)." *Journal of Food Composition and Analysis* 49 (2016): 19–34.

Kisiel, W. "Flavonoids from *Lactuca quercina* and *L. tatarica*." *Acta societatis botanicorum Poloniae* 67 (1998): 247.

Kisiel, W., and B. Barszcz. "A Germacrolide Glucoside from *Lactuca tatarica*." *Phytochemistry* 48 (1998): 205–6.

Kisiel, W., and B. Barszcz. "Minor Sesquiterpene Lactones from Lactuca virosa." *Phytochemistry* 46, no. 7 (1997): 1241–3.

Kisiel, W., and D. Gromek. "Sesquiterpene Lactones from Lactuca saligna." *Phytochemistry* 34, no. 6 (1993): 1644–6.

Kisiel, W., and K. Michalska. "Lignans and Sesquiterpenoids from *Lactuca sibirica*." *Fitoterapia* 79 (2008): 241–4.

Kisiel, W., and K. Zielińska. "Sesquiterpenoids and Phenolics from *Lactuca perennis*." *Fitoterapia* 71 (2000): 86–7.

Kisiel, W., B. Barszcz, and E. Szneler. "Sesquiterpene Lactones from *Lactuca tatarica*." *Phytochemistry* 45 (1997): 365–8.

Kisiel, W., A. Stojakowska, J. Malarz, and S. Kohlmüzer. "Sesquiterpene Lactones in Agrobacterium rhizogenes—Transformed Hairy Root Culture of *Lactuca virosa*." *Phytochemistry* 40, no. 4 (1995): 1139–40.

Konstantopoulou, E., G. Kapotis, G. Salachas, S. A. Petropoulos, I. C. Karapanos, and H. C. Passam. "Nutritional Quality of Greenhouse Lettuce at Harvest and after Storage in Relation to N Application and Cultivation Season." *Scientia Horticulturae* 125 (2010): 93.e1–93.e5.

Koopman, W. J. M. "Zooming in on the Lettuce Genome: Species Relationships in Lactuca sl, Inferred from Chromosomal and Molecular Characters." Ph.D. diss., Wageningen University and Research, 2002.

Koudela, M., and K. Petříková. "Nutrients Content and Yield in Selected Cultivars of Leaf Lettuce (*Lactuca sativa* L. var. crispa)." *Horticultural Science* 35 (2008): 99–106.

Kpodar, M. S., S. D. Karou, G. Katawa, K. Anani, H. E. Gbekley, Y. Adjrah, T. Tchacondo, K. Batawila, and J. Simpore. "An Ethnobotanical Study of Plants Used to Treat Liver Diseases in the Maritime Region of Togo." *Journal of Ethnopharmacology* 181 (2016): 263–73.

Křístková, E., I. Doležalová, A. Lebeda, V. Vinter, and A. Novotná. "Description of Morphological Characters of Lettuce (*Lactuca sativa* L.) Genetic Resources." *Horticultural Science* 35 (2008): 113–29.

Lans, C. "Do Recent Research Studies Validate the Medicinal Plants Used in British Columbia, Canada for Pet Diseases and Wild Animals Taken Into Temporary Care?" *Journal of Ethnopharmacology* 236 (2019): 366–92.

Lebeda, A., I. Dolezalová, V. Feráková, and D. Astley. "Geographical Distribution of wild Lactuca Species (Asteraceae, Lactuceae)." *The Botanical Review* 70 (2004): 328–56.

Lebeda, A., I. Doležalová, E. Křístková, M. Kitner, I. Petrželová, B. Mieslerová, and A. Novotná. "Wild Lactuca Germplasm for Lettuce Breeding: Current Status, Gaps and Challenges." *Euphytica* 170 (2009).

Lebeda, A., E. Křístková, I. Doležalová, M. Kitner, and M. P. Widrlechner. "Wild Lactuca Species in North America." *North American Crop Wild Relatives Volume 2: Important Species* (2019): 131–94.

Lee, J. H., P. Felipe, Y. H. Yang, M. Y. Kim, O. Y. Kwon, D.-E. Sok, H. C. Kim, and M. R. Kim. "Effects of Dietary Supplementation with Red-pigmented Leafy Lettuce (*Lactuca sativa*) on Lipid Profiles and Antioxidant Status in C57BL/6J Mice Fed a High-fat High-cholesterol Diet." *British Journal of Nutrition* 101 (2009): 1246–54.

Lee, J.-S., and D. Chandra. "Effects of Different Packaging Materials and Methods on the Physical, Biochemical and Sensory Qualities of Lettuce." *Journal of Food Science and Technology* 55 (2018): 1685–94.

Li, Z., X. Zhao, A. K. Sandhu, and L. Gu. "Effects of Exogenous Abscisic Acid on Yield, Antioxidant Capacities, and Phytochemical Contents of Greenhouse Grown Lettuces." *Journal of Agricultural and Food Chemistry* 58 (2010): 6503–9.

Liu, X., S. Ardo, M. Bunning, J. Parry, K. Zhou, C. Stushnoff, F. Stoniker, L. Yu, and P. Kendall. "Total Phenolic Content and DPPH Radical Scavenging Activity of Lettuce (*Lactuca sativa* L.) Grown in Colorado." *LWT-Food Science and Technology* 40 (2007): 552–7.

Llorach, R., A. Martínez-Sánchez, F. A. Tomás-Barberán, M. I. Gil, and F. Ferreres. "Characterisation of Polyphenols and Antioxidant Properties of Five Lettuce Varieties and Escarole." *Food Chemistry* 108 (2008): 1028–38.

López, A., G.-A. Javier, J. Fenoll, P. Hellín, and P. Flores. "Chemical Composition and Antioxidant Capacity of Lettuce: Comparative Study of Regular-sized (Romaine) and Baby-sized (Little Gem and Mini Romaine) Types." *Journal of Food Composition and Analysis* 33 (2014): 39–48.

López-Gálvez, F., A. Allende, P. Truchado, A. Martínez-Sánchez, J. A. Tudela, M. V. Selma, and M. I. Gil. "Suitability of Aqueous Chlorine Dioxide versus Sodium Hypochlorite as an Effective Sanitizer for Preserving Quality of Fresh-Cut Lettuce While Avoiding by-Product Formation." *Postharvest Biology and Technology* 55 (2010): 53–60.

López-Gálvez, G., M. Saltveit, and M. Cantwell. "Wound-Induced Phenylalanine Ammonia Lyase Activity: Factors Affecting Its Induction and Correlation with the Quality of Minimally Processed Lettuces." *Postharvest Biology and Technology* 9 (1996): 223–33.

Luna, M. C., J. A. Tudela, A. Martínez-Sánchez, A. Allende, A. Marín, and M. I. Gil. "Long-Term Deficit and Excess of Irrigation Influences Quality and Browning Related Enzymes and Phenolic Metabolism of Fresh-Cut Iceberg Lettuce (*Lactuca sativa* L.)." *Postharvest Biology and Technology* 73 (2012): 37–45.

Lüthje, P., D. N. Dzung, and A. Brauner. "Lactuca Indica Extract Interferes with Uroepithelial Infection by *Escherichia coli*." *Journal of Ethnopharmacology* 135 (2011): 672–7.

Mai, F., and M. A. Glomb. "Isolation of Phenolic Compounds from Iceberg Lettuce and Impact on Enzymatic Browning." *Journal of Agricultural and Food Chemistry* 61 (2013): 2868–74.

Mai, F., and M. A. Glomb. "Lettucenin Sesquiterpenes Contribute Significantly to the Browning of Lettuce." *Journal of Agricultural and Food Chemistry* 62 (2014): 4747–53.

Malejane, D. N., P. Tinyani, P. Soundy, Y. Sultanbawa, and D. Sivakumar. "Deficit Irrigation Improves Phenolic Content and Antioxidant Activity in Leafy Lettuce Varieties." *Food Science & Nutrition* 6 (2017): 334–41.

Mañez, S., M. C. Recio, R. M. Giner, M. J. Sanz, M. C. Terencio, J. B. Peris, G. Stübing, and J.-L. Rios. "A Chematoxonomic Review of the Subtribe Crepidinase Based on Its Phenol Constituents." *Biochemical Systematics and Ecology* 22 (1994): 297–305.

Martín-Diana, A. B., D. Rico, and C. Barry-Ryan. "Green Tea Extract as a Natural Antioxidant to Extend the Shelf-Life of Fresh-Cut Lettuce." *Innovative Food Science & Emerging Technologies* 9 (2008): 593–603.

Martínez, J. A., and F. Artés. "Effect of Packaging Treatments and Vacuum-Cooling on Quality of Winter Harvested Iceberg Lettuce." *Food Research International* 32 (1999): 621–27.

McKeehen, J. D., D. J. Smart, C. L. Mackowiak, R. M. Wheeler, and S. S. Nielsen. "Effect of CO2 Levels on Nutrient Content of Lettuce and Radish." *Advances in Space Research* 18 (1996): 85–92.

Michalska, K., A. Beharav, and W. Kisiel. “Sesquiterpene Lactones from Roots of *Lactuca georgica*.” *Phytochemistry Letters* 10 (2014): 10–12.

Michalska, K., and W. Kisiel. “Chemical Constituents from *Lactuca inermis*, a Wild African Species.” *Biochemical Systematics and Ecology* 55 (2014): 104–6.

Michalska, K., and W. Kisiel. “Root Constituents of *Lactuca sibirica* and a Comparison of Metabolite Profiles of *L. sibirica* and *L. tatarica*.” *Acta Societatis Botanicorum Poloniae* 78 (2009): 25–7.

Michalska, K., and W. Kisiel. “Sesquiterpene Lactones from Roots of *Lactuca aculeata*.” *Biochemical Systematics and Ecology* 38 (2010): 830–2.

Michalska, K., and W. Kisiel. “Structural Diversity of Sesquiterpene Lactones in Roots of *Lactuca viminea*.” *Biochemical Systematics and Ecology* 51 (2013): 16–18.

Michalska, K., W. Kisiel, and A. Stojakowska. “Chemical Constituents of *Lactuca dregeana*.” *Biochemical Systematics and Ecology* 2015, no. 59 (2015): 302–4.

Michalska, K., O. Michalski, and A. Stojakowska. “Sesquiterpenoids from Roots of *Lactuca sativa* var. *angustana* cv. “Grüner Stern.”” *Phytochemistry Letters* 20 (2017): 425–8.

Michalska, K., A. Stojakowska, and W. Kisiel. “Phenolic constituents of *Lactuca tenerrima*.” *Biochemical Systematics and Ecology* 42 (2012): 32–4.

Michalska, K., A. Stojakowska, J. Malarz, I. Doležalová, A. Lebeda, and W. Kisiel. “Systematic Implications of Sesquiterpene Lactones in *Lactuca* Species.” *Biochemical Systematics and Ecology* 37, no. 3 (2009): 174–9.

Michalska, K., E. Szneler, and W. Kisiel. “*Lactuca altaica* as a Rich Source of Sesquiterpene Lactones.” *Biochemical Systematics and Ecology* 38 (2010): 1246–9.

Michalska, K., E. Szneler, and W. Kisiel. “Sesquiterpene Lactones from *Lactuca canadensis* and Their Chemotaxonomic Significance.” *Phytochemistry* 90 (2013): 90–4.

Michalska, K., M. Żylewski, and W. Kisiel. “Structure Elucidation and Complete NMR Spectral Assignments of Two New Sesquiterpene Lactone Xylosides from *Lactuca triangulata*.” *Magnetic Resonance in Chemistry* 46, no. 12 (2008): 1185–7.

Morshedi, A., M. H. Dashti-Rahmatabadi, and A. Rafati. “A Comparison Between the Analgesic Effect of Ethanolic Extract of *Lactuca sativa* Seeds and Morphine Sulphate in Mice.” *European Journal of Pain* 10 (2006): S64c–S64.

Motti, R., and P. Motti. “An Ethnobotanical Survey of Useful Plants in the Agro Nocerino Sarnese (Campania, Southern Italy).” *Human Ecology* 45 (2017): 865–78.

Mou, B. “Genetic Variation of Beta-carotene and Lutein Contents in Lettuce.” *American Society for Horticultural Science* 130, no. 6 (2005): 870–6.

Mou, B. “Nutritional Quality of Lettuce.” *Current Nutrition & Food Science* 8 (2012): 177–87.

Mou, B., and E. J. Ryder. “Relationship between the Nutritional Value and the Head Structure of Lettuce.” In *XXVI International Horticultural Congress: Advances in Vegetable Breeding 637* (2004): 361–7.

Myszka, K., M. T. Schmidt, M. Majcher, W. Juzwa, and K. Czaczyk. “β-Caryophyllene-Rich Pepper Essential Oils Suppress Spoilage Activity of Pseudomonas Fluorescens KM06 in Fresh-Cut Lettuce.” *LWT - Food Science and Technology* 83 (2017): 118–26.

Neocleous, D., A. Koukounaras, A. S. Siomos, and M. Vasilakakis. “Assessing the Salinity Effects on Mineral Composition and Nutritional Quality of Green and Red “Baby” Lettuce.” *Journal of Food Quality* 37 (2014): 1–8.

Nicolle, C., N. Cardinault, E. Gueux, L. Jaffrelo, E. Rock, A. Mazur, P. Amouroux, and C. Rémésy. “Health Effect of Vegetable-based Diet: Lettuce Consumption Improves

Cholesterol Metabolism and Antioxidant Status in the Rat." *Clinical Nutrition* 23 (2004): 605–14.

Nishimura, K., T. Miyase, A. Ueno, T. Noro, M. Kuroyanagi, and S. Fukushima. "Sesquiterpene Lactones from *Lactuca laciniata*." *Phytochemistry* 25 (1986): 2375–9.

Ordidge, M., P. García-Macías, N. H. Battey, M. H. Gordon, P. Hadley, P. John, J. A. Lovegrove, E. Vysini, and A. Wagstaffe. "Phenolic Contents of Lettuce, Strawberry, Raspberry, and Blueberry Crops Cultivated under Plastic Films Varying in Ultraviolet Transparency." *Food Chemistry* 119 (2010): 1224–7.

Pepe, G., E. Sommella, M. Manfra, M. De Nisco, G. C. Tenore, A. Scopa, A. Sofo, et al. "Evaluation of Anti-inflammatory Activity and Fast UHPLC–DAD–IT-TOF Profiling of Polyphenolic Compounds Extracted from Green Lettuce (*Lactuca sativa* L.; Var. Maravilla De Verano)." *Food Chemistry* 167 (2014): 153–61.

Pérez-López, U., J. Miranda-Apodaca, A. Muñoz-Rueda, and A. Mena-Petite. "Lettuce Production and Antioxidant Capacity Are Differentially Modified by Salt Stress and Light Intensity under Ambient and Elevated CO_2." *Journal of Plant Physiology* 170 (2013): 1517–25.

Pinto, E., A. A. Almeida, A. ARM Aguiar, and I. MPLVO Ferreira. "Changes in Macrominerals, Trace Elements and Pigments Content during Lettuce (*Lactuca sativa* L.) Growth: Influence of Soil Composition." *Food Chemistry* 152 (2014): 603–11.

Pomeranz, C., and F. Sperling. "Ueber Lactucerylacetat (On the Lactucon)." *Monatshefte für Chemie und verwandte Teile anderer Wissenschaften* 25, no. 2 (1904): 785–92.

Postu, P. A., J. A. K. Noumedem, O. Cioanca, M. Hancianu, M. Mihasan, M. Ciorpac, D. L. Gorgan, B. A. Petre, and L. Hritcu. "*Lactuca capensis* Reverses Memory Deficits in Aβ1-42-induced an Animal Model of Alzheimer's Disease." *Journal of Cellular and Molecular Medicine* 22 (2017): 111–22.

Pour, Z. S., A. Hosseinkhani, N. Asadi, H. R. Shahraki, H. Vafaei, M. Kasraeian, K. Bazrafshan, and A. Faraji. "Double-blind Randomized Placebo-controlled Trial on Efficacy and Safety of *Lactuca sativa* L. Seeds on Pregnancy-related Insomnia." *Journal of Ethnopharmacology* 227 (2018): 176–80.

Qin, X.-X., M.-Y. Zhang, Y.-Y. Han, J.-H. Hao, C.-J. Liu, and S.-X. Fan. "Beneficial Phytochemicals With Anti-Tumor Potential Revealed Through Metabolic Profiling of New Red Pigmented Lettuces (*Lactuca sativa* L.)." *International Journal of Molecular Sciences* 19 (2018): 1165.

Quartacci, M. F., C. Sgherri, and S. Frisenda. "Biochar Amendment Affects Phenolic Composition and Antioxidant Capacity Restoring the Nutraceutical Value of Lettuce Grown in a Copper-Contaminated Soil." *Scientia Horticulturae* 215 (2017): 9–14.

Radhakrishnan, R., and I.-J. Lee. "Gibberellins Producing Bacillus Methylotrophicus KE2 Supports Plant Growth and Enhances Nutritional Metabolites and Food Values of Lettuce." *Plant Physiology and Biochemistry* 109 (2016): 181–9.

Rajičić, T. S., T. van Hintum, A. Lebeda, and K. J. Dehmer. "Analysis of Wild Lactuca Accessions: Conservation and Identification of Redundancy." *Plant Genetic Resources* 6 (2008): 153–63.

Rätsch, C. *The Encyclopedia of Psychoactive Plants: Ethnopharmacology and Its Applications*. Simon and Schuster, 2005.

Rees, S., and J. Harborne. "Flavonoids and Other Phenolics of Cichorium and Related Members of the Lactuceae (Compositae)." *Botanical Journal of the Linnean Society* 89 (1984): 313–19.

Ribas-Agustí, A., M. Gratacós-Cubarsí, C. Sárraga, J.-A. García-Regueiro, and M. Castellari. "Analysis of Eleven Phenolic Compounds Including Novel P-coumaroyl Derivatives in Lettuce (*Lactuca sativa* L.) by Ultra-high-performance Liquid Chromatography with Photodiode Array and Mass Spectrometry Detection." *Phytochemical Analysis* 22, no. 6 (2011): 555–63.

Ribeiro, R. V., I. G. C. Bieski, S. O. Balogun, and D. T. de Oliveira Martins. "Ethnobotanical Study of Medicinal Plants Used by Ribeirinhos in the North Araguaia Microregion, Mato Grosso, Brazil." *Journal of Ethnopharmacology* 205 (2017): 69–102.

Romani, A., P. Pinelli, C. Galardi, G. Sani, A. Cimato, and D. Heimler. "Polyphenols in Greenhouse and Open-air-grown Lettuce." *Food Chemistry* 79 (2002): 337–42.

Samuolienė, G., R. Sirtautas, A. Brazaitytė, and P. Duchovskis. "LED Lighting and Seasonality Effects Antioxidant Properties of Baby Leaf Lettuce." *Food Chemistry* 134 (2012): 1494–9.

Santos, J., M. T. Oliva-Teles, C. Delerue-Matos, and M. B. P. P. Oliveira. "Multi-elemental Analysis of Ready-to-eat "Baby Leaf" Vegetables Using Microwave Digestion and High-resolution Continuum Source Atomic Absorption Spectrometry." *Food Chemistry* 151 (2014): 311–16.

Sayyah, M., N. Hadidi, and M. Kamalinejad. "Analgesic and Anti-inflammatory Activity of *Lactuca sativa* Seed Extract in Rats." *Journal of Ethnopharmacology* 92 (2004): 325–9.

Serafini, M., R. Bugianesi, M. Salucci, E. Azzini, A. Raguzzini, and G. Maiani. "Effect of Acute Ingestion of Fresh and Stored Lettuce (*Lactuca sativa*) on Plasma Total Antioxidant Capacity and Antioxidant Levels in Human Subjects." *British Journal of Nutrition* 88 (2002): 615–23.

Serna, M., F. Hernández, F. Coll, and A. Amorós. "Brassinosteroid Analogues Effect on Yield and Quality Parameters of Field-Grown Lettuce (*Lactuca sativa* L.)." *Scientia Horticulturae* 143 (2012): 29–37.

Sessa, R. A., M. H. Bennett, M. J. Lewis, J. W. Mansfield, and M. H. Beale. "Metabolite Profiling of Sesquiterpene Lactones from *Lactuca* Species: Major Latex Components Are Novel Oxalate and Sulfate Conjugates of Lactucin and Its Derivatives." *Journal of Biological Chemistry* 275 (2000): 26877–84.

Shalaby, T., Y. Bayoumi, T. Alshaal, N. Elhawat, A. Sztrik, and H. El-Ramady. "Selenium Fortification Induces Growth, Antioxidant Activity, Yield and Nutritional Quality of Lettuce in Salt-Affected Soil Using Foliar and Soil Applications." *Plant and Soil* 421 (2017): 245–58.

Shinozaki, J., T. Nakane, N. Onodera, A. Takano, and K. Masuda. "Composite Constituent: Lactucenyl Acetate, a Novel Migrated Lupane Triterpenoid from *Lactuca indica* Revision of Structure of Tarolupenyl Acetate." *Chemical and Pharmaceutical Bulletin* 59 (2011): 767–9.

Simpson, J. C. E. "The Triterpene Group. Part XI. Triterpenes from Lactuca virosa." *Journal of the Chemical Society* (1944): 283–5.

Singh, B., P. Sultan, Q. P. Hassan, S. Gairola, and Y. S. Bedi. "Ethnobotany, Traditional Knowledge, and Diversity of Wild Edible Plants and Fungi: A Case Study in the Bandipora District of Kashmir Himalaya, India." *Journal of Herbs Spices & Medicinal Plants* 22 (2016): 247–78.

Song, Q., M. L. Gomez-Barrios, E. L. Hopper, M. A. Hjortso, and N. H. Fischer. "Biosynthetic Studies of Lactucin Derivatives in Hairy Root Cultures of *Lactuca floridana*." *Phytochemistry* 40 (1995): 1659–65.

Stojakowska, A., and J. Malarz. "Bioactive Phenolics from In Vitro Cultures of *Lactuca aculeata* Boiss. et Kotschy." *Phytochemistry Letters* 19 (2017): 7–11.
Stojakowska, A., K. Michalska, N. Kłeczek, J. Malarz, and A. Beharav. "Phenolics and Terpenoids from a Wild Edible Plant *Lactuca orientalis* (Boiss.) Boiss.: A Preliminary Study." *Journal of Food Composition and Analysis* 69 (2018): 20–4.
Stojakowska, A., K. Michalska, J. Malarz, A. Beharav, and W. Kisiel. "Root Tubers of *Lactuca tuberosa* as a Source of Antioxidant Phenolic Compounds and New Furofuran Lignans." *Food Chemistry* 138 (2013): 1250–5.
Takasugi, M., S. Kawashima, T. L. Graham, T. Shimada, H. Takazawa, T. Masamune, and N. Katsui. "Isolation and Structure of Lettucenin A, a Novel Guaianolide Phytoalexin from Lactuca sativa var. capitata (Compositae)." *Journal of the Chemical Society, Chemical Communications* 10 (1985): 621–2.
Terencio, M. C., M. J. Sanz, M. L. Fonseca, S. Máñez, and J. L. Ríos. "Phenolic Compounds from Lactuca viminea L." *Zeitschrift für Naturforschung C* 47 (1992): 17–20.
Touloun, O. *Les peuplements de scorpions du sud ouest marocain: écologie, biogéographie et épidémiologie des envenimations*. Editions universitaires europeennes, 2012.
Tsioutsiou, E. E., P. Giordani, E. Hanlidou, M. Biagi, V. De Feo, and L. Cornara. "Ethnobotanical Study of Medicinal Plants Used in Central Macedonia, Greece." *Evidence-Based Complementary and Alternative Medicine* 2019 (2019): 1–22.
Varga, F., I. Šolić, M. J. Dujaković, Ł. Łuczaj, and M. Grdiša. "The First Contribution to the Ethnobotany of Inland Dalmatia: Medicinal and Wild Food Plants of the Knin Area, Croatia." *Acta Societatis Botanicorum Poloniae* 88 (2019).
Varoquaux, P., J. Mazollier, and G. Albagnac. "The Influence of Raw Material Characteristics on the Storage Life of Fresh-Cut Butterhead Lettuce." *Postharvest Biology and Technology* 9 (1996): 127–39.
Viacava, G. E., and S. I. Roura. "Principal Component and Hierarchical Cluster Analysis to Select Natural Elicitors for Enhancing Phytochemical Content and Antioxidant Activity of Lettuce Sprouts." *Scientia Horticulturae* 193 (2015): 13–21.
Viacava, G. E., S. I. Roura, L. A. Berrueta, C. Iriondo, B. Gallo, and R. M. Alonso-Salces. "Characterization of Phenolic Compounds in Green and Red Oak-leaf Lettuce Cultivars by UHPLC-DAD-ESI-QToF/MS Using MSE Scan Mode." *Journal of Mass Spectrometry* 52 (2017): 873–902.
Viacava, G. E., S. I. Roura, D. M. López-Márquez, L. A. Berrueta, B. Gallo, and R. M. Alonso-Salces. "Polyphenolic Profile of Butterhead Lettuce Cultivar by Ultrahigh Performance Liquid Chromatography Coupled Online to UV–visible Spectrophotometry and Quadrupole Time-of-flight Mass Spectrometry." *Food Chemistry* 260 (2018): 239–73.
Wang, S.-Y., H.-N. Chang, K.-T. Lin, C.-P. Lo, N.-S. Yang, and L.-F. Shyur. "Antioxidant Properties and Phytochemical Characteristics of Extracts from *Lactuca indica*." *Journal of Agricultural and Food Chemistry* 51 (2003): 1506–12.
Wang, X.-X., X. Gao, and Z.-J. Jia. "Sesquiterpenoids from *Lactuca tatarica*." *Fitoterapia* 81 (2010): 42–4.
Wei, Z., S.-X. Zhu, R. G. Van den Berg, F. T. Bakker, and M. E. Schranz. "Phylogenetic Relationships within Lactuca L. (Asteraceae), Including African Species, Based on Chloroplast DNA Sequence Comparisons." *Genetic Resources and Crop Evolution* 64 (2017): 55–71.

Wieczyńska, J., and I. Cavoski. "Antimicrobial, Antioxidant and Sensory Features of Eugenol, Carvacrol and Trans-Anethole in Active Packaging for Organic Ready-to-Eat Iceberg Lettuce." *Food Chemistry* 259 (2018): 251–60.

Wießner, S., B. Thiel, J. Krämer, and U. Köpke. "Hygienic Quality of Head Lettuce: Effects of Organic and Mineral Fertilizers." *Food Control* 20 (2009): 881–6.

Witkowska, I. M., and E. J. Woltering. "Storage of Intact Heads Prior to Processing Limits the Shelf-Life of Fresh-Cut Lactuca Sativa L." *Postharvest Biology and Technology* 91 (2014): 25–31.

Yadava, R. N., and J. Jharbade. "New Antibacterial Triterpenoid Saponin from Lactuca scariola." *Fitoterapia* 79 (2008): 245–9.

Yadava, R. N., and J. Jharbade. "A New Bioactive Triterpenoid Saponin from the Seeds of *Lactuca scariola* Linn." *Natural Product Research* 21 (2007): 500–6.

Yang, X., X. Cui, L. Zhao, D. Guo, L. Feng, S. Wei, C. Zhao, and D. Huang. "Exogenous Glycine Nitrogen Enhances Accumulation of Glycosylated Flavonoids and Antioxidant Activity in Lettuce (*Lactuca sativa* L.)." *Frontiers in Plant Science* 8 (2017).

Zdravković, J., N. Pavlović, R. Pavlović, P. Mašković, J. Mladenović, M. Đurić, and G. Aćamović-Đoković. "Antimicrobial Activity of Lettuce (*Lactuca sativa* L.) Extract Grown in Plastic and Glasshouses." *Acta Horticulturae* 960 (2012): 299–303.

Zhao, L., Y. Huang, C. Hannah-Bick, A. N. Fulton, and A. A. Keller. "Application of Metabolomics to Assess the Impact of Cu(OH)2 Nanopesticide on the Nutritional Value of Lettuce (Lactuca Sativa): Enhanced Cu Intake and Reduced Antioxidants." *NanoImpact* 3–4 (2016): 58–66.

Złotek, U., and M. Świeca. "Elicitation Effect of Saccharomyces Cerevisiae Yeast Extract on Main Health-promoting Compounds and Antioxidant and Anti-inflammatory Potential of Butter Lettuce (*Lactuca sativa* L.)." *Journal of the Science of Food and Agriculture* 96 (2016): 2565–72.

Złotek, U., M. Świeca, and A. Jakubczyk. "Effect of Abiotic Elicitation on Main Health-Promoting Compounds, Antioxidant Activity and Commercial Quality of Butter Lettuce (*Lactuca sativa* L.)." *Food Chemistry* 148 (2014): 253–60.

Zohary, D. "The Wild Genetic Resources of Cultivated Lettuce (*Lactuca sativa* L.)." *Euphytica* 53 (1991): 31–5.

Part IV

Indigenous Communities

Concept of Health, Illness, Beliefs, and Practices

14

Indigenous Medicines and Rituals

The Traditional Indian Medicine System

Shruti Chattaraj*

Department of Botany, Ananda Mohan College, Kolkata, West Bengal, India

*Corresponding Author's Email: shrutichattaraj@gmail.com

Introduction

Indigenous medicines or the traditional medicine system has a very long history. For human beings, health and illness have always been a primary concern. To treat or address different types of illness and to maintain good health and well-being, people across different countries have turned to traditional healers, home remedies, different rituals, and ancient medicinal knowledge for centuries. The aim of every medicine system is to meet the health care needs. Indigenous medicine combines the medical aspects of traditional knowledge derived over generations with the spiritual teachings and various rituals of indigenous peoples which strengthen the spiritual well-being as well as helps in balancing the patient's physical, mental, emotional, and spiritual health and well-being (Liu et al. 2005). Every developing country and many societies have two different treatment or medicine systems that are totally different and are not integrated. The first one is the modern treatment system, that is, Western-style medicine, which includes vaccination, medication, advanced medical technology, and diagnosis. The second medicine system, developed before the era of modern medicine, is a nonformal system called Indigenous medicine, also known as traditional medicine or alternative medicine system, which relies on the knowledge of different herbs, the medicinal value of plants and mineral-based medicines, spiritual therapies, manual techniques, and exercises, applied singularly or in combination to treat, diagnose, and prevent illnesses or maintain well-being (Fokunang et al. 2011).

During the course of the development of indigenous medicine, different civilizations have arisen and persisted, but the medicine systems developed by these ancient indigenous people in various parts of the world are still believed in and practiced. In most Asian and African countries, indigenous people developed their own medicine systems, and most of the population in these countries relies on their traditional medicine systems for primary healthcare treatments and needs. Among the most popular indigenous medicine systems, few include traditional Chinese medicine, traditional European medicine, traditional African medicine, traditional Korean medicine, traditional Iranian medicine, traditional Japanese medicine, traditional Brazilian medicine, traditional Mongolian medicine, traditional Cambodian medicine, traditional Indian medicine systems, and many more (Matsuomoto, Inoue, and Kajii 1999; Patwardhan et al. 2005; Park et al. 2012). Although there might be huge differences in the basic principles and philosophy of these traditional medicine systems, it cannot be denied that they have served humanity for centuries in the management and treatment of illnesses and diseases. Compared to modern or Western medicine systems, indigenous medicines are cheaper and are much more preferred for being safe and lacking side effects as they depend on drugs of natural origin (Kamboj 2000).

Objectives and Methods

India has a long history of medicine. In other words, India is also a leader in modern medicine, offering a wide range of advanced medical procedures. It has expertise in areas ranging from cardiac and orthopedic surgeries to dental and eye procedures, along with organ transplants. These diverse medical offerings cater to varied healthcare needs. On the other hand, the oldest and most widely used medicine system in traditional Indian medicine is Ayurveda. Ayurveda emphasizes holistic medicine, which takes the body, mind, and spirit as a whole. It is also based on the idea that the body and mind are closely connected, and that an imbalance in one area can affect another. Ayurveda is a Sanskrit term that means "science of life." It originated in India more than 3,000 years ago. It's considered by many scholars to be the oldest healing science. In this present study, an overview of the Ayurveda's diagnosis method, various techniques, therapies, drugs and rituals used for the treatment of the individuals are discussed for providing the preliminary idea and understanding of Indigenous medicine system and various rituals of Indian Ayurveda.

Indigenous Medicines and Rituals

For centuries, indigenous and traditional medicine has been an integral resource for healthcare needs in society and communities. On the other hand, the World Health Organization (WHO) recognizes the value and diversity of the cultures of indigenous peoples and local communities, along with their traditional knowledge. The cultures of traditional medicine are still used today. It is based on knowledge, beliefs, and practices that are unique to different cultures. Traditional medicine has contributed to modern medicine in many ways, such as providing the basis for many pharmaceutical products, including aspirin and artemisinin; helping to develop effective treatments for health conditions; and providing a source of culturally acceptable care. The WHO is working to integrate traditional medicine into national health systems. The WHO has a Global Traditional Medicine Centre that aims to provide evidence and data to support the safe and equitable use of traditional medicine.

Thus, over time, indigenous people in various parts of the world developed their own medicine system and traditional healing practices which use herbal medicines, yoga, acupuncture, indigenous therapies, and other forms of traditional medicines (Singh and Rastogi 2018). Along with this, they believe in different healing powers and follow different rituals for the treatment of certain illnesses. The indigenous medicine systems are based on different principles and theories; for example, traditional Chinese medicine (TCM), one of the oldest and most popular medicine systems, aims to restore or maintain yin and yang balance to prevent or heal disease. Yin and yang are opposing energies like happiness and sadness, heat and cold, earth and heaven, and they believe that when yin and yang are balanced, everyone feels energized and relaxed, but when it is imbalanced, it affects health.

TCM practitioners also believe that along with yin and yang, qi (life force or energy) must be balanced and freely flowing in every body for a healthy body (Che et al. 2024). Most commonly used healing practices in TCM are acupuncture, medicinal herbs, Qi gong, diet, and massage (Sivin 1987). Chinese herbal mixtures have been used to treat many disorders, including irritable bowel syndrome and Tourette syndrome (Zhang et al. 2019). African traditional medicine (TAM) is another holistic health care system that relies on principles that are divided into three levels, namely divination, spiritualism, and herbalism (Ozioma and Chinwe 2019). The TAM healing practice is based on the concepts of divination, animal sacrifice, incarnations, culture, knowledge, attitudes, religious background, exorcism, herbs, and their community beliefs to cure various diseases (Chaitanya et al. 2022). Some common traditional healing methods practiced in various indigenous medicine systems are discussed in Table 14.1.

Indigenous Medicine System of India

Indigenous medicine of India is one of the oldest healing practices in the world. It believes that a harmonious coexistence or balanced relationship with nature results in physical, mental, and emotional well-being (Liu et al. 2005). The traditional Indian medicine, commonly known as the AYUSH system of medicine, is divided into six different recognized branches, namely Ayurveda, Yoga, Unani, Siddha, Naturopathy, and Homeopathy. Although all these six indigenous medicine systems are not of Indian origin, all of them assimilated into Indian culture through the amalgamation of influences from other civilizations, be it Greece or Germany or our own scriptures. Ayurveda is called the science of life; it is an age-old medicine system that originated and developed in India between 2500 and 500 BC (Jaiswal and Williams 2016). The Siddha system of medicine, which is one of the ancient medicine systems, originated from

Table 14.1. List of Some Common Healing Techniques and Rituals in Traditional Medicine

Traditional Medicine	Healing Techniques	Used for Treatment
Traditional Chinese medicine	**Acupuncture:** A thin needle is inserted through the skin to stimulate specific acupoints on the body.	Pain, nausea and vomiting, headaches, respiratory disorders, tennis elbow, dental pain, osteoarthritis (Che et al. 2024)
	Tai Chi: Tai chi is a type of gentle and slow exercise that includes body movement and focused breath work. It has been described as "meditation in motion" and "medication in motion."	Osteoarthritis, helps increase flexibility and strength, improves cardiovascular fitness, promotes weight loss, and provides aerobic benefits (Che et al. 2024)
	Cupping: Also called cupping therapy, a practitioner uses warm cups or glass jars that create suction on the skin on certain body areas (usually the back, stomach, arms, and legs). Cupping pulls your skin into the jar, breaks open tiny blood vessels beneath the skin, and works by creating this setting for blood to flow to the area and stimulate the injury-healing process.	Helping with chronic pain, high blood pressure, and other ailments like breathing issues, carpal tunnel syndrome and skin issues (Che et al. 2024).
	Herbs: Herbs are prepared in capsule form, teas or extracts, and powders, in traditional or custom formulas.	Herbs are used to treat the whole person and their symptoms. Many herbs may help with hard-to-diagnose or -treat syndromes, including allergies, infertility, and menopause (Che et al. 2024).
	Moxibustion: It is performed by burning small cones of dried leaves on certain designated points of the body.	Helps in pain relief, improves digestion, and improves blood circulation (Zhang et al. 2019)
Traditional Japanese medicine system	**Shinrin-Yoku (Forest Bathing):** Process of therapeutic relaxation by encouraging individuals to immerse themselves in nature through mindful walk in the forest.	Reduces blood pressure by decreasing stress hormone level (Sreedhar, Watanabe, and Arumugam 2017).
	Ikebana (Flower Arranging): are of arranging flowers	Boosts mental state, regulate mood and physical well-being.
Traditional African medicine system	**Ngoma, umxhentso, intlombe:** is the ritual drumming and dancing with rhythms.	The rhythmic beats and movements are believed to induce trance-like states and alter consciousness, allowing people to connect with their inner selves and helps release emotional blockages.
	Kaiy (Cauterization): ancient medical therapy in which a red hot iron or coal is placed on the skin.	Relieves pain and stops bleeding, destroying pathogenic substances within the body (Haddabi and Williamson 2023).
Traditional Indian medicine system	**Rasashastra:** ancient tradition of healing that uses medicines incorporated with metals like gold and mercury.	Stops or slows the process of aging (Liu et al. 2005).

Dravidian culture in Tamil Nadu, South India. The term Siddha means achievements, and Siddhars are those who have achieved perfection in medicine. In ancient times, the "Siddhargal" or Siddhars were the foremost scholars of this system.

On the other hand, Unani medicine (Yünäné Nizäm-i Öibb or Öibb) originated in Greece (Yünän); it is also known as Greco-Egyptian medicine, as Greeks adopted medical knowledge from Egypt and Mesopotamian civilization. This was further adopted by Arabs and was developed, improved, and popularized by Arabic scholars like Ibn Sina (Avicenna). The theoretical framework of this system is based on the teachings of Hippocrates and Galen, later developed into an elaborate Medical System by Arabs. In the twelfth century, it arrived in India after the establishment of the Delhi Sultanate. Unani medicine is based on the concept of the four humors: Phlegm (Balgham), Blood (Dam), Yellow bile (Ṣafrā'), and Black bile (Saudā'). Thus, the Unani system of medicine emphasizes diagnosing a disease through Nabz (pulse), Baul (wine), Baraz (stool), and so on. Besides, it gives due importance to the surroundings and the ecological conditions on the state of health of humans.

Yet again, the word "Yoga" originated from "yuj," a Sanskrit word meaning "to unite or integrate." Yoga originated in the Indus-Sarasvati civilization in Northern India over 5,000 years ago, with scriptures present in the Rig Veda and Upanishads. It is primarily a way of life, first propounded by Maharshi Patanjali in systematic form in Yogsutra (Adhikari and Paul 2018). Naturopathy is rooted in the healing wisdom of many cultures and times based on the principle of natural healing. Naturopathy promotes healing by stimulating the body's inherent power to regain health with the help of the five elements of nature—Earth, Water, Air, Fire, and Ether. Homeopathy is a specialized system of therapeutics, developed by Dr. Samuel Christian Friedrich Hahnemann (1755–1843), a German physician. Homeopathy was brought by European missionaries into India around AD 1810 and is now an established indigenous system of medicine in India. It is based on the natural law of healing: *Similia Similibus Curantur*, which means "Likes are cured by, likes" (Loudon 2006).

Ayurveda: The Indian Medicine System

The word Ayurveda means *Ayur* meaning life and *Veda* meaning science, so Ayurveda means the science of life. Ayurved is accepted as one of the oldest documented comprehensive medical systems, nurtured between 2500 and 500 BC in India. According to Indian Hindu mythology, the different knowledge, thoughts, and legends in the Vedic era were documented by Aryans in four major collections: the *Rigveda*, *Samaveda*, *Yajurveda*, and *Atharvaveda* (Adhikari and Paul 2018). The Ayurveda is considered an *Upaveda* that is part of the *Atharvaveda*. The knowledge and concepts of Ayurveda were comprehensively recorded in Ayurvedic literature, *Charak Samhita* (1900 BC) and *Sushruta Samhita* (600 BC). *Charak Samhita*, written by Charak, contains the concept of the practice of Ayurveda and describes the medicinal value and uses of 341 plants and their products. The second Ayurvedic literature, *Sushruta*

Samhita, written by Sushruta, documented 395 medicinal plants, 57 animal origin drugs, and 4 minerals and metals used in therapeutic agents. It also gave special emphasis on surgery, describing eight surgical methods: resection, stab, incision, puncture, puncture and collaterals extraction, suturing, and bandaging (Singh 2017).

(a) **Ayurvedic Principles:** Ayurveda is based on the five element theory and the three humoralism theory. The five element theory says that everything in this universe that is all objects and living bodies are composed of basic five elements called Pancha Mahabhutas which include prithvi (earth), jala (water), Agni (fire), vayu (air), and akash (ether). Therefore, a fundamental harmony develops between the universe and the individuals. The pancha mahabhutas are present in the living individual as the doshas, dhatus, and malas. The three humoralism theory believes that the human body contains three humors or doshas called tridosha (Figure 14.1). Tridoshas are vata (gas), pitta (bile), and kapha (mucus), and the balance of these dosha determines the health or illness of the human body. The different body areas are predominated by the tridoshas: vata (ether + air) in the large intestine, pitta (fire) in digestive organs, and the chest for kapha (earth + water). The vata represents the movement and sensation felt in the body, which is the function of the autonomous and central nervous system. The functions of the endocrine gland, like digestion, tissue formation, blood pigmentation, and so on, are representative of pitta. The factors responsible for strengthening the stomach and the joints, providing firmness to the limbs, and refreshing the sense organs are the representatives of kapha. According to Ayurveda, the basic body structure contains Sapta Dhatus, namely *rasa* (chyle),

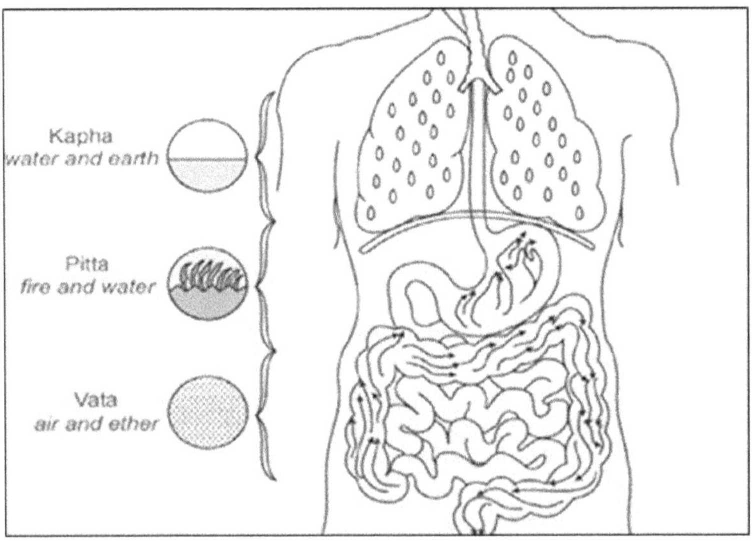

Figure 14.1. The three humors or tridosha of the human body. Source: Author.

rakta (blood), *mamsa* (muscle tissue/flesh), *medas* (fat tissue), *asthi* (bone tissue), *majja* (bone marrow), and *shukra* (semen); all of these are derived from food. All the saptadhatus, after the process of digestion, are partly used by the body and the remaining part is eliminated as excreta or waste product called malas. Malas are the waste products produced in the living body, and two main types of mala are listed in Ayurveda, that is Ahara mala and Dhatu mala. Ahara mala is the waste from food, which is again of three types purisha(feces mainly composed of earth), mutra (urine composed of jal and agni), and sveda (sweat consisting of jal). The dhatu mala are the waste products developed from cells and tissue, and it includes secretion from eyes, nose, ears, and elements like nails, hair, lactic acid, and carbon dioxide. A perfect balance and equilibrium in elements like doshas, dhatus, and malas ensures a healthy body. Any imbalance in dosha and dhatu elements of the body causes abnormality in quantity and quality of malas and results in an unhealthy and diseased body (Pandey, Rastogi, and Rawat 2013; Jaiswal and Williams 2016).

(b) **Diagnosis Method in Ayurvedic System:** In Indian society, the Ayurveda practitioners believe that disease develops when the balance between the doshas (bodily humors) and dhatus (tissues) is disturbed and is influenced by the environment. Ayurvedic diagnosis involves assessment of an individual's physical, mental, and emotional constitution. Diagnosis of illness in Ayurveda is called ashtasthana pariksha or eight-point diagnosis used for rogi pariksha. It includes Nadi pariksha (pulse), mutra pariksha (urine examination), mala pariksha (stool examination), jihva pariksha (tongue examination), sparsha pariksha (touch, skin, or tactile sense assessment), Druk pariksha (assessment of eyes and vision), akriti pariksha (general body build assessment), and shabda pariksha (examination of voice and speech of patient) (Deli and Li 2008).

(c) **Treatment in Ayurveda Medicine:** Ayurvedic treatment or therapy is administered as herbal concoctions and lifestyle changes that help in balancing the three principal energies of the body, the tridoshas that is vata, pitta, and kapha. Ayurvedic treatment includes eight specialties Kaya chikitsa (medicine), Shalya tantra (surgery), Salakya tantra (ENT treatment), Kaumarabhrtya (gynecology and pediatrics), Bhutavidya (Ayurvedic psychology), Agada Tantra (toxicology), Rasayana shastra(rejuvenation and anti-aging), and Vajikarana (eugenics and expediting). Ayurvedic treatment or therapy starts with shodhana, then shaman, and finally rasayana. Shodhana is the process of cleansing in which toxins, both emotional and physical, are removed or neutralized. After shodhana, shaman (palliative treatment) is done to restore the balance of doshas and reduce the disease intensity. Finally, health is maintained and negative effects of disease are reduced by rejuvenation therapy or rasayana. In Ayurvedic treatment, different therapies are used like drug therapy, psychotherapy, and surgical therapy (Shi, Zhang, and Li 2020). In drug therapy, drugs prepared from plants, animals, and minerals are used in single or compound form which stimulates the natural healing power of the body. In Indian herbal therapy, oil obtained from herbs is used to eliminate toxins from the body to regain the natural balance of the body. In psychotherapy, the three fundamental mental attributes or trigunas, Sattva (tendency toward selfless service), Rajas (tendency toward ambition), and Tamas (tendency toward lethargy) are maintained in harmony to keep the mind calm. In psychotherapy, music meditation, yoga with pranayama and meditation, concentration, sattvic diet, and self-study are used for the treatment and to bring a healthy body and harmonious interpersonal relationships. In Ayurveda, eight types of surgical methods were used: resection, incision, stab, puncture, extraction, puncture and collaterals, suturing, and bandaging (Singh 2017). In traditional Indian medicine, the herbal medicines, massage, and dietary interventions are mentioned. The primary ingredients of Ayurvedic drugs are plants, herbs, and different metals (e.g., gold, silver, copper, tin, iron, mercury, lead etc.), minerals, substances, organic matters, elements from earth (like arsenic, sand, lime, antimony), and marine drugs. Ayurveda mentioned many plants with healing and medicinal values and some of these plants are mentioned in Table 14.2.

Table 14.2. Some Common Medicinal Plants and Their Use in Traditional Medicine

Medicinal Plants	Common Name	Medicinal Properties/Uses
Achillea millefolium L.	Biranjasipha	Simulative and carminative are used to eliminate gas from intestine and stomach.
Argyreia speciosa Sweet	Vridha daraka, Elephant creeper	Leaves are used to treat skin diseases, roots help in controlling inflammation, anemia, diabetes, cerebral disorders, syphilis, and ulcer wounds. Plant also used as aphrodisiac, brain tonic, cardiotonic, expectorant, and appetizer.
Asparagus racemosus Wild	Shatavari, Wild asparagus	A potent Ayurvedic rejuvenative. It supplies many female hormones and is recommended for women having hysterectomies. It helps to maintain the urinary tract and strengthens the immune system and purifies the blood.
Capparis spinosa L.	Himsra, Capers	Hepatic stimulant used for improving the functional efficiency of the liver. Also used for treatment of rheumatism, hypertension, diabetes, dysentery.
Cichorium intybus Linn	Kasani, Wild Chicory	Hepatic stimulants help in increasing bile secretion, increase digestive power. Aqueous root extract used as a remedy for malaria.

Table 14.2 (Continued)

Medicinal Plants	Common Name	Medicinal Properties/Uses
Commiphora mukul Engl.	Guggul	A major ingredient in joint and immunocare and regarded as a remedy in Ayurvedic medicine; it increases white blood cell count to possess strong immune-modulating properties. It also protects against the common cold and is used in various other conditions, such as lowering cholesterol and triglycerides, while maintaining the HDL to LDL ratio.
Crocus sativus L.	Kumkuma, Saffron	In Ayurvedic therapies, it is used as a promoter of immune defense and a mild stimulant. Used in treating depression, Alzheimer's disease, menstrual cramps, cardiovascular ailments.
Cyperus scariosus Br.	Nagarmusta, Umbrella's edge	Anti-inflammatory, antimicrobial, hypotensive, stimulant of central nervous system, antidiabetic and analgesic.
Didymocarpus pedicellata	Shilapushpa	Diuretic effect used in Ayurvedic medicine for the treatment of renal diseases like kidney stone and bladder stone.
Garcinia cambogia Desr	Garcinia	Helps in improving cholesterol level by lowering triglycerides and LDL and raising HDL. Used as a heart tonic and contains a high amount of vitamin C.
Glycyrrhiza glabra L.	Yashti-madhu, Licorice	Digestive Disorders, Ulcers, Bronchitis, Skin health. It is rich in flavonoids and antioxidants.
Gymnema sylvestre R.Br.	Meshashringi, Gurmara	Antidiabetic as it increases insulin production by regenerating pancreas cells and the site of insulin production. It neutralizes the sweet craving by abolishing the taste of sugar.
Melia azadirachta L.	Persian lilac	Ayurvedic medicine for centuries due to its detoxifying properties, antispasmodic action. Tonic and astringent that promotes healing. Beneficial for digestive, respiratory, circulatory, and urinary systems.
Momordica charantia L.	Karela, Bitter melon	Widely used in Ayurvedic medicine for diabetic patients as it suppresses the neural response to sweet taste stimuli. Anti-inflammatory and anticancer properties.
Moringa pterygosperma Gaertn	Shigru, Horseradish tree	Rich in vitamin A and C, calcium, iron. Leaves contain sulphur, amino acids, methionine and cystine. Flowers and roots contain pterygospermin compounds having powerful antibiotic and fungicidal effects.
Mucuna pruriens Baker	Kapikachchhu, Cow-itch plant	Ayurvedic healers claim that it is an effective tonic for the nervous system as it contains L-DOPA, a direct precursor of dopamine.
Nardostachys jatamansi DC.	Jatamansi, Musk root	Ayurvedic practitioners include it in formulations to treat anxiety and mental health. It has been shown to be effective in maintaining restful sleep and alleviating many menopausal symptoms.

(Continued)

Table 14.2 (Continued)

Medicinal Plants	Common Name	Medicinal Properties/Uses
Piper longum L.	Pippali	Treatment of asthma, cough, indigestion, diarrhea, epilepsy, insomnia, rheumatoid arthritis, and tuberculosis. Used as immunostimulant, analgesic, carminative, and contraceptive.
Piper nigrum L.	Maricha, Black pepper	It contains an alkaloid piperine that has been widely used to amplify the body's ability to absorb nutrients contained in the food and aid the digestive process.
Rubia cordifolia L.	Manjishta, Indian Madder	Best Ayurvedic blood-purifying herb. Used as an immune regulator, supports heart health, regulates blood pressure and blood vessel constriction.
Saxifraga ligulata Wall	Pasanavheda	In Ayurveda, pashanabheda drug is made from its rhizomes used to treat kidney stones. Roots used for liver disease, pulmonary infection, diarrhea, and tuberculosis.
Terminalia arjuna W. and A.	Arjuna	Have cardioprotective effects, regulates blood pressure and heart rate.
Terminalia chebula Retz.	Haritaki	One of the components of Ayurvedic medicine "triphala," promoting health by purification and detoxification. Have anti-mutagenic activity.
Tinospora cordifolia Miers	Guduchi	Anti-inflammatory, antidiabetic, antioxidant, antimicrobial, anti-osteoporotic, antiulcer, and immunomodulatory properties.
Tribulus terrestris L.	Gokshura	Widely used in Ayurveda for many purposes. It is diuretic, boosts digestive health, improves heart function, and is anthelmintic.
Withania somnifera (Linn.) Dunal	Ashwagandha	Ashwagandha is one of the best Ayurvedic herbs. Stress Tolerance, Immunity, Joint Pains, Skin health. It is one of the best health tonics and restorative agents that have been used to treat general debility, exhaustion, stress induced fatigue, and insomnia.
Zingiber officinale Rosc	Sunthi, Ginger	Ayurvedic medicine to improve digestion and to prevent nausea. Helps in cancer prevention, anti-inflammatory, antioxidant, and antiplatelet effects.

Source: Pandey, Rastogi, and Rawat 2013.

Ritualistic Practices of India for Healing

A unique and distinctive feature of Indian traditional healing methods is ritualism. In Ayurveda, healthcare is delivered by the Ayurvedic practitioner through both ritualistic and non-ritualistic practices. One of the famous traditional healing practices is sacred therapy. The sacred may be evoked in different forms, such as spirits of ancestors and demons or local versions of God. The sacredness of the healing practices is further reinforced by the legends associated with the healer and/or healing center.

The sacredness of these healing centers is maintained by the priests, swāmis, fakirs, tāntrics, and gurus. In spiritual practices, the Hindus wear a mark (tilak or pottu) on their forehead, and they believe that tilak or pottu cools the forehead and prevents energy loss. Sometimes chandan or bhasma (the holy ash) is applied on the forehead with the belief that it helps in fast healing from any illness. There is a ritual of keeping holy flowers from the bed of God or Goddesses in touch with the patients for fast recovery from illness. In spiritual healing, restoration of health is achieved through meditation, some types of movements of the body, maintenance of hygiene, and water sanitation.

Again, the ritual of upavasa or fasting on special occasions like festivals is considered very good for the digestive system, and it helps to cultivate control over the senses, sublimate our desires, and guide our minds to be poised and at peace. In some small villages and towns, Shamanic healing (a healing process) is practiced for healing psychic distress like depression, anxiety, conversion symptoms, and psychosomatic symptoms. Here, shamanic practitioners known as baba, ojha, or tantric often conduct rituals such as chanting of sacred verses, mantras, sprinkling of holy water, or preparing a talisman infused with special healing qualities. Some rituals are mentioned in the ancient scripts related to birth and death, such as a religious ceremony or ritual related to birth in Hindu families called "The Sixth." This ritual is performed on the sixth day after delivery, in which the newborn is placed on a religious blanket, red powder mixed with water is applied on the soles and palms of the infant, and mantras and prayers are recited with the belief that a holy spirit blesses the newborn's life. During the cradle ceremony on the eleventh day after delivery, the baby is officially named (Kirmayer 2012).

Conclusion

Among the various indigenous medicine systems, Indian traditional medicine, Ayurveda, is the most ancient and popular medicine system in India and the world. Indian traditional medicine is not only a holistic medical system but also a healthy way of life. The ancient Indian civilization was very much close to nature and was aware of the importance of the maintenance of our natural environment. In modern society, there is an ever-growing disconnection from the natural world. Ancient people enhanced their own health by going closer to nature, engaging in mental and physical exercise, and eating fresh and healthy foods, including herbs. Today, Western medicine, or modern or allopathic medicine, occupies the mainstream position, but alongside this, people are worried about the side effects of synthetic modern drugs. Meanwhile, herbal drugs are gradually evolving again from the edge to the mainstream. Indian medicine has a good scientific background, but in developed countries, herbal medicine promotion still faces many challenges.

In Western countries, Ayurvedic aromatherapy and essential oil therapy are becoming very popular. Indian medicine is becoming more attractive as it is regarded as an "alternative therapy" to Western modern medicine in other countries, especially Europe and America. Some Europeans and Americans even take life courses in Indian medicine and experience the regimen of a full Ayurvedic medicine system, which includes different lifestyle rituals, diet, meditation, still sitting, yoga practice, different massage therapies, and spiritual lectures. Ayurveda puts a great amount of emphasis on the deterrence and encouragement for the healthy maintenance of one's life by maintaining a balanced lifestyle with a proper diet.

References

Adhikari, P. P., and S. B. Paul. "History of Indian Traditional Medicine: A Medical Inheritance." *Asian Journal of Pharmaceutical and Clinical Research* 11 (2018): 421.

Chaitanya, M. V., H. G. Baye, H. S. Ali, and F. B. Usamo. *Traditional African Medicine.* IntechOpen eBooks, 2022.

Che, C. T., V. George, T. P. Ijinu, P. Pushpangadan, and K. Andrae-Marobela. "Traditional Medicine." In *Pharmacognosy*, 2nd ed., 11–28. London: Academic Press, 2024.

Deli, Y., and K. Li. "Traditional Indian Medicine and Traditional Chinese Medicine." *International Journal of Traditional Chinese Medicine* 30 (2008): 314–16.

Fokunang, C., V. Ndikum, O. Tabi, R. Jiofack, B. Ngameni, N. Guedje, E. Tembe-Fokunang,, P. Tomkins, S. Barkwan, F. Kechia, E. Asongalem, J. Ngoupayou, N. Torimiro, K. Gonsu, V. Sielinou, B. Ngadjui, I. Angwafor, A. Nkongmeneck, O. Abena, and J. Lohoue. "Traditional Medicine: Past, Present and Future Research and Development Prospects and Integration in the National Health System of Cameroon." *African Journal of Traditional Complementary and Alternative Medicines* 8, no. 3 (2011): 284–95.

Haddabi, A. A., and E. D. Williamson. "H23 Traditional Healing by Skin Cauterization (kaiy)." *British Journal of Dermatology* 188 (2023).

Jaiswal, Y., and L. Williams. "A Glimpse of Ayurveda – the Forgotten History and Principles of Indian Traditional Medicine." *Journal of Traditional Complementary Medicine* 7 (2016): 50–3.

Kamboj, V. P. "Herbal Medicine." *Current Science* 78 (2000): 35–9.

Kirmayer, L. "Cultural Competence and Evidence-Based Practice In Mental Health: Epistemic Communities and the Politics of Pluralism." *Social Science and Medicine* 75 (2012): 249–56.

Liu, X. M., J. Q. Zou, Z. X. Shen, and G. Q. Su. "Overview of Traditional Indian Medicine." Modernization of Traditional Chinese Medicine *World Science and Technology* 7 (2005): 86–8

Loudon, I. "A Brief History of Homeopathy." *Journal of the Royal Society of Medicine 99* (2006): 607–10.

Matsuomoto, M., K. Inoue, and E. Kajii. "Integrating Traditional Medicine in Japan: The Case of Kampo Medicines." *Complementary Therapies in Medicine* 7 (1999): 254–5

Ozioma, E. J., and O. A. N. Chinwe. *Herbal Medicines in African Traditional Medicine.* IntechOpen eBooks, 2019.

Pandey, M. M., S. Rastogi, and A. K. S. Rawat. "Indian Traditional Ayurvedic System of Medicine and Nutritional Supplementation." *Evidence-based Complementary and Alternative Medicine* 2013 (2013): 1–12.
Park, H., H. Lee, B. Shin, J. Liu, Q. Shang, H. Yamashita, and B. Lim. "Traditional Medicine in China, Korea, and Japan: A Brief Introduction and Comparison." *Evidence-based Complementary and Alternative Medicine* 2012 (2012): 1–9.
Patwardhan, B., D. Warude, P. Pushpangadan, and N. Bhatt. "Ayurveda and Traditional Chinese Medicine: A Comparative Overview." *Evidence-Based Complementary and Alternative Medicine* 2 (2005): 465–73.
Shi, Y., C. Zhang, and X. Li. "Traditional Medicine in India." *Journal of Traditional Chinese Medical Sciences* 8 (2020): S51–5.
Singh, R., and S. Rastogi. "WHO ICD-11 Showcasing of Traditional Medicine: Lesson from a Lost Opportunity." *Annals Ayurvedic Med* 7 (2018): 66–71.
Singh, V. "Sushruta: The Father of Surgery." *National Journal of Maxillofacial Surgery* 8 (2017): 1–3.
Sivin, N. *Traditional Medicine in Contemporary China*. Ann Arbor: University of Michigan, Center for Chinese Studies, 1987.
Sreedhar, R., K. Watanabe, and S. Arumugam. "Introduction to Japanese Kampo Medicines." In *Japanese Kampo Medicines for the Treatment of Common Diseases: Focus on Inflammation*. Academic Press, London, 2017: pp. 1–11.
Zhang, J., Q. Zhang, G. Liu, and N. Zhang. "Therapeutic Potentials and Mechanisms of the Chinese Traditional Medicine Danshensu." *European Journal of Pharmacology* 864 (2019): 172710
Zhang, R., X. Zhu, H. Bai, and K. Ning. "Network Pharmacology Databases for Traditional Chinese Medicine: Review and Assessment." *Frontiers in Pharmacology* 10 (2019).

15

Indigenous Healing, Social Beliefs, and Practices among the Onges of Little Andaman of Andaman Archipelagos

Satyaki Paul[1] and Sabatini Chatterjee[2*]

[1]Dr. Ambedkar Chair (Dr. Ambedkar Foundation, Ministry of Social Justice & Empowerment, Govt. of India), KISS Deemed to be University, Bhubaneswar, Odisha, India

[2]Andaman & Nicobar Regional Centre, Anthropological Survey of India (Ministry of Culture, Govt. of India), Port Blair, Andaman & Nicobar Islands, India

*Corresponding Author's Email: sabatinichatterjee11@gmail.com[2]

Introduction

The Andaman and Nicobar archipelagos are made up of around 572 islands, islets out of which only some spaces are habitable (Reddy 2007). The islands are located between the Bay of Bengal and the Andaman Sea. They feature diverse landscapes, including rainforests, beaches, hills, and coral reefs. The islands' marine ecosystems are vital to life above and below water. In the Andaman archipelago, the Great Andaman and Little Andaman were mostly occupied by the original inhabitants of the regions (Cipriani 1966). The Duncan Passage separates South Andaman from Little Andaman while the Ten Degree Channel separates the Andaman archipelago from the Nicobar archipelago. Focusing back on Little Andaman, it can be observed that, since time immemorial, it has been home to a sole tribe, that is, Onges, who are surrounded by sea and dense forest. Radcliffe-Brown (1922) first stated that the indigenous populace entered the Andamans from the Lower Burma (present Myanmar) region. Cipriani (1966) in his research on midden sites observed that Onges were the first group to arrive in the Andaman region which was rich in fish, turtles, crabs, dugongs, and other fauna. Intriguingly, it was devoid of any ferocious animal or even monkeys.

The first contact of Onges can be recorded in T. E. Alexander's report, which detailed a gruesome fight between both parties in 1825. M. V. Portman became the first to establish long-term contact with them from 1885–7 (Basu 1990). Apart from these contacts, other earlier accounts highlighted their tradition of cutting all body pieces, which were later thrown into fire. This instilled fear among outsiders regarding the fierceness of Onges. However, several scholars have noted that this is a superstitious social rite which Onges followed to circumvent any evil spirits in the region (Portman 1899; Radcliffe-Brown 1922). The Little Andaman was opened to refugees in 1967, which led to the resettlement of Onges. Initially, the Onges were spread across the entirety of Little Andaman, and they were resettled into the Dugong Creek in 1976, and another group was settled in South Bay Settlement (Basu 1990). The area was declared a tribal reserve covering around 520 square kilometers due to their seminomadic nature, which is embedded in their hunting and gathering lifestyle.

In general, the Onges are one of the most primitive tribes in India. They belong to the Negrito racial stock, and they have been relegated to the reserved pockets both at Dugong Creek and South Bay of Little Andaman Island. They are also diminishing in number. They are exogamous groups and live close to nature and they seek to receive their food and other items for mundane sustenance. They call themselves as *en-iregale* (perfect man), which is even accepted by the Great Andamanese folks (Singh 1992). They separate themselves into different partitions like *tetaje*, *beriedalu*, *ingotijalo*, *inge*, and so on, who reside in communal huts (Basu 1990). Their skeletal features show strong zygomatic bones and broad flat-nasal roots. The zygomatic bones are characteristically supported by strong teeth with good biting strength, which they use to extract nuts and even open up coconuts. They are small in stature in comparison to their neighboring cohort tribal groups and share similar soft elastic skin with scanty body hair. There is also the presence of steatopygia among males and females due to the amassing of fat in the gluteal region (Cipriani 1966). Their palate is unusually arched with white teeth and no caries.

The colonial administrators of the then British Raj introduced dogs along with tea and clothes. The Onges accepted the dogs due to their love for hunting. The Duncan Passage created a vacuum which separated the Onges from other tribal cohorts. They resided in deep forests and chiefly relied on meats of wild boar, turtle, dugong, wild fruits, and honey. These were usually roasted or boiled while green vegetables were absent from their initial diet. They were aloof from the modern world much like the Sentinelese until the beginning of the nineteenth century (Basu 1990). Portman (1899) noted that they had lived thousands of years without any communication with the outside world except for a few contacts during shipwrecks. The use of iron was initiated with the subsequent contacts of Malay and Chinese sailors, which was apparent through the artifacts obtained from the midden sites (Basu 1990; Cipriani 1966). The territories are denoted by the presence of a communal hut (*beyras*) in a region wherein the exchange of women is considered a medium of communicative exchange between various groups (Basu 1990). They had also a temporary hut called *korale* due to their seminomadic nature.

The tsunami of 2004 had caused severe psychological stress and trauma to the said tribe (Anthropological Survey of India 2007). Although there were no deaths, the incident still haunts them. In due course of time, they have now experienced the impact of outsiders, as efforts at befriending them have proved successful. They have also been provided with pucca houses, food, clothes, and medicine by the Andaman Adim Janjati Vikas Samiti (AAJVS) of the Andaman and Nicobar Administration.

Objectives and Methods

The Onges are scarcely found in the Great Andaman region or even in other areas of Little Andaman. Even at the turn of the twenty-first century, they prefer to stay in their designated tribal reserve area in Dugong Creek. The Andaman & Nicobar Protection of Aboriginal Tribes (PAT) Regulation, 1956, limits the entry of outsiders/non-locals in the reserve area due to them being a part of sensitive Particularly Vulnerable Tribal Groups (PVTGs) regulated by the AAJVS of A&N administration. Their docile nature and fragile sociocultural contours are significant reasons for which fieldwork is restricted by the Tribal Welfare Department of the Andaman & Nicobar Administration. There are previous research works conducted by the Andaman & Nicobar Tribal Research Institute (ANTRI); however, now it is nonoperational due to a lack of staff and funding issues.

This particular study provides a unique outlook on the Onges community by systematically and methodically analyzing the secondary sources of data on indigenous healing, social beliefs, and practices among the Onges of Little Andaman of Andaman archipelagos. Moreover, this study is an addition to the part of the documentation of the indigenous knowledge system of the Onges community and the greater whole, that is, the traditional knowledge system of our Indian culture. The resettlement of 1974 had somewhat affected the community; however, with the aid of AAJVS of the A &N administration, the Onges have bounced back and are continuing their age-old traditions practiced by the community since time immemorial. All of these are vividly discussed in the following sections of the present study to enable the readers to understand the contemporary status quo of the Onges residing in Dugong Creek of Little Andaman, Andaman archipelagos.

Outline of the Onges

In the 1790s, Lt. Colebrooke observed that the term Onge or Ungee as they pronounced it, was used during his first contact with the said community (Basu 1990). However, this is debatable, as the Onges themselves never recognized the term and rather they call themselves as *en-iregale* or the perfect man (Cipriani 1966). The Onges consider their origin in the Great Spirit *onkobowkwe*'s wishes residing in the sky (Singh 1992). Another myth is there which states that two persons, that is, *engigegi* and his wife, had their genesis from a monitor lizard (*eiyugey*) who planted seedlings of the *lukwe-gelako* tree before going to hunt, and after their return, they saw that those seeds transformed into man and woman.

The Onges were resettled in 1974; however, prior to that, they used to roam in bands due to their seminomadic nature. Onges call their home *guabolambe* or the Little Andaman. They used to reside in beehive-shaped communal huts (*beyras*), which are now present in the Dugong Creek settlement. A replica of the same hut was built following authentic traditional design, materials, and participation of the said community at the Andaman & Nicobar Regional Centre, Anthropological Survey of India, Sri Vijaya Puram (erstwhile Port Blair) (Singh 2022). The second author is working as a junior research fellow at the same center during the construction of the hut, wherein she noted its features. The said center also has the Nicobarese hut, Jarawas hut, and Shompen hut within its premises, which act as an open museum for the tourists and researchers coming to visit the Zonal Anthropological Museum. The hut used to house more than eighteen individuals in real time (Singh 1992). However, the names of the huts varied as per their ecological ambience, as noted by Basu (1990) wherein some of the names were *tongalange*, *totiboye*, *butumogo*, *kawateokoi*, and so on. There is also the presence of temporary huts (*korale*) within the community, which are used to date, even after the construction of pucca houses by the local administration. Monogamy is practiced with family as the present constituent unit of an Onges band. An exogamous egalitarian band mainly encompassed an extended family, along with the prevalence of remarriage, which enabled stepsons and stepdaughters to become part of the same band. However, there is an absence of property, ownership, inheritance, and succession within the said community.

Their socio-religious practices involve spirits, the afterlife, and *onkobowkwe*, who is their supreme spirit guarding them from any form of harm. The Onges also believe that the spirits of their dead ancestors who are buried inside their communal huts roam around them and also protect them from harm. However, they do not worship any kind of idol, nor do they have any kind of sacrificial rites. The sole art form practiced by the said community is the drawing of the geometrical pattern of white clay and red clay on the body and face. There is a presence of making crude pottery, especially cooking pots also known as *tobuchue* in the said community, which seems to have perished (Singh 1992). The pots are first baked under direct sun and then are dried in fire (Basu 1990). There is an abundance of potsherds in the sites where communal huts are present across the Little Andamans (Singh 1992; Chander and Vijayachari 2018). A well-preserved pot is present in the Zonal Anthropological Museum of the Andaman and Nicobar Regional Centre, Anthropological Survey of India.

There are no special individuals who act as craftsmen; rather, everyone crafted things as and when required by them. *Nakuinyage* or traditional tassel dress is used by women to cover their lower abdomen region. Most of the ceremonial dresses, that is, *keye* (dance apparel), loincloths, headbands, chest bands, wristlets, armlets, and so on, are crafted from cane strips, barks, bark fiber, palm leaves, and other items locally available. These are worn by both men and women, wherein in ceremonies they spontaneously sing folksongs which might be linked to their mundane activities such as hunting or gathering or ceremonies or rituals, but the tonalities may be monotonous. There is an absence of any form of musical items accompanying such traditional dances in the said community.

In terms of socio-demography, the Onges were counted as 672 in 1901, 631 in 1911, 346 in 1921, 250 in 1931, 150 in 1951, 129 in 1961, 112 in 1971, and so on (Basu 1990). The present number is 126 after the birth of a baby boy from Andaman's Onge tribe King Totoko and Queen Priya (PTI 2024). There is a high inclination toward procreation wherein Onge women believe that they become pregnant as per the wishes of the Great Spirit, *onkobowkwe*. The women from the said community enjoy equal status and they chiefly fetch water, collect firewood and rear their children. Apart from these, they also gather edible materials from the forest and collect fish from the shallow waters. Tattooing and hair grooming are carried out by the women members of the Onges. Presently, the women also work as daily wage laborers in coconut plantations and contribute to the socioeconomic stability of their family. Moreover, they also receive allowances, free medical treatment, education, and other social services as a part of governmental assistance provisioned by the AAJVS of A & N administration.

Indigenous Healing, Social Beliefs, and Practices

The Onges have a name for every island, islet, and even Sentinel Island, which points toward the fact that they are wanderlusts from the beginning. The Onges travel in bands that usually break plants, make scratches on the trunks, and so on to create markers of their presence in the area. They also have great eyesight, which adds a feather to their seminomadic nature following the sun's (tenculu) position and their arm movement (Cipriani 1966). In earlier times, Cipriani (1966) observed that Onges had no form of hygiene, which also extends to their cooking utensils. Their nakedness often came in handy in protecting them from various skin-related illnesses, which later got altered due to the introduction of modern clothes. The consumption of tobacco and alcohol has also greatly affected the morale of the said community (Sekhsaria 2001).

There are rituals and ceremonies linked with the initiation of boys into adulthood known as *tanagiru* wherein the boy has to demonstrate his hunting skills (Singh 1992). The rituals at the onset of puberty for girls are also significant wherein a girl consumes wild jackfruit (buludange) for 4–5 days. The birth rituals are not very complex in comparison to their cohort tribes. During delivery, a woman is attended by her mother or other women of affinal and consanguineal relation. As soon as a child is born in a new hut (*kordle*), the placenta is buried on the spot where the baby was born (Basu 1990). There are some restrictions imposed on the mother concerning the food she eats after delivery. However, as discussed earlier, the Onges now visit G.B. Pant Hospital, Sri Vijaya Puram (erstwhile Port Blair) during their stay at Adi Basera or visit the hospital at Dugong Creek settlement or Hut Bay.

Marriage rituals are also conducted in a modest manner. After the conventional method of greeting, the bride sits on the lap of the bridegroom, followed by reciprocated hugging (Singh 1992). This is a significant aspect of the Onges socio-culture. A banquet is held on the occasion to honor the couple and the guests. As for the ritual of the dead, the Onges bury the dead inside the hut, under the cot/bed of the deceased person.

These rituals are done by *gallankare* or *gultarandi* that is a person who shares a putative relation with the individual. According to their traditional practice, they exhume the lower jaw (*innibirangey*) of the corpse after some period in a discreet manner, and outsiders are prohibited in such events.

Their small stature is the reason that they travel in a band. The Onges fear another spirit named *eiuga* (lizard-like and bigger than a crocodile). They consider themselves to be tactful in deceiving their spirits by stealing tubers from the soil. To evade their dead ancestors, they carry *ibidanghe* (necklace of human jaws) on their necks, which also aids them in hunting, fishing, and gathering food for daily sustenance. They also contribute to death, disease, and childbirth as part of the activities of supernatural beings or their dead ancestors. In earlier times, the Onges used to practice a common remedy as a part of their indigenous healing, which involved smearing the entire body with a mixture of ochre, turtle fat, and honey. Another remedy is smoking the infected region, wherein a person suffering from fever might be placed near a low-lit fire. A person would spit on the hair and skin along with the massaging of the patient's head. Ochre is heated in water and is also massaged on the chest, throat, and neck. All of these are considered to relieve an individual from high fever.

The Onges use a specific plant *Orophea katschalica* (*tonjoghe*) in the process of extracting honey from the hives of rock bees. It is a very effective bee repellent and is harmless to humans. The remarkable use of endemic flora by them proves the richness of the Indigenous knowledge system which needs to be documented and protected. (see Table 15.1). In a similar vein, in 1993, Debaprasad Chattopadhyay, a microbiologist, observed that the Onges were surrounded by mosquitoes but they hardly got infected with malaria. They used to consume a medicinal brew which gave them immunity against malaria (Bhargava 1983; McGirk 1998). The plant *Alstonia macrophylla* is used by Onges to concoct medicine having the power to fight against malaria and its Plasmodium falciparum variant which is effective on seven patients. The discovery is a paradigm-shifting one; however, it was soon entangled in an antagonistic patent dispute, in due course overshadowing its academic significance and immense potential (Sekhsaria 2001). This hullabaloo epitomized a profound assault on the Indigenous knowledge system, particularly the Indigenous knowledge systems of the Onges.

The idea of giving back to the community can be observed as often nonexistent among the researchers. The Onges have often been easily persuaded to share their ancestral knowledge with outsiders, sometimes to their loss. Such exposure has had calamitous costs—not only for the delicate coastal ecosystem of the islands but also for the well-being of the tribal population. Yet, perhaps the most devastating impact has stemmed from insensitive administrative policies, which have relentlessly pursued ill-conceived development projects. These interventions have led to rampant deforestation, the degradation of vital mangrove forests, and the alarming erosion of coral reefs, inflicting irreversible damage on both the natural environment and the cultural heritage of the Onges (Dasgupta 1996). The present administration is working to reverse all the past damages but only time will tell how effective the "arms-length approach" is considering the turn of the twenty-first century.

Table 15.1. Endemic Plants Used by the Onges of Little Andaman for Indigenous Healing and Social Practices (Source: Pandey and Diwakar 2008; Chander and Vijayachari 2018).

Sl. No	Scientific and Family Name	Local Name	Type	Usage
1	*Donax cannaeformis* Family: Marantaceae	Kagle, Tambowka	Shrub	The leaves are boiled in water and the paste is used to cure abdominal and spinal aches. The stems are also utilized in basketry (Toleh). The leaves are also considered to soothe pain in prenatal and postnatal periods.
2	*Daemonorps manii* Family: Arecaceae	Tamoyen, Tomoje	Tree	The shoot is used to cover and protect the female genitalia from mosquito bites
3	*Mailkara littoralis* Family: Sapotaceae	Mohwa	Tree	The wood is used to make bows. And the fruits are also consumed as a part of diet.
4	*Heritiera littoralis* Family: Stericuliaceae	Moro, Sundri	Tree	The leaves in a concoction with leaves of Hibiscus tiliaceus are mixed to make tea. The roasted seeds of the fruits are also consumed
5	*Pavetta sp* Family: Rubiaceae		Tree	The tree trunks are used as pillars in the building of Onge huts.
6	*Adrisia sp* Family: Rhizophoraceae	Daboja	Tree	The leaves are crushed to create a paste used to cure chest pain.
7	*Horsefieldia sp* Family: Myristicaceae	Jugane	Tree	The fruits are considered to be a cure for abdominal pain.
8	*Thespesia populnea* Family: Malvaceae	Tebokala	Tree	The raw leaves are considered to be a cure for constipation-related problems.
9	*Leea sp* Family: Leeaceae	Elegai, Kototo	Tree	The leaves are utilized as bed sheets in Onge huts.
10	*Scaevola sericea* Family: Goodeniaceae	Yae	Shrub	The fruits are considered to be a cure for fever, common colds, and headaches. The fruit is also considered to be a cure for diarrhea.
11	*Pongamia pinnata* Family: Fabaceae	Oicunae	Shrub	The paste prepared from pulverizing the bark is considered to be a cure for malaria.
12	*Desmodium umbellatum* Family: Fabaceae	Damle	Shrub	The raw leaves are considered to be a cure for fever.
13	*Mallotus peltatus* Family: Euphorbiaceae	Patage	Shrub	The raw leaves are considered to be a cure for abdominal aches.
14	*Garcinia andamanica* Family: Clusiaceae		Tree	The tree trunks are used as pillars in the building of Onge communal huts.
15	*Calophyllum sp* Family: Clusiaceae		Tree	The trunk of the tree is utilized to create canoes (*Danges*).

(*Continued*)

Table 15.1 (Continued)

Sl. No	Scientific and Family Name	Local Name	Type	Usage
16	*Canarium euphyllum* Family: Burseraceae	Dhup	Tree	The seared resin acts as a mosquito repellent.
17	*Wedelia biflora* Family: Asteraceae	Takunkala	Herb	The leaves are crushed to create a paste, that is used to treat wounds.
18	*Orophea katschallica* Family: Annonaceae	Tonyoge	Tree	The leaves are crushed to create a paste which is used during honey collection as a bee repellent.
19	*Desmos dasymaschalus* Family: Annonaceae		Shrub	The branches of the shrub are used to craft arrows for fishing. The tree trunks are used as pillars in the building of Onge huts.
20	*Calophyllum inophyllum* Family: Clusiaceae	Tebae	Tree	The latex of the tree is considered to be a cure for earaches.
21	*Drypetes assamica* Family: Euphorbiaceae	Torelulu	Shrub	The leaves of the shrub are used to treat dental caries.
22	*Annona squamosa* Family: Annonaceae	Tonya-ong	Tree	The leaves of the tree are crushed to make a paste which treats menstrual disorders.
23	*Mallotus repandus* Family: Euphorbiaceae	Chinatigale	Tree	The leaves are crushed to create a paste which treats cough.
24	*Miliusa andamanica* Family: Annonaceae	Kobotilabe	Tree	The bark is considered to cure headaches. And is often tied in fractured regions.
25	*Premna corymbosa* Family: Verbanaceae	Thhamoza	Shrub	The leaves are pasted and applied on the skin which is considered to be a cure for back pain.
26	Zingiber squarrosum Family: Zingiberaceae	Toetonai	Herb	The leaves are considered to be a cure for malaria, cough, fever, and skin injuries (topical application in most cases). The stem is tied to the fractured region as a cure.
27	*Cycas rumphii* Family: Cycadaceae	Ameene	Tree	The seeds of the fruit are cooked and consumed as a part of the diet.
28	*Oroxylum indicum* Family: Bignoniaceae	Talaralu	Tree	The fruits are consumed raw as a part of the diet.
29	*Trichosanthes bracteata* Family: Cucurbitaceae	Onto, Tulero	Climber	The seared fruits are consumed as a part of the diet.
30	*Abrus preatorius* Family: Fabaceae	Gunci	Climber	The ripe seared pods are consumed as a part of the diet.
31	*Hibiscus tiliaceus* Family: Malvaceae	Koibo	Tree	The leaves in a concoction with leaves of *Hibiscus littoralis* are mixed to make a special tea.
32	*Rhizophora apiculata* (Rhizophoraceae)	Daboja	Tree	The fruits are boiled and then consumed as a part of the diet.

(*Continued*)

Table 15.1 (Continued)

Sl. No	Scientific and Family Name	Local Name	Type	Usage
33	*Guettarda speciosa* Family: Rubiaceae	Toikutto	Tree	The flowers are worn in the hair.
34	*Licuala peltate* Family: Arecaceae	Selai Pathi, Tamru	Tree	The leaves were earlier used to craft umbrellas to be used in the rainy season.
35	*Crinum latifolium* Family: Amaryllidaceae	Takule	Shrub	The flowers are worn in the hair.
36	*Dioscorea glabra* Family: Dioscoreaceae	Teetakorel	Climber	The boiled tubers are consumed as a part of the diet.
37	*Flagellaria indica* Family: Flagellariaceae	Tambokacha	Climber	The stem is chewed like sugarcane and is consumed as a part of the diet.
38	*Dracaena augustifolia* Family: Dracanaceae	Buckripathi	Tree	The seared fruits are consumed as a part of the diet.
39	*Gloriosa superba* Family: Liliaceae	Kurabo	Climber	The flowers are worn in the hair.
40	*Pandanus tectorius* Family: Pandanaceae	Bali, Mane, Keora	Tree	The fruits are considered to be favorite among the Onges.
41	*Zingiber squarrosum* Family: Zingiberaceae	Kumbabe	Herb	The petioles are considered to quench the thirst of the Onges.
42	*Barringtonia asiatica* Family: Lecythidaceae	Cigola	Tree	The seared fruits are rarely considered as it is poisonous.
43	*Ficus hispida* Family: Moraceae	Boikwe	Tree	The seared fruits are consumed as a part of the diet.

Conclusion and Recommendation

The age-old time-tested ancestral knowledge which was passed down from one generation to another is a testament to their belief in such healing practices. For generations, their knowledge systems have guided them in matters of health, spirituality, and communal well-being, shaping their unique way of life which can be observed in the form of a nature-human-spirit complex. However, the intrusion of globalization has led to the steady erosion of these invaluable Indigenous knowledge systems. The indigenous healing practices falling into disuse and the younger generations increasingly disconnected from their roots, the passing of the older folk signals not just the loss of individuals deemed PVTGs but the evanescing of an entire repository of Indigenous knowledge systems.

This issue is a significant crisis of our twenty-first century which is exacerbated by the community's growing dependence on tobacco and alcohol, which has significantly deteriorated their health and further distanced them from their indigenous healing practices. The Onges, once resilient people who thrived on their deep knowledge of medicinal plants, holistic treatments, and spiritual healing, now face an existential threat—not only from external influences but also from the neglect of their own cultural identity. To deal with these issues, Auxiliary Nurses and Midwives (ANM), Pharmacists, and male Health Workers have been posted at the Sub-Centre of Dugong Creek and are working round the clock. Moreover, the Directorate of Health Services under the Andaman & Nicobar Administration organizes frequent Multispecialty Tribal Health Camps and gives in situ treatment to the Onges to avoid infant mortality. The effect of Pradhan Mantri Janjati Adivasi Nyaya Maha Abhiyan (PM-JANMAN) on such tribes also needs to be assessed to meet their needs rather than providing amenities not required by them. The Andaman and Nicobar Tribal Research Institute (ANTRI), Tribal Welfare Department of the Andaman & Nicobar Administration can initiate some kind of research in this domain to better meet the needs of Onges.

Apart from these, the Onges stand at a crossroads—either their knowledge systems fade into oblivion, or they experience a resurgence that ensures their cultural and physical survival. The Onge Reserve is roughly 30 percent smaller (more than 200 square kilometers of forest have been handed over for settlements, plantations, and agriculture). The choice is ours to make. The Onges have adopted the modern way of living but still profess their traditional skills of hunting, gathering, food collection, and medicines. The role of practicing anthropologists (especially the Anthropological Survey of India) and scholars becomes crucial. The responsibility to give back to the community is not one that can be deferred; it is a call to action that demands immediate and committed intervention. The need of the hour is cultural revitalization—a concerted effort to document, preserve, and revive the traditional knowledge of the Onges. This can be achieved through community-driven initiatives, the integration of indigenous healing into contemporary healthcare approaches, and the promotion of intergenerational knowledge transmission. Such revitalization must also extend beyond mere documentation; it should empower the Onges to reclaim their heritage with pride. Encouraging Indigenous education, fostering self-sustaining health practices, and creating platforms where elders can share their wisdom with the younger generation are essential steps toward cultural resurgence through enabling specially tailored awareness programs and policies that support indigenous well-being, considering their vulnerability characterized by distinctive culture and relatively simple socio-techno-economic background.

References

Anthropological Survey of India. *Tsunami in South Asia: Studies on Impact of Tsunami on Communities of Andaman and Nicobar Island.* Kolkata: Allied Publishers Private Limited, 2007.

Basu, B. *The Onge.* Kolkata: Seagull Publishers on behalf of Anthropological Survey of India, 1990.

Bhargava, N. "Ethnobotanical Studies of the Tribes of Andaman and Nicobar Islands." *Economic Botany* 37 (1983): 110–19.

Chander, M., and P. Vijayachari. "Ethnomedicinal Knowledge among the Tribes of Little Andaman Island, Andaman and Nicobar Island, India." *Pharmacognosy Magazine* 14 (2018): 488–93.

Cipriani, L. *The Andaman Islanders*. New York: Frederick A. Praeger Publishers, 1966.

Dasgupta, S. "No Penny for the Onges?" *Down To Earth*, January 15, 1996.

McGirk, T. "Gene Piracy." *Time*, November 9, 1998.

Portman, M. *History of Our Relations with the Andamanese (Vol I and II)*. Calcutta: Office of the Superintendent Government Printing India, 1899.

Radcliffe-Brown, A. R. *The Andaman Islanders*. Cambridge: Cambridge University Press, 1922.

Reddy, S. "Mega Tourism in Andaman and Nicobar Islands: Some Concerns." *Journal of Human Ecology* 21 (2007): 231–9.

Sekhsaria, P. "Deforestation in Andaman and Nicobar: Its Impact on Onge." *Economic and Political Weekly* 36 (2001): 3643–8.

Singh, K. S. *People of India: Andaman & Nicobar Islands (Vol – XII)*. New Delhi: Affiliated East-West Press, 1992.

Singh, S. "Anthropological Survey of India Builds Tribal Hut Replicas to Promote Unique Heritage." *The Hindu*, November 07, 2022.

Perception of Health and Traditional Health-Seeking Behavior among the Tai Ahom, Tai Khamte, and Tai Phake Communities of Northeastern Part of India

Yikham Gogoi[1] and Satyaki Paul[2*]

[1] Andaman & Nicobar Regional Centre, Anthropological Survey of India (Ministry of Culture, Govt. of India), Port Blair, Andaman & Nicobar Islands, India

[2]Dr. Ambedkar Chair (Dr. Ambedkar Foundation, Ministry of Social Justice & Empowerment, Govt. of India), KISS Deemed to be University, Bhubaneswar, Odisha, India

*Corresponding Author's Email: satyakipaul54@gmail.com[2]

Introduction

In historical terms, Assam was known as *Pragjyotish* or *Kamrupa* in various ancient Indian texts (Bal 2021). The state is located in the northeast part of our nation. It constitutes around 12.45 percent of the total tribal population of our nation (Census of India 2011), wherein most of the populace, that is, around 94.4 percent, inhabits the rural areas (Neer Nirmal Pariyojana, Assam 2016). There are fourteen tribes inhabiting the hilly regions and nine tribes inhabiting the valley regions of Assam (Sarmah and Dutta 2018). These indigenous populaces due to their varied geographical locales practice diverse forms of ritualistic practices including divination and ethnomedicines as a part and parcel of their knowledge systems (Sadir 1914; Kar 2016; Gogoi 2021). These traditional knowledge systems are pertinent considering their sustainable nature and their successful application since time immemorial. The foresight and wisdom gained by such a populace are through experience, and such experience is passed down from one generation to the next (Behera and Patel 2000). This can be associated with traditional knowledge systems and such populaces usually survive in adverse conditions due to the nature-man spirit complex (Rao 2021).

The definition of health-seeking behavior can be assessed as any action undertaken by people who self-perceive themselves to have some health-related issues and purposefully find some apt remedy to address such illness (Oberoi et al. 2016). As per World Health Organization (1948), "Health is a state of complete physical, mental and social well-being and not merely the absence of disease or infirmity." Most of the tribes of India, even though inhabiting remote locations, can maintain sustainable and healthy lifestyles due to their closeness to Mother Nature and their knowledge about the endemic ecological niches.

In the recent past, a few studies were conducted to document the ethnomedicinal practices utilized to treat varying degrees of maladies among several communities residing in Assam, especially in Tai-speaking communities (Das and Tag 2006; Buragohain 2011; Bailung and Puzari 2016; Borah 2016; Borah and Sengupta 2018; Baruah 2020; Dutta 2023). In the entirety of research in ethnomedicinal practices in India, a gigantic research gap persists as these are just pieces of knowledge about the entire traditional knowledge system. These knowledge systems, although small in parts, but in a collective sense, are capable enough to alleviate inequalities, enable social justice, and redress challenges pertaining to global health presaged by the sixth extinction in the Holocene era (Janes and Corbett 2009).

However, at present, due to the prevalence of allopathic practices, there is a decline in ethnomedicinal practices chiefly due to mental reformation, even though they are quite aware of its side effects (Kumar et al. 2021). These practices might snowball and cause untimely evanescence of ethnomedicinal practices, which is one of the core components of traditional knowledge systems (Kunwar 2008). The coronavirus pandemic taught us the necessity of alternative medicinal practices (Paudyal et al. 2021) and how such practices can aid the government of the day in sustainably battling such virulent diseases (Kumar et al. 2021). Thus, it is quintessential to culturally revitalize such practices by documenting, preserving, and promoting them in the mainstream populace. It is essential that such oral traditions would be lost in the sands of time considering their delicate sociocultural fabric denoting their traditional knowledge systems and their health-seeking behaviors. In a similar vein, in the later part of the chapter, it can be observed that a nature-spirit-man complex is at play within the Ahom people, which is yet to be fully explored, and this book chapter is like a singular piece to the entire puzzle in the purview of indigenous knowledge systems possessed by them.

Objectives and Methods

The initial leg of research was carried out from June to July 2009 and October to November 2009 among the Tai Ahom people of Assam. The second leg was carried out from August to September 2010 and December 2010 among the Tai Phake people of Assam. And the last leg of research was carried out from January to February 2011 and October to November 2011 among the Khamti people of Arunachal Pradesh. The central maxim of the study revolved around the notion of "Differential Fertility and

Infant Mortality in Three Tai Mongoloid Population Groups of North East India: A Study on Biosocial Correlates." For this study, convenient sampling was employed to select three Tai-speaking groups from Napam, Dhemaji, Manmow, Nanam, Khamti, Sensup, Borphake, Pomung, Phaneng, Munglang, Longtong, Ningam villages of Assam and Arunachal Pradesh. The snowball method was employed as a recruitment method to accept voluntary participants in the research frame (Paul and Bagchi 2022).

The primary data were collected employing open-ended schedules from a total of 744 individuals belonging to all the age groups and in due course, the answers to such questions were triangulated and inconsistencies were removed during data cleaning. Nonetheless, for the present study, the health perception and health-seeking behavior of Tai Ahom, Tai Phake, and Tai Khamte are being discussed. Apart from this, it is also to be noted that both oral and written consent were taken during the survey.

About the Tai People

The "Ahom / Asom" are the most renowned group of people who migrated to Assam in the thirteenth century (Sadir 1914). Even the term Assam comes from the word "Asama / Asamiya," which means "Peerless" in the socioculturally evanesced Ahom language (Sarma 1976). The medieval history of Assam correlates to the Ahom kingdom, wherein the Mughals were unable to defeat them in battles due to their prowess (Bal 2021). In the contemporary pan-Indian context, members of the Tai community mostly reside in Assam, Arunachal Pradesh, and Meghalaya in the northeastern part of India. Ahom is the most dominant group among all other groups such as Phake, Khamti, Khamyang, Turung, Aiton, and Mann (Figure 16.1).

In terms of historical advent, Ahoms were the first Tai-speaking people to invade Assam, establishing their dynasty in the upper Brahmaputra valley of Assam in AD 1228, governed by Chaolung Sukapha for around 600 years (Doley 2014). The Khamtis are also Tai-speaking people who reside in the upper regions of Assam and Arunachal Pradesh. The members of the Khamti community journeyed to Assam between AD 1750 and 1850. The Khamtis' original home is called Khamtilong or Mung Khamtilong, and the site is situated adjacent to Delta in the Ayeyarwady region of present-day Myanmar. The Phakes, another Tai-speaking clan, migrated to Assam through the Patkai hills from Mong Kong (Mogaung) province in Northern Myanmar in the latter half of the eighteenth century. Often Assamese people refer to Phakes as "Phakial" in their native Assamese language. According to their oral history, the Phakes had their genesis in Mung Mao in *Lak li kat hao* (AD 1215) and built a Phake principality in the Hukwang Valley of northern Burma (Pukhan 2015). They fled their principality in *Lak-li kat kao* (AD 1775) for Assam because of Burmese tyranny (Gogoi 1996). On the whole, the Phakes are progressive individuals. In terms of religion, they follow Theravada Buddhism and have a high level of culture. However, due to close contact with the mainstream populace, these three Tai-speaking communities are somewhat assimilated and might lose their values due to acculturation along with a certain degree of xenocentric attitude present within them.

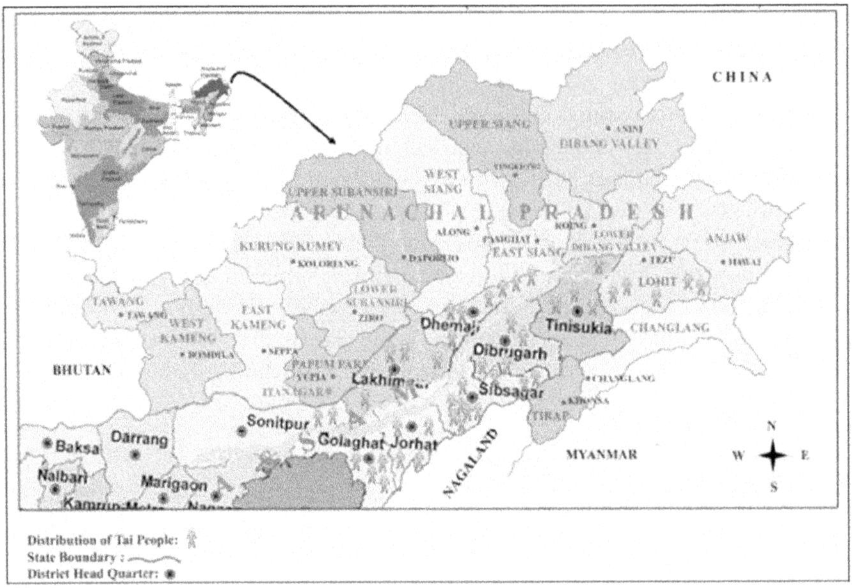

Figure 16.1. Distributions of Tai people residing in Assam and Arunachal Pradesh. Source: Author.

Perception of Women among the Tai People

In terms of macro-cultural settings, Indian men consider themselves to be superior to their female counterparts among Tai people. Such a form of negative discrimination is kind of taken for granted in most of the rural settings across the board. The women of the Tai group still believe in magico-religious practices, especially divination for treating illness. They believe in evil eyes/*drishtidosham*, ancestral spirits, and supernatural activities manifested in the form of diseases. So, whenever a woman is unable to perform mundane activities, she is considered to be sick and is affected by evil spirits. Even expectant mothers are to observe taboos during this period. For example, among Tai people, in the case of pregnancy, there is usually an inclination toward a male child rather than a female one; herein, when a male child is born, a celebration is carried out in a village with the beating of *dhol/tasha* (trumpets) along with the distribution of sweets to commemorate the occasion.

There is a certain degree of preferential treatment among the Tai people regarding such rites de passage stage. In this vein, in the case of the birth of a female child, usually the birth is announced with a less pronounced celebration in the family (Joseph 1986). Everything is regulated by the head of the family, which even involves seeking advice on health-related matters from the *bejes/bejnis* (medicine man/woman in Tai Ahom communities), which affects their health in the long run (Kalita and Phukan 2010). The members of the Tai community have faith in the understanding that childbirth is the gift of God or a natural phenomenon, and regular medical checkups or taking medicines are prohibited during such periods. Herein, such facts align with the data on the overall life expectancy and male-female ratio across India (Basu 2004).

Even in politics, the power remains in the hands of *sarpanch-pati* or *devar* and this is noted as *Sarpanch-patism* (Sarin 2023). This was also observed in a latent manner among the Tai people where the decision was somewhat influenced by her spouse and other male members of the family. Herein women are just used as rubber and stamp by the husband even after interventions at various levels by the Indian courts (Sarin 2023). The women typically adapt to become oppressed while her husband becomes the oppressor considering the values and mores of a patriarchal society. However, as homemakers, the decisions are well respected and women hold a significant position in the family. She is relatively free in making decisions and is firm in those decisions unlike those of non-tribal societies. Nonetheless, it was observed that the status of tribal women is comparatively lower than that of tribal men.

Concepts of Health, Medicinal Knowledge, and Practices

The remote communities are usually closely linked with their sociocultural and environmental contexts, which can be seen through their nature-man-spirit complex (Mann 1981). However, they also suffer from various kinds of diseases due to their environments. For example, anemia is quite prevalent in the northeastern part of India, which also affects their psyche and bodily functions (Basu 1969; Basu, Jindal, and Kshatriya 1994). Anemia impairs the body and exacerbates vulnerability to diverse diseases which affect the human body, especially among would-be mothers. Maternal health conditions are affected, especially among those experiencing frequent and shorter intervals of pregnancies (Basu, Jindal, and Kshatriya 1994). The food security of pregnant women has a direct effect on their reproductive outcomes, as well as on the survival, growth, and development of their offspring.

The Tai people are patrilineal, with men occupying a dominant social position; the senior male in the household is highly respected, and his directives are rarely challenged. In spite of this hierarchical structure, women in these groups are recognized for their handling of personal responsibilities; they manage domestic duties, engage in agricultural work, and so on. Their role as both providers and caregivers is integral to their households and communities, underscoring the significant contribution of women's reproductive labor. In the said communities, young women are generally considered marriageable upon reaching menarche, with procreation viewed as a natural progression after nuptials. The belief in divine connection at the commencement of pregnancy is strong, with the view that new life is given by God. Even though limited care is given to pregnant women, they observe certain taboos and limitations intended to protect the well-being of the unborn child. Pregnant women face no prohibitions on household tasks and continue to engage in daily chores such as cooking, cleaning, and washing, in addition to agricultural labor. As gatherers, Khamti and Phake women also collect vegetables and firewood from nearby forests, while Ahom women frequently fish even during pregnancy. These errands are seen as typical, and no distinct spaces are generally made for expectant mothers in these three communities.

The nourishment regimens of pregnant women in the Khamti and Phake communities are characteristically the same as those of other family members, with few supplementary dishes provided lest the family is socioeconomically better off. In some instances, a pregnant woman's desire for certain foods may be met by her husband, provided that the foods are believed to be innocuous for pregnancy. Among the Ahoms, nourishing items such as eggs, meat, fish, fruits, and milk are occasionally included in a pregnant woman's diet. Some particular food items, however, are circumvented across all three communities during this period; unripe papayas and pineapples, for example, are believed to induce miscarriage. Furthermore, the Ahom community restricts a traditional dish called *Khar*, an alkaloid preparation made from black gram or banana pith, as well as excessive sour fruits, strong spices, and hot chilies during pregnancy, due to concerns over their potentially harmful effects. Bamboo shoots, also known as *Khorisa* or *Nam mai chum*, a common food item in these groups, are also restricted as they are thought to have abortive properties. These exhibit their knowledge regarding commonly available endemic floras at their disposal.

The *Khamti* community observes a variety of taboos and restrictions for pregnant women wherein they are barred from attending funeral rites, visiting burial grounds, or walking under old, large trees. At night, they avoid distant locations to prevent encounters with malevolent spirits. During festivals, these women refrain from touching items used in religious rituals, gathering vegetables from kitchen gardens, or entering granaries. Furthermore, pregnant Khamti women are in the habit of spitting through an opening in the bamboo floor as a practice believed to ensure an easier delivery. They are also forbidden from consuming food prepared for monks at the *Buddha Vihara* (Buddhist Monasteries), a socio-religious ceiling shared with Phake women, who also evade carrying meals to abbots.

The Phake women adhere to numerous restrictions from early pregnancy through childbirth. Even though they can continue with most diurnal errands, they avoid activities such as using needles and thread, stepping on brooms, or touching ropes tied around a cow's neck, mirroring customs in the Ahom community. Furthermore, Phake women are restricted from entering homes where a recent death occurred until after the final funeral rites. Like their husbands, they are also barred from killing animals or birds during pregnancy. Other customs include avoiding nailing walls or sitting on doorsteps.

Among Tai-speaking groups in Assam and Arunachal Pradesh, miscarriage is not uncommon due to its rare occurrence. The demanding physical labor many women undertake during pregnancy, along with limited access to medical care, likely contributes to this phenomenon. Even though natural pregnancy loss is frequent, induced abortion is rare. In urban areas, Khamti women characteristically give birth in hospitals, frequently seeing doctors and taking prescribed supplements. This is in contrast to the rural regions, where healthcare access is minimal, and women seldom seek expert medical care. Instead, they rely on ethnomedicinal treatments and the aid of *dais*, knowledgeable older women who serve as midwives.

In these communities, *Dais* plays an indispensable role in childbirth, especially among the Ahom and Phake groups, where they are often called upon to assist as the mother faces contractions. In Khamti and Phake societies, a trained nurse may assist the *dai*, with doctors consulted only in case of complications during childbirth. In most Ahom relations, however, the "dai" stereotypically supervises the delivery process without help. For a smoother and less painful birth, Khamti women are given sufficient hot water to drink once labor starts, and they adopt a crouching position, which is supposed to ease the delivery process. The Ahom and Phake also practice squatting deliveries for a quicker, less painful experience. The umbilical cord is cut with any sharp implement available, whether a sickle, knife, blade, or bamboo shard.

In due course, after childbirth, mothers are routinely seated near a specifically prepared fireplace for more than a few days. The balminess from the fire is believed to aid the womb's recovery and to ward off malevolent spirits that might harm the mother and newborn. This social practice, intended for both healing and safety, is experientially detected across the Khamti, Ahom, and Phake communities. Following delivery, Khamti mothers follow dietary restrictions, consuming primarily boiled foods while avoiding oily and spicy dishes. They are typically served chicken (*kai*) boiled with black pepper (*mak phit lom*) and papaya (*mak chang phu*). There are some foods, such as sticky rice (*khao no*), sugar (*ku wan*), and pork (*mue*), that are prohibited as these are thought to cause gastric problems.

The Ahom community has distinct rituals associated with life events, such as birth, menarche, marriage, and death. For the well-being of an expected infant, the family takes part in a special ritual in the mother's fifth month of gestation (seventeen to twenty weeks). At this time, the mother of the pregnant woman, or every so often her mother-in-law, offers her a mixture of ghee, honey, milk, sugar, and curd, a ritual known as *Panchamrit*. This custom, characteristically made for a first pregnancy, is supposed to endorse the child's health.

The Ahom expectant mothers observe numerous guidelines to safeguard their health and that of the unborn child. They refrain from stepping over ropes around cows' necks, answering nature's call under large trees, climbing elevated places, crossing rivers, or lifting heavy items. Foods that are intensely bitter, sour, spicy, alkaline, or overly sweet are avoided, and neither the expectant mother nor her husband may kill animals or birds. These customs and restrictions aim to ensure the overall well-being of both mother and child. The family members, especially women, sustain a close watch over the pregnant woman during the initial three months and the final two months of her term, keeping her from going out alone. A small iron knife is often kept beside her, sometimes placed under her bed, as a means of protection against supernatural forces. She also avoids walking beneath raised bamboo structures to prevent the child from developing a weak physique symbolized by bamboo.

In cases of delivery at home with the help of *dais*, the entire household rallies to prepare for childbirth when labor pains commence. The womenfolk organize the designated delivery room, exposing all storage cabinets, which is believed to smooth the birth process. Often a knowledgeable elderly woman from the family or community supports the mother during delivery, tethering a cloth around her abdomen to release severe pain by thwarting its upward movement. The male family members, plus the husband, are barred from entering the delivery room. A fire, made from dry firewood, is lit to guard against infections and harmful spiritual influences. After birth, as per customs, a knowledgeable woman who has had children herself archetypically cuts the umbilical cord using a sterilized piece, such as scissors, a fresh blade, or a bamboo strip. In the immediate postpartum period, the mother is given a simple meal of rice accompanied by a curry made with black pepper, often with chicken prepared in a similar vein, to aid her recovery.

Taking place on the third day following childbirth among the Ahoms, the mother is customarily served a distinct dish called *Kachu Jaal Hkuwa*, prepared with tender colocasia shoots and seasoned with black pepper. In more affluent families, this curry may consist of chicken or duck meat. Ethnomedicinal aromatic plants such as *Manimuni* (*Centella asiatica*), young shoots of *Tezmuri* (*Zanthoxylum nitidum*), *Malkathi* (*Spilanthes clava*) flowers, shoots of *Bihlongoni* (a type of fern), and *Bonjaluk* (*Oldenlandia corymbosa*) are often added. These ingredients are believed to alleviate body aches and promote uterine healing. Fish varieties like *Singi* (*Heteropneustes fossilis*), *Sol* (*Channa striata*), *Senga* (*Channa stewartii*), and *Sengeli* (*Channa gachua*), as well as a unique curry made from mud eel (*Amphipnous cuchia*) with similar herbs and black pepper, are also given to invigorate the mother's health. One more ethnomedicinal practice includes boiling or roasting young shoots of *Hugloti* (*Premna integrifolia*) enfolded in banana leaves, which are consumed daily for up to a month to aid in uterine recovery among the Ahoms in Assam.

Right after birth, thorny plum branches are hung over each door and window to protect the newborn from harmful spirits. The Ahoms also place protective amulets on the infant, such as a fishbone from *Borali*, a small piece of *Boch* root (*Acorus calamus*), a *Latumoni* seed (*Abrus precatorius*), a dried piece of garlic (*Allium cepa*), or a red bead, to guard against black magic and evil influences. A piece of an old fishing net is hung near the mother's room, and mustard seeds in a cloth are placed under the bed or on the wall, all believed to repel malevolent spirits. Visitors are not permitted to enter the mother's room unless they have thoroughly cleansed and consecrated themselves with fire to remove any lingering spirits.

In the survey, it was discovered that maternal health challenges among the Ahom, Khamti, and Phake communities are prejudiced by premature child marriages and high birth rates. These marriages stereotypically occur soon after menarche, particularly in less well-off or rural people, leading to early childbearing. This societal pattern, coupled with a cultural preference for male children, results in high fertility rates that strain women's health. Furthermore, inadequate maternal care in rural areas, where expectant mothers engage in household and agricultural work, exacerbates these health issues. Even though traditional practices remain dominant in these communities, socioeconomic status, educational achievement, and other variables play roles in the maternal health of women in these societies, with women in Northeast India enjoying fairly higher social status than in other parts of India.

Table 16.1. Medicinal Plants Used by the Tai People

Scientific Name, Family Name, and Parts Used	Local Name	Procedure	Dosage and Medicinal Uses	Community
Aerva Sanguinolenta (L.) Family: Amaranthaceae Parts Used: Shoot	Bhung ma ya ja noi (Khamti) Saru Arokson (Assamese)	A decoction is given to nursing mothers as a galactagogue.	About 25 ml once daily for a fortnight.	Khamti
Alpinia galanga(L.) wild Family: Zinziberaceae Parts Used: Rhizome	Heo chang (Khamti) Korphul (Assamese)	The rhizome is cooked with rice and given to the mother after childbirth as a tonic	Once on every alternative day for a month. Used for General weakness	Ahom Khamti Phake
Amaranthus spinosus L. Family: Amaranthaceae Parts Used: Shoot	Phak hon Phak Khun (Ahom) Pu-Lon (Khamti) Pu lum nam (Phake)	A tender shoot is given to nursing as lactagogue.	Several times as vegetable.	Ahom Khamti Phake
Ananaas comosus (A.) Merr. Family: Bromeliaceae Parts Used: Leaf, Unripe fruit	Mak-king-hom (Ahom) Mak-Maha-Nat (Phake)	Leaves are crushed and soaked in water and liquid is given to hasten childbirth. Paste of unripe fruit with black pepper Decoction with black pepper	About 30 ml once or twice within a gap of one hour. 100 ml once daily for a week, used as abortifacient, and griping pain of the abdomen	Ahom, Phake Ahom Khamti Phake
Arundo donax L. Family: Poaceae Parts Used: Rhizome	Mai-oo (Ahom, Khamti, Phake)	Paste with root of *Saccharum spontanerum* (Kuhiar) and rhizome of Alpinia allughus, black pepper is given as lactifuge.	About 10 ml twice daily for a fortnight	Khamti Ahom Khamti Phake

(*Continued*)

Table 16.1 (Continued)

Scientific Name, Family Name, and Parts Used	Local Name	Procedure	Dosage and Medicinal Uses	Community
Alstonia scholaris (L) B.Br. Family: Apocynaceae Parts Used: Tree	Mai dong (Phake) Tun tong (Khamti) Chatiana (Assamese)	Nursing mothers used to pray under the tree to increase breast milk. Or The tender leaves are used for the treatment of mother after childbirth.	Almost every day for a month	Ahom, Phake, Khamti,
Alipinia allughas (Retz.) Rosc. Family: Zinziberaceae Parts Used: Rhizome	Phak bun hyeo (Ahom) Mun hyeo (Khamti) Tora (Assamese)	Paste made from the cooked entrails of kandulifish (*Notopterus notopterus*) is given to eat with rice to women in gripping pain after childbirth. Steamed rice cooked by wrapping with leaves is given to the mother for general health.	Once a day or twice, used for gripping pain Once daily for fifteen days at least, used for General weakness	Ahom Khamti Phake
Bambusa balcooa Family: Poaceae Parts Used: Tender shoot	Mai chang	By making paste	200 gm. Once daily for two days on an empty stomach, used as abortifacient	Khamti
Caryota urens L. Family: Arecaceae Parts Used: Root	Mak buo, Tun buo (Ahom) Cham-chip (Khamti), Chewa goch (Assamese)	Decoction with black pepper is given to nursing mothers lactagogue.	About 25 ml once daily during the nursing period for several days.	Ahom Khamti
Croton-joufra Roxb. Family: Euphorbiaceae Parts Used: Stem bark	Tun-mai-khao-che (Ahom, Khamti) Goch Mahudi (Assamese)	Stem bark juice is boiled with flesh *Mastocembelus pancalus* (chirika fish) with a little common salt is given in postnatal diarrhea	About 30 ml twice daily till cure)	Ahom Khamti

Curcuma longa Family: Zingiberaceae Parts Used: Rhizome	Khao maen	Juice	15 ml daily on an empty stomach for a fortnight, used for blood purifier	Khamti
Calotropis gigantea (L.) R. Br. Family: Asclepiadaceae Parts Used: Leaf	Yang-ken-tha (Ahom) Houng Phouk (Khamti, Phake) Boga Akon (Assamese)	Leaf smeared with mustard oil and used for dry fomentation in cases of body pain and the poultice is also applied to the lower abdomen of women after childbirth, which is said to help in the contraction of the uterus.	Applied everyday upto fifteen days	Ahom Khamti Phake
Carica papaya L. Family: Caricaceae	Mak Chang Phu (Ahom, Phake, Khamti)	Latex of tender fruit is given as abortifacient	About 15 gm is administered thrice daily for a week. It is effective only when given at around eight weeks of pregnancy), used for pregnancy	Ahom Khamti Phake
	Mak Ma La Ka, Mak Mu Lita	Young tender fruit is given as an abortifacient which is said to be effective only for six to seven weeks.		
Celtis tetrandra Roxb. Family: Ulmaceae Parts Used: Tender leaf and shoot	Tun-su-ku-ta (Khamti), Sukuta (Assamese)	Tender leaves and shoots are used as vegetables, which are also said to be useful in loss of appetite and also to relieve the pains, of mothers after childbirth.	Given in curry, useful in loss of appetite and also to relieve pain especially after childbirth	Khami
Clerodandrum viscosum Vent Family: Verbenaceae Parts Used: Root	Tong ping khoum	a piece of root is tied with a black thread around the loin of the expectant mother	One piece, for easy delivery	Khamti
Centella asiatica (L.) Urban Family: Apiaceae	Phe-om-hoi Phak-om-oi-lung (Ahom) Phak-nang (Khamti) Bormanimuni (Assamese) Paste is given in dysmenorhoea	The plant is cooked with mud water fishes like Clerius batrachus (Pla-duk-nam or Pa muk-nam) or Heterupneustes fossilis (Pk-duk ni or Pa muk hi) in general weakness and also given to women during postnatal period, which is said to act as a general tonic and also help in the contraction of the uterus.	Approximately 50 grams are used during a woman's menstrual period to help manage menorrhoea over several days.	Ahom Khamti
Curculigo orchidiodes Gertn (Amary) Family: llidaceae Parts Used: Tuber	Tun-Khang lai (Khamti) Nagini (Assamese)	Tuber paste is given in impotency.	A piece of tuber is tied on the left arm of the pregnant woman and it is said to ensure a male child.	Ahom Khamti

(*Continued*)

Table 16.1 (Continued)

Scientific Name, Family Name, and Parts Used	Local Name	Procedure	Dosage and Medicinal Uses	Community
Cajamus cajan (L.) Millsp. Family: Fabaceae Parts Used: Seed and leaf	Tho-nyeng (Khamti) Rohar mah (Assamese)	The paste is applied over the mammae as lactifuge	Once in every alternative day	Khamti
Colocasia esculenta Family: Araceae Parts Used: Stem	Man (Ahom)	Cooked with black pepper powder sometimes also add chicken or duck meat	used after childbirth for quick healing of the mother	Ahom
i)*Centela asiatica* Family: Apiaceae ii)*Xanthoxylum nitidum* Family: Rutaceae iii) *Hautunia cordata* Family: Saururaceae iv) *Spilanthes clava* Family: Asteraceae v) *Cyclosorus exelca* Family: Thelypteridaceae vi) *Hedyotis corymbosa* Family: Rubiaceae	i)Manimuni ii)Tezmuri iii) Mosundori iv) Malkathi hurbs v) Bihlongoni vi) Bonjaluk (Pa-ta-pa)	Cooked with black pepper powder	used for relief from body ache along with accelerating the healing of the womb after childbirth	Ahom
Dioscorea esculenta (Lour.) Bunk. Family: Dioscoreaceae Parts Used:	Pao man (Khamti) Japani alu (Assamese) Bulb	The roasted bulb is given to women suffering from abdominal gripe during menstruation.	Roasted in open fire and about 50 gm. Bulbil given twice daily, used for the treatment of suffering from abdominal grip during menstruation	Ahom Khamti Phake
Euphorbia hirta L. Family: Euphorbiaceae Parts Used:	Pe-Khep (Khamti) Phak-Khep (Ahom) Gakhiroti bon (Assamese)	Given in curries to nursing mothers to improve lactation.	Once daily at least for one month.	Ahom Khamti

Euphorbia antiquorum Family: Euphorbiceae Parts Used:	Yang kin (Ahom) Li ngu (Khamti, Phake) Siju (Assamese) Stem	Pounded and fried with egg delivered by black hen is given to menorrhagia.	About 20 gm. Stem with two eggs once daily for three days of menses, used for menstrual problem	Ahom Khamti Phake.
Flemigia strobilifera R.Br. Family: Fabaceae Parts Used:	Tun Mung lying (Ahom) Tun ma lam (Khamti) Makhiloti (Assamese) Root	A decoction is given for menstrual irregularity.	About 20 gm. Stem with two eggs once daily for three days of menses, used for menstrual problem	Ahom Khamti
Ipomea aquatic Family: Convolvulaceae Parts Used:	Phak pung Shoot	Curry prepared with lentils (Lens esculentus)	Once daily from the sixth day of childbirth for ten days, used as galactogogue to nourishing mother	Khamti
Ipomea agnatica Forsk. Family: Convolvulaceae Parts Used:	Phak-in nam, Phak- Pung (Ahom, Khamti, Phake) Kolmou (Assamese) Young shoots	Decoction with water in (*Gallinula choloropus*) with black pepper mixed with Musa balbi siana is given to women for contraction of the uterus after childbirth.	About 20 ml once daily for a fortnight.	Ahom Khamti Phake
Jatropha gossipifolia Family: Euphorbeace Parts Used: Root	Tun Khru Khram (Ahom) Tun Kong Nyeng (Phake, Khamti)	Decoction with root of *Sida cordifolia*, sprouted seed of *Vigna mungo*, black pepper, and head of *Pharatima posthuma* with little common salt is given to women after childbirth for contraction of the uterus.	About 100 ml twice daily for a fortnight, used for contraction of uterus	Ahom Khamti Phake
Justicia adhatoda L. Family: Acanthaceae Parts Used: Root and Leaf	Cha-lung Khao (Ahom) Mow la (Khamti) Boga Bahok (Assamese)	Juice is applied as a liniment on the abdomen to hasten childbirth; Warm juice is applied as a massage on the lower abdomen after childbirth for contraction of the uterus.	Several times a day, used for contraction of uterus Twice daily for a fortnight.	Ahom Khamti

(*Continued*)

Table 16.1 (Continued)

Scientific Name, Family Name, and Parts Used	Local Name	Procedure	Dosage and Medicinal Uses	Community
Lagenaria siceraria (Molina) Family: Cucurbitaceae Parts Used:	Mak moup Ahom Khamti Khamyang Aiton Jati Lao (Assamese) Fruit	Juice of roasted fruit is given in gripping pain and body care during menstruation.	50 ml juice is given twice daily for three consecutive days, used for menstrual problem	Ahom Khamti Phake
Murraya koenigii Family: Rutaceae Parts Used: Leaf	Tun phi phan	Garlic with bulbs of ginger is given to children	To protect from evil spirit and prevent fever	Khamti, Khamyang
Mussaenda roxburghii Hook. F. Family: Rubiaceae Parts Used: Leaf and Root	Nai Ya huk kai (Ahom) Yanai (Khamti), Hug Loti (Assamese)	Boiled or roasted in fire wrapping with banana leaf Decoction	Once or twice daily and continue up to one month A cup, boiled and diluted with water, used for quick healing of the womb after childbirth as well as quick healing after delivery	Ahom, Khamti
Musa balbisiana Colla Family: Musaceae Parts Used: Inflorescence	Kui Huin Jang (Aiton) Tun Kui Huin (Ahom) Tun Kui (Phake) Kui Huin (Khamti) Athia kol (Assamese)_	Abnormal inflorescence of non-setting fruits with black pepper is given to women as an antifertility remedy.	Cooked and given to eat, in curry, used as anti fertility	Ahom Khamti Phake
Morus australis Poir. Family: Moraceae Parts Used: Leaf	Nuni (Assamese) Block leng (Ahom) Mo Mun Kai (Khamti, Phake, Aiton, Khamyang)	Decoction with long pepper, black pepper, and flesh of *Ompok pabo* is given in anemia	About 25 ml twice daily for a fortnight, used to treat anemia	
		Paste with *Alpinia galanga* fruit (Korphul) and shoots of *Meyna laxiifolia* is given as general tonic after childbirth.	About 15 gm twice daily for a week, used to treat Weakness About 15 gm Twice daily for a week.	Ahom Phake Khamti

Mimosa pudica L. Family: Mimosaceae Parts Used: Root	Mai ja rap (Ahom) Ya-non (Khamti) Ni-Lajibon (Assamese)	A decoction is given in dysmenorrhoea.	About 15 ml twice daily for three days.	Ahom Khamti
Natasiatus herpeticum Buch. Ham.ex. Arn. Family: Icacinaceae Parts Used: Root	Chik kon them (Khamti)	Juice is applied as a liniment on breasts of women at the time of first childbirth. Make the breast longer and improve lactation.	At least twice daily, used to improve lactation	Ahom Khamti.
Nyctanthes arbor-tristis L. Family: Oleaccae Parts Used: Root	Block-oo- no-cha (Ahom, Khamti) Sewali Phul (Assamese)	Paste mixed with honey is applied to the vagina and is said to help in the conception of barren women.	It is applied from the third day of menses and should continue for a week or more, used for Childlessness	Ahom Khamti Phake
Ocimum basilicum L. Family: Lamiaceae Parts Used: Leaf	Im Khim Phuk (Ahom, Phake, Khamti, Khamyang)	A decoction is given as an emmenagogue after childbirth it is also said to be useful in menorrhagia.	About 15 ml once daily for a fortnight, used for menorrhagia	Ahom Phake Khamti
Piper betle L. Family: Piperaceae Parts Used: Tender	Thao-mao-pu	Decoction	100 ml once daily for three days from the first day of menses, used for menorrhaea	Khamti
Ricinus communis Family: Euphorbiaceae Parts Used:	Tun Khong (Ahom) Tun Po Khong (Aiton) Tun Kung (Khamti) Era goch. (Assamese)	Leaves heated with smeared mustard oil are used to place over the lower abdomen to heal womb after childbirth.	The practice is followed during postnatal period for at least twelve days.	Ahom Khamti Phake.
Rubus rugosus Sm. Family: Rosaceae Parts Used: Root	Nya-tao-lio (Ahom) Mak Pu Khamti Phake Khamyang	Extract is given to relieve pain in dysmenorrhoea.	About 5 ml twice daily for three days from the first day of menses. Used for menstrual problem	Ahom Phake Khamti

(*Continued*)

Table 16.1 (Continued)

Scientific Name, Family Name, and Parts Used	Local Name	Procedure	Dosage and Medicinal Uses	Community
Smilax perfoliata lour. Family: Smilaceae Parts Used: Root	Thao malung rau (Ahom) Nam Kang hang (Khamti, Phake) Tikani Boruah (Assamese)	Juice mixed with black pepper is given with cow's milk for dysentery in women after childbirth.	About 5 ml of juice in 20 ml of milk twice daily till cure. Used for dysentery in women after childbirth	Ahom Khamti Phake
Saraca asoca (Roxb.) Family: Caesalpiniaceae Parts Used: Flower	Tun mok ngong (Khamti)	Paste is given in menorrhagia	About 30 grams twice. Used for menstrual problem	Khamti
Vitex negundo L. Family: Verbenaceae Parts Used: Leaf	Ya Pan (Ahom) Yang Pan (Khamti) Ya pan (Phake) Pocho tia (Assamese)	Roasted leaves in banana leaves in a fire pit are given to the mother after childbirth for contraction of the uterus and to relieve pain.	About 200 grams. Once daily for a fortnight. Used for pain after childbirth	Ahom Khamti Phake.

Source: Authors.

Conclusion and Recommendation

The anthropological efforts form the foundation of current medical anthropology (Janes and Corbett 2009). The study on the three Tai-speaking communities reaffirms that they are still practicing their age-old ethnomedicinal practices even at the turn of the twenty-first century. Even the ones who are highly educated follow the suit of amalgamating the traditional knowledge systems with that of the modern knowledge systems. The infusion of sociocultural and socio-biological practices in the Tai-speaking people showcases their strong connections with their cultural roots. The use of herbs, roots, leaves, and so on, as medicine showcases its potent effectiveness which needs to be promoted as a part of cultural revitalization which is a very important positive aspect of the said community residing in Assam and Arunachal Pradesh. However, the sociocultural aspects of taboos and superstitions are also prevalent variables which act as the determinants of health-seeking behavioral trends in the communities.

The womenfolk of Ahom, Khamte, and Phake are more inclined toward ethnomedicinal practices and also give due significance to undertaking magico-religious practices to recuperate from diverse illnesses under the guidance of *bejes* and *bejnis*. The strong presence of belief in divination, black magic, and white magic is considered to be part and parcel of the social causes of certain diseases among the three communities. As discussed earlier, when a woman becomes incapacitated or unable to perform work, she is usually considered to be affected by the evil eye of bad spirits. Even expecting mothers are not allowed to get checked up at neighboring primary health centers due to their superstitions that modern practices might hamper childbirth, which is considered an act of God by them.

The taboos are strictly observed by them as it is also considered a pollution period. Nevertheless, a social change was observed in the mindset of young mothers who are now availing themselves of basic treatments from primary health care centers in their vicinity frequently. The delivery is also being done in such centers. Moreover, the government of the day employed numerous ASHA (Accredited Social Health Activists) workers to disseminate awareness regarding maternal and child health-related issues among the Tai-speaking women in remote parts of Assam and Arunachal Pradesh. Herein, more and more reliance on institutional delivery practices is a good thing as they are a part of tried and tested modern knowledge systems. In a similar vein, their traditional knowledge systems are also being maintained in the community parallelly, which needs to be lauded.

In the contemporary context, to protect and preserve such oral traditional practices, large-scale research must be done to document their ethnomedicinal practices in their entirety. The present book chapter did document the ethnomedicinal practices of the three Tai-speaking communities in Assam and Arunachal Pradesh. However, such practices are required to be promoted by the government of the day on a large scale so that they are available for all masses and classes. An ethnomedicinal garden can be developed as a part of a newly thought Botanical Garden which would be maintained by the Botanical Survey of India, Govt. of India. Even a specially tailored project on the nature-man-spirit complex can be developed by the Anthropological Survey of India, Govt. of India, which would document social, cultural, and economic facets of such practices which would revitalize and globalize such practices on a larger scale considering the need for harmless alternative medicines as potential solutions in contrast to allopathic medicines which have definite side effects on the human body in the long run.

References

Bal, T. "Relation of Koch and Mughals on Political Realm: From Akbar to Aurangzeb." *International Journal of History* 4 (2021): 48–51.

Baruah, H. "Health Perceptions and Ethnomedicinal Practices among the Tai Khamti in Namsai District of Arunachal Pradesh, India." *Antrocom Journal of Anthropology* 16 (2020): 223–34.

Basu, A. M. *Culture, the Status of Women, and Demographic Behaviour: Illustrated with the Case of India*. Oxford: Clarendon Press, 2004.

Basu, A. "The Pahira: A Population Genetical Study." *American Journal of Physical Anthropology* 31 (1969): 399–416.

Basu, S., A. Jindal, and G. Kshatriya. "Perceptions of Health and Pattern of Health Seeking Behaviour among the Selected Tribal Population Groups of Madhya Pradesh and Orissa." In *Tribal Health in India*, edited by S. Basu. New Delhi: Manak Publications Pvt. Ltd., 1994.

Behera, D. K., and P. Patel, P. "Resource Management through Indigenous Knowledge." *A Special Issue of Journal of Social Sciences* 4, no. 4 (2000): 233–334.

Borah, J., and S. Sengupta. "A Study of Awareness Concerning Reproductive Healthcare Practices: Experience from the Dibongiya Deoris of Assam." In *Indigenous Health Practices among the People of North East India*, edited by S. Sengupta, 137–46. New Delhi: Kalpaz Publications, 2018.

Borah, P. "Indigenous Knowledge and Practices of the Phakeyals: A Study in Barphake Village of Margherita." *The Clarion-International Multidisciplinary Journal* 5 (2016): 98–101.

Buragohain, J. "Ethnomedicinal Plants Used by the Ethnic Communities of Tinsukia District of Assam, India." *Recent Research in Science and Technology* 3 (2011): 31–42.

Das, A., and H. Tag. "Ethnomedicinal Studies of the Khamti Tribe of Arunachal Pradesh." *Indian Journal of Traditional Knowledge* 5 (2006): 317–22.

Doley, P. "Role of Sukapha in Founding Ahom Kingdom in Assam." *Pratidhwani the Echo* 3, no. 1 (2014): 54–7.

Dutta, D. "Some Traditional Plants Used by the Ahoms in Health Management and Medicine in Upper Assam, India." *Antrocom Online Journal of Anthropology* 19 (2023): 197–200.

Gogoi, P. *Tai of Northeast India*. Dhemaji, Assam: Chumphra Printers and Publishers, 1996.

Gogoi, S. "Divination as an Indigenous Practice among the Ahom and the Lua: A Comparative Study." *The South East Asian Review* 46 (2021): 173–85.

Janes, C., and C. Kitty. "Anthropology and Global Health." *Annual Review Anthropology* 38 (2009): 167–83.

Joseph, T. *Tribal People of India*. New Delhi: Indian Social Institute, 1986.

Kalita, D., and B. Phukan. "Some Ethnomedicines Used by the Tai Ahom of Dibrugarh District, Assam, India." *Indian Journal of Natural Products and Resources* 1 (2010): 207–511.

Kar, B. "What Is Ethno-medicine and Why Does It Matter Today?" *Adivasi* 56, no. 1 (2016): 8–16.

Kumar, P., S. Singh, A. Sharma, et al. "Arundo donax L.: An Overview on Its Traditional and Ethnomedicinal Importance, Phytochemistry and Pharmacological Aspects." *Journal of Herbmed Pharmacology* 10 (2021): 269–80.

Mann, R. S. "Animism, Economy, Ecology and Change among Negrito Hunters and Gatherers." In *Nature-Man-Spirit Complex in India*, edited by Rann Singh Mann, 179–208. New Delhi: Concept Publishing Company, 1981.

Oberoi, S, N. Chaudhary, S. Patnaik, and S. Amarjit. "Understanding Health-seeking Behavior." *Journal of Family Medicine and Primary Care* 5 (2016): 463–4.

Paudyal, V., S. Sun, R. Hussain, A. Mohammed, and E. Hedima. "Complementary and Alternative Medicines Use in COVID-19: A Global Perspective on Practice, Police and Research." *Research in Social and Administrative Pharmacy* 18 (2021): 2524–8.

Paul, S., and B. Subrata. *Fieldwork for All*. Kolkata: Dasgupta & Co. Pvt. Ltd, 2022.

Pukhan, S. *Tai Phakes: A Historical & Cultural Study*. EBH Publishers (India), 2015.

Puzari, M., and B. Bailung. "Traditional Use of Plants by the Ahoms in Human Health Management in Upper Assam, India." *Journal of Medicinal Plants Studies* 4 (2016): 48–51.

Rao, V. Srinivasa. *Tribal Livelihood and Governance: Regional Concerns*. Jaipur: Rawat Publications, 2021.

Ripu, K., and R. Bussmann. "Ethnobotany in the Nepal Himalaya." *Journal of Ethnobiology and Ethnomedicine* 24 (2008): 1–8.

Sadir, M. "The Ahoms: Their Origin, Manners and Customs." *Journal of the Royal Society of Arts* 62 (1914): 338–40.

Sarin, J. "'Pradhanpatis' Using Wives as Rubber Stamps Will Frustrate Aim of Women Empowerment: Allahabad HC." *Hindustan Times*, Prayagraj, November 28, 2023.

Sarma, S. N. "Assamese Literature." In *A History of Indian Literature*, edited by Jan Gonda. Wiesbaden: Otto Harrassowitz, 1976.

Sarmah, U., and B. Dutta. "Health Seeking Behaviour and Access to Health Care Services: A Study With Special Reference to Tangsa Tribal Women of Margherita Sub-Division, Assam." *Journal of the Anthropological Survey of India* 67 (2018): 256–66.

World Health Organization. *Summary Reports on Proceedings Minutes and Final Acts of the International Health Conference held in New York from 19 June to 22 July 1946*. World Health Organization, 1948.

17

Indigenous Knowledge Systems of the Great Andamanese Community Residing in Port Blair and Strait Island of Andaman Archipelagos

Sabatini Chatterjee,[1*] Satyaki Paul,[2*] and Jurol[3]

[1]Andaman & Nicobar Regional Centre, Anthropological Survey of India (Ministry of Culture, Govt. of India), Port Blair, Andaman & Nicobar Islands, India

[2]Dr. Ambedkar Chair (Dr. Ambedkar Foundation, Ministry of Social Justice & Empowerment, Govt. of India), KISS Deemed to be University, Bhubaneswar, Odisha, India

[3]Port Blair, Andaman & Nicobar Islands, India

*Corresponding Author's Email: satyakipaul54@gmail.com

Introduction

In the early eighteenth century, surveyors under the then British Raj scouted the Andaman archipelago to create a safe spot for ships in the region during turbulent weather conditions. This particular geographic locale is home to several original inhabitants, including the Andamanese tribal group. The references to Andaman and its populace can be found in the writings of various Arab and Chinese scholars (Cooper 2002). Earlier scholars even linked the original inhabitants with Ramayana, insinuating that they might be the *vanar sena* because the Malays were already calling the place Pulo Handuman (Cadell 1889; Portman 1899; Cooper 2002). The geographic niche was ecologically rich without the presence of any monkeys, and the space was often visited to capture people as slaves, sea slugs, and so on (Cadell 1889). In 1789, the space was first colonized by Captain Archibald Blair with a massive uprising from the local Andamanese populace at Chatham Island (Radcliffe-Brown 1948). The settlement was later shifted to Port Cornwallis (current Diglipur) in the North Andaman region, which was soon abandoned in 1796 owing to inhospitable conditions and attacks from the tribal people (Chakraborty 1990; Saini 2020). In 1858, another massive effort was carried out by the colonial administrators of the then British Raj to create a penal settlement for keeping the prisoners of the First War of Indian Independence away from the mainland. This led to the creation of penal settlements in the region.

Andamanese Homes, colloquially known by the then Great Andamanese as *Góp-l'ăka-báng*, was an initiative started by the colonial administrators to understand the local populace, which would enable them to easily subjugate the tribal masses (Sen 2009; Saini 2020). Several efforts were made wherein the Andamanese populace was divided into two groups for convenience, that is, the Great Andaman Group encompassing the Northern group: *Aka-Cari*, *Aka-Kora*, *Aka-Bo*, *Aka-Jeru*, and Southern group: *Aka-Kede*, *Aka-Kol*, *Oko-Juwoi*, *A-Pucikwar*, *Akar-Bale*, and *Aka-Bea*; and the Little Andaman Group encompassing the Onges of Little Andaman, Jarawas of South Andaman, and the residents of North Sentinel Island (Portman 1899; Radcliffe-Brown 1948). In due course, Aka-Bea was the one who became the first one to come in contact with the British people (Radcliffe-Brown 1948). The *Aka-Bea-Da* subgroup was an intermixture of longshore (*Ar-yauto*) men, creek (*Adajig*) dwellers, and forest dwellers (*Eremtaga*) (Cipriani 1966). In addition, they also became the first ones to become extinct by the beginning of the twentieth century (Radcliffe-Brown 1948). Initially, the numbers of Jarawas were higher than those of other Andamanese groups, which reduced in due course due to punitive expeditions undertaken by the colonial administrators to capture land from the local tribal populace.

In this vein, Portman (1899) observed that "it appears to me quite possible that some disease was introduced among the Jarawas by the people of Lieutenant Blair's Settlement which reduced this tribe considerably in numbers, and this enabled the Aka-Bea-da to obtain the upper hand." Furthermore, Radcliffe-Brown (1922) laments that

> During the last fifty years the numbers of the Andamanese have been greatly diminished. This has been the result of the European occupation of the islands, and is chiefly due to new diseases that have been introduced amongst them. Syphilis was introduced among the tribes of the South Andaman about 1870, and this has now spread among all the Great Andaman tribes that are, excluding the hostile Jarawas. A large number of natives are infected, and the disease is responsible directly and indirectly for a considerable increase in the death-rate.

In due course, the Andamanese were labeled as Great Andamanese to easily differentiate from other tribal populace such as Onges, Jarawas, and Sentinelese (Srivastava et al. 2020).

In addition, the name Great Andamanese stems from their inhabitation of the Great Andaman geographical region which is further subdivided into North Andaman, Middle Andaman, and South Andaman, who are now classified as Particularly Vulnerable Tribal Groups (PVTGs) by the government of the day residing in a specially allotted 6.02 square kilometer reserve area in Strait Islands. Most of the younger generation is now residing in Sri Vijaya Puram (erstwhile Port Blair) to benefit from educational, vocational, and other facilities, creating a unique space for the tribes to socially integrate with the mainstream populace. At present, *Aka-Cari* (Sare) and *Aka-Jeru* are the only two subgroups that have survived out of the original ten subgroups, and in the 1990s, the populace was dwindling at twenty-three to thirty (Dutta 1978;

Chakraborty 1990), now after positive interventions of the Andaman & Nicobar Administration, the number has improved to fifty-eight in 2023–4 (Directorate of Economics & Statistics 2023–4).

The said positive interventions have ameliorated their socioeconomic conditions on one hand; conversely, such close contact with the mainstream has made the Great Andamanese tribal populace overdependent on modern-day traditional knowledge systems and less dependent on their earlier hunter-gatherer lifestyle and culture, factoring in the devastating effects of the Tsunami of 2004 (Khatua 2022). The knowledge systems of the Great Andamanese are evanescing due to disuse and even due to the xenocentrism now developing in the minds of the said people due to the rapid changes in technoscape. The aged populace residing in the Strait Islands is still somewhat following their traditional lifestyle; however, a significant social change is evident among the individuals residing in Sri Vijaya Puram and other parts of the Great Andaman region due to globalization at the turn of the twenty-first century. This study tries to document their knowledge systems and status quo regarding social identity as members of the Great Andamanese. An emic perspective is also presented by the third author, who seeks to throw light on the social customs and practices currently at play among the individuals residing in Sri Vijaya Puram (erstwhile Port Blair) and the Strait Islands of the Andaman Archipelagos.

Objectives and Methods

The Andaman & Nicobar Administration has resettled the Great Andamanese on Strait Island. Accordingly, the elder generation of the Great Andamanese populace resides in the Strait Islands while the younger generation resides in various pockets of the Great Andaman region. However, the Andaman & Nicobar Protection of Aboriginal Tribes (PAT) Regulation, 1956, restricts interaction with the native tribes of Andaman and Nicobar Islands; this also includes the Great Andamanese tribal people who are also considered to be Particularly Vulnerable Tribal Groups (There are five Particularly Vulnerable Tribal Groups in the Andaman Islands such as Great Andamanese, Jarawas, Onges, Sentineles, and Shom Pens. In 1858, the Great Andamanese were estimated at nearly 3,500, and in 1901, their number declined to 625) (Man 1885).

Consequently, conducting full-fledged conventional Malinowskian fieldwork is not possible without the approval of the Tribal Welfare Department of the Andaman & Nicobar Administration. In this situation, this particular study traverses into a different direction by meticulously analyzing already available pieces of literature, including research papers, reports, news articles, and so on, with respect to the Indigenous knowledge systems of the Great Andamanese tribal populace, which is again being conformed and checked by our third author to reaffirm the authenticity of such oral knowledge that still might be in practice among the said community.

Furthermore, this study has added to the repository of profound Indigenous Knowledge with special reference to endemic plants among the Great Andamanese, highlighting the ecological niche as a biodiversity hotspot that needs to be preserved (Table 17.1). The traditional practices and ethnobotanical knowledge for future

Table 17.1. Knowledge Systems and Different Endemic Plants Used by the Great Andamanese

Sl. No	Scientific and Family Name	Local Name	Plant Type	Current Usage Pattern
1	*Dinochloa scandens* Family: Poaceae	Baurat	Shrub	This is used to create fire. Two dry stems are rubbed together to create fire. The smaller stems are also used as a part of a spear that is later used for fishing activities.
2	*Pandanus odoratissimus* Family: Pandanaceae	Oro	Tree	The leaves are used to make cigar-like products.
3	*Pandanus leram* Family: Pandanaceae	Toto	Tree	The girls from the said community create skirts (*totokhudiuye*) from this tree's leaves. The skirt covers from omphalion to the knee region.
4	*Pandanus andamanensium* Family: Pandanaceae	Toto	Tree	The fruits are considered to be their favorite snack and are also cooked with fish. In earlier times, the leaves were also used to make waist girdles which were worn by men during their ceremonial dances.
5	*Musa sapientum* Family: Musaceae	Keofo	Herb	These are used as vegetables and are cooked with other items.
6	*Dendrobium formosum* Family: Orchidaceae	Ekhu	Epiphyte	The stems are used to create waistbands (*chirbele*).
7	*Rinorea bengalensis* Family: Violaceae	Tavo	Shrub	The bark of this shrub is crushed to create a paste-like substance that is rubbed on the chest for chest pain, common colds, coughs, and even dysentery. The leaves are crushed to create a mixture that is used as a cure for headaches.
8	*Rinorea macrophylla* Family: Violaceae	Gene, Takhko	Shrub	The bark and leaves are crushed to create a paste which is applied on the breast to promote lactation.
9	*Premna serratifolia* Family: Verbenaceae	Charo	Shrub	The leaves are crushed to create a paste which is applied to the body to get relief from body aches.
10	*Sterculia macrophylla* Family: Sterculiaceae	Pocho	Tree	The tree trunks are hollowed to create dugout canoes.
11	*Citrus medica* Family: Rutaceae	Miyae	Shrub	The shrub has fruits which is crushed to extract its juice which is effective for the treatment of constipation-related ailments.
12	*Ficus sp. (sur, sycomorus)* Family: Moraceae	Rengo	Tree	The roots are tied to a fractured region of the body.
13	*Ficus nervosa* Family: Moraceae	Kurvo	Tree	These are sweet fruits that are consumed by the said community.

14	*Artocarpus gomeziana* Family: Moraceae	Koeto	Tree	The trunks are used to create dugout canoes.
15	*Haematocarpus Validus* Family: Menispermaceae	Khino	Liana	The flexible stems are used to create traps to capture deer and wild boards. The same stem was also used in hut construction in early times.
16	*Erythrina orientalis* Family: Fabaceae	Laro	Bark	The bark is boiled and the extract is used as a cure for high fever.
17	*Azadirachta indica* Family: Meliaceae	Suruk	Tree	The leaves are boiled and the extract is used to wash wounds of the body.
18	*Pongamia pinnata* Family: Fabaceae	Theep	Shrub	The bark is boiled and the extract is mixed in bath water as a cure for high fever. The twigs are also used as brushes for toothaches.
19	*Ocimum sanctum* Family: Lamiaceae	Tulsi	Shrub	The sap is taken as a cure for common colds.
20	*Thespesia populnea* Family: Malvaceae	Ramo	Tree	In earlier days, the logs are used as fuel during rainy seasons.
21	*Pterocarpus delbergoides* Family: Fabaceae	Chawleke	Tree	The tree trunks are carved into sounding boards (*buamoh*). This is the only musical instrument among all the communities of the Andaman archipelago.
22	*Argyreia hookeri* Family: Convolvulaceae	Bilikhhu	Climber	The leaves are boiled and the extract is applied to reduce swelling. It is also used to cure hydrocele among the males of the said community.
23	*Antidesma coriaceum* Family: Euphorbiaceae	Rae	Shrub	The extract obtained from chewing the leaves is sprayed over the body during honey collection. It is a very effective bee repellent.
24	*Phyllanthus amarus* Family: Euphorbiaceae	Katai	Herb	The leaves are crushed to create a paste which is then applied to snake bites or centipede bites.
25	*Canarium denticulatum* Family: Burseraceae	Dhup	Tree	The trunks are used to create dugout canoes.
26	*Anodendron peniculatum* Family: Apocynaceae	Pharako	Climber	The leaves of this plant have abortive properties and are used by the said community.
27	*Phaeanthus andamanicus* Family: Annonaceae	Berechhell	Tree	The tree's wood is carved out to make bows (*coh*). The same wood is also used to create rudders of a dugout canoe.
28	*Annona squamosa* Family: Annonaceae	Kona	Tree	The leaves of this particular tree are thrown into fire in stormy weather. This local belief is said to have calmed down the stormy weather.

(*Continued*)

Table 17.1 (Continued)

Sl. No	Scientific and Family Name	Local Name	Plant Type	Current Usage Pattern
29	*Semecarpus prainii* Family: Anacardiaceae	Bop	Tree	The plant's flower name is added to a Great Andamanese girl when they have attained puberty (*boptalo*).
30	*Polyalthia jenkinsii* Family: Annonaceae	Khibirtes	Tree	The extract obtained from chewing the leaves is sprayed over the body during honey collection. It is a very effective bee repellent.
31	*Sargassum wightii* Family: Sargassaceae	Chawpo	Seaweed	This is used to treat malarial fever.
32	*Eupatorium odoratum* Family: Asteraceae	Chalechechemo	Herb	The leaves are pulverized and the extract is applied to wounds to stop bleeding.
33	*Tamarindus indica* Family: Caesalpiniaceae	Meo	Tree	The pods are cooked with fish to give it a unique umami flavor.
34	*Carica papaya* Family: Cariacaceae	Pipita	Tree	The leaves are dried and crushed that is later used as a substitute for tobacco.
35	*Calophyllum inophyllum* Family: Clusiaceae	Ta	Tree	The flowers are presented to God as offerings.
36	*Hibiscus tiliaceus* Family: Malvaceae	Bole	Tree	The leaves are crushed and the extract is used to treat stomach disorders.
37	*Macaranga tanarius* Family: Euphorbiaceae	Pharango	Tree	The leaves are used to wrap meats which can increase the life span of the meat for a few days.
38	*Acacia pennata* Family: Mimosaceae	Kamo	Tree	The fruits are eaten as a part of a daily diet.
39	*Ficus retusa* Family: Moraceae	Rengo	Tree	The fiber extracted from the bark is often used to create bow string and even harpoon lines.
40	*Cissus repens* Family: Vitaceae	Gitarafir	Climber	The flexible stems are used to tie down wild boards after hunting.
41	*Tetrastigma lanceolarium* Family: Vitaceae	Girabalo	Climber	The stems are used as a map that directs the way through a jungle.

Source: Authors.

generations to come consider the balance of literature reviews and well-rounded informed analysis being carried out with the aid of our third author, which is therefore creating a confirmative knowledge base. Apart from these, the integration of various perspectives and scholarly discussions with other experts possessing knowledge of endemic flora by the first author as Junior Research Fellow at the Anthropological Survey of India during her stay in the Andaman & Nicobar Islands has thus been instrumental in molding the present work, offering a meticulous understanding of the Great Andamanese community's knowledge systems within the broader sociocultural and ecological landscape.

Profile of the Great Andamanese

In relation to the prior discourse, the Great Andamanese formerly encompassed around ten distinct groups which were divided in accordance with their language and inimitable social-cultural practices (Chakraborty 1990). The 1901 census provides an estimate of around 625 individuals from all ten groups (Radcliffe-Brown 1948). Later, the head count further decreased from 455 in 1922 to 207 in 1921 due to the vices the Great Andamanese community had accrued due to their prolonged contact with the then Britishers (Saini 2020). However, it is estimated that there were around 5,000 to 8,000 able-bodied Great Andamanese individuals who resisted forceful encroachment of the then British Raj during 1788–9. The reinstitution of the settlement at Port Blair in 1858 was naturally begrudged by the Great Andamanese. From April to May 1859, the Great Andamanese launched some premeditated strikes at the British encampments. The first attack took place on April 6, 1859, and the second attack took place on April 14, 1859, wherein 1,500 able-bodied Great Andamanese men participated in the strike with knives and small adzes to disrupt the British occupation in the region (Mathur 1968).

The Battle of Aberdeen is a historic fight that took place on May 17, 1859, which was thwarted by the then British due to a betrayal of Doodhnath Tewarry (Sasikumar 2023). It was one of the most significant premeditated freedom struggles carried out by the Great Andamanese community against the then British colonial administrators.

> In the fight at Aberdeen in the year 1859 several tribes were present such as the Port Campbell South Tribe, the Port Mouat North and South Tribes, and the Labyrinth and Rutland Island Tribes, about 250 men in all. Most of the Andamanese that took part in it are yet alive, and are now living peacefully at the Home. The Port Mouat South Tribe led the fight, of whom Maia Ria-lola was the Chief. (Portman 1899)

However, the defeat caused the deaths of numerous able-bodied Great Andamanese men which reduced the gene pool of the total population in due course of time (Chakraborty 1990).

Since then, the socio-demography of the Great Andamanese populace has started a downward spiraling effect. The Andaman Homes initiative also depopulated the said community as they were forced to stay in contact with outsiders, wherein they had to succumb to unknown diseases such as influenza, measles, and so on (Radcliffe-Brown 1948). In 1949, after two years of Indian independence from the then British Raj, the Great Andamanese community was resettled in Bluff Island, where the ecological niche was appropriated to meet the daily livelihood of the tribal populace (Avtans 2012; Saini 2020). The populace further shrank to nineteen by 1961, wherein in 1969, they were again resettled in Strait Island, which led to the present booming figure of fifty-eight in 2023–4 (Directorate of Economics & Statistics 2023–4). These resettlements also led to a degree of change in their hunting-gathering lifestyle to waiting for financial assistance toward present sedentary mainstream livelihood options. Nevertheless, such a change in livelihood cannot be compared to the last straw, which led to the serious collision to exterminate the then British settlement in the Battle of Aberdeen, leading to increased pacification of the then colonial administrators. The ire led to the total evanescing of the *Aka-Bea* group at the beginning of the twentieth century, who were considered to be the first groups to come in contact with the then colonial administrators (Sen 2010). Such a kind of pacification led to the cultural ethnocide of most of the groups of the Great Andamanese tribal community.

In the recent past, *Adi Basera* was set up in Port Blair (currently Sri Vijaya Puram) which acts as a home away from home, considering the distance in sea routes and the havoc caused by the tsunami of 2004. In early 2010, the *Aka-Bo* dialect and *Aka-Kora* died with their last speakers (Majumdar 2021). The *Aka-Cari* (*Sare*) is also considered to be lost considering the death of the last speaker Licho, but the third author claims that there are still some practitioners of the Sare language from the Great Andamanese community. Currently, the locals including the Great Andamanese are still reliving the horrors of the tsunami of 2004 and the death of *Jirake* in 2005. The death of *Jirake* in 2005 led to the coronation of his wife as Queen *Surmai* (Majumdar 2005) which was also new for them. The incumbent queen is growing old and now the question is who is going to succeed her as the new king. And will he try to opt for a cultural revitalization of the community is the million-dollar question considering the tepid state of awareness regarding their Indigenous knowledge systems.

Knowledge Systems of the Great Andamanese

The Great Andamanese were born hunter-gatherers, and they could easily understand their ecological niche due to their lived experiences that molded the Indigenous knowledge system which they possessed since time immemorial and was passed down from one generation to another in the form of oral traditions. The trial and error method is innate to their closeness with nature, wherein they would differentiate between rainy (Jeichar), summer (Khirnu), and cold (Thow) seasons. They usually recognize these seasons through the appearance of seasonal fruits and flowers, where *jillital* (*jilli* flower) indicates the advent of summer, *tipak* flower denotes mid-summer, while *fuchotal* is seen when the rainy season starts, *reyetal* during the season, and *pedak* indicates full rainy season (Chakraborty 1990). They even recognize spaces with good fish to catch and when it will be most tasty using flowers and fruits.

As per their knowledge on garjan, jikar, tochol flower blooms, they ensure the right time to catch fish on shore (sardines) and creek (*katla*) and in shallow waters (for *red bhetki*). The perfect fishing time was post-ebb (*charejeo*) conditions and from dusk to dawn, they used to look for turtles and dugongs. The dugong was an important animal for them to hunt, as it was believed that one who hunted dugong would be considered a fine warrior among all male Great Andamanese. They also consume locally available wild boar during the rainy season, which is the best time because these animals accumulate fat during this period. In contrast, hunting turtles is omitted in the rainy season due to low-fat content in that specific season.

In the past, there was *akachaphan* (eldest member of the group who acted as leader of the whole tribe) who was also considered to be the traditional healer. He/she used to administer medicine by using ethnomedicinal plants for curing an individual in the group (Awasthi 1991). The Great Andamanese differentiate soil types into different types like *khar* (sandy), *keyeb* (red clay), *kaat* or *bung* (mud), *maaw* (hard), *lim* (soft), odu (white clay), and *tal* (powdery white clay). The knowledge systems of the Great Andamanese considered that soil to be an important part of traditional healing practices. In *Jeru* dialect, the third author points out that the following healing practices are still in use amid the said community:

(a) Itching (*Yaoh*): A paste of red clay (*keyeb*) is applied to the body;
(b) Vomiting: The white clay (*odu*) is mixed with water which is later drunk by the individual;
(c) Snakebite: A cord is tied above the snake bite and white powdery clay (*tal*) is applied to the region. However, the concept of poison is unknown to them;
(d) Stomachaches: The white clay (*odu*) is mixed with water which is later drunk by the individual.

Apart from *akachaphan*, there was a concept of *erjum* (leader of the hunting and gathering group) who had the power to ward off evil spirits (*lau*). The person used to chant *khiyanchebem khuyalanthiktefak marakayech* (you are not part of us, go away from here). And before venturing out to open seas, the *erjum* used to chant *mime bawrbetang para bothe thhuthirekho natchlebam thhibitai siralive* (make the air soothing, my boys are going to hunt, do not deceive them) (Chakraborty 1990). At present, Queen Surmai is leading the Great Andamanese after the death of her husband King Jirake, which presents a unique turn where for the first time a queen was appointed as leader of the Great Andamanese community (Majumdar 2005). Before Jirake, Loka was the king of the Great Andamanese (Chakraborty 1990). There was also a prevalence of ultimogeniture which is now reversed to primogeniture similar to what the mainstream populace follows; this may be the result of years of acculturation (Khatua 2022).

The concept of ebb (*charejeo*) and high tide (*charebefile*) is also present in their Indigenous knowledge system wherein *eno* (master of water) resides in the sea and emits or takes in water which causes it to rise and ebb (Chakraborty 1990). The idea of building a canoe was from visualizing the rainbow (*billiro*) which is used by evil spirits (*lau*) to move from one place to another. It is also thought that evil spirits (*lau*) collectively shake the earth which leads to earthquakes (*thizit*), which is an interesting theory. It can be noted that in the statement the Great Andamanese people knew that a tsunami was coming wherein late *Licho* (who died in 2020) observed that "Jirake was a great king, and he told us two days in advance that the sea was getting warm and there would be a flood. How right he was!" (Majumdar 2005).

The Great Andamanese also used to divide jungle regions by judging: the closeness to shore, an area affected by the tide, the area with underwater rocks, and deep-sea regions. They used to understand the depth of water using the changes in sound produced by the boat on the water, which is unique. The day was also divided into the degree of heat, and they used to believe that the sun that had risen was different from the one that is setting down. The nighttime is also divided into parts where the time and date were calculated from one full moon (*baradul*) to a new moon (*lechar*). The concept of minute and hour was not present, and they never used to start to obtain direction. The long rope (*luremo*) that was used for hunting turtles was earlier used as a measure of distance. Furthermore, in terms of death rituals in the past, it can be observed that sun burial and cremation were carried out wherein warriors were cremated while sun burial was considered to be the most prestigious one that was reserved for the *akachaphan* (leader) of the said community. Nowadays, the members of the Great Andamanese community are usually cremated at a crematorium or sometimes they follow traditions of other religions in case of marrying into other communities.

In the contemporary context, the third author noted that some changes are being made to ease the tasks associated with several social rites. Herein in the recent past, the third author had undergone the puberty stage where she noted that there was a certain degree of changes in the turtle eating ceremony. A girl has to sit for three days at her parents' house with folded arms and legs stretched out in front with two big toes touching each other. The individual has to face the sea in such a manner that a fireplace would also be present near her/his body. The person is also massaged with turtle fat (*choukvi*). The next day a turtle is caught which is boiled in an aluminum pot. The body of the person is decorated with white clay (tolo odu) in a zigzag pattern. Once the ritual is completed, then yellow leaves (*boltaich*) are tied around the waist of the person. The person is fed turtle meat along with tea, which is a newer addition to the ceremony (Chakraborty 1992). In due course of feeding, the person who feeds the concoction chants *odanta auphil taraf thui jaitocha aifefuro kotrai thuijoitachefol* (the meat is offered to you in the same manner as it is offered during the funeral). The entire family starts wailing in remembrance of all the ancestors or family members who are now not present in this particular life-changing ritual. The third author notes that Hindi is now the main language which is used to communicate with everyone. Nevertheless, they are now trying to relearn their own language bit by bit and most of the social rites are in disuse. But this ceremony continues to be a significant part of their life-changing rituals considering other evanescing social rites.

Conclusion and Recommendation

The innate closeness to nature is evident in the knowledge system of the Great Andamanese community. This can be further linked to the concept of a nature-man-spirit complex which the cultural ethos showcases due to their mundane interaction with the sea, forest, flora, and fauna for their sustenance considering the harsh climatic conditions of the sea. The tribe was shifted multiple times considering their first contact with the British people to the postindependence shift to Bluff Island to Strait Island at present. The cultural ethnocide was initiated by the then colonial administrators of the British Raj and began with the evanescing of the Aka-Bea subgroup. Later, numerous social interventions were undertaken to recuperate the numbers in this tribe. Later, a few islands were scouted and prepared to meet the needs which include their basic needs (to satisfy their cultural institutions), instrumental needs (like their socioeconomic needs), and their integrative needs (their religion, myth, morals, values, etc.). This is how Strait Island was selected as a suitable space for their stay. At present, the government of the day is trying to preserve and conserve once-thriving oral traditions, medicinal practices, ecological wisdom, and social customs which are now at risk of fading into obscurity due to close contact with the mainstream.

However, not all social change is erroneous, because the selection of *Surmai* as Queen in 2005 after the death of the then King *Jirake* is a welcome move which symbolizes the adaptability of the community to meet modern times. Their traditional ecological knowledge—encompassing sustainable hunting and gathering techniques, the medicinal properties of native flora, and intricate knowledge of marine and terrestrial ecosystems—holds immense value, particularly in an era of global environmental crises. The wisdom embedded in their folklore, rituals, and social organization offers invaluable insights into human resilience, coexistence with nature, and the preservation of biodiversity. If these knowledge systems are allowed to vanish, the world will lose an irreplaceable repository of wisdom that has survived several eras. The Directorate of Health Services, A&N administration is trying to counsel youths against the ill effects of tobacco and alcohol. Special de-addiction camps are also organized at Straight Island; for skin problems, a dermatologist has been deputed on duty-cum-tour to Straight Island, and the children are provided quality education and sports facilities (the third author along with another female Phigar is receiving training in archery). Along with said interventional activities, medical camps are also being organized from time to time.

At this critical juncture, the urgency of documentation cannot be overstated. A systematic effort must be undertaken to record, preserve, and revitalize the indigenous knowledge of the Great Andamanese before it is lost forever. This necessitates the formation of a dedicated committee constituted by the Andaman & Nicobar Administrators comprising anthropologists, ethno-historians, and, notably, community elders who are the true knowledge bearers of tangible and intangible aspects of Great Andamanese culture. The role of such a committee should not be limited to mere documentation but should extend to fostering intergenerational knowledge transmission within the community itself. Educational initiatives, storytelling programs, and cultural workshops can serve as vital tools to reignite interest and pride among younger generations in their ancestral legacy. Furthermore, any effort to preserve indigenous knowledge must be undertaken with the utmost sensitivity and respect for the community's agency.

Historically, Indigenous communities across the world have been subjected to exploitative documentation practices, where their knowledge was extracted without their consent and appropriated for external purposes. To avoid repeating such injustices, the Great Andamanese themselves must play a central role in the documentation process, ensuring that their narratives are recorded through their perspectives and voices. The inward gaze is important to enable in-depth documentation of pieces of information in relation to the culture and its subcultures. In addition to documentation, active cultural revitalization efforts must be pursued by Andaman Adim Janjati Vikas Samiti (AAJVS)—Andaman & Nicobar Administration.

Language, which serves as the vessel of cultural memory, is a crucial aspect of indigenous knowledge. Moreover, with the Great Andamanese languages dwindling in use, there is an urgent need to develop language preservation programs, including the creation of digital atlases, digitized dictionaries, online accessible oral history archives, and educational materials that encourage linguistic continuity. Traditional practices, such as ethnomedicinal plant usage and artisanal craftsmanship (*buamoh* making), should be revived through community-led initiatives that integrate Indigenous knowledge into contemporary livelihoods. To end, if proactive measures are taken now in mission mode, there remains hope that the rich sociocultural remains of this tribe will not be relegated to books but will continue to flourish as a living tradition. If ignored, however, we risk allowing a time-tested Indigenous knowledge system to disappear, leaving future generations bereft of the knowledge that was once an innate part of Andaman & Nicobar Islands.

References

Avtans, A. "The Rise and Fall of the Great Andamanese." *Linguistica Indica*, April 8, 2012.

Awasthi, A. "Ethnobotanical Studies of the Negrito Islanders of Andaman Islands, India: The Great Andamanese." *Economic Botany* 45 (1991): 274–80.

Cadell, T. "The Andamans and Andamanese." *Scottish Geographical Magazine* 5 (1889): 57–73.

Chakraborty, D. *The Great Andamanese*. Calcutta: Seagull Books, 1990.

Chakraborty, D. "The Turtle Eating Ceremony among the Great Andamanese." *Journal of Anthropological Survey of India* 41 (1992): 11–17.

Cipriani, L. *The Andaman Islanders*. London: Weinfeld & Nicolson, 1966.

Cooper, Z. *Archaeology and History: Early Settlements in the Andaman Islands*. New Delhi: Oxford University Press, 2002.

Directorate of Economics & Statistics 2023–4. *Basic Statistics: Demographic – A&N Islands*. Directorate of Economics & Statistics Andaman & Nicobar Administration, 2024.

Dutta, P. *The Great Andamanese: Past and Present*. Kolkata: Anthropological Survey of India, 1978.

Khatua, N. "Anthropology Vanishing Tribal Culture: A Case of Great Andamanese Tribe of Andaman Islands." *Journal of the Andaman Science Association* 27 (2022): 196–203.

Majumdar, A. "Disappearing Dialects." *Millenium Post*, June 05, 2021.

Majumdar, B. "Tribals Defy Custom, Bow to Queen – Great Andamanese Gear Up to Coronate First Woman." *The Telegraph*, December 12, 2005.

Man, E. *On the Aboriginal Inhabitants of the Andaman Islands*. London: Royal Anthropological Institute of Great Britain and Ireland, 1885.

Mathur, L. *History of the Andaman and Nicobar Islands (1756–1966)*. New Delhi: Sterling Publishers, 1968.

Portman, M. *History of our Relations with the Andamanese (Vol I and II)*. Calcutta: Office of the Superintendent Government Printing India, 1899.

Radcliffe-Brown, A. R. *The Andaman Islanders: A Study in Social Anthropology*. Cambridge: Cambridge University Press, 1922.

Radcliffe-Brown, A. R. *The Andaman Islanders*. Illinois: The Free Press, 1948.

Saini, A. "As COVID-19 Reaches the Andaman Islands, the Story of the Great Andamanese Tribe Should be a Wake-up Call for Administrators." *The Hindu*, July 18, 2020.

Sasikumar, M. *The Sentinel Islanders*. New Delhi: Manohar, 2023.

Sen, S. "Savage Bodies, Civilized Pleasures: M.V. Portman and the Andamanese." *American Ethnologist* 36 (2009): 364–79.

Sen S. *Savagery and Colonialism in the Indian Ocean: Power, Pleasure and the Andaman Islanders*. New York: Routledge, 2010.

Srivastava, V., U. Kumar, M. Sasikumar, V. Pulamaghatta, S. Patel, and P. Goyal. "Draft of the Policies for Great Andamanese and Sentinelese." *Journal of the Anthropological Survey of India* 69 (2020): 165–76.

Part V

Indian Knowledge System and Ethnomedicinal Values

18

Concept of Ayurveda, Siddha, and Unani in Indian Traditional Knowledge System and Ethnomedicinal Values

Gour Gopal Satpati*

Department of Botany, Bangabasi Evening College, University of Calcutta, Kolkata, India

*Corresponding Author's Email: gour_satpati@yahoo.co.in

Introduction

According to the World Health Organization (WHO), 80 percent of people in developing nations receive all of their primary medical care from traditional medicine. The word "traditional" refers to a historical, cultural, and folk medical system that would be considered "alternative" in a Western setting; it does not mean conventional or allopathic (Rupani and Chavez 2018). India is renowned for its Ayurvedic, Siddha, and Unani ancient medical systems. Even the ancient Vedas and other texts make reference to medical systems (Pandey, Rastogi, and Rawat 2013). Traditional medicine uses different plants and preparation methods depending on the location. Additionally, traditional medicines, particularly herbal ones, are becoming more and more accepted in the developed world. Due to their creative qualities, reduced toxicity, and negligible side effects, traditional medical systems have greatly increased in popularity worldwide.

Ayurveda: Holistic System of Medicine

One of the world's oldest medical specialties is traditional Indian medicine. The most popular system of ancient Indian medicine, Ayurveda, places a strong emphasis on holistic treatment, which considers the body, mind, and spirit as one. Ayurveda literally means "science of life," as the ancient Indian medical system was centered on understanding human nature and ailment. It has been noted that people with good health have well-balanced metabolisms. It is predicated on the idea that peaceful living with nature is how humans attain physical, mental, and emotional well-being (Shi, Zhang, and Li 2021). Ayurveda is not a diet plan for people looking for a way out or a reason to continue mistreating their bodies or minds. It is a system of long life, independence, and empowerment. Over the course of more than two millennia, Ayurvedic treatments have changed and developed. Herbal remedies, specific diets, massage, yoga, meditation, laxatives, enemas, and medical oils are examples of therapies. Usually, complex plant compounds, minerals, and metal components serve as the basis for Ayurvedic remedies (perhaps influenced by early Indian alchemy or rasashastra). Surgical procedures such as rhinoplasty, lithotomy, sutures, cataract surgery, and the removal of foreign objects were also taught in ancient Ayurvedic writings.

(a) **History and Concepts:** From the middle of the first millennium BC onward, there is historical evidence for Ayurvedic writings, vocabulary, and concepts. The primary classical books on Ayurveda start with stories of how the gods passed down medical knowledge to sages, who in turn passed it on to human doctors. The Sushruta Samhita, also known as Sushruta's Compendium, is presented in printed form as the teachings of Dhanvantari, the Hindu Ayurvedic deity who took on the form of King Divodāsa of Varanasi, to a group of doctors, among them Sushruta. However, the earliest versions of the text do not include this frame and instead attribute the work to King Divodāsa. Baba Hari Dass in the 1970s and Maharishi Ayurveda in the 1980s were two notable figures who modified Ayurveda for Western consumption. The three fundamental ideas, known as doshas (vata, pitta, and kapha), are based on five aspects of Indian philosophy. The doshas of Ayurveda can be recognized as regulatory control factors for basic physiological processes in living systems that have maintained their identity throughout biological history: pitta and its subdoshas regulate throughput, turnover, and thus energy; kapha and its subdoshas regulate storage, structure, and lubrication; and vata and its subdoshas regulate input/output processes and motion (Kumar, Dobos, and Rampp 2016).

(b) **Plant-Based Remedies:** Plants are the basis for 90 percent of Ayurvedic treatments. Plant-based remedies in Ayurveda can be made from roots, leaves, fruits, bark, or seeds; cardamom and cinnamon are two examples of plant-based ingredients (Kumar, Dobos, and Rampp 2016). Hundreds of plant-derived medications were compiled by William Dymock and others in the nineteenth century, together with information on their use, microscopic makeup, chemical makeup, toxicology, common myths and stories, and connection to British Indian trade. A popular herbal remedy is triphala, which is a mixture of three fruits: amalaki, bibhitaki, and haritaki. (Peterson, Denniston, and Chopra 2017). In Ayurveda, the herbs *Ocimum tenuiflorum* (tulsi) and *Withania somnifera* (ashwagandha) are also frequently utilized. Table 18.1 highlights the plant-based substances and remedies used in the Indian Ayurvedic system.

(c) **Diagnosis:** Ayurveda categorizes illnesses into two groups: those that can be treated medically or surgically and those that cause mental and physical "pain" for the three reasons listed above. Instead of the disease itself, diagnosis and therapy are typically human traits. Prior to making a diagnosis, the doctor should take into account the patient's age, living situation, social and cultural

Table 18.1. Plant-Based Substances or Plants Used in the Indian Ayurvedic System. Source: Author.

Plants/Plant-Based Substances Used in Ayurveda	Remedies
Cardamom—*Elettaria cardamomum*	Detoxification, digestion, and cure respiratory health issues
Cinnamon—*Cinnamomum verum*	Cure muscle and joint pain, joint aches, arthritis
Triphala: Polyherbal formulation Amalaki—*Phyllanthus emblica* Bibhitaki—*Terminalia bellirica* Haritaki—*Terminalia chebula*	Used to treat digestive problems including stomach ulcers, hyperacidity; skin-related disorders and arthritis
Ashwagandha—*Withania somnifera*	Stress management, anxiety, improves immunity, memory development, inflammation, muscle strength
Tulsi—*Ocimum tenuiflorum*	Used to treat asthma, cough, and cold
Opium—*Papaver somniferum*	Used as antispasmodic, analgesic, and antitussive agents
Achira/Edible canna/ Indian shot—*Cannabis indica*	Used to treat diarrhea, dysentery, fever, dropsy, and malaria

background, and constitution. Seeing the disease's symptoms and indicators is the primary method of diagnosis. Skin tone, eyes, urine, feces, and tongue coating can all serve as diagnostic markers. Three categories of mental energy—Satwa, Rajas, and Tamas—may be distinguished in Ayurvedic treatment, which can also help patients relax. These three types of energy working in harmony can protect people from illness and interference, awaken their senses, and inspire them to pursue peace. According to Indian medical professionals, mental health is the most important aspect of human health since it has a direct impact on physical health.

Siddha: Achievement and Perfection

"Siddha" is a Sanskrit term meaning "one who is accomplished" or "perfected," often referring to a spiritual master who has attained a high level of enlightenment or mastery. It is derived from the Sanskrit word "siddhi," which means "achievement" or "perfection." It is used in Hinduism and Jainism to describe a person who has reached spiritual liberation. Siddha Medicine also refers to a traditional Indian medical system originating in Tamil Nadu, often associated with the teachings of the "Siddhars." Thus, the Siddha medicinal system not only focuses on treating the disease but it also takes into account the patient's behavior, environmental aspects, age, habits, and physical condition.

(i) **History and Concepts:** The ancient Indian traditional healing method known as siddha originated in South India, primarily in Tamil Nadu. The Hindu god

Shiva is claimed to have introduced the system of this treatment to his consort Parvati, according to ancient Siddha literature. Afterward, Parvati gave it to Nandi, who informed nine Devtas about it. Siddhar Agasthyar is regarded as the founder of this medicinal system, despite the fact that its origin is thought to be divine. The primary contributions to this medical system are eighteen well-known Siddhars. The original Siddha writings and treatises were composed in Tamil. One of the world's first systems of traditional medicine, it treats the mind and soul in addition to the body. The Tamil term Siddhi, which means "an object to be attained," "perfection," or "heavenly bliss," is where the word Siddha originates. According to Siddha, illness results from a disruption in the normal balance of the three humors, which are collectively referred to as mukkuttram: vaadham (airy), pittham (fiery), and kapam (watery). The environment, climate, food, exercise, and stress are thought to have an impact on this balance. The ratios of Vaadham, Pittham, and Kapam are 4:2:1 under typical circumstances. The Siddha system states that the five elements of nature—earth, water, fire, air, and ether—are the fundamental building blocks of all physical objects. It is thought that the microcosm of the physical body and the macrocosm of the outside world are closely related. Bone, flesh, nerves, skin, and hair are the elements of earth; blood, semen, glandular secretions, and sweat are the elements of water; hunger, thirst, sleep, beauty, and indolence are the elements of fire; contraction, expansion, and motion are the elements of air; and the interstices of the stomach, heart, neck, and head are the elements of ether.

(ii) **Plant-Based Remedies:** Plant-based, mineral, and animal products are used in Siddha medicine, an age-old traditional medical system from South India that focuses on treating the underlying causes of illnesses rather than just their symptoms (Joseph Thas 2008). Most commonly used herbs in the Siddha medicine system are highlighted in Table 18.2.

(iii) **Diagnosis:** The Siddha medical system employs a number of techniques to identify illnesses, such as assessing the patient's voice, body color, digestion, pulse, tongue, and eyes. The patient's traits, surroundings, and other elements are taken into consideration when making the diagnosis. A range of therapeutic approaches is used in Siddha medicine, including herbal remedies, dietary and lifestyle advice, yoga, meditation, massage, and detoxification treatments. Several methods of diagnosis include Naa (Tongue examination), Naadi (Pulse examination), Niram (Examination of body complexion), Malam (Stool examination), Neer (Urine examination), and so on. Factors responsible for the treatment considerations are age, race, sex, habits, habitats, physical and mental state, and so on.

Table 18.2. Plant-Based Remedies in Siddha. Source: Author.

Plants/Plant-Based Substances Used in Siddha	Remedies
Ashwagandha—*Withania somnifera*	Stress management, anxiety, improves immunity, memory development, inflammation, muscle strength
Triphala: Polyherbal formulation Amalaki—*Phyllanthus emblica* Bibhitaki—*Terminalia bellirica* Haritaki—*Terminalia chebula*	Used to treat digestive problems including stomach ulcers, hyperacidity; skin-related disorders and arthritis
Bael—*Aegle marmelos*	Used to cure inflammation, digestive problems, asthma, fever, diabetes with potential antioxidant and antimicrobial properties
Neem—*Azadirachta indica*	Used for skin disorders, fever, skin ailments, dental problems
Brahmi—*Bacopa monnieri*	Powerful antioxidants, reduces stress and anxiety, inflammation and boost brain function
Amla—*Phyllanthus emblica*	Used to cure diabetes, skin and hair problems, anemia, digestion and heart problems
Turmeric—*Curcuma longa*	Powerful antioxidant, boost immunity, cure inflammation, cancer and liver health issues, skin disorders
Chyawanprash—Polyherbal formulation including clove (*Syzygium aromaticum*), cardamom (*Elettaria cardamomum*), cinnamon (*Cinnamomum verum*)	Boost digestion and immunity, cure respiratory health, enhance vitality, delaying aging process
Atis/Patis/Mohra—*Aconitum heterophyllum*	Used to treat diarrhea, dyspepsia, diabetes, and abdominal pain

Unani: Humoral System of Medicine

Unani medicine is a traditional medical system that originated in Greece and is based on the teachings of Hippocrates. It is practiced in South Asia and Central Asia. Unani medicine recognizes the mental, emotional, spiritual, and physical causes of illness or health and believes that each individual should take responsibility for their own well-being. Thus, Unani is a humoral system that seeks to balance the four humors—Dam, Balgham, Ṣafrā, and Saudā.

a. **History and Concepts:** Unani medicine, also known as Yunani medicine, is Perso-Arabic traditional medicine used in Muslim communities in South Asia and contemporary Central Asia. Unani medicine is not really science that is, pseudoscientific. Early Unani medicine was influenced by Arab and Persian elaborations of the Greek medical system by individuals such as Ibn Sina and al-Razi. During Alexander's invasion of India, Unani medicine and Indian Buddhist medicine collaborated. The similarities between the two systems' fundamental conceptual frameworks demonstrate the extensive knowledge interchange that took place at the time. With the founding of the Delhi Sultanate in the twelfth century, the Islamic medical legacy was brought to India. During the Mughal Empire, it developed on its own, influenced by Sushruta and Charaka's Indian medical teachings. At his royal courts, Alauddin Khalji (d. 1316) had a number of distinguished physicians, or Hakims. The growth of Unani in India and the production of Unani literature were both influenced by this royal sponsorship. Greco-Arab medicine, another name for Unani medicine, is an ancient medical system that has its roots in Greece. It has a long-standing idea and set of drug management principles and is more prevalent in the Indian Subcontinent. This medical technique is even regarded by some authorities as holistic. It contains medications with a natural identity and origin. If not appropriately detected, isolated, processed, and administered, it could be dangerous (Rahman, Khan, and Latif 2008). Although Unani medicine has been influenced by Indian and Chinese traditional systems, its Hellenistic roots are still evident in its foundation in the ancient four humors: phlegm (balgham), blood (dam), yellow bile (ṣafrā), and black bile (saudā').

b. **Plant-Based Remedies:** The Unani medical system is acknowledged by the WHO as an alternative method of meeting the population's medical needs. In the Unani medical system, medications originating from plants, animals, and minerals are the main sources of medication (Kamartaha, Kavi, and Vinay 2021). Numerous herbs, such as costus, atis/patis (Greenish Himalayan Monkshood), calamus, and khubazi, are utilized in Unani medicine. Table 18.3 shows some important medicinal plants in the Unani system.
c. **Diagnosis:** In the Unani medical system, the three most crucial components for disease diagnosis are the examination of the baul (urine), the stool (baraz), and the pulse (nabz). A person's health is greatly influenced by their environment and the ecological conditions. A patient's pulse, urine, and stool are examined, together with their temperament and humors, in order to

Table 18.3. Common Plants Used in the Unani System. Source: Author.

Plants Used in Unani	Remedies
Costus/Insulin plant—*Costus speciosus*	Lower blood sugar levels, Cure asthma, fever, and inflammation
Calamus—*Calamus tenuis, C. erectus*	Restore blood glucose level, Cure stomach disorders, inflammation, piles and, fevers
Khubazi/Khubbazi—*Malva sylvestris*	Used to treat injuries, inflammation and, urinary problems
Atis/Patis/Greenish Himalayan Monkshood—*Aconitum heterophyllum*	Used to treat abdominal pain, cough, fever
Bhuiamla/Bhuiavla/Kiru Nelli—*Phyllanthus amarus*	Rich in antioxidant, Cure diabetes, stomach disorders, inflammation, skin infection, viral infection
Ajwain/Bishop's weed—*Trachyspermum ammi*	Improve digestion by secreting gastric juices

identify illness in Unani medicine. The full personality of the patient is also taken into account by Unani medicine, including their physical characteristics, means of self-defense, response to their surroundings, and preferences. Other methods commonly used include inspection, palpation, questioning, occlusion, and percussion.

Conclusion and Future Directions

Herbal medications are progressively making their way from the fringe to the mainstream market as more and more individuals turn to complementary treatment and become concerned about the negative effects of synthetic drugs. A WHO survey indicates that 80 percent of people worldwide feel hopeful about the advancement of traditional medicine and are open to using herbal remedies as their primary form of treatment. More than 3,000 types of medicinal plants and over 6,000 types of herbs are utilized by people in India, which has abundant herbal plant resources. Approximately 75 percent of herbal species in developing nations are produced in more than 1,000 factories. Indian medicine has a strong scientific foundation and has recently gained recognition. Nonetheless, there are still a lot of obstacles to overcome in the promotion of herbal therapy, particularly in affluent nations.

1. Acknowledgments: The author is thankful to the Department of Botany, Bangabasi Evening College for working facilities.

References

Joseph Thas, J. "Siddha Medicine-background and Principles and the Application for Skin Diseases." *Clinics in Dermatology* 26, no. 1 (2008): 62–78.

Kamartaha, S., O. Kavi, and R. Vinay. "Diversity of Unani Medicinal Plants of Northwest Gujarat." *International Journal of Unani and Integrative Medicine* 5, no. 2 (2021): 188–95.

Kumar, S., G. J. Dobos, and T. Rampp. "The Significance of Ayurvedic Medicinal Plants." *Journal of Evidence-Based Complementary & Alternative Medicine* 22, no. 3 (2016): 494–501.

Pandey, M. M., S. Rastogi, and A. K. S. Rawat. "Indian Traditional Ayurvedic System of Medicine and Nutritional Supplementation." *Evidence-Based Complementary and Alternative Medicine* 376327 (2013): 1–12.

Peterson, C. T., K. Denniston, and D. Chopra. "Therapeutic Uses of Triphala in Ayurvedic Medicine." *Journal of Alternative and Complementary Medicine* 23, no. 8 (2017): 607–14.

Rahman, S. Z., R. A. Khan, and A. Latif. "Importance of Pharmacovigilance in Unani System of Medicine." *Indian Journal of Pharmacology* 40, no. Suppl1 (2008): S17–S20.

Rupani, R., and A. Chavez. "Medicinal Plants with Traditional Use: Ethnobotany in the Indian subcontinent." *Clinics in Dermatology* 36, no. 3 (2018): 306–9.

Shi, Y., C. Zhang, and X. Li. "Traditional Medicine in India." *Journal of Traditional Chinese Medical Sciences* 8, no. 1 (2021): S51–5.

19

Ethnomedicinal Practices and Traditional Healthcare Systems of the Nicobarese Tribe of Nicobar Archipelagos

Satyaki Paul,[1] Anstice Justin,[2] and Sabatini Chatterjee[2*]

[1]Dr. Ambedkar Chair (Dr. Ambedkar Foundation, Ministry of Social Justice & Empowerment, Govt. of India), KISS Deemed to be University, Bhubaneswar, Odisha, India

[2]Andaman & Nicobar Regional Centre, Anthropological Survey of India (Ministry of Culture, Govt. of India), Port Blair, Andaman & Nicobar Islands, India

*Corresponding Author's Email: sabatinichatterjee11@gmail.com

Introduction

The Nicobarese is the dominant tribal population with an estimated number of 27,780 residing in the entire Andaman & Nicobar Islands (Directorate of Economics & Statistics 2023–4). They resided on twelve islands in the Nicobar Archipelagos and Little Andaman in the Andaman Archipelagos (Justin 1990). The label "Nicobar" is Tamil in origin from the word *Nakkavaram* or Land of the Naked as mentioned in the Tanjore inscriptions (A&N Gazetteer 1909; Whitehead 1924). There are even mentions in ancient texts such as *Ramayana* wherein Lord Rama passed through the islands while he was in exile (Mathur 1967) along with Somdev's *Kathasaritsagar*'s account of Nicobars being called *Narikel Dweep* and several other written historical records (Justin 1990). There is an intricate relationship between the populace and their environment, especially with their flora (Mann 1981). The etymology of the name "Nicobarese" comes from their residence on the Nicobar Archipelagos; however, the term "Nicobarese" was first given by Reverend Bishop John Richardson (Justin 1990).

The islands and their islanders are peace-loving people who have a traumatized past during the Japanese invasion during the Second World War from 1942–5, which was later recaptured again by the then British Raj until the independence of our nation

(Justin 1990). The Nicobar Archipelagos became an integral part of independent India, and it became a regulated space after the promulgation of the Andaman and Nicobar Islands (Protection of Aboriginal Tribes) Regulation in 1956, wherein entry to Nicobar Archipelagos became strictly prohibited to non-domiciled persons. However, in the 1960s, the then government settled a few non-tribals, including ex-defense personnel, in the region. In the 1970s, some Tamil people from the mainland also started working in banana plantations located in the Katchal islands. After that, some Car-Nicobari families were resettled to Little Andamans in 1973–74 due to a lack of space and an increasing population. In terms of geographical separation, the Nicobar Archipelagos are separated from the Andaman Archipelagos via a 145 km wide 10-degree channel. A special terrestrial bird, Nicobar megapode, is also endemic to Great Nicobar Island (Kumari 2024). In total, there are twenty-two islands in the Nicobar group of islands, with innumerable undiscovered flora and fauna (Khullar 2017) wherein only twelve are populated (Justin 1990).

The Nicobar Archipelagos received the status of a separate district on August 1, 1974, with its headquarters in Car Nicobar (*Pu*) where one-third of its population resides. The people of Car Nicobar call themselves "the people," "men," or "*ta-rik*" (Whitehead 1924). The Nicobarese are quintessentially horticulturalists and pig herders mostly residing near the seashore lines. They are quite well-known for their copra trade with the outside world since time immemorial. They have their *el-panam* or spaces such as a cemetery, traders' quarters, and village hall on the beach (Whitehead 1924). Their tribe can be divided into six groups that is, the residents of Car Nicobar (ta-rik), Chowra (som pai), Teressa (som lurro), Katchal-Kamorta-Trinket (som ita), Pulo Milo (sop piheun), Little Nicobar (sop Panjang), Kondul (sop la mongshe), Pulo Bhabi of Long/Great Nicobar (sop kanalo) (Justin 1990). In addition, there is another single interiorly located remote seminomadic tribe of the Shompen on Great Nicobar who are quite elusive (Whitehead 1924). On a broader territorial sense, the islands can be divided into three divisions that is, northernmost or Car Nicobar (Pu), Central group or Chowra (Sane nyo), Teressa (Luroo), Bompuka (Pohat), Katchal (Tinhyu), Kamorta (Kalat or Kinlaha), Nancowry (Muot), Trinket (Laful), and Southern group or Pulo Milo (Piheun), Little Nicobar (Panjang or Ong or Tokuo-no Long), Kondul (Lamongshe), and Great Nicobar (To Kirong Long) in their native language (Justin 1990). These groups have varying sociocultural rites, languages, ethnomedicinal knowledge, magico-religious practices, and so on (Whitehead 1924; Man 1932; Justin 1990; Nandan 1993).

The Nicobarese populace has been exposed to the external influences of outside cultures since time immemorial. The sociocultural fabric kept on evolving with the acculturation of various cultures such as that of Chinese, Malaysian, Burmese, Portuguese, Danish, and so on. These acculturations were carried out to sustain their way of living, which can be considered a direct response to ecological adaptation (Justin 1990). At present, the traditional knowledge system is somewhat disappearing due to integration with the mainstream. The tsunami of 2004 wreaked havoc on the Nicobar villages, and it also made an everlasting impact on the minds of the Nicobarese people (Verma, Bhatia, and Srivastava 2010; Prasad 2013). This led to a sudden shift from observing the traditional knowledge systems to modern allopathic practices. However, still, there is a good presence of the mundane use of folk medicine in treating basic maladies. The Nicobarese people are very superstitious and believe in self-medication; herein, such ethnomedicinal practices and other magico-religious practices are vividly discussed in this study.

Objectives and Methods

This study consists of a secondary analysis of assorted research articles, books, reports, and so on. The conventional on-site Malinowskian fieldwork is naturally improbable due to restrictions of the Andaman & Nicobar Protection of Aboriginal Tribes (PAT) Regulation, 1956, on the entry of non-domicile persons into the Nicobar district of the Andaman & Nicobar Islands. However, the emic perspectives such as lived experience and knowledge of folk medicine of the second author, who also belongs to the Nicobarese community, add value to this chapter. The secondary data were amassed based on the rationale and nature of the outline for this chapter. In this pulse, we mainly explored the ethnomedicinal knowledge and magico-religious practices followed among the Nicobarese residing in Andaman & Nicobar Islands (Figure 19.1).

The Nicobarese community is the only Scheduled Tribe of the Union Territory of Andaman & Nicobar Island which is in contrast to the Great Andamanese, Jarawas, Sentinelese, Onges, and Shompens, who are considered Particularly Vulnerable Tribal Groups (PVTGs) in the same space (Directorate of Economics & Statistics 2023–4). Through this chapter, we would like to note that the Nicobar district of Andaman & Nicobar Islands has a rich heritage of ethnomedicinal plants. In this context, diverse medicinal papers from multifaceted and interdisciplinary perspectives on the same region have also been recognized as crucial secondary information for the compiling of this present study.

About the Nicobarese People

The Nicobarese folklore itself consists of various lores among distinct groups which showcase their external origin either from Malaysia, Indonesia, or Myanmar (Justin 1990). The material culture of the Nicobarese people developed in a much later phase. In general, the Nicobarese people are very superstitious; for example, they regard pregnancy as the work of an evil spirit or *shaitan* (Nandan 1993). They are patrilineal and have communal huts near seashores called *tuhet* (principal homestead) where festive occasions take place (Whitehead 1924; Man 1932; Justin 1990; Nandan 1993). In terms of residence style, they had a matrilocal form of residence which evanesced from their customs in due course of time (Nandan 1993). The Nicobarese language belongs to the Austro-Asiatic subfamily language grouped with the Munda language and the Mon-Khmer languages (Das 1977). There is also a certain degree of distinctness

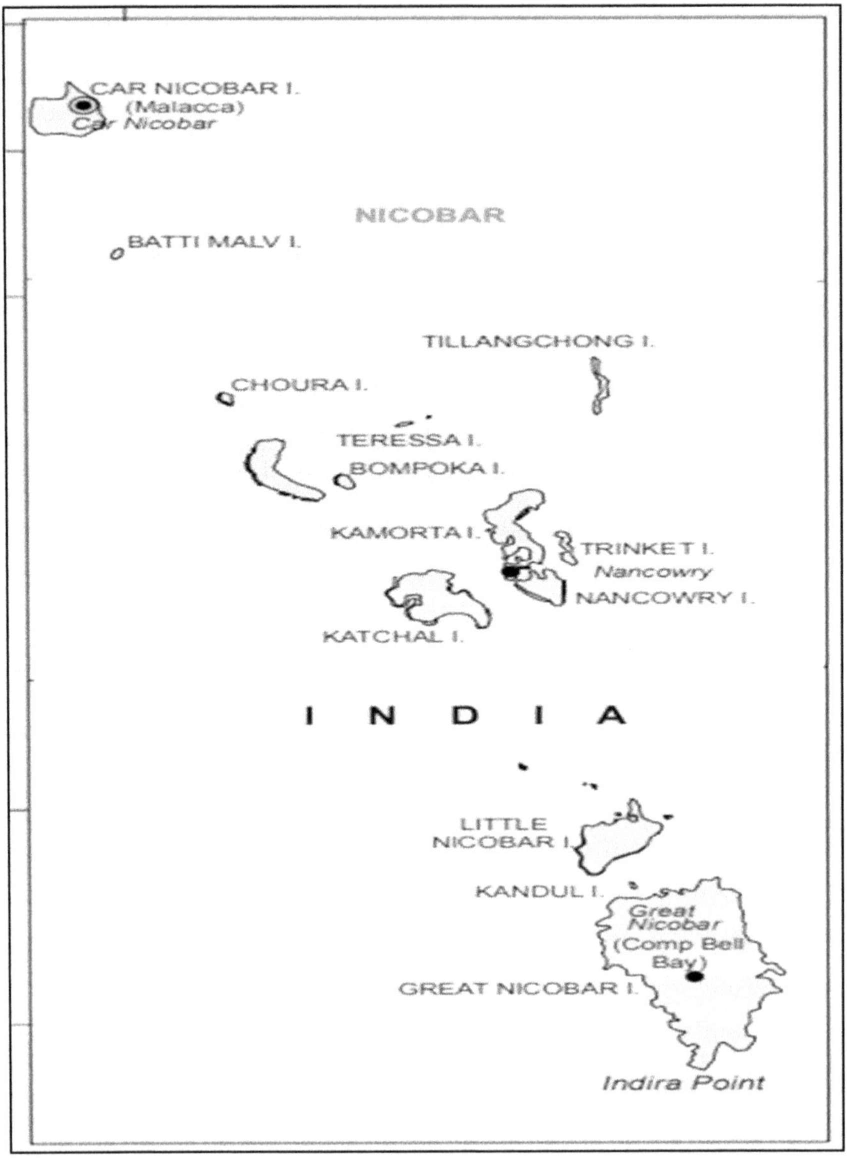

Figure 19.1. Map of the Nicobar district in Andaman and Nicobar Islands. Source: Author.

between various groups of Nicobarese people, wherein the Car Nicobarese language is somewhat incoherent to central and southern groups of islands (Justin 1990).

There are two types of families (*haidechiye*) observed among the Nicobarese populace, that is, nuclear and joint family (Nandan 1993). There is a presence of joking relationships and teknonymy observed amid the populace. The couvade practice during childbirth was also observed (Man 1932). Apart from that, they are toddy (*tari*) loving individuals who live a very simple and peaceful life, which is also reflected in their earlier clothing style that is, *neng* or loin cloth (Man 1932). Some people have started making *handia* (fermented rice beer) due to their close contact with the Ranchiwalas (Justin 1990). The *neng* was worn by men in the omphalion/waist region and was made up of colored cloth which they used to procure from traders. It was folded to a width of between 3–4 inches except at its ends; it was passed around the waist and between the legs, and secured at the posterior region, leaving the ends hanging loose. Man (1932) noted that even Shompens had started wearing *nengs*. This might be a case of visual adaptation (Paul, Justin, and Chatterjee 2024). However, in earlier times, the Nicobarese from different groups were identified using the style of neng and the color of it (Man 1932). At present, several individuals have adopted a pair of shorts or *paijam* and people at Campbell Bay or Kondul Island wear shirts along with pants colloquially called *kanha tahia* (Nandan 1993). The women wear sewn white *lungi* (forming a long skirt) called *loie hulen* along with a blouse called *kanjut*. These are all modern clothing styles integrated with traditional clothing which points toward the fact that they are becoming somewhat assimilated in the mainstream (Justin 1990). They used to make rain gear out of lean known as *dani patti* but they are obsolete and are out of use due to modern clothes available across the board, especially after the boom of Flipkart and Amazon.

In terms of hygiene, they used to utilize *alahui sabun*, a locally available leaf which is also now replaced with modern-day soaps (Nandan 1993). In terms of mundane consumption, the Nicobarese people commonly preferred coconut milk and toddy as beverages (Whitehead 1924; Man 1932). The pandanus or *larop* (*pandanus leram*) fruit was indispensable to them which also became a part extensively of their diet during lean seasons, except on Chowra island (Justin 1990). During the rule of the British Raj, the advent of Christianity with *Vedappan Solomon* in 1906 and the advent of Muslims with *malikku beepori altered* the religious contours of the Nicobarese which had its roots in the practice of animism (Justin 1990). At present, the number of Nicobarese individuals who practice Christianity outweighs all others who practice Islam and Animism (Census of India 2011). In terms of relationships with the outside world, it can be seen that in the twentieth century, the Nicobarese people used to trade in oil, fiber, copra, birds' nests, split cane, areca nuts, sea slugs, ambergris, tortoise shells, parrots and even monkeys (Man 1932). In return, they used to accept items such as ornaments, beads, silverware, glass, salt, tobacco, colored cloth/calico, and so on (Man 1932). They are now mostly engrossed in agricultural activities mainly dealing with coconut (*kao*), arecanut (*yeh*), and banana plantations.

The Nicobarese people have kept alive their traditions and customs even at the turn of the twenty-first century as observed through their practice of *haka ap* (live sacrifices to canoes) during the ossuary festival (*kanaha-un*) and *kiolo* (semireligious festival). They have a nuclear or joint family (Justin 1990). Nevertheless, as per the accounts of the second author, there is a decrease in trust in folk medicine, *Menluana* (priest doctor) and *Tamiluono* or *Totarong* (traditional healers) in general. In the contemporary context, they are engrossed in the processing of copra, coconut plantation, banana plantation, and supply of areca nuts to the mainstream populace which is an ode to their past as documented by numerous ethnologists and even modern researchers (Whitehead 1924; Man 1932; Justin 1990; Tripathi 2016; Prasad 2016).

Medicinal Knowledge among the Nicobarese

The Nicobarese are very superstitious individuals, and their superstitions are intertwined with the use of endemic flora to treat maladies (Justin 1990). They used to believe in the powers of *to-mi-luo-no* or Medicine Man or Wise Man, who is usually contacted once a person falls sick (Whitehead 1924). The same person is also called *menluana* in several other texts, who are called *ma* (masters) (Man 1932) and also serves as the head of sacred affairs (Nandan 1993). The concept of health is associated with the level of work that one can undertake, and failure to do so due to some symptoms in parts of the body (like limbs, eyes, and tongue) can be considered sickness or associated with certain diseases (Verma, Bhatia, and Srivastava 2010; Prasad 2013). A wooden artifact called *Kareau* was also kept in communal spaces or *goal-ghars*, which acted as a medium to be in touch with the spiritual realm. These statues also protected against malevolent spirits; however, they are now in decline due to the tsunami of 2004, which wreaked havoc in the region, thereby altering some vital socio-religious practices among the Nicobarese people.

In general, the traditional medicine men usually possessed powers to subjugate the evil spirits (even divination) and had higher degrees of intelligence wherein they could adjudge whether a person was guilty or not just by observing their hands (Man 1932). The medicine man is aided by the Headman or chief of the village and *ma-a-fai* or aspirants of the priesthood (Man 1932) after drinking toddy (Nandan 1993). The ethnomedicinal practices are essentially oral traditions that are transmitted from *to-mi-luo-no* to *ma-a-fai* orally as there is no particular written document regarding such practices (Nandan 1993). Whitehead (1924) observed that Nicobarese used to procure a bunch of leaves from a plant which they colloquially called *to-ki-teuiny* to capture spirits. Along with this, song and dance were carried on by *ma-a-fai* till midnight wearing garlands of young banana leaves (1924). To ward off evil spirits from a sick person's body, *intakoi* (magical performance) was carried out by offering pig's meat, pandanus paste, coconut, boiled rice, and toddy to the effigies of spirit and its partner (Nandan 1993). A charm called *henta-koi* or ornate shields was prepared by Nicobarese people who acted as charms to recuperate from sickness as deemed by the priest doctor.

Furthermore, blood therapy is also quite popular among the Nicobarese populace wherein they consider that pig blood has medicinal value (Justin 1990). They smear their face and body with the blood of a live pig or one slaughtered for this purpose. Fowl's blood is also applied to the forehead for relief from nausea and headache. It has a soothing effect on pregnant women. Also, it can revitalize the nerves of persons recuperating from an extended period of some ailment (Justin 1990). In a similar vein, in the case of a child who is two or three months old, an unripe coconut is boiled in a Chowra pot which is rubbed all over with a concoction of fowl's blood mixed with turmeric and other crushed leaves provided by the to-mi-luo-no (Whitehead 1924). However, the traditional witch doctors and their novices had no official connection with *Kun-seu-ro* (thanksgiving festival) or any other. They usually take part as inhabitants of the village (Whitehead 1924).

In the native language, the diseases are colloquially named as fever (*punkayo* or *vmoi*), snake bite (*kapo* or *pcch*), tuberculosis (*to chionp-ngo*), stomach pain (*ellonreinyab*), cough (*ehe*), injury (*to-suktore*), eye and ear ache (*chok mat* and *elnang*), and so on that are usually treated by the *to-mi-luo-no* (Prasad 2013). Apart from these, the Nicobarese people of Car Nicobar also practice a traditional method of fishing known as *neulo* wherein individuals sprinkle a paste in shallow water or during low tide or ankle-deep waters (Justin 1990) which makes the fish unconscious. The paste is prepared by mixing *kinyav* seeds and mashed kernel. The Nicobarese people usually place a fishing basket or *tamatu* before sprinkling the paste which knocks them out (Justin 1990). Some fish die and fall to the bottom, and others seem to float. These are caught easily by the Nicobarese people, and such kinds of drugs available among the said tribe enable easy fishing and often in surplus quantities (Justin 1990). Therefore, from all the above-discussed contexts, it can be observed from all these social practices that the local medicinal plants are quite an integral part and parcel of the lives of the said populace wherein it is not just used to cure ailments but also used for daily sustenance.

Medicinal Plants Used by Nicobarese People

The most common list of maladies among the Nicobarese populace is cough and fever, vomiting and nausea, headache, body aches, and so on (Verma, Bhatia, and Srivastava 2010; Prasad 2013; Chander et al. 2015). These maladies are cured by medicine men who use endemic ethnomedicinal plants to cure sick persons. The processed medicine is administered often orally, topically (application on the skin), or as eye or ear drops by the medicine man. The plants used to treat such maladies can be classified into groups based on disorders. All these medicinal uses of these plants are given here in detail; these are:

(a) **Cough and Fever:** In case of cough, medicinal plants such as *Abrus precatorius* (Fabaceae), *Ocimum tenuiflorum* (Lamiaceae), *Lepinsanthes rubiginosa* (Sapindaceae), *Ganophyllum falcatum* (Sapindaceae), *Tylophora indica* (Asclepiadaceae), *Senna occidentalis* (Caesalpiniaceae), *Ipomoea gracilis* (Convolvulaceae), *Citrus medica* (Rutaceae), *Achyranthes aspera* (Amaranthaceae), *Zingiber officinale* (Zingiberaceae) are used as remedies for cough. These are often administered through oral medium, while *Ocimum tenuiflorum*, *Tylophora indica*, *Senna occidentalis*, and *Ipomoea gracilis* are applied to the skin. In case of fever, medicinal plants *Leea indica* (Leeaceae), *Ficus rumphii* (Moraceae), *Phyllanthus amarus* (Euphorbiaceae), *Colubrina asiatica* (Rhamnaceae), *Cajanus Cajan* (Fabaceae), *Wattakaka volubilis* (Asclepiadaceae), *Callicarpa arborea* (Verbenaceae), *Physalis minima* (Solanaceae), *Alstonia macropylla* (Apocynaceae), *Glochiodion calocarpum* (Phyllanthaceae), *Ipomea pescaprae* (Convolvulaceae), *Jasminum syringifolium* (Oleaceae) are used as remedies. These are often administered through the oral medium, while *Alstonia macropylla*, *Glochiodion calocarpum*, *Ipomea pescaprae*, and *Jasminum syringifolium* are applied on the skin of sick Nicobarese individuals.

(b) **Blood vomiting, giddiness, and nausea:** In case of blood vomiting, medicinal plants such as *Lepisanthes rubiginosa* (Sapindaceae), *Cyclea peltata* (Menispermaceae), *Phyllanthus amarus* (Euphorbiaceae), *Leea grandifolia* (Leeaceae), *Passiflora foetida* (Passifloraceae), *Punica granatum* (Punicaceae), *Gossypium barbadense* (Malvaceae), *Abutilon indicum* (Malvaceae) are orally administered to persons who are vomiting blood. In case of giddiness, vomiting, and nausea, medicinal plants such as *Scaevola taccada* (Goodeniaceae), *Ipomoea pescaprae* (Convolvulaceae), *Claoxylon indicum* (Euphorbiaceae), *Clerodendrum paniculatum* (Verbenaceae) are applied on the skin of a nauseating or vomiting Nicobarese individual.

(c) **Headaches and Body Aches:** In case of body aches, medicinal plants such as *Annona reticulata* (Annonaceae), *Datura metel* (Solanaceae), *Morinda citrifolia* (Rubiaceae), *Ehretia laevis* (Boraginaceae), *Sida acuta* (Malvaceae), *Jasminum syringifolium* (Olanaceae), *Ficus rumphii* (Moraceae), *Leea* indica (Leeaceae) are administered to the skin of a Nicobarese person having severe body aches. In case of headaches, medicinal plants such as *Claoxylon indicum* (Euphorbiaceae), *Datura metel* (Solanaceae), *Colubrina asiatica* (Rhamnaceae), *Lantana camara* (Verbanaceae), *Sterculia guttata* (Sterculiaceae), *Gossypium barbadense* (Malvaceae), *Piper betle* (Piperaceae) are administered to the forehead skin of a Nicobarese person having severe headaches.

(d) **Abdominal Pain:** In case of abdominal pain, medicinal plants such as *Sterculia guttata* (Sterculiaceae), *Momordica charantia* (Cucurbitaceae), *Annona reticulata* (Annonaceae), *Ricinus communis* (Euphorbiaceae), *Phyllanthus amarus* (Euphorbiaceae), *Leea indica* (Leeaceae), *Blachia andamanica* (Euphorbiaceae), *Tabernaemontana crispa* (Apocynaceae), *Vernonia patula* (Asteraceae), *Leea grandifolia* (Leeaceae), *Macaranga peltata* (Euphorbiaceae), *Brenia vitisidaea* (Euphorbiaceae), *Dillenia andamanica* (Dilleniaceae), *Tournefortia argentea* (Boraginaceae), *Cordia subcordata* (Boraginaceae), *Psychotria montana* (Rubiaceae), *Cassia fistula* (Caesalpiniaceae), and so on, are used as remedies. Most of these are orally administered, while *Tournefortia argentea*, *Cordia subcordata*, *Psychotria montana*, and *Cassia fistula* are applied on the skin of the Nicobarese individual who is having abdominal pain.

(e) **Fracture of Bones:** In case of bone fracture, medicinal plants such as *Morinda citrifolia* (Rubiaceae), *Clerodendrum inerme* (Verbenaceae),

Annona reticulata (Annonaceae), *Callicarpa arborea* (Verbenaceae), *Scaevola taccada* (Goodeniaceae), *Ipomoea pescaprae* (Convolvulaceae), *Datura metel* (Solanaceae), *Sida acuta* (Malvaceae), *Capsicum annuum* (Solanaceae), *Calamus nicobaricus* (Arecaceae), *Tamarindus indica* (Caesalpiniaceae), and *Curcuma longifolia* (Zingiberaceae) are applied on the skin of the Nicobarese individual who has fractured their bones for steady recuperation.

(f) **Snakebite:** In the case of snake bites which are quite prevalent, medicinal plants such as *Capsicum annuum* (Solanaceae), *Clerodendrum inerme* (Verbenaceae), *Cnesmone javanica* (Euphorbiaceae), *Dischidia benghalensis* (Asclepiadaceae), *Sida acuta* (Malvaceae), Ipomoea gracilis (Convolvulaceae), *Euphorbia pallens* (Euphorbiaceae), *Barringtonia racemosa* (Barringtoniaceae), *Alstonia macrophylla* (Apocynaceae), *Urena lobata* (Malvaceae), and *Clerodendrum paniculatum* (Verbenaceae) are used as remedies. Most of these medicines are administered orally while only *Clerodendrum paniculatum* is directly applied to the skin of the Nicobarese person who suffered from a snake bite.

(g) **Skin Allergies:** In case of severe skin allergies such as eczema, medicinal plants such as *Citrus medica* (Rutaceae), *Curcuma longifolia* (Zingiberaceae), *Lawsonia inermis* (Lythraceae), *Annona reticulata* (Annonaceae), and *Azadirchta indica* (Meliaceae) are used as remedies. All of these medicinal plants are applied on the skin of Nicobarese individuals who have skin allergies or severe cases of eczema.

(h) **Menstrual Problems:** In case of menstrual problems faced by Nicobarese women, medicinal plants such as *Claoxylon indicum* (Euphorbiaceae), *Ficus rumphii* (Moraceae), *Ipomoea pescaprae* (Convolvulaceae), Annona reticulata (Annonaceae), Jasminum syringifolium (Oleaceae), Ganophyllum falcatum (Sapindaceae), and Dillenia andamanica (Dilleniaceae) are used as remedies. These are orally administered to Nicobarese women.

(i) **Contraception:** In the case of contraceptives, medicinal plants such as *Psychotria montana* (Rubiaceae), *Stachytarpheta jamaicensis* (Verbenaceae), Drymoglossum heterophyllum (Polypodiaceae), and *Leea indica* (Leeaceae) are used as remedies. All of them are orally administered by the Nicobarese women as natural contraceptives.

(j) **Ethnomedicinal Plants used to treat Dental Problems:** In the case of dental problems, medicinal plants such as *Cajanus cajan* (Fabaceae), *Albizia retusa* (Mimosaceae), *Moringa oleifera* (Moringaceae), *Tylophora indica* (Asclepiadaceae), *Sida acuta* (Malvaceae), and *Ficus rumphii* (Moraceae) are used as remedies. Most of them are orally administered, while *Sida acuta* and *Ficus rumphii* are directly applied to the teeth by the Nicobarese men and women.

(k) **Diarrhea:** In case of diarrhea, medicinal plants such as *Lepisanthes rubiginosa* (Sapindaceae), *Sterculia guttata* (Sterculiaceae), *Morinda citrifolia* (Rubiaceae), *Tabernaemontana crispa* (Apocynaceae), *Ganophyllum falcatum* (Sapindaceae), and *Urena lobata* (Malvaceae) are used as remedies. All of these medicinal plants are orally administered to individuals suffering from diarrhea.

(l) **Infertility:** In case of infertility, medicinal plants such as *Ipomoea pescaprae* (Convolvulaceae), *Ricinus communis* (Euphorbiaceae), *Senna occidentalis* (Caesalpiniaceae), Premna corymbosa (Verbenaceae), Callicarpa longifolia (Verbenaceae), Commelina benghalensis (Commelinaceae), Ipomea gracilis (Convolvulaceae), Macaranga peltata (Euphorbiaceae), Ganophyllum falcatum (Sapindaceae), and Colubrina asiatica (Rhamnaceae) are used as remedies. Most of the medicinal plants are orally administered while *Ipomoea pescaprae, Ricinus communis*, and *Senna occidentalis* are applied on the skin of Nicobarese persons who are suffering from infertility.

(m) **Open Wounds and Cuts:** In case of open wounds, medicinal plants such as *Lindsaea ensifolia* (Lindsaeaceae), *Lepisanthes rubiginosa* (Sapindaceae), *Dillenia andamanica* (Dilleniaceae), *Vernonia divergens* (Asteraceae), *Curcuma longifolia* (Zingiberaceae), *Annona reticulata* (Annonaceae), *Ipomoea gracilis* (Convolvulaceae), *Premna corymbose* (Verbenaceae), *Ficus rumphoo* (Moraceae), *Urena lobata* (Malvaceae), *Areca catechu* (Arecaceae), *Thysanolaena maxima* (Poaceae), and *Clerodendrum paniculatum* (Verbenaceae) are used as remedies. All of the abovementioned plants are applied to the skin as a paste especially where there are cuts or wounds to treat them.

(n) **Tuberculosis:** In case of individuals suffering from Tuberculosis, medicinal plants such as *Ganophyllum falcatum* (Sapindaceae) and *Lepisanthes rubiginosa* (Sapindaceae) are used as remedies. These are orally administered to Nicobarese men and women.

(o) **Malaria:** In the case of malaria, medicinal plants such as *Phyllanthus amarus* (Euphorbiaceae), *Guettarda speciosa* (Rubiaceae), *Pandanus leram* (Pandanaceae), *Catharanthus roseus* (Apocynaceae), *Guettarda speciosa* (Rubiaceae), *Pemphis acidula* (Lythraceae), *Azadirachta indica* (Meliaceae), *Ehretia laevis* (Boraginaceae), and *Senna tora* (Caesalpiniaceae) are used as remedies. Most of the plants are applied on the skin while *Phyllanthus amarus* is only taken orally by the person suffering from malaria.

(p) **Filariasis:** In the case of filariasis, medicinal plants such as *Azadirachta indica* (Meliaceae), *Memecylon edule* (Memecylaceae), *Glochidion calocarpum* (Phyllanthaceae), and *Adenostemma lavenia* (Asteraceae) are used as remedies. All of them are applied to the skin directly.

The above-discussed medicinal plants are taken after the direction of *to-mi-luo-no* or medicine men. Nevertheless, there are social customs ingrained in the life of Nicobarese; for example, a pregnant woman is not allowed to visit a garden, as her visit might alter the quality and quantity of fruits, or they are prohibited from going near a weed called *bachop*, as according to their accounts it has properties that cause stillbirth (Nandan 1993). Thus, it can be determined from the results and discussions section that all of the magico-religious mores had somewhat ethnomedicinal facets that became a part of the ever-evolving sociocultural contours of the Nicobarese tribe. The tribe still practices all forms of ethnomedicinal remedies linked with their traditional knowledge system due to their apparent distrust of allopathic medicines because of their side effects, as per the second author (Prasad 2013). Such continuance of ethnomedicinal practice is essential for the survival of a delicate oral tradition.

Conclusion and Recommendation

In today's world of modernization and globalization, the inevitability of change is the universal constant. The Nicobarese contacts with outsiders have enabled a wave of development in the Nicobar district, and the social transformations that have taken place are unparalleled in the last twenty to thirty years (Justin 1990). There is a change in the housing pattern from beehive hives to sloping roof models. Earlier, bamboo was used to construct houses; nowadays, it has been replaced with cemented structures. Since 1978, an election mechanism has also been put in place wherein individuals or captains are selected through secret ballot. There are always pros and cons to everything, so now, with the increased contact with the modern world and its modern knowledge systems, there is a rise in unemployment among Nicobarese. These unemployed youths are getting addicted to alcohol and all other vices. The specific barter system between Nicobarese and Shompen, wherein they used to trade for honey or *tagani* (Nandan 1993), has now evanesced and is a thing of the distant past.

The Nicobarese people used to make fire by using stems of *Arcocarpus chaplash* earlier, which has now been altered to matchbox. The process of all its use has now been forgotten due to disuse. There is an urgent need to culturally revitalize the Nicobarese sects on traditional vocation and associated environmental niche to enable sustainability and the right way of livelihood. In terms of preserving and promoting ethnomedicinal practices, even though numerous research works have been carried out, it is essential to correctly document every social aspect associated with the endemic flora of the region. There are several medicinal plants such as *Leea indica* (used to treat cough, body aches, and abdominal pain, along with its use as contraceptives), *Ficus rumphii* (used to treat cough, body aches, and menstrual problems, along with its use to resolve dental problems), *Datura metel* (used to treat headaches, abdominal pain, and treatment of fractured bones), and numerous other plants, as discussed above, can be promoted by the Ministry of AYUSH.

There are some rare endemic medicinal plants like *Begonia andamanensis*, *Dillenia andamanica*, *Glochiodion Calocarpum*, *Pandanus leram*, and *Leea grandifolia* which can be increased through plant propagation in medicinal gardens. The Andaman & Nicobar Administration is trying its level best to protect the tribes and endemic flora/fauna but more proactive steps need to be taken to ensure sustainable development in the region. This can be only possible through transdisciplinary research. Herein the possibilities of research and possible contribution are limitless; however, it is essential to act now because it is now or never. The complete assimilation of the Nicobarese community and devalorization of the traditional knowledge system might lead to the existence of the said community in its outlook per se; without its knowledge and oral tradition of local ecological niche, a community cannot survive in such proximity to nature as a natural calamity might wipe away the entire existence without such knowledge.

References

Chander, P., K. Paluru, Chinnaiah and P. Vijayachari. "Herbal Medicine & Healthcare Practices among Nicobarese of Nancowry Group of Islands – an Indigenous Tribe of Andaman & Nicobar Islands." *Indian Journal of Medical Research* 141 (2015): 720–44.

Das, A. *A Study of the Nicobarese Language*. Calcutta: Anthropological Survey of India, 1977.

Government of India. *Imperial Gazetteer of India, Provincial Series, Andaman and Nicobar Islands.* Calcutta: Superintendent of Government Printing, 1909.

Justin, A. *The Nicobarese.* Kolkata: Seagull Publishers, 1990.

Khullar, B. "The First Official Record of Animal Diversity of the Great Nicobar." *Mongabay*, Andaman and Nicobar Islands, December 29, 2017.

Kumari, K. "A Mascot in Peril: How a Massive Development Project Threatens the Nicobar Megapode." *Frontline*, Andaman and Nicobar Islands, May 07, 2024.

Man, E. *The Nicobar Islands and Their People.* Royal Anthropological Institute of Great Britain and Ireland: Billing and Sons Ltd, 1932.

Mann, R. S. "The Andaman and Nicobar Islanders — Some Ecological Perspectives." *Man in India* 61, no. 1 (1981): 61–8.

Mathur, K. *Nicobar Islands.* New Delhi: National Book Trust, 1967.

Nandan, A. *The Nicobarese of Great Nicobar: An Ethnography.* New Delhi: Gyan Publishing House, 1993.

Paul, S., A. Justin, and S. Chatterjee. "Sentinelese Contacts: Anthropologically Revisiting the Most Reclusive Masters of the Terra Incognita North Sentinel Island." *Humanities and Social Sciences Communications* 11, no. 1512 (2024): 1–10.

Prasad, D. "Ethno-medicine And Indigenous Therapeutic Practices of the Nicobarese of Katchal Island." *Journal of the Andaman Science Association* 18 (2013): 96–101.

Prasad, D. "Post-tsunami Rehabilitation and Resettlement in Nicobar Islands: An Anthropological Approach." *The Researchers* 2 (2016): 46–59.

Tripathi, P. "Tribes of Andaman and Nicobar Islands: A Comparative Study of Great Andamanese and Nicobarese." *Salesian Journal of Humanities and Social Sciences* 7 (2016): 26–48.

Verma, C., S. Bhatia, and S. Srivastava. "Traditional Medicine of the Nicobarese." *Indian Journal of Traditional Knowledge* 9 (2010): 779–85.

Whitehead, G. *In the Nicobar Islands: The Record Of a Lengthy Sojourn In Islands Of Sunshine & Palms Amongst a People Primitive in Their Habits & Beliefs & Simple in Their Manner of Living, with a Description of Their Customs & Religious Ceremonies & an Account of Their Superstitions, Traditions & Folklore.* London: Seeley Service and Co. Limited, 1924.

20

Elements and Wellness Application of Botany and Medicinal Plants in Ancient India

A Systematic Review

Arun Makal*

Department of Anthropology, Bangabasi Evening College, University of Calcutta, Kolkata, India

*Corresponding Author's Email: arunmakal6@gmail.com

Introduction

The beginning of the relationship between humans and plants can be traced back to prehistoric times. Evidence specifies that plants have been cultivated as drugs approximately 60,000 years ago. The scripts about medicinal plants date back to almost 5,000 years ago in India, China, and Egypt and at least 2,500 years in Greece and Central Asia (Solecki 1975; Ang-Lee, Moss, and Yuan 2001; Fatemeh, Zahra, and Hossein 2018). Accordingly, the medical botany or the study of medicinal plants and their traditional uses has been a part of Indian culture for thousands of years, with evidence in the Rig Veda, the Artharvaveda, and other ancient texts. The Rig Veda, which is a repository of human knowledge written between 4500 and 1600 BC, describes the medicinal properties of plants. On the other hand, the Artharvaveda, dating back to 2000 BC, is a basis of Ayurvedic medicine. In addition, the Sushruta Samhita and Charaka Samhita, written in 1000 BC, describe therapeutics and Materia Medica, a branch of medical science that deals with the sources, nature, properties, and preparation of drugs (Ravishankar and Shukla 2007; Makal 2024).

In relation to the various ancient texts, the Indus Valley Civilization, also known as the Harappan civilization, dates back to around 3300 BC and lasted until around 1300 BC. It is considered advanced for its time. They were also skilled at medical science with evidence of proto-dentistry, brain surgery, and usage of herbs for treatment. They used drugs and medical interventions like trephination and tooth drilling. They were also skilled in sanitation and water management. Besides, the evidence suggests that the Harappans were sophisticated in their use of plants for vegetables, culinary, and medicinal purposes (Mohanty and Panda 2020; Makal 2024). Evidence also suggests the Indus Valley people primarily used plants like wheat, barley, peas, lentils, mustard seeds, sesame, rice, and cotton for agriculture. They worshipped trees, glazed their pottery with the juice of plants, and painted them with a large number of plant designs. They also knew the commercial value of plants and plant products. They considered the Peepal tree to be the most sacred. One of the seals shows a god standing between the branches of a Peepal tree, and the god is being worshipped by a devotee on his knees.

Besides the Indus Valley Civilization, there are sufficient indications to show that agriculture, medicine, and horticulture developed to a great extent during the Vedic period. Vedic literature used a large number of terms in the description of plants and plant parts. Even the Rig Veda mentions that Vedic Indians had knowledge about food manufacture, the action of light on the process, and storage of energy in the bodies of plants. In other words, the Vedic period was a time when people used plants for medicine, rituals, and sacrifices. The Vedas, Upanishads, and epics like the Ramayana and Mahabharata mention many plants and their medicinal properties (Kalpana and Sitaram 2016; Makal 2024). Thus, the Vedas are a collection of hymns and other religious texts composed in India long ago. They are the Rigveda, Yajurveda, Samaveda, and Atharvaveda. The Atharvaveda is an encyclopedia for medicine. It was a collection of spells, prayers, charms, and hymns. Again, in the Vedic Samhitas, there are references to many plants including Artu, Asvattha, Apamarga, Amula, and Soma; water plants and weeds like lotus, lily, pundarika, and puskara, as well as herbs and grasses like isika, ulapa, darbha, and satamba, along with their medicinal features and properties.

With respect to Vedic medical systems, the post-Vedic Indian literature demonstrates that botany flourished as a separate scientific discipline, with texts like the "Vrksayurveda" by Parasara highlighting detailed knowledge about plant anatomy, classification, and medicinal properties, indicating a well-developed understanding of plant life beyond just practical applications in agriculture and medicine. Moreover, the post-Vedic texts like the "Vrikshayurveda" provide intricate descriptions of various plant parts, including roots, stems, leaves, flowers, and fruits, showcasing a deep understanding of plant morphology. These texts also demonstrate early attempts at classifying plants based on their characteristics, with specific terminology used to identify different plant groups (Balkrishna et al. 2019; Makal 2024).

Objectives and Methods

The ancient science of studying plants in India was called Vrikshayurveda, which means "tree care" or "arboreal medicine." It was a comprehensive and detailed treatise on plant life. It covered topics like how to procure, preserve, and treat seeds; how to prepare pits for planting saplings; how to select soil and water plants; how to nourish and fertilize plants; how to protect plants from diseases; how to lay out a garden; and

groundwater resources. This Vrikshayurveda was written around 400 BC by Salihotra. It is considered one of the earliest texts to describe various branches of botany. It exemplifies a comprehensive understanding of plant biology, ailments, and treatments. It highlights the role of trees in health and spirituality. Thus, this Vrikshayurveda also enunciated the Indian ethos on plants and trees, environment, and ecology. Keeping all the considerations of use of botany, the scientific study of plants, the arboreal medicine of Vrikshayurveda and medicinal herbs of the Indus Valley Civilization, Vedic and post-Vedic period in mind, the present chapter has tried to examine the elements and wellness application of botany and medicinal plants in ancient India by extensive review and reflections from the available secondary evidence. Besides, it has explored the application of plants, plant parts, and plant products of Indus Valley Civilization and Vedic period as well as science of ethnomedicine developed in the post-Vedic times.

Medical Botany in Ancient India

Medical botany in ancient India was primarily concerned with identifying and classifying plants as sources of drugs. This was an important part of Ayurvedic medicine, an ancestral Indian medical discipline. Ancient Indian botanists discussed concepts like the movement of sap within plants, the role of sunlight in photosynthesis, and the impact of environmental factors on plant growth, indicating a grasp of plant physiology. In ancient India, the knowledge of botany was directly applied to fields like medicine (in the "Charaka Samhita" and "Sushruta Samhita") and agriculture ("Krishi Parasara"), further establishing it as an independent scientific discipline. Besides, in India, the study of taxonomical rank classification and naming of plants in the Sanskrit language is much older than that of Latin and Greek languages, and the study dates back to Vedic period from 2500 BC to 600 BC. In the Rig Veda, three groups of plants have been recognized, namely, trees (*Briksha*), herbs (*Osadhi*), and creepers (*Virudh*). These are further classified into flowering, nonflowering, fruit bearing, and fruitless plants. The Atharva Veda also contains descriptions of many medicinal plants.

In the ancient Indian texts, the nomenclature of the plants was generally based on the plants, botanical characters, and their therapeutic properties. Different ancient written records in the form of manuscripts, are available in Sanskrit and several other Indian languages. Sanskrit literature includes the Vedas, the Upanishads, and epics like the Ramayana and the Mahabharata. The common literature available includes prose, poetry, and drama of a number of Sanskrit authors like Kalidasa, Magha, and Bhavabhuti, in whose works the information on plants is incidental and given by way of comparison. Technical literature on medicinal plants with complete detail of morphology and pharmacology is described in works like the Charaka Samhita and Sushruta Samhita, lexicons like Medinikosa and Amarakosa, as well as encyclopedic works like Arthasastra and Brihat Samhita are also there. In addition, there is an exclusive Sanskrit and plants related work under the title of Vrikshayurveda. Parasara's

Vrikshayurveda is supposed to be the most ancient work in actual botany; it was composed during first century BC and first century AD. From the literary evidence it is clear that even in the First Millennium BC, botany was fully systematized and taxonomy was well developed in India (Jain 2013; Balkrishna et al. 2019; Sahu 2023; Makal 2024).

The significant examples of ancient Indian medicinal plants include Senna (which comes from the *Cassia angustifolia* plant and has laxative, antibacterial, and anti-inflammatory properties) and Neem (*Azadirachta indica* which has been used medicinally from prehistoric times to the present). The study of medicinal plants and their traditional uses in India is called medical ethnobotany. Plants have been used in the Indian subcontinent for thousands of years to maintain health and treat disease. Some examples of ancient Indian medical botany are given here:

(a) **Vrikshayurveda:** A science that developed in post-Vedic India and was the basis for medicine, agriculture, and arbori-horticulture. The Charaka and Susruta Samhitas are examples of medical texts based on Vriksayurveda.
(b) **Siddha:** An ancient Tamil medicine system dating back to 4,000–10,000 BC. Siddhars used about 13,000 plants in their system, which were classified into three groups: herbal products, inorganic substances, and animal products.
(c) **Unani:** A medicine system that originated in Greece and was introduced to India by the Arabs around the eleventh century. Unani medicine incorporated elements from other traditional medicine systems, including those of India, China, Egypt, Persia, Iraq, and Syria.
(d) **Ayurvedic Medicine:** This system of medicine, documented in the Atharva Veda, Rig Veda, and Sushruta Samhita, uses hundreds of herbs and spices, including turmeric.

Role of Medicinal Plants in Ancient India

Medicinal plants were a vital part of ancient Indian healthcare and culture. These medicinal plants were used to treat a variety of health issues and were also used for cultural reasons. The ancient Rishis (Sages) of India developed Ayurveda, a holistic system of natural healing based on plants. On the other hand, the Vedic literatures like Rigveda and Atharvaveda describe the properties of medicinal plants and are among the earliest written documents on Indian medicine. Again, healers and practitioners of traditional medicine prepared their own recipes and dispensed them to patients. Besides, the medicinal plants used in ancient India were used to treat a variety of health issues and also used for cultural reasons. Ancient Indians considered biodiversity to be an inseparable part of their life and culture. Even presently, many people in India still use traditional Ayurvedic medicine, which is based on plants. In addition, medicinal plants are an important part of indigenous medical systems around the world.

Plant-based products used to treat diseases or to maintain health are called herbal products, botanical products, or phytomedicines. In other words, herbal medicine, also called botanical medicine or phytomedicine, refers to using a plant's seeds, berries, roots, leaves, bark, or flowers for medicinal purposes. Herbalism has a long tradition of use outside conventional medicine. The major use of herbal medicines is for health promotion and therapy for chronic, as opposed to life-threatening, conditions. However, the usage of traditional remedies increases when conventional medicine is ineffective in the treatment of disease, such as in advanced cancer and in the face of new infectious diseases. Accordingly, medicinal plants have many uses, including treating ailments, improving health, and making perfumes. In such a way, many plants were used as medicinal remedies in ancient India, including Aloe vera, Garlic, Tulsi, Shatavari, and more. The common medicinal plants used in ancient India include Ashwagandha, Giloe, Turmeric, Ginger, Cinnamon, Tulsi, Black Pepper, Black Cumin, Amla, Garlic, and Flaxseeds. These plants have been traditionally used as herbal remedies for multiple diseases since ancient times. Besides, these herbs have been utilized in food preparations and traditional medicines in several countries. The history, medicinal uses, and properties of these common medicinal plants of ancient India are described in Table 20.1.

Use of Plants in Indus Valley Civilization

The Indus Valley Civilization was the first known mature civilization of ancient India, located around the Indus River in present-day Pakistan. It flourished from approximately 2500 to 1500 BC. The Indus Valley Civilization people used plants for food, fiber, and other purposes. There is concrete evidence of the cultivation of barley, bread wheat, field pea, jujube, rice, green gram, linseed, and cotton from the southern region of the Harappan civilization. Evidence also suggests that Indus Valley people consumed cereals (barley, wheat, millets, and rice were grown in large quantities); pulses (peas, lentils, and green gram were grown); fruits (jujubes, melons, and bananas were grown); oilseeds (linseed was grown); and spices (well-spiced foods were likely eaten). Besides, in the cities of Harappa and Mohenjodaro, leftovers of large granaries were found that suggest that they produced more than their requirements. Barley and wheat were grown by them on a large scale. They also grew some other crops such as pulses, cotton, cereals, dates, melons, and peas. On the other hand, the discovery of the preserved structure of jute fibers on an artifact securely dated to 2200–1900 BC is the earliest evidence for the use of this plant for textiles in the Indus civilization (Agrawal 2007; Bates 2019).

Thus, Indus Valley people grew a variety of crops, including wheat, barley, cotton, cereals, and dates. They were the first to cultivate cotton. They also domesticated animals like cows, buffalo, sheep, goats, dogs, and cats. The Indus Valley people domesticated buffaloes to plow fields and transport goods. Furthermore, the evidence suggests that the Indus Valley people used a variety of medicinal plants including cannabis, ephedra,

Table 20.1. Common Medicinal Plants Used in Ancient India

Local Name	Scientific and Family Name	History	Medicinal Uses and Properties
Ashwagandha	*Withania somnifera* Family: Solanaceae	Ashwagandha is pharmacologically a significant medicinal plant of the Indian subcontinent, used in Ayurvedic and indigenous systems of medicine for more than 3,000 years. It's also known as Indian ginseng.	Ashwagandha is commonly used to treat stress, anxiety, and insomnia. Other potential uses include improving sleep, increasing energy, improving sexual health, reducing blood sugar, improving brain function, and reducing inflammation.
Giloe	*Tinospora cordifolia* Family: Menispermaceae	Giloy has been used in India since ancient times for its many health benefits. In Ayurvedic texts, Giloy is considered a potent and important medicinal product. In Hindu mythology, "giloe" refers to a heavenly elixir that keeps celestial beings young.	Giloy has anti-inflammatory, antioxidant, antidiabetic, antipyretic, and immunomodulatory properties. It is used to treat various ailments and diseases, including diabetes, hypertriglyceridemia, stress, and anxiety. It is also used to increase platelet count in dengue.
Turmeric	*Curcuma longa* Family: Zingiberaceae	Turmeric was used in ancient India for cooking, medicine, and religious rituals. It was also used as a natural dye and perfume. The use of turmeric dates back nearly 4,000 years to the Vedic culture in India, where it was used as a culinary spice and had some religious significance.	Used to treat digestive issues, joint pain, arthritis, intestinal problems and also used to treat coughs, respiratory ailments, anorexia, rheumatism, dysentery, abdominal pain, dental disorders, liver disease, acidity, dyspepsia, ulcers, indigestion, and flatulence.
Ginger	*Zingiber officinale* Family: Zingiberaceae	Ginger has been used in India for thousands of years as a spice and medicinal herb. Ginger was used as a tonic root and flavoring agent in ancient India. It was exported from India to the Roman Empire over 2,000 years ago.	Used to treat many ailments, including headaches, nausea, stomach problems, and colds. It was also used as a tonic for the memory and digestive system.

Cinnamon	*Cinnamomum verum* Family: Lauraceae	Cinnamon was mentioned in India as early as 1180. The first mention of cinnamon growing in India was in Maimonides's Mishneh Torah around 1180. Cinnamon originated in Sri Lanka, which was known as Ceylon in ancient times. Cinnamon was used in traditional European medicine. The Dutch destroyed cinnamon trees along the coast of India to maintain their monopoly on the spice. The Portuguese eventually established control over the cinnamon trade.	Cinnamon has many potential medicinal uses for its antioxidant, anti-inflammatory, antidiabetic, and antimicrobial properties. It may help reduce inflammation, pain, and joint tenderness and swelling. It may help lower blood sugar and reduce the risk of type 2 diabetes. It may improve insulin sensitivity and may be beneficial for the aging brain. It may help treat digestive issues. It plays a role in traditional medicine for treating bronchitis.
Tulsi	*Ocimum tenuiflorum* Family: Lamiaceae	Tulsi is known as holy basil. In the Rig Veda, Tulasi is mentioned and that is generally dated around to 1500 BC. Prakash and Gupta (2011) assert that Tulasi has been used in India for around 5,000 years and is acclaimed for its healing properties of the mind, body, and spirit. Tulsi is a sacred plant in Hinduism. The Lord Krishna, an avatar of Vishnu, is said to wear a garland of holy basil leaves and flowers around his neck.	Tulsi has been used for its therapeutic properties since around 5000–4000 BC. It is revered as the "Queen of Herbs" in the Ayurvedic tradition. Tulsi is used in Ayurvedic medicine to treat respiratory ailments, digestive problems, and more. Tulsi is also used in granny's remedies.
Black Pepper	*Piper nigrum* Family: Piperaceae	Black pepper (*Piper nigrum*) has been used in Indian cooking since at least 2000 BC. It originated in the Western Ghats region of India, and was especially prized in the Malabar Coast, which is now part of Kerala. The Yajur Veda, one of the oldest Vedas, mentions the use of pipali (pepper in Sanskrit). Black pepper was so valuable that it was known as "black gold" by merchants. The finest Indian pepper continues to come from the Malabar region. In Ayurveda, black pepper is called maricha. In Assamese, black pepper is called jalook or gulmorich.	Black pepper has many medicinal uses including anti-inflammatory, antimicrobial, and antioxidant properties. It stimulate the stomach to secrete acids that help with digestion. It stimulate leucocytes, which increase immunity against pathogens. It improve the iron supplements. It boost melanocyte proliferation, which can bring back pigmentation to depigmented skin. It regulate blood sugar levels. It may also increase high-density lipoprotein (good cholesterol). It helps to treat dry coughs, relieve nasal congestion, nerve degeneration.

(*Continued*)

Table 20.1 (Continued)

Local Name	Scientific and Family Name	History	Medicinal Uses and Properties
Black Cumin	*Nigella sativa* Family: Ranunculaceae	Black cumin was an ancient spice and medicine in India. It was used as a condiment, in herbal medicines, and as a spice in cooking. It is native to the Indian subcontinent, the eastern Mediterranean, northern Africa, and West Asia. It has been used in ancient Greek, Roman, and Hebrew texts. A bottle of black cumin oil was found in the tomb of King Tutankhamen. It is mentioned in religious books of Islam and Christianity. In India, it is used as a spice in cooking, and as a garnish on bread and vegetable curries. In Bengal, it is used as Phanchphorn in many vegetable preparations. It is also used in pickle preparation. Black cumin is also known as kalonji, kala jeera, Himali Jira, fennel flower, black caraway, nutmeg flower, and Roman coriander.	Black cumin in traditional Indian medicine was used to treat a variety of diseases, including asthma, bronchitis, fever, and inflammation. Black cumin has been used in traditional Chinese medicine, Arabian medicine, and Ayurveda. Black cumin has many health benefits including antioxidant, anti-inflammatory, antimicrobial, immunomodulatory, hepatoprotective, neuro-protective, gastroprotective properties. Black cumin may help with Alzheimer's disease, Parkinson's disease, stroke, brain injury, anxiety, depression, and epilepsy. It helps to treat acne, psoriasis, eczema, and vitiligo. It is also used to treat, rheumatoid arthritis, diarrhea, indigestion, dyspepsia, hypertension, high blood pressure, diabetes, metabolic syndrome.
Amla	*Phyllanthus emblica* Family: Phyllanthaceae	Amla is known as Indian gooseberry. It has been used in ancient Indian medicine, culture, and folk remedies. According to Hindu mythology, the Amla tree grew from tears shed by Brahma while he meditated on Vishnu. The twenty-first Buddha, Phussa Buddha, is said to have achieved enlightenment under an amla tree. Amla is also used in Siddha, Unani, Tibetan, Sri Lankan, and Chinese medicine. It is used to make Chyawanprash, an Ayurvedic preparation that is said to restore health and longevity.	Amla is a key ingredient in Ayurvedic medicine and is considered a super berry. It is used to treat bleeding disorders and hyperacidity. It is a rich source of vitamin C, minerals, and amino acids. It contains carbohydrates, fiber, protein, iron, calcium, and phosphorous. It is used in folk remedies to treat constipation, gastric ulcers, and inflammatory bowel disease. Besides, it is also used to promote longevity, strengthen immunity, and purify the blood. Amla is considered a "Rasayana" bestowed with anti-aging effects.

Garlic	*Allium sativum* Family: Amaryllidaceae	Garlic has been used in India since ancient times as a food and medicine. Garlic was used in the Indus Valley Civilization. The Sanskrit word for garlic is lasuna. Fresh garlic was eaten while it was still tender and immature, and before the bulb separated into cloves. Garlic was used in the ancient medical traditions of Tibbi, Unani, and Ayurveda. The Charaka Samhita, a leading surviving medical text, recommended garlic to treat heart disease and arthritis.	In ancient India, garlic was used to treat ailments such as arthritis, parasites, leprosy, and heart disease, as well as symptoms like fatigue and indigestion. The Sanskrit word for garlic is mahoushudh, which means panacea, or "cure-all." Even before the development of germ theory, garlic was used to ward of germs.
Flaxseeds	*Linum usitatissimum* Family: Linaceae	Flaxseeds were a vital crop in ancient India, valued for their nutritional benefits and for making textiles. Flaxseeds were also known as alsi in Hindi. Flaxseeds were used in Ayurvedic practices for centuries. Flaxseeds can help reduce the risk of heart disease by lowering cholesterol and triglycerides. It can help with weight loss by suppressing hunger and cravings.	Flaxseeds are high in fiber, which can help with constipation and maintain bowel health. It contains soluble fiber, which traps cholesterol and fat in the digestive system, making it difficult for the body to absorb. It contains omega-3 fatty acids, fiber, lignins, and antioxidants, which can help reduce the risk of heart disease. It contains soluble fiber, which becomes sticky when mixed with water, which can help suppress hunger and cravings. It can help with skin health.
Shatavari	*Asparagus racemosus* Family: Asparagaceae	Shatavari is a medicinal plant that has been used in Ayurvedic medicine since ancient times. It is native to the Indian subcontinent and is also found in Africa, Sri Lanka, China, and the Himalayas. The name "Shatavari" translates to "she who possesses a hundred husbands." It has been used to promote women's health and vigor. It is also used to support the digestive system. It is sometimes used as a rejuvenative tonic to help women transition through various phases of life, including menopause.	Shatavari is an adaptogenic herb that can manage stress. It is also used to support the female reproductive system. It is commonly used to boost milk production during breastfeeding. Shatavari powder treats gastric ulcers and might prevent future ulcers from forming. Supports lactation. Some breastfeeding mothers use shatavari powder to increase their milk production. In Bengali, it is called Śatmali. In Marathi and Gujurati, it is called Śatāvarī. In Tamil, it is called Śimāi-sadāvarī.

(*Continued*)

Table 20.1 (Continued)

Local Name	Scientific and Family Name	History	Medicinal Uses and Properties
Gurmar	*Gymnema sylvestre* Family: Apocynaceae	Gurmar is a shrub native to India that has been used in Ayurvedic medicine for thousands of years. It's also known as "sugar destroyer." The ancient literature on Indian medicine, Sushruta, describes gurmar as a destroyer of madhumeha (glycosuria) and other urinary disorders.	Gurmar is used to treat diabetes by inhibiting sugar absorption and stimulating the pancreas to metabolize excess sugar. Gurmar is also used to treat jaundice, constipation, cardiopathy, asthma, bronchitis, and more. The root juice of the plant is used to treat snakebites.
Senna	*Cassia angustifolia* Family: Fabaceae	Senna has been used in India since ancient times as a laxative and purgative. It is also known as "Tirunelvelly Senna." It is believed to have been used in Tirunelvelle, Tamil Nadu, around the eleventh century. It is a native of Pakistan, India, North Africa, and Sudan. It is grown in semi-arid regions of Gujarat, Rajasthan, and Tamil Nadu. It is also used in Unani system of medicine.	Senna is used on a short-term basis to treat constipation. It also is used to empty the bowels before surgery and certain medical procedures. Senna is in a class of medications called stimulant laxatives. It works by increasing activity of the intestines to cause a bowel movement. It is used to cleanse the body and blood by purging "obstructions," melancholy, and phlegm.

Source: Author.

ginger, turmeric, and garlic. Besides, the dental evidence suggests that cattle in the Indus Valley Civilization consumed ginger and turmeric. Again, garlic cloves were used in the Indus Valley Civilization. Other evidence of medical practices suggests that the Indus Valley Civilization used earth and clays internally and externally such as for treating wounds and in surgery. Also, other evidence suggests that the Indus Valley Civilization had knowledge of bone structure and performed brain surgery. Again, the Indus Valley Civilization had healing practices with victims surviving for a substantial period of time following operations. As a final point, the Indus Valley Civilization is considered to be advanced for its time. They were also skilled at medical science with evidence of proto-dentistry, brain surgery, and usage of herbs for treatment.

Renowned Plants, Practice, and Classification in Vedic Period

The Vedic period, or the Vedic age (*c*. 1500–*c*. 500 BC) is the period in the late Bronze Age and early Iron Age of the history of India. So, the Vedic period was a time between 1500 and 500 BC when the Vedas were composed. The Vedas are the oldest sacred texts of Hinduism. The Vedic period is significant because it helped establish the social, political, and religious foundations of India. The Vedic period saw a transition from a seminomadic lifestyle to settled agriculture. The Vedic society was patriarchal and patrilineal. The Vedic economy was based on a combination of pastoralism and agriculture. The Vedas were composed and orally transmitted by speakers of an Old Indo-Aryan language. Some of the Vedas are Rig Veda (one of the oldest Vedic Sanskrit texts, composed during the Early Vedic age), Yajur Veda (contains formulas and mantras for rituals and sacrifices), Sama Veda (the shortest of all Vedas and consists of hymns used for rituals), and Aranyakas (also called forest books as they were written chiefly by hermits residing in the forests for their students). The Vedic age is divided into the Early Vedic period (1500–1000 BC) and the Later Vedic period (1000–600 BC). These periods are distinguished by the significant social changes that occurred between the writing of the first Vedas and the emergence of later Vedic scriptures (Bloomfield 1908).

The most renowned plant that finds frequent mention in the Rig Veda and later Samhitas is the Soma plant. The Vedic Indians hail the Soma plant as the Lord of the forest (Vanaraja). The botanical identity of the Soma plant has not been decided till today. The probable candidates are Ephedra (a Gymnosperm), Sarcostemma (flowering plant), and mushroom (a fungus). The second most mentioned plant was Peepal or the Asvattha (*Ficus religiosa*) during the Vedic period. The Rig Veda refers to utensils and vessels fashioned out of the wood of the Asvattha tree. Some of the other trees that find mention in the Vedas are (i) Silk cotton (*Salmalia malabaricum*) (ii) Khadira (*Acacia catechu*) (iii) Simsupa (*Dalbergia sissoo*) (iv) Vibhitaka (*Terminalia bellerica*) (v) Sami (*Prosopis* sp.) (vi) Plaksa (*Ficus infectoria*), and (vii) Iksu or sugar cane (*Saccharum officinarum*) finds a mention as a cultivated plant in the Atharvaveda, Maitaryani Samhita, and other texts. The Vedic Indians knew about many flower-bearing and fruit-bearing plants like Palasa (*Butea monosperma*) and two varieties of lotus that is white (pundarika) and blue (puskara), white lily (kumuda), cucumber (urvaruka), jujuba (*Zizypus jujuba*), udumbara (*Ficus glomerata*), kharjura (*Phoenix dactylifera*), and bilva (*Aegle marmelos*).

The written records, in the form of manuscripts, are available in Sanskrit and several other Indian languages. Sanskrit literature includes the Vedas, the Upanisads, and epics like the Ramayana and the Mahabharata. The lay literature includes prose, poetry, and drama of a number of Sanskrit authors like Kalidasa, Magha, and Bhavabhuti, in whose works the information on plants is incidental and given by way of comparison. On the other hand, the methodological literature comprises medical works like the Charaka Samhita and Susruta Samhita, lexicons like Medininighantu and Amarakosa, and encyclopedic works like Arthasastra and Brhatsamhita are also there. In addition, there is an exclusive Sanskrit and plants related work under the title of Vrksayurveda. Parasara's Vrksayurveda is supposed to be the most ancient work in actual botany. It was composed during first century BC and first century AD. From the literary evidence, it is clear that even in the First Millennium BC, botany was fully systematized and taxonomy was well developed in India. The naming of plants and study of classification in India is even older than those of Greeks and Romans, and dates back to Vedic period (2500 BC to 600 BC).

The Rig Veda recognized three groups of plants, namely, trees (Vriksha), herbs (Osadhi), and creepers (Virudh). These are further classified into flowering, nonflowering, fruit bearing, and fruitless plants. Atharvaveda also contains descriptions of many medicinal plants. Casual references to different parts of the plant are found scattered throughout the Rig Veda, and almost complete details of plants are found in the Atharvaveda. The Atharvaveda is perhaps the earliest recorded authority on plant morphology. It presents an account of eight types of growth habits of trees. These are Visakha (spreading branches), Manjari (leaves with long clusters), Sthambini (bushy plants), Prastanavati (which expands), Ekasrnga (those with monopodial growth), Pratanavati (creeping plants), Amsumati (with many stalks), and Kandini (plants with knotty joints). The Taittiriya Samhita and the Vajasenayi Samhita explain that plants are comprised of Mula (root), the Tula (shoot), the Kanda (stem), the Valsa (twigs), Puspa (flowers), and Phala (fruits). On the other hand, the trees have Skandha (the crown), Sakha (branches), and Parna (leaf).

In addition, various types of plants are renowned, namely, Vriksa, Vana, and Druma (trees), Visakha (shrubs with spreading branches), Sasa (an herb), Amsumali (a spreading or deliquescent plant), Vratati (a climber), Stambini (a bushy plant), Pratanavati (a creeper), and Alasala (those spreading on the ground). The Vriksayurveda of Parasara deals comprehensively with the morphology of plants. According to Parasara, the Vriksangas (parts of plant) are Patra (leaf), Puspa (flowers), Phala (fruits), Mula (root), Tvak (bark), Kanda (stem), Sara (heartwood), Svarasa (sap), Niryasa (exudation), Kantaka (spines), Bija (seed), and Praroha (shoot). Thus, the ancient literature classified the roots on the basis of their growth behavior and structures like Sakha, Sipha (root originating from the branches), Krsnamuli (black colored root), Sveta muli (colored root), Bahumuli (many roots), Tripadi (plant with three main roots), Asta-padi (plant with eight roots), Sthulamula (thick root), Suksmamula (thin root), and Jatamula (fasciculated root).

During the Vedic period, people extensively used a variety of plant products for food, medicine, religious rituals, and even agriculture, demonstrating a deep understanding of botany and plant properties, with evidence found in Vedic texts like the Rig Veda where specific plants are mentioned and their usage described in detail; key practices included using grains like rice, barley, and lentils as staple food, utilizing plants for medicinal purposes, and incorporating plant parts into religious ceremonies as offerings to deities. The key aspects of plant product usage in the Vedic period are given below:

(i) **Food crops:** The Vedic people cultivated a range of grains like rice, barley, millet, sesame, lentils, and pulses, which formed the basis of their diet.
(ii) **Medicinal plants:** Vedic texts mention various plants with medicinal properties, used for treating ailments with knowledge about different parts of the plant like roots, leaves, and bark.
(iii) **Religious rituals:** Plants played a crucial role in Vedic rituals, with specific plants used as offerings to gods, for decorating the sacrificial altar, and in various ceremonial practices.

Some important plant examples of the Vedic period which are used in religious practices are Darbha grass (used to cover the sacrificial altar during rituals); Soma plant (considered a sacred plant, believed to provide divine power and used in religious ceremonies); Ashoka tree (associated with fertility and used in rituals); and Banyan tree (considered a sacred tree, often used as a place of worship). Besides, the Vedic texts demonstrate a detailed understanding of different plant parts and their specific uses, including leaves, flowers, fruits, seeds, and roots. Various evidence suggests that the Vedic people practiced crop rotation and used manure to improve soil fertility, indicating an advanced level of agricultural knowledge.

Botany and Medicinal Plants in Post-Vedic Time

The post-Vedic period, also known as the Later Vedic period, was a time in India from about 1000 to 600 BC. It was a time of significant social, economic, and cultural change. The post-Vedic period in India was a time of significant change, including the rise of new religions, literary developments, and social shifts. In post-Vedic India, botany developed into an independent science that was used in medicine, agriculture, and horticulture. The ancient Indian texts categorized plants into groups like herbs, trees, and creepers, and documented their medicinal properties. The important ideas about post-Vedic Indian botany are given here:

(a) **Botany and Medicine:** Botany and medicine are related through the study of medicinal plants and their use in treating disease. The study of plants and medicine is called medicinal botany, and the use of plants for medicinal purposes is called herbal medicine. The texts of Charaka and Susruta Samhitas embody the science of medicine based on botany. On the other hand, the ancient Vrikshayurveda text deals with various tree and plant species including herbs, shrubs, and trees. It also covers agrihorticulture, home gardening, intercropping, and storage.

(b) **Botany and Agriculture:** Botany is the study of plants, while agriculture is the practice of growing crops and raising animals for food. Agricultural botany is the study of plants used for farming and food production. The text of Krsi-Parasara embodies the science of agriculture based on botany. On the other hand, the text of Upavana-vinoda illustrates the branch of botany known as arbori-horticulture.

(c) **Botany and Ritual:** Botany and ritual are closely linked in many cultures, with plants used in ceremonies, worship, and to ward off evil spirits. In Hinduism, plants like mango, banana, coconut, banyan, holy basil, peepal, rice, and black gram are used in rituals. Different trees are associated with different gods and goddesses. Conversely, in Buddhism, the plants like Rubia manjith, Zea mays, Pinus bhutanica, and Pinus roxburghii are used in rituals. They are used to make smoke offerings, burnt as incense, and to ward off evil spirits. In a similar way, the Vedas describe the plants and trees used in ritualistic activities or yajñas. The Yajur Veda Saṃhitās and Brāhmaṇās describe the names of plants, trees, and their products used in the yajñas, yāgās, hōmās, and iṣṭis.

(d) **Botany and Holistic Development:** Botany and holistic development refers to the idea that studying botany, the science of plants, can contribute to a person's overall well-being and development by fostering a deeper connection with nature, promoting environmental awareness, and understanding the vital role plants play in the ecosystem, thus impacting not only intellectual growth but also emotional and social aspects of a person's life. In a similar way, the renowned ancient text Vrikshayurveda suggests that tree planting is one of the means to attain the four broad aims of life that is Dharma, Artha, Kama, and Moksha.

Many medicinal plants were used in post-Vedic times including herbs, grasses, water plants, and weeds. The herbs mentioned in the Vedic texts are Ishika and Ulapa. On the other hand, the grasses mentioned in the Vedic texts are Darbha and Satamba. Moreover, the water plants mentioned in the Vedic texts are Lotus, Lily, Pundarika, and Puskara. Many other medicinal plants mentioned in post-Vedic times include *Eclipta alba* (a plant that promotes hair growth and is hepatoprotective), *Emblica officinalis* (A fruit, i.e., an antioxidant and adaptogen), *Eugenia jambolana* (A plant, i.e., anti-inflammatory, hypoglycemic, antidiarrheal, and antipyretic), *Ficus religiosa* (a plant that is anti-inflammatory, hypoglycemic, and antiulcer), *Camomile* (A plant, i.e., used to treat wounds, burns, stings, and ulcers).

Science of Ethnomedicine in Ancient India

The medical ethnobotany of India is the study of Indian medicinal plants and their traditional uses. Plants have been used in the Indian subcontinent for the treatment of disease and health maintenance for thousands of years and remain important staples of health and folk medicine for millions. Thus, ethnomedicine in ancient India primarily refers to the traditional medical practices based on the knowledge of indigenous plants and animals used by various tribal communities across the Indian subcontinent, with the most prominent example being the well-documented system of Ayurveda, which is considered a comprehensive and codified form of this knowledge, drawing from ancient Indian scriptures like the Vedas and Puranas for its practices and plant-based remedies. The significant points about the ethnomedicine in ancient India are given here:

(i) **Ayurveda as the Central System:** Ayurveda is considered the most well-known example of ethnomedicine in India, with its focus on holistic healing using herbal remedies, dietary adjustments, and lifestyle practices like yoga and meditation.
(ii) **Source of Knowledge:** The knowledge of ethnomedicine in ancient India was passed down orally through generations within tribal communities and was often closely linked to their cultural beliefs and practices.
(iii) **Plant-based Remedies:** The primary source of medicine in ancient Indian ethnomedicine was plants, with different parts of the plants like leaves, bark, roots, and fruits being used for various ailments.
(iv) **Role of Traditional Healers:** Specialized healers within communities, often called Vaidya in Ayurveda, held the knowledge of identifying and utilizing medicinal plants.
(v) **Spiritual Aspects:** Ethnomedicine in ancient India often intertwined with spiritual beliefs, where healing practices were seen as a way to restore balance within the body and the cosmos.

Thus, many medical systems are mentioned in the ancient Vedas and other scriptures. But Ayurveda is the most recognized example of ethnomedicine in ancient India. The Ayurvedic concept appeared and developed between 2500 and 500 BC in India. The literal meaning of Ayurveda is "science of life," because ancient Indian system of health care focused on views of man and his illness. Specifically in India, Ayurveda is considered not just as an ethnomedicine but also as a complete medical system that takes into consideration physical, psychological, philosophical, ethical, and spiritual well-being of mankind.

Holistic Healing Using Ayurvedic Medicinal Plants

The use of medicinal plants in Ayurveda is based on the science of "Herbs and Plants." However, there are some controversies surrounding the use of medicinal plants in Ayurveda, including the lack of a taxonomic system and the use of common names for different plants. Acharya Charak, who was born around 300 BC, was a vital contributor to Ayurveda's ancient art and science, medicine, and lifestyle system that originated in ancient India. Acharya Charak was designated as the Father of Indian Medicine. His well-known book, the "Samhita Charak," is regarded as an Ayurvedic encyclopedia. The Charaka Samhita is the oldest known Hindu text on Ayurveda (life sciences) followed by the Sushruta Samhita and Ashtanga Hrdaya. It is believed that Dhanvantari is the Hindu God of Ayurveda, the traditional Indian system of medicine. He is also known as the physician of all Gods and Goddesses. This Ayurveda is a holistic healing system that uses natural remedies, including medicinal plants, to promote health and wellness. Ayurveda treatments may include diet, exercise, lifestyle changes, herbal formulations, massages, and medicinal preparations. Besides, this Ayurveda is based on the belief that health and wellness depend on a balance between the mind, body, spirit, and environment.

The bulk of the Ayurvedic medicines belong to the plant kingdom. Each plant or herb has a specific quality and can be used to treat a multitude of ailments and diseases. Medicinal plants like aloe, turmeric, tulsi, pepper, elachi, and ginger are commonly used in a number of Ayurvedic home remedies and are considered to be the best aid in fighting ailments. Besides, all the Ayurvedic texts deal with botanical aspects, mainly the identification and categorization of plants as sources of drugs. The Charaka Samhita has a chapter titled Vibhagavidya, dealing with the classification of plants and animals. The Sushruta Samhita, the second Ayurvedic classic, also deals with several aspects of botany such as morphology and taxonomy. Susruta also provides classification of plants on the basis of medicinal properties. Thus, early Indian texts, like the Vedas, mention plants with magical properties. The Sushruta Samhita describes over 700 plants used for medicinal purposes. This text reflects a level of medical knowledge and practice comparable to ancient Egypt.

These Ayurvedic medicinal plants are used in a traditional Indian healing system and are considered safe and nontoxic. They are often recommended for their therapeutic value and are said to treat the root cause of disease, which can help keep you healthy in the long run. Ayurvedic herbs are also said to balance doshas, improve vitality, and boost immunity. Different Ayurvedic medicinal plants like Ghrit-Kumari (*Aloe barbadensis*), Sarpgandha (*Rauwolfia serpentina*), Brahmi (*Bacopa monnieri*), Tulsi (*Ocimum sanctum*), Gugglu (*Commiphora mukul*), Amla (*Emblica officinalis*), Ashwagandha (*Withania somnifera*), Arjun (*Terminalia Arjuna*), Turmeric (*Curcuma longa*), Neem (Azadirachta indica), and so on, are some examples out of the list of the medicinal plants which were part of our ancient medicinal system, and surprisingly, it has been shown that the phytochemicals found in these plants were able to fight a number of diseases, as shown in Figure 20.1.

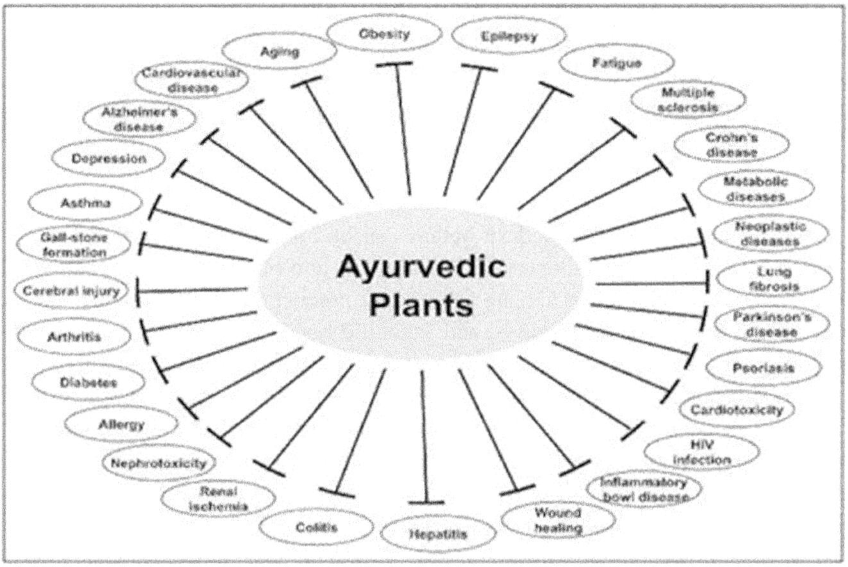

Figure 20.1. Ayurvedic medicinal plants able to fight with a number of diseases. Source: Author.

Conclusion and Recommendation

This study has concluded that the common medicinal plants used in ancient India include Ashwagandha, Giloe, Ginger, Cinnamon, Tulsi, Black Pepper, Black Cumin, Amla, Turmeric, Garlic, and Flaxseeds. In addition, this study shows that the Ayurvedic system of medicine or Ayurveda is an indigenous ancient medical science of India. Again, the ancient texts like Atharva Veda, Rig Veda, and Sushruta Samhita used hundreds of herbs and spices for the treatment of various illnesses. Again, on the basis of historical periods of ancient India, it may be concluded that the study of plants (plant taxonomy and study of medicinal plants) had been developed during the Vedic period (2500 BC to 600 BC). Our ancient Doctors, Healers, and Sages like Sushruta and Shastrakarma (Father of Indian Surgery), Atreya and Agnivesa (Master and the disciple together compiled Ayurveda), Sage Agasthya and Patanjali had vast knowledge of plants with their botanical characteristics and medicinal value.

Therefore literature related to botanical descriptions and information in the Vedas are available in Rig Veda, Yajur Veda, and Atharva Veda, but they are mostly in discrete form. Accordingly, an attempt has been made to accumulate it in one place for the benefit of interested scholars, readers, and students. For this reason, this systematic review has described in detail the medical botany in ancient India; the role of medicinal plants in ancient India; the use of plants in the Indus Valley Civilization; renowned plants, practice, and classification in the Vedic period; botany and medicinal plants in post-Vedic time; the science of ethnomedicine in ancient India; and holistic healing using Ayurvedic medicinal plants. It is clearly evident from the discussion that the morphology, taxonomy, classification of plants, anatomy, physiology, and the agricultural and botanical terminologies are revealed in the Vedas with a specific purpose. In post-Vedic India, botany developed into an independent science that was used in medicine, agriculture, and horticulture. The ancient Indian texts categorized plants into groups like herbs, trees, and creepers, and documented their medicinal properties.

In fact, many aspects of modern botany can be traced back to Vedas and other derived Sanskrit literature. The detailed taxonomies and classifications also happened in the Charaka Saṃhita and Susruta Saṃhita. Consequently, we understand that the ancient Scientists, Doctors, Healers, and Sages did realize the need to classify plants according to their various characteristics and properties. In most cases, they come close to modern classifications. To further conclude, there is an urgent need to protect the traditional knowledge such as Vedic botany and agriculture for future generations. Vedic botany can be adopted as part of the syllabus at higher levels of education in order to propagate our traditional knowledge among the later generations. Finally, this study has recommended that India should develop a health policy with a strong emphasis on promoting and integrating the traditional or ancient medicinal system into modern healthcare to resolve the health issues of Indian people. Improving research and conservation of traditional and ancient Indian medicinal knowledge are significant to discourse the health of Indian populations.

References

Agrawal, D. P. *The Indus Civilisation: An Interdisciplinary Perspective.* Delhi: Aryan Books International, 2007.

Ang-Lee, M. K., J. Moss, and C. S. Yuan. "Herbal Medicines and Perioperative Care." *JAMA* 286, no. 2 (2001): 208–16.

Balkrishna, A., R. K. Mishra, A. Srivastava, B. Joshi, R. Marde, and U. B. Prajapati. "Ancient Indian Rishi's (Sages) Knowledge of Botany and Medicinal Plants Since Vedic Period Was Much Older Than the Period of Theophrastus, A Case Study-Who Was the Actual Father of Botany?" *International Journal of Unani and Integrative Medicine* 3, no. 3 (2019): 40–4.

Bates, J. "Oilseeds, Spices, Fruits and Flavour in the Indus Civilization." *Journal of Archaeological Science: Reports* 24 (2019): 879–87.

Bloomfield, M. *The Religion of the Veda: The Ancient Religion of India, from Rig-Vēda to Upanishads.* New York: Knickerbocker Press, 1908.

Fatemeh, J. K., L. Zahra, and A. K. Hossein. "Medicinal Plants: Past History and Future Perspective." *Journal of Herbmed Pharmacology* 7, no. 1 (2018): 1–7.

Jain, A. K. "Traditional Botanical Knowledge in Ancient India." *Journal of Traditional and Folk Practices* 1, no. 1 (2013): 31–8.

Kalpana, R. M., and B. Sitaram. "Indication of Vedic Plants Available in the Present Era." *International Journal of Ayurveda and Pharma Research* 4, no. 11 (2016): 22–37.

Makal, A. *Indian Knowledge System: Outlines, Concepts and Applications.* Kolkata: Techno World Publishers, 2024.

Mohanty, R. B., and T. Panda. "Plant Domestication in Indus Valley Civilization." *Indian Journal of History of Science* 55, no. 4 (2020): 349–53.

Prakash, S., and N. Gupta. "Tulasi: The Wonder Herb: Pharmacological Activities of *Ocimum Sanctum*." *Asian Journal of Pharmaceutical and Clinical Research* 4, no. 3 (2011): 29–32.

Ravishankar, B., and V. J. Shukla. "Indian Systems of Medicine: A Brief Profile." *African Journal of Traditional, Complementary and Alternative Medicines* 4, no. 3 (2007): 319–37.

Sahu, S. C. "Holy Basil: A Medicinal Plant in India from Ancient Vedic Times." *Annals of Clinical Case Studies* 5 (2023): 41–2.

Solecki, R. S. "Shanidar IV, a Neanderthal Flower Burial in Northern Iraq." *Science* 190, no. 4217 (1975): 880–1.

Part VI

Current Healthcare Sector and Benefits of Medicinal Plants

21

Benefits and Contributions of Medicinal Plants to Health Sector

Piyasa Ghosh, Shinjini Dey, and Srijita Ghosh*

Post Graduate Department of Botany, Scottish Church College, Kolkata, WB, India

*Corresponding Author's Email: srijita.ghosh@scottishchurch.ac.in

Introduction

Throughout history, humans have depended on nature for mental and physical well-being, underscoring the deep connection between health and the natural world.[1] Plants, as essential elements of nature, play a crucial role in supporting life and nurturing all living organisms (Jamshidi-Kia, Lorigooini, and Amini-Khoei 2017). Early humans recognized the vital role of plants in meeting their essential needs for food, shelter, and clothing, while also turning to medicinal plants for healing. Ancient civilizations such as those in China, Egypt, Greece, and India documented the significance of these plants in early scientific practices, highlighting their role as the primary treatment option for thousands of years (Mosihuzzaman, 2012). In modern times, the rising popularity of herbal products has encouraged healthcare sectors to embrace plant-based therapeutics as viable alternatives. The health benefits of medicinal plants arise from their secondary metabolites, which, through coevolution with biological targets, enhance their efficacy in promoting human health and defending against environmental challenges (Pant, Pandey, and Dall'Acqua 2021). Traditional herbal medicine employs whole plants or their parts, either raw or processed, to address various health conditions. Polyherbal formulations leverage the synergistic effects of active compounds from multiple medicinal herbs to deliver targeted health benefits. Additionally, a wide range of plant-derived products—including herbal teas, health drinks, tablets, lozenges, essential oils, and cosmetics—are increasingly valued for their contributions to overall well-being (Li and Weng 2017). Traditional medicinal

[1] Acknowledgments: Authors are supported financially by the fund received from DST-FIST Programme-SR/ FST/College-/2023/1486 (G).

plants possess various health-promoting and disease-preventive properties, including antimicrobial, anti-inflammatory, and anticancer effects, making them a valuable source for effective medicines. Remarkably, around half of the pharmaceutical drugs used globally have their origins in these traditional herbal remedies (Zahn et al. 2019). Approximately, 10,000 medicinal plants out of 250,000 higher plant species worldwide have a record of traditional medicinal use, and about 200 species among them have been developed into conventional Western pharmaceuticals (Reid et al. 2018). To address the high costs, drug resistance, and side effects of synthetic drugs, scientists are exploring medicinal plants and their active compounds for novel formulations with improved efficacy and extended shelf life. This involves isolating bioactive compounds by analyzing their chemical and pharmaceutical properties, which have been integral to traditional remedies. Additionally, researchers review existing literature to substantiate the disease-preventive activities of these compounds (Patra et al. 2018). The herbal medicine market, including phytomedicines, pyrotherapeutic agents, and dietary supplements, has seen substantial global growth as consumers increasingly favor these products for their perceived safety and cost-effectiveness compared to synthetic pharmaceuticals (Bareetseng 2022). According to the WHO, approximately 80 percent of the global population relies on herbal medicines as their primary healthcare option, with around 250 plant-derived drugs used for essential health needs (WHO 2019). While in vitro and preclinical studies have highlighted the potential health benefits of bioactive compounds in medicinal plants, further research is essential to assess their safety, efficacy, and medical applications. Well-designed clinical trials with adequate sample sizes are critical to generating sufficient evidence for regulatory approval and clinical practice (Dar et al. 2023).

Conceptual Framework

A medicinal plant is defined as any plant that contains biologically active compounds in its leaves, roots, or other parts, which can be used in therapeutic treatments or for developing valuable medicines. Both the whole plant and specific parts can exhibit pharmacological potency (Rungsung et al. 2015). Medicinal plants are garnering growing interest as a source of new therapeutic compounds, driving the development of innovative medicines and serving essential roles in both conventional and traditional healthcare systems. Beyond novel drug synthesis, these plants include a diverse array of species used as spices, flavoring agents, fragrances, and cosmetic ingredients. Their multifunctional applications highlight their importance in health and wellness (Astutik, Pretzsch, and Ndzifon Kimengsi 2019).

(a) **Ancient use of medicinal plants:** Ancient written records reveal that medicinal substances have been used for healing for millennia. According to ancient Babylonian records, plants have been used as medicine for 60,000 years (Qazi and Molvi 2016). The ancient Egyptians harnessed natural sources to create various healing substances between 3,000 and 6,000 years ago, utilizing medicinal plants for analgesics, sedatives, and remedies for gastrointestinal and urinary tract disorders. They were pioneers in the medicinal use of castor oil, wine, opium, mints, marijuana, and the brewing of beer from barley and wheat. Following this, ancient Greece saw the therapeutic use of medicinal plants emerge around 3,000 years ago. Hippocrates, the father of Greek medicine, along with his pupil Aristotle, employed these plants to treat various ailments. Their practices laid the foundation for herbal medicine in Western healthcare (Rosso 2023). Ancient cultures in China, India, and Tibet engaged in extensive plant experimentation for medicinal purposes thousands of years ago. Traditional Chinese Medicine (TCM) has roots dating back to 2700 BC, utilizing herbs and holistic approaches for healing. Ayurveda, established over 5,000 years ago by Hindu healers, features a comprehensive "materia medica" that includes around 1,500 herbs and 10,000 formulations. These systems highlight the deep connection between nature and wellness in early civilizations, showcasing a rich legacy of herbal knowledge that continues to influence modern practices (Jindal and Seth 2022).

(b) **Primary and secondary metabolites:** Plants contain two main types of metabolites: primary and secondary metabolites. Primary metabolites are essential for normal growth, development, and reproduction. They include polysaccharides, carbohydrates, sugars, proteins, amino acids, and lipids. Additionally, fermentation products like ethanol, acetic acid, citric acid, and lactic acid also fall under this category, playing crucial roles in supporting the plant's life processes. These metabolites ensure the overall health and vitality of the plant (Cooper and Nicola 2014). Secondary metabolites (phenolic, steroid, lignans, etc.) on the other hand are not associated with normal growth and development directly. Generally, they are produced in appropriate conditions when there is a need for their activity. For instance, they provide defense response in plants when exposed to herbivory, pathogen invasion, and interspecific competition and protect the plants from a number of abiotic stresses such as changes in temperature, water quantity, and light intensity, exposure to UV, metal toxicity, and mineral deficiency. In addition, they serve as attractants for beneficial organisms like symbionts and pollinators. At the cellular level, these secondary metabolites are involved in signal transduction, modification of gene expression, and regulation of plant growth (Stéphane et al. 2021). The unique medicinal properties of a plant are often linked to the specific combination of secondary metabolites it contains. These compounds can vary significantly between different plant species or families, contributing to their distinct therapeutic effects. This diversity in secondary metabolites is key to the plant's medicinal potential (Wink 1999). The ecological function of secondary metabolites in plants may be related to their potential to have biological effects on humans. For example, cytotoxic secondary products of plants that defend against microbial pathogens could be useful as antimicrobial drugs for humans, provided they are less toxic. Similarly, secondary metabolites with neurotoxic activity against herbivorous animals could be developed into medicines that have potent sedative, antidepressant, muscle relaxant, or anesthetic properties (Briskin 2000). Secondary metabolites have evolved with the molecular targets in the cells or tissues of competing pathogens and animals, thereby effectively imparting their action to facilitate defense response and ecological adaptation of plants (Ramawat and Goyal 2020). Some secondary metabolites in plants closely resemble endogenous hormones, neurotransmitters, and signaling molecules found in humans. This structural similarity allows these plant compounds to interact effectively with specific target sites in the body, such as the endocrine and central nervous systems. As a result, they can exert beneficial medicinal effects, mimicking the actions of natural biological molecules. This intriguing phenomenon, known as "evolutionary molecular modeling," was described by Wink (1999). It suggests that over time, certain plant secondary metabolites have evolved to share characteristics with the molecules in other organisms, enhancing their therapeutic potential. This connection underscores the intricate relationship between plant chemistry and human physiology.

(c) **Bioactive compounds:** Bioactive compounds are chemicals that exhibit specific biological activities and have the potential to impact human health. These compounds can be classified as essential, like vitamins, or nonessential, such as polyphenols and alkaloids. They are derived from a variety of natural sources, including plants, animals, marine organisms, and microorganisms. The diverse range of bioactive compounds plays a crucial role in nutrition and health, contributing to disease prevention and overall well-being. Their potential therapeutic effects make them a focus of research in health and medicine (Swamy and Akhtar 2019). A plant extract typically contains one or more active compounds, which can be extracted by treating plant tissues with specific solvents. To isolate the desired substances, further processing of the extract is often necessary. These active compounds are produced in limited amounts and can vary in concentration across different parts of the plant, including roots, barks, leaves, woods, tubers, gums, oleoresin exudates, flowers, fruits, rhizomes, twigs, and the whole plant. This variability emphasizes the importance of selecting the appropriate plant part for extraction to maximize the yield of beneficial compounds. Understanding these dynamics is crucial for effective utilization in herbal medicine and natural product development (Patel, Panchal, and Ingle 2019).

Health Benefits of Medicinal Plants

Medicinal plants represent the most ancient form of medication, used for thousands of years in traditional medicine in many countries around the world. Thus, medicinal plants, also known as herbs, have many potential health benefits, including reducing inflammation, fighting infection, and treating pain. These medicinal plants have many properties including antioxidant, antimicrobial, anti-inflammatory, and anticancer properties, which are described here.

(i) **Antimicrobial properties of medicinal plants:** The rise of multidrug-resistant microorganisms has significantly increased the rate of infectious diseases worldwide. As a result, the medical community is now largely dependent on natural substances with antimicrobial properties. The bioactive compounds in plant-derived substances are primarily secondary metabolites, which often exhibit inhibitory effects on the growth of microorganisms. Existing scientific literature on plant extracts, combined with traditional herbal knowledge, can guide the discovery of new medicinal agents. This integration of ancient wisdom and modern research holds significant potential for developing effective therapies from plants (Solanki, Sultana, and Singh 2021). The mechanism by which various compounds from medicinal plants exert their antimicrobial effect can vary considerably. Some compounds induce bacterial cell lysis by destabilizing the bacterial plasma membrane. Some bioactive compounds inhibit the activity of enzymes involved in bacterial metabolism, effectively hindering their growth. Additionally, certain specific compounds enhance immune function, empowering the body to combat microbial diseases. This dual action, that is, both inhibitory and immunomodulatory, highlights the therapeutic potential of plant-derived substances in fighting infections (Sen and Samanta 2015).

(ii) **Antibacterial activity:** Many medicinal plants serve as rich sources of bioactive compounds with strong antibacterial activity. Alkaloids derived from these plants, such as berberine from *Berberis* spp. and sanguinarine from the *Papaveraceae* family, demonstrate significant antibacterial properties against various bacterial strains. These compounds have been studied for their effectiveness in treating infections and inhibiting bacterial growth. Their mechanisms of action often involve disrupting bacterial metabolism and cellular integrity. The exploration of such plant-derived alkaloids continues to offer promising avenues for the development of new antimicrobial therapies. This underscores the importance of traditional medicine in modern pharmacology (Vuddanda, Chakraborty, and Singh 2010; Nostro et al. 2000). Berberine is an isoquinoline alkaloid which intercalates DNA molecules and suppresses the growth and proliferation of bacterial cells by interfering with RNA polymerase, topoisomerase IV, and gyrase (Kim et al. 2002). *Camellia sinensis* (tea) and *Allium cepa* (onion) contain flavonoids such as kaempferol and quercetin, which play a role in inhibiting essential enzymes in bacteria. These compounds also disrupt bacterial cell membranes, contributing to their antibacterial effects. Their dual action enhances the potential of these plants as natural remedies against microbial infections (Cushnie, Cushnie, and Lamb 2014; Cushnie and Lamb 2005). Researchers are currently investigating globally for plant sources with antitubercular properties due to emerging incidents of multidrug resistance of *Mycobacterium tuberculosis*. The plant *Fatuoa pilosa* contains secondary metabolites such as chalcones and coumarin (Scopoletin) which are active against mycobacteria (Shukla et al. 2017). The essential oil present in *Daucus carota* interacts with the intracellular cytoskeleton of *Helicobacter pylori* and *Mycoplasma pneumoniae* and inhibits their growth (Wangchuk et al. 2011).

(iii) **Antifungal activity:** The bioactive compounds found in medicinal plants are crucial therapeutic agents against fungal pathogens. Research has shown that epigallocatechin gallate (EGCG), a polyphenol present in *Camellia sinensis* (tea), effectively prevents the growth of *Aspergillus* spp. and *Candida* spp. These findings highlight the antifungal properties of EGCG, which may disrupt fungal cell function and inhibit proliferation. The use of such plant-derived compounds offers a promising approach to developing natural antifungal treatments. Continued exploration of these bioactive compounds can enhance our understanding of their mechanisms and therapeutic applications (Munoz et al. 2017; Zhang et al. 2011). The antifungal activities of tea tree oil, derived from *Melaleuca alternifolia*, and oregano oil from *Origanum vulgare* are well-documented in various studies. Both oils exhibit significant efficacy against a range of fungal pathogens, making them valuable in natural therapeutic applications. Their active compounds contribute to their potent antifungal properties, supporting their use in traditional and alternative medicine (Roana et al. 2021; Nostro et al. 2007). The antifungal potential of flavonoids extracted from *Mangifera indica* (mango) possesses significant growth-retarding activity against *Aspergillus* sp. and a variety of fungal species (Disegha and Akani 2017). The essential oils from *Mentha suaveolens* contain piperitone oxide and pulegone, which are powerful antifungal agents against vaginal candidiasis (Pietrella et al. 2011).

(iv) **Antiviral activity:** Certain medicinal plants produce compounds that specifically interfere with viral replication, helping to prevent the spread of viral infections. Flavonoids like hesperidin and quercetin have shown promise in inhibiting common viral infections caused by the influenza virus, herpes simplex virus (HSV), and human immunodeficiency virus (HIV). These plant-based compounds may disrupt various stages of the viral life cycle, enhancing their potential as natural antiviral agents. Research into their mechanisms of action continues to shed light on their therapeutic benefits. This underscores the importance of traditional herbal remedies in developing effective treatments for viral infections (Kim, Narayanan, and Chang 2010; Chiang et al. 2005). Flavonoids such as chrysin, glycyrrhizin from licorice, and swertifrancheside have shown potential antiviral properties against HIV. These compounds may inhibit viral replication and support immune function. Their efficacy highlights the importance of natural compounds in HIV research and treatment strategies (Mamedov and Egamberdieva 2019). Green tea (*Camellia sinensis*) and pomegranate (*Punica granatum*) are rich in tannins, which have demonstrated the ability to disrupt the replication of hepatitis C virus (HCV) and respiratory syncytial virus (RSV). These compounds may help inhibit viral activity and support overall health. Their potential as natural antiviral agents is an area of growing interest in research (Salles et al. 2021; Wang et al. 2009). The Covid-19 pandemic, caused by SARS-CoV-2, has profoundly impacted global health, leading to thousands of daily deaths and overwhelming healthcare systems. Despite the urgent need for effective treatments, researchers have made significant strides in understanding the virus and its mechanisms. Pure extracts from various plants, such as *Agastache rugosa*, *Artemisia annua*, and *Cassia alata*, have shown promising antiviral properties against SARS-CoV-2. Additionally, numerous active compounds isolated from medicinal plants—such as acacetin, allicin, curcumin, zingerone, and taxifolin—have demonstrated inhibitory effects on the virus. These compounds may work by disrupting viral replication or modulating immune responses. The exploration of these natural extracts and compounds is critical in the ongoing search for effective therapies and preventive measures against Covid-19. Continued research could unveil new avenues for treatment and contribute to the global fight against the pandemic (Adhikari et al. 2021).

Medicinal Plants with Anti-inflammatory Properties

In response to tissue damage or infection, the body initiates an inflammatory response characterized by swelling, redness, pain, heat, and loss of function. This complex reaction helps to isolate the affected area and promotes healing. All these characteristic symptoms are called tissue inflammation. During the inflammatory response, various mediators of inflammation (cytokines, chemokines, eicosanoids, vasoactive amines, and different proteolytic enzymes) are expressed and regulated by coordinated activation of many signal transduction pathways. Severe, prolonged inflammation can contribute to the development of chronic diseases such as inflammatory bowel disease, arthritis, and cancer. This persistent inflammatory response disrupts normal tissue function and can lead to long-term health complications (Gusev and Zhuravleva 2022). Natural bioactive substances from plants fight against inflammation by inactivating enzyme function, regulating signaling cascade of inflammatory pathways, or reducing the synthesis of proinflammatory molecules. Numerous compounds from medicinal plants with documented anti-inflammatory properties offer potential therapeutic benefits for managing inflammation-related conditions (Mir and Masoodi 2020).

Gingerol, a bioactive compound from ginger, may help control the inflammatory response by reducing the production of inflammatory cytokines like tumor necrosis factor-alpha (TNF-α) and interleukin-6 (IL-6) (Yucel et al. 2022). *Curcuma longa* contains curcumin, a potent anti-inflammatory agent that inhibits the activation of the key inflammatory regulator nuclear factor-kappa B (NF-κB) (Wang et al. 2015). On the other hand, the plant *Evodia rutaecarpa* is well-known for its anti-inflammatory features and the two alkaloids from this plant, evodiamine and rutaecarpine, are capable of in vitro inhibition of PGE2. Additionally, they have been shown to inhibit COX expression via suppression of NF-kB (Jeong et al. 2021). Ligunstrazine, an alkaloid extracted from *Ligusticum wallichii*, prevents membrane depolarization triggered by ATP by targeting and inhibiting P2X3 (Soares-Bezerra et al. 2013). In addition, the plant *Phyllanthus amarus*, belonging to the Euphorbiaceae family, contains various lignan compounds, including nirtetralin, phyltetralin, phyllanthin, and niranthin. Notably, nirtetralin has demonstrated inhibitory action on IL-1β production in inflamed tissue (see Figure 21.1). Additionally, the intact extract from this plant significantly reduces paw edema induced by platelet-activating factor (PAF), bradykinin, and endothelin-1. These properties highlight its potential as an anti-inflammatory agent (Kassuya et al. 2005).

The flavone (Luteolin) present in the leaves of *Perilla nankinensis* not only has anti-inflammatory effects but also possesses antioxidative and antiallergic properties (Seelinger, Merfort, and Schempp 2008). The well-known plant marigold (*Tagetes erecta*) from the family Compositae is a rich source of carotenoids like Luteins, which have been found to exhibit powerful anti-inflammatory activity, resulting from their superoxide radical-scavenging capabilities (Meurer et al. 2019). Thymohydroquinone, thymoquinone, and dithymoquinone are secondary metabolites derived from the seeds of *Nigella sativa*. These compounds have demonstrated inhibitory action against COX-1 and COX-2 enzymes, which play key roles in inflammation and pain pathways. Their potential as anti-inflammatory agents makes them a subject of interest in therapeutic research (Marsik et al. 2005). Leaves of *Smallanthus sonchifolius* (the Yacon tree) contain sesquiterpenes that have been observed to suppress NO generation and thereby have strong anti-inflammatory effects (Hong et al. 2008). Hinkitiol, a tropolone derivative sourced from the heartwood of Cupressaceae family plants, has

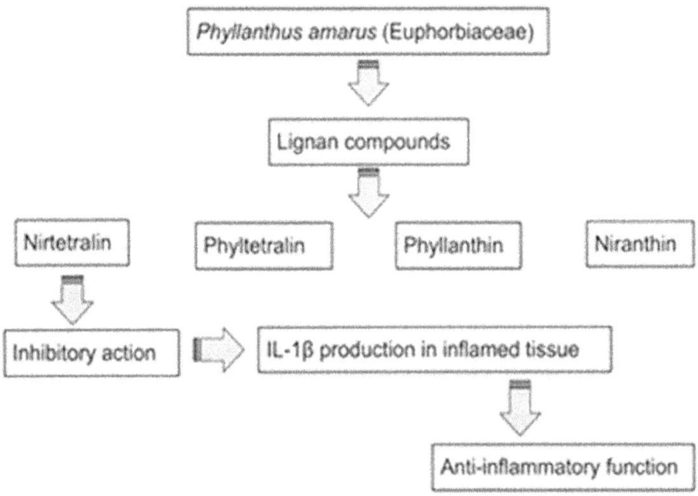

Figure 21.1. Lignan compounds of *Phyllanthus amarus* and anti-inflammatory function of nirtetralin. Source: Author.

demonstrated notable anti-inflammatory activity. It inhibits tumor necrosis factor-alpha (TNF-α) in LPS-induced macrophage cell lines. This highlights its potential for therapeutic applications in managing inflammatory conditions (Byeon et al. 2008).

Effects of Medicinal Plants for Treatment of CVDs

Cardiovascular diseases (CVDs) have emerged as a leading cause of health issues and fatalities globally, impacting both developed and developing nations in recent decades. A range of critical risk factors has been identified, including elevated levels of low-density lipoprotein (LDL) cholesterol, smoking, and chronic stress. Additionally, renal disorders, hypertension, endocrine dysfunctions, obesity, and diabetes significantly contribute to CVD risk. Lack of regular physical activity and excessive alcohol consumption further exacerbate these risks. Understanding these factors is essential for prevention and management strategies aimed at reducing the burden of cardiovascular diseases. Public health initiatives focused on lifestyle modifications can play a crucial role in combating this epidemic (Ho 2018). Active constituents from medicinal plants can significantly influence heart diseases by targeting multiple pathways and mechanisms. These compounds act as potassium channel activators, enhance nitric oxide (NO) generation, and influence the cGMP pathway, promoting vasodilation. They also inhibit voltage-gated calcium channels and modulate the PGI2 and cAMP pathways, which are critical for cardiovascular function. Additionally, phosphodiesterase inhibitors (PDE5) and inhibitors of protein kinase C (PKC) play roles in regulating vascular tone and cardiac function. Furthermore, the activation of endothelial transient receptor potential (TRP) channels and the scavenging of free radicals contribute to their cardioprotective effects. By addressing these diverse targets, medicinal plants offer promising avenues for preventing and treating heart diseases (Tachjian, Maria, and Jahangir 2010).

Garlic (*Allium sativum*) has been utilized in traditional medicines to improve cardiovascular health for centuries. The bioactive compounds (allicin, flavonoids, and sulfur compounds) in garlic have antiplatelet and antioxidant properties that have been employed in medicines to reduce levels of LDL cholesterol, lower blood pressure, and enhance the function of endothelium (Alali et al. 2017). Conversely, the medicinal plant *Crataegus* spp., commonly known as Hawthorn, has certain cardioprotective benefits. The key biologically active compounds of this plant are procyanidins and flavonoids, which improve heart function by lowering blood pressure and enhancing blood flow (Lu et al. 2023). In addition, curcumin, a characteristic active compound of turmeric (*Curcuma longa*), exhibits anti-inflammatory, antioxidant, antithrombotic, and antiplatelet properties. Additionally, this particular compound has proven to lower inflammatory indicators, enhance endothelial function, and stop atherosclerosis development, suggesting its potent medicinal power against cardiovascular diseases (Li et al. 2020).

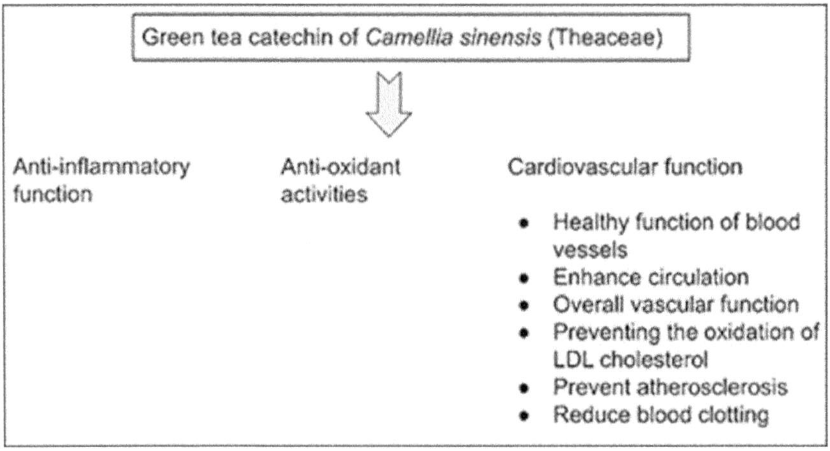

Figure 21.2. Bioactivities of catechin. Source: Author.

Green tea (*Camellia sinensis*) is a rich source of catechins, particularly epigallocatechin gallate (EGCG), which have been shown to offer numerous benefits for heart health. These compounds possess significant anti-inflammatory and antioxidant activities, helping to protect cardiovascular health. By supporting the healthy function of blood vessels, catechins enhance circulation and improve overall vascular function. They also play a crucial role in preventing the oxidation of low-density lipoprotein (LDL) cholesterol, which is a key factor in the development of atherosclerosis (see Figure 21.2). Additionally, green tea catechins help reduce blood clotting, further lowering the risk of cardiovascular diseases. Regular consumption of green tea may contribute to better heart health and a decreased likelihood of heart-related issues. Overall, the health benefits of green tea make it a valuable addition to a heart-healthy diet (Fang et al. 2019). Moreover, the cardiac glycoside digoxin, derived from *Digitalis* spp., has been recognized for its therapeutic effects for thousands of years. Its pharmacological properties help improve cardiac output and regulate heart rhythm, making it effective in treating congestive heart failure. Digoxin enhances the strength of heart contractions, which is crucial for patients with weakened hearts. When used at optimal levels, it can significantly improve symptoms and quality of life. Its long-standing use highlights its importance in cardiovascular medicine (Virgadamo et al. 2015).

Anticancer Activities of Medicinal Plants

Cancer has become a widespread and serious health problem in today's world, with many surveys that report the prevalence of different types of cancer in different regions of the world (Wang and Feng 2022). The identification of vinca alkaloids, such as vincristine and vinblastine, along with podophyllotoxins in the 1950s, paved the way for further research into plant-derived anticancer compounds. These discoveries sparked interest in exploring a broader range of bioactive molecules with potential anticancer properties. As a result, many therapeutic agents have since been developed from various plant sources (Martino et al. 2018). Phytomolecules exert their anticancer activity by interacting with various cellular mechanisms, including the regulation of apoptosis and the cell cycle. They modify signaling pathways involving nuclear factor-kappa B (NF-κB), p38/MAPK, and PI3/Akt, as well as influence cyclooxygenase enzyme activity. Additionally, these compounds can modulate various epigenetic mechanisms, contributing to their potential as cancer therapies (Schnekenburger, Dicato, and Diederich 2014).

Bioactive compounds like polyphenols are abundant in medicinal plants. Resveratrol, mostly found in grapes and berries, is one such polyphenol that has potent anticancer properties and acts by suppressing metastasis and angiogenesis, activating apoptosis and reducing cell proliferation of cancer cells (Kulkarni and Canto 2015). The epigallocatechin gallate (EGCG) present in green tea can also prevent the spread of cancer by regulating signaling pathways of cell proliferation, angiogenesis, and cell survival (Gan et al. 2018). On the other hand, the medicinal plant-derived alkaloids have demonstrated significant anticancer activity, with vinca alkaloids like vincristine and vinblastine being prominent examples. Isolated from *Catharanthus roseus*, these compounds are widely used in chemotherapy for treating cancers such as lymphoma and leukemia. Their ability to inhibit cell division makes them effective against rapidly dividing cancer cells. The successful application of these alkaloids highlights the importance of plant sources in cancer treatment (Taher et al. 2019). Camptothecin, an alkaloid derived from the plant *Camptotheca acuminata*, targets and inactivates the enzyme topoisomerase I, which plays a crucial role in DNA replication and repair. By disrupting this enzyme's function, camptothecin effectively hinders cancer cell proliferation. This mechanism has led to its use in treating various cancers, underscoring the therapeutic potential of plant-derived compounds (Fan et al. 2022).

In addition, terpenoids are a class of bioactive substances present in several medicinal plants, showing their potential power against cancer. The major terpenoid (paclitaxel) found in *Taxus brevifolia* (Pacific yew tree) activates apoptosis and inhibits proliferation of cancer cells (Barbuti and Chen 2015). *Betula* spp. contains betulinic acid which has strong anticancer effects (Aswathy et al. 2022). Accordingly, the medicinal plants which are rich sources of sulfur-containing compounds are extensively utilized to treat a number of cancers. Allyl isothiocyanate is a common sulfur compound in *Allium* species like garlic and onion, and they have been found to slow down the process of tumor development and reduce the spread of cancer (De Gianni and Fimognari 2015). Sulforaphane, found abundantly in vegetables like cauliflower and broccoli, significantly reduces the growth and spread of cancer cells. Its potent antioxidant and anti-inflammatory properties contribute to its protective effects against cancer development (Zhou et al. 2022).

Use of Medicinal Plants for Traditional Herbal Medicines

Traditional medicine is the earliest form of healthcare, rooted in the skills and knowledge developed over generations within various cultures. This system encompasses theories and beliefs about health, drawing from extensive therapeutic practices passed down through generations. It is utilized for the prevention, diagnosis, and treatment of both physical and mental ailments. In addition to addressing specific health issues, traditional medicine plays a significant role in maintaining overall health and well-being. Practices may include herbal remedies, acupuncture, massage, and dietary therapies, reflecting the diverse approaches to healing. The integration of traditional medicine into modern healthcare systems can enhance patient care and provide holistic treatment options. As interest in alternative therapies grows, traditional medicine continues to be a valuable resource for promoting health (Vecchiato 2019). Traditional Chinese medicine (TCM) has emerged as the leading traditional medical system worldwide, with Indian Ayurvedic medicine coming in second in terms of popularity.

In Western nations, "Oriental Medicine" generally refers to the traditional medical practices of China, Japan, and Korea introduced by Korean immigrants, while "Asian Medicine" is a broader term that usually includes Traditional Chinese Medicine (TCM), Ayurveda from India, and Tibetan medicines (Liu 2011). In remote and disadvantaged areas, traditional home remedies and folk medicine are the primary healthcare choices due to distance, financial constraints, and skepticism toward medical professionals. Most remedies (85 percent) use plant materials to treat health issues, with tribal groups relying on their knowledge and experience to apply wild plant species for common health problems (Staub et al. 2015). Among the various treatments in traditional medicine, the use of medicinal plants remains the most prevalent method for healing and health maintenance. With regard to this, herbal medicine is one such specific type of traditional medical practice that focuses on the treatment of health conditions using medicinal plant-based remedies (Skalli and Jordan 2017).

According to the World Health Organization (WHO), herbal medicine encompasses the use of herbs, herbal materials, preparations, and finished products that contain active ingredients derived from plants. This practice leverages the therapeutic properties of various plant materials for health benefits. Herbal medicine is widely utilized across cultures for the prevention and treatment of various ailments (WHO 2019). Herbal drugs are comprised of active constituents (flavonoids, alkaloids, tannins, terpenoids, saponins, glycosides), which are derived from whole plant or plant parts in their raw or processed form and are often combined with additional substances such as diluents, solvents, or preservatives to enhance their stability or efficacy (Bent 2008).

In herbal treatment, some medicinal plants or their parts have been shown to be effective when consumed directly without any prior modifications. However, in certain cases, the plants are prepared in a particular way before their application (Mosihuzzaman 2012). The herbalists carefully follow the specific methods associated with the collection, processing, storage, and preservation of the plants. They choose their target plant for medicinal preparations by considering the plants habitat, latitude and longitude of the geographical area, level of exposure to sun and shade, amount of rainfall, quality of soil, variation in temperature, pollution level, and biotic interactions (Niemiec and Trzepieciński 2018). Various techniques are employed to extract bioactive compounds from selected plant species, with boiling in water or other liquid media being one of the most commonly used methods. This approach is tailored for the specific extraction of desired active compounds, optimizing their yield and efficacy. Heating raw plant parts in liquid material ensures the production of pure extraction and concentrated therapeutic substances, as well as removes the chances of obtaining poisons and impurities in the medicines (Azwanida 2015).

Most plant-based medicines exert their therapeutic effect by a combined action of multiple phytochemicals. This concept of multiple chemicals working together to produce a strong effect on single or multiple target sites has probably originated from the way plants use secondary metabolites to promote their survival. When secondary metabolites function as defense chemicals, multiple compounds often work synergistically, enhancing protection against various herbivores and pathogens. This additive effect not only increases the effectiveness of the plant's defense mechanisms but also reduces the likelihood of these organisms developing resistance. By employing a diverse array of chemical defenses, plants can maintain their resilience in the face of threats. This complexity in defense strategies highlights the evolutionary adaptations of plants to survive and thrive in their environments (Richards et al. 2016). Individual plants generally contain only small amounts of bioactive chemicals, which limits their ability to exert potent therapeutic effects.

Therefore, most herbal remedies rely on the concept of synergism, combining multiple herbs to develop a potent cure for various health conditions. This blending of herbs increases their efficacy in achieving desired medicinal outcomes compared to using a single herb or cumulative effect of individual plants. Certain active constituents in herbs have been found to exhibit significant pharmacological effects only when combined with other herbs but do not produce noticeable effects when used individually (Parasuraman, Thing, and Dhanaraj 2014). Research has found two possible mechanisms for the synergistic action of multiple herbs: pharmacokinetic synergy and pharmacodynamic synergy (Spinella 2002). Pharmacokinetic synergy refers to the possible role of herbs in aiding the bioavailability and elimination of other herbs, whereas pharmacodynamic synergy describes the combined action of bioactive compounds that share a common health benefit and target similar cellular receptors or biological processes. Combined herbal remedies can target multiple pathways simultaneously, offering relief from diseases that present both visible and hidden symptoms. This multifaceted approach enhances their therapeutic potential and overall effectiveness in treatment (Choi, oh, and Jerng 2017).

The physical properties of the preparation and the specific health condition being targeted are the two key factors that are usually considered in order to administer herbal medications. Tea or any other drinks are commonly used for the oral consumption of herbal remedies where the ingredients are present in either diluted or concentrated form. Infusion and decoction are the two common ways of producing herbal teas which ensure the proper release of medicinal components in the water-soluble form (Poswal et al. 2019). Apart from consuming plant-based medicines as tea, various levels of processing and refinement of plant extract are performed to produce therapeutic syrups, tablets, tinctures, oral sprays, sauces, snuffs, sublingual lozenges, and encapsulated powders. In many cultures, tonics and potions are consumed regularly to maintain general health, increase resistance to disease, revitalize the body, and accelerate recovery from sickness or injury (Dores et al. 2023).

Furthermore, botanical products can be ingested through various non-oral methods including inhalation of plant-based aerosols, essential oils, and vapors as well as absorption through rectal and vaginal suppositories. Chewing of solid and raw plant parts such as roots, barks, gums, berries, and so on, has been found to be beneficial for healing purposes (Balekundri and Mannur 2020). Globally, various cultures utilize organic plant material by applying it externally. A poultice is created by grinding or crushing herbs and mixing them with a liquid, such as hot water, along with a binding agent like flour or cornmeal to form a therapeutic paste. This paste can be applied directly to the skin for localized treatment. Herbal poultices are effective for a variety of conditions, including wounds, bruises, cuts, sprains, and strains. They can also alleviate arthritic joint pain, insect bites, discoloration, and other dermatological issues. This traditional remedy harnesses the healing properties of plants for targeted relief (Yadav et al. 2021). Additionally, medicinal herbs have also been utilized in producing products for personal care such as creams, balms, lotions, powders, and oils, which are used to promote hygiene, soothe, and protect the skin (Hussain et al. 2022).

Common Medicinal Plants Utilized in Herbal Medicine

Echinacea has been used as a medicinal plant in traditional medicine for centuries, valued for its immune-boosting properties. The common species *Echinacea purpurea* contains an array of secondary metabolites, including alkamides, derivatives of caffeic acid, polysaccharides, and glycoproteins. This herb is used in herbal remedies to effectively treat infections, wounds, toothache, skin disorders, bowel pain, cancer, syphilis, and is also used as an antitoxin for snake bites. Despite having several therapeutic benefits, this herb can cause severe adverse effects like nausea, abdominal pain, urticaria, erythematous, and allergic reactions in particular individuals (Manayi, Vazirian, and Saeidnia 2015). On the other hand, the biologically active compounds in *Ginkgo biloba*, particularly its leaf extract, have been demonstrated to enhance blood flow and improve cognitive function. The seeds are used for respiratory problems, serving as a natural expectorant, cough suppressant, and asthma reliever, while the leaves are utilized to alleviate cardiovascular disease and asthma. The side effects of using this herb are headache, dizziness, vomiting, restlessness, diarrhea, nausea, and dermal sensitivity. By inhibiting platelet-activating factor, *Ginkgo* may alter the time of bleeding, which could amplify the anticoagulant properties of warfarin and aspirin (Shahrajabian, Sun, and Cheng 2022).

In addition, the plant *Hypericum perforatum*, commonly known as St. John's wort, possesses sedative and astringent properties due to its active compounds, including hypericin, hyperforin, and melatonin. These compounds contribute to its use in managing mood disorders and promoting relaxation. Mental health conditions like anxiety, depression, and menopausal neurosis, various wounds, nerve-related problems such as sciatica, neuralgia, and fibrositis are cured by using this herb. Common adverse effects associated with this herb are constipation, fatigue, nausea, dry mouth, vomiting, headaches, and photosensitivity (Canenguez Benitez et al. 2022). Moreover, the Ginseng, or *Eleutherococcus senticosus*, is a popular Chinese medicinal herb and is believed to enhance the body's resilience to stress, maintain good health, and provide relief from conditions like depression, diabetes, and high blood pressure. Ginseng's multiple active compounds, including ginsenosides, exhibit pharmacological properties that sometimes interact with each other, so the entire root is typically used in herbal preparations to balance the effect. Dehydrated roots are usually used to make products like tablets, tea, capsules, extracts, and elixirs. Overuse of the herb may lead to high blood pressure, vaginal bleeding, insomnia, agitation, and mastalgia (Jung, Lee, and Paik 2017).

Garlic (*Allium sativum*) has been used in traditional medicine to treat coughs, colds, influenza, and chronic respiratory diseases such as bronchitis and asthma. Additionally, it is recognized for its benefits in managing hypercholesterolemia and hypertension. In herbal preparation, the crushing of garlic leads to the activation of compound allicin by the action of alliinase enzymes in the absence of heat or acid. Allicin gives rise to both lipid-soluble (ajoene, sulfides) and water-soluble (cysteine) sulfur compounds which are mostly involved in its biological activity. Garlic can be administered through various forms, including oil-filled capsules, condensed dried powder, enteric-coated tablets, and aged aqueous alcoholic solutions. These methods enhance its bioavailability and therapeutic effects. Garlic extract may cause a burning sensation in the digestive tract, skin irritations, nausea, and diaphoresis, and excessive use leads to severe and spontaneous spinal epidural hematoma, a potentially fatal condition (Ansary et al. 2020).

Piper methysticum, commonly known as Kava, is possessed of anxiolytic, stomachic, and diuretic properties and has been proven to be beneficial for multiple illnesses including nervous disorders, fatigue, fever, headaches, urinary tract infections, rheumatism, asthma, gonorrhea, and syphilis. Oral ingestion of this herb has been reported to cause side effects such as headaches, dizziness, localized numbness, and gastrointestinal discomfort (Bian et al. 2020). Additionally, the *Valerian* (*Valeriana officinalis*) is a plant used in herbal medicine for its calming effects, reducing anxiety and promoting relaxation. The root of the plant contains various compounds, with valerenic acid and valerena-4,7(11)-diene identified as key contributors to its sedative properties. While generally considered safe, valerian can cause side effects like agitation, headaches, and digestive issues in some individuals. In some cases, excessive consumption may trigger abdominal pain, exhaustion, lightheadedness, chest tightness, and tremors (Lanje, Patil, and Wankhade 2020). Furthermore, the *Ephedra sinica* (Ma huang) is a traditionally used medicinal herb that is abundant in alkaloids, ephedrine, and pseudoephedrine. The herb therapeutically improves cold, cough, bronchial asthma, hay fever, rheumatism, enuresis, narcolepsy, and myasthenia gravis. Ma huang is recognized as a risky herb due to its potential side effects, which include stroke, hypertension, psychosis, and seizures. Additionally, it may cause irritability and insomnia, raising concerns about its safety in medicinal use. Caution is advised when considering ma huang for therapeutic purposes (Al Dhamen et al. 2019).

Current Status of Medicinal Plants in Conventional Medicine

A significant portion of the populations in China and India, as well as many developed countries, rely heavily on traditional herbal medicine for their primary healthcare needs. This practice is rooted in centuries of cultural heritage and knowledge. As interest in holistic and natural remedies grows, herbal medicine continues to play a vital role in health and wellness globally (Silveira et al. 2018). The Himalayan alpine and subalpine regions are a vital source of wild medicinal plants, providing around 90 percent of the plant species needed by the pharmaceutical industry. This biodiversity supports both traditional medicine and modern pharmaceutical development (Negi et al. 2018; Snow, Leach, and Clare 2017). Herbal medicine has seen a surge in global acceptance as a form of complementary and alternative medicine (CAM) over the past two decades. Herbal medicines are often used alongside conventional treatment without substituting it. Medicinal plants, utilized as CAM, have the ability to cure mild health conditions, prevent the occurrence of diseases, and promote overall health (Enioutina et al. 2017).

CAM has gained popularity in the Western world with over 40 percent of Americans and a substantial proportion of Europeans utilizing it (Adhikari and Paul 2018). The natural product market constitutes 35 percent of the overall industry, with plants representing 25 percent of this segment. These plants serve as a direct source of raw materials for developing therapeutic products. Additionally, they play a crucial role in generating lead bioactive molecules essential for drug discovery and development (Calixto 2019). The 2015 Nobel Prize in Physiology or Medicine awarded to Tu Youyou for her discovery of artemisinin from *Artemisia annua* highlights the increasing integration of herbal products in modern medicine. This ancient herb, used in Chinese medicine since the East Jin Dynasty, was effectively isolated through a traditional low-temperature technique (Wang, Wong, and Liao 2018). Research into traditional plant-based medicines has significantly contributed to the development of early pharmaceuticals. Key compounds include Digoxin, derived from Foxglove, and Quinine from the Cinchona tree. Morphine, sourced from the Opium poppy, along with Aspirin from willow bark and Pilocarpine from the Maranham Jaborandi plant, has played crucial roles in medical advancements. These discoveries have laid the foundation for modern chemical, clinical, and pharmaceutical studies (Jamshidi-Kia, Lorigooini, and Amini-Khoei 2017).

Subsequently, more pharmaceutical companies formulated medicines based on traditional knowledge. For instance, Acheflan, a product with analgesic and anti-inflammatory properties, is developed from the essential oils of *Cordia verbenacea*. Sintocalmy, a marketed product used for insomnia and anxiety, is derived from the leaves of *Passiflora incarnata*. Similarly, the leaves of *Mikania glomerata* are used to synthesize a product named Melagrião, which is marketed by a Brazilian company, Catarinense Pharma and used in the treatment of cough and asthma (Calixto 2019). There are even more products available in the market that are made from plant sources, such as VP-Precip, which is formulated by combining extract of bilberry and oils of evening primrose and flaxseed. The commercial product OraMagic Rx, a cure for psoriasis and cold sore, is derived from Aloe vera. Vitadirect Turmeric Plus harnesses the anti-inflammatory properties of turmeric curcumin and curcuminoids. Additionally, Ellura, made from berry fruits, is effective in treating urinary tract infections (Kesharwani, Misra, and Singh 2019).

Methods for Discovering Novel Drugs from Medicinal Plants

Developing new medicines from plants involves a complex process that utilizes various approaches and techniques. The traditional method of drug discovery generally tests the plant materials for the presence of pharmaceutical properties and uses techniques such as chromatography and spectroscopy for the separation and analysis of bioactive components. If the activity of any active compound is detected, the plant extract is subsequently fractioned for the isolation of the active compound (Koparde, Doijad, and Magdum 2019). The process of breaking down and isolating plant compounds is typically directed by biological testing, a technique known as bioassay-guided fractionation, which helps guide each step of the process (Mani et al. 2022). An alternative approach involves isolating plant compounds without initial screening for bioactivity, yielding a range of natural substances that can subsequently be evaluated for their biological properties (Altemimi et al. 2017). Modern techniques, such as high-throughput screening (HTS), enable the rapid testing of hundreds of molecules using automated systems, requiring minimal amounts of compounds. To harness the potential of natural products in these modern screening programs, a comprehensive library of natural compounds must be established (Ayon 2023). Surveying ethnobotany across different cultures is a valuable method for identifying the potential medicinal value of plants. This approach explores and investigates the folk remedies utilized by indigenous communities. By documenting traditional knowledge, researchers can uncover insights into plants that may offer therapeutic benefits (Suntar 2020; Hilal and Hilal 2017).

Advantages of Using Herbal Medicines over Synthetic Drugs

Even though diseases across the world are frequently being dealt with conventional medicines which are synthesized scientifically in laboratories and have shown great contributions toward disease management, repeated use of such synthetic medicines has particular limitations. Challenges in modern medicine, including antibiotic resistance, adverse reactions, emerging diseases, and high treatment costs, have increased interest in medicinal plants as alternative remedies. This trend reflects a search for more sustainable and effective healthcare solutions (Catalano et al. 2022). Medicinal plant products have undergone a natural process of selection over time, refining their molecular interactions to precisely target specific biological pathways, resulting in minimal toxicity and adverse effects (Pengelly 2020). Natural products have a range of structural variation; for example, chiral centers, aromatic rings, complex rings (phenols and their oxygen-substituted derivatives), the number of heteroatoms, and the degree of saturation are important factors for the biosynthesis of chemically and structurally diverse secondary metabolites (Dhami and Mishra 2015). Evolution in plants is a probable reason behind the increased amount of chemical variety in secondary metabolites, and this variation in chemical compounds is not much greater in artificially constructed chemical libraries (Merillon and Ramawat 2020).

The chemical diversity in medicinal plants offers numerous beneficial properties that enhance their use as curative medicines. One key advantage is the reduced level of disease resistance, attributed to the presence of various phytochemicals in a combined form within the cells. This synergistic effect can enhance the efficacy of these plants against various ailments. By leveraging this natural complexity, researchers can develop more effective treatments with fewer side effects (Mundy, Pendry, and Rahman 2016). The diverse range of secondary metabolites in plants facilitates the discovery of novel lead compounds, templates, and scaffolds. This rich chemical diversity provides opportunities for innovation that are often unattainable within the constraints of synthetic combinatorial chemical libraries. By exploring these natural compounds, researchers can uncover unique structures with potential therapeutic applications. Ultimately, this approach enhances the development of new drugs and treatments that leverage the complexity of plant chemistry (Egbuna et al. 2019). Having co-evolved with living organisms, natural secondary metabolites often possess a higher degree of drug-likeness and biological adaptability than synthetic compounds, which are designed in the laboratory. Further research into the synthetic pathways and protein engineering associated with these natural compounds can unlock their full potential (Nguyen-Vo et al. 2019).

Challenges and Future Directions

While the adoption of herbal medicine as a primary healthcare option is gaining widespread acceptance, concerns about the efficacy and reliability of these plant-based remedies persist in the medical field. Several challenges related to the quality, standardization, and therapeutic performance of herbal medicines must be addressed. Issues such as variability in plant composition, potential contamination, and lack of rigorous clinical evidence hinder their integration into mainstream healthcare.

Overcoming these obstacles is essential to fully harness the benefits of herbal medicines for safe and effective patient care (Bhardwaj, Verma, and Gupta 2018).

Standardizing and maintaining the quality of products derived from medicinal plants poses significant challenges. Factors such as variations in growing seasons, pathogen infections, and heavy metal contamination can affect the levels of active constituents within the plants. These fluctuations may lead to the formation of synergistic compounds, which could result in unexpected adverse effects. Ensuring consistent quality and safety is crucial for the effective use of herbal medicines in healthcare (Caesar and Cech 2019). Furthermore, the way plants are harvested and processed can also hamper the composition and concentration of bioactive compounds. These issues can be managed if a standardized protocol for each process, from the cultivation of individual plants to the extraction of bioactive components and the formulation of medicinal drugs, can be developed (Gu and Pei 2017; Sahebkar et al. 2015).

The proportion of a medicinal substance that reaches the bloodstream and exerts its desired effects in the body is termed bioavailability of that medicinal drug. Limited effectiveness of bioactive compounds from medicinal plants is largely due to their poor bioavailability, which arises from factors like low solubility, rapid metabolic degradation, and inadequate absorption. These challenges hinder the therapeutic potential of plant-derived compounds in clinical applications (Mukherjee, Harwansh, and Bhattacharyya 2015). Experimental approaches like the formation of prodrugs, delivery techniques using nanoparticles, and using adjuvants for better absorption can be utilized to overcome this problem (Sabuj and Islam 2020; Chakraborty, Shivakumar, and Ramachandran 2016).

Combining multiple bioactive compounds from medicinal plants can enhance the therapeutic value of herbal drugs. The synergistic actions of these compounds facilitate improved absorption and selective delivery to target cells or tissues. This multifaceted approach can lead to more effective medicinal effects, optimizing the overall efficacy of the treatment (Karole et al. 2019). The use of pharmacogenomic techniques can help identify genetic variations that affect individual responses to the active compounds in medicinal plants. This can aid in the development of personalized medication systems for each individual based on their unique genetic composition that causes differences in drug metabolism and effectiveness within the body (Sahoo and Brijesh 2019).

Often individuals using herbal medicines or dietary supplements do not share this with their health care providers, considering herbal products as a safer option than conventional medications. However, in reality, herbal medicines may pose potential risks, as reported in several studies where a substantial number of emergency visits and hospitalization cases were attributed to consuming herbal medicines (Geller et al. 2015). Several active compounds in a multi-herbal formulation can interact synergistically or antagonistically to either enhance or diminish the effectiveness and toxicity of the combined compounds (Hemaiswarya, Prabhakar, and Doble 2022). Using herbal products as complementary medicine with conventional medications may lead to negative herb-drug interactions, affecting the absorption and metabolism of conventional drugs (Gouws and Hamman 2020). In addition, if consumed at a high dose or used for a prolonged period, plant-based medicines can cause harmful impacts in the body. Extensive toxicological research, covering both short-term and long-term effects of herbal drugs, is essential to establish safe dosage limits. This research also evaluates potential drug interactions to ensure patient safety and efficacy (Jitareanu et al. 2022).

Medicinal plants are increasingly threatened by unregulated exploitation, resulting in the extinction of valuable species. According to the International Union for Conservation of Nature, between 50,000 and 80,000 flowering plant species are utilized globally in pharmaceutical industries. Alarmingly, around 15,000 of these species are at high risk of extinction due to habitat destruction and overharvesting. This loss not only diminishes biodiversity but also jeopardizes the future availability of important medicinal resources. Sustainable practices and conservation efforts are crucial to protect these plants and ensure their continued use in medicine. Addressing these threats will help preserve both ecological balance and the potential for new drug discoveries (Chen et al. 2016). The rising human population and excessive consumption of plants are contributing to a decline in approximately 20 percent of the world's wildlife resources. This decline threatens biodiversity and disrupts ecosystems, highlighting the urgent need for sustainable practices (Mir et al. 2021). Integrating an environmental code of ethics into the exploitation and utilization of medicinal plants is essential for conserving biodiversity. This approach promotes sustainable practices that balance human needs with the preservation of ecological integrity (Kadam and Pawar 2020).

Conclusion

Medicinal plants have been used since ancient times, and their therapeutic properties continue to play a crucial role in modern medical treatments. The bioactive compounds found in these plants offer significant potential for developing innovative pharmaceuticals and enhancing healthcare outcomes. While many health conditions and chronic diseases have been effectively treated with herbal remedies, concerns about the safety and efficacy of these products persist, necessitating extensive future research. Additionally, as demand for medicinal plants increases, conservation efforts are vital to prevent overexploitation and ensure their long-term sustainability. Protecting these valuable resources not only safeguards biodiversity but also maintains the availability of effective natural treatments. Striking a balance between utilization and conservation is essential for the continued benefits of medicinal plants in healthcare.

References

Adhikari, B., B. P. Marasini, B. Rayamajhee, B. R. Bhattarai, G. Lamichhane, K. Khadayat, A. Adhikari, S. Khanal, and N. Parajuli. "Potential Roles of Medicinal Plants for the

Treatment of Viral Diseases Focusing on COVID19: A Review." *Phytotherapy Research* 35, no. 3 (2021): 1298–312.
Adhikari, P. P., and S. B. Paul. "History of Indian Traditional Medicine: A Medical Inheritance." *History* 11, no. 1 (2018): 421.
Alali, F. Q., T. El-Elimat, L. Khalid, R. Hudaib, T. Saleh Al-Shehabi, and A. H. Eid. "Garlic for Cardiovascular Disease: Prevention or Treatment?" *Current Pharmaceutical Design* 23, no. 7 (2017): 1028–41.
Al Dhamen, M., R. Ahmad, N. Ahmad, and A. A. Naqvi. "Clinical Uses and Toxicity of *Ephedra sinica*: An Evidence-based Comprehensive Retrospective Review (2004–2017)." *Pharmacognosy Journal* 11, no. 2 (2019).
Altemimi, A., N. Lakhssassi, A. Baharlouei, D. G. Watson, and D. A. Lightfoot. "Phytochemicals: Extraction, Isolation, and Identification of Bioactive Compounds from Plant Extracts." *Plants* 6, no. 4 (2017): 42.
Ansary, J., T. Y. Forbes-Hernández, E. Gil, D. Cianciosi, J. Zhang, M. Elexpuru-Zabaleta, J. Simal-Gandara, F. Giampieri, and M. Battino. "Potential Health Benefit of Garlic Based on Human Intervention Studies: A Brief Overview." *Antioxidants* 9, no. 7 (2020): 619.
Astutik, S., J. Pretzsch, and J. Ndzifon Kimengsi. "Asian Medicinal Plants' Production and Utilization Potentials: A Review." *Sustainability* 11, no. 19 (2019): 5483.
Aswathy, M., A. Vijayan, U. D. Daimary, S. Girisa, K. V. Radhakrishnan, and A. B. Kunnumakkara. "Betulinic Acid: A Natural Promising Anticancer Drug, Current Situation, and Future Perspectives." *Journal of Biochemical and Molecular Toxicology* 36, no. 12 (2022): e23206.
Ayon, N. J. "High-throughput Screening of Natural Product and Synthetic Molecule Libraries for Antibacterial Drug Discovery." *Metabolites* 13, no. 5 (2023): 625.
Azwanida, N. N. "A Review on the Extraction Methods Use in Medicinal Plants, Principle, Strength and Limitation." *Medicinal and Aromatic Plants* 4, no. 3 (2015): 1–6.
Balekundri, A., and V. Mannur. "Quality Control of the Traditional Herbs and Herbal Products: A Review." *Future Journal of Pharmaceutical Sciences* 6 (2020): 1–9.
Barbuti, A. M., and Z. S. Chen. "Paclitaxel through the Ages of Anticancer Therapy: Exploring Its Role in Chemoresistance and Radiation Therapy." *Cancers* 7, no. 4 (2015): 2360–71.
Bareetseng, S. "The Worldwide Herbal Market: Trends and Opportunities." *Journal of Biomedical Research and Environmental Sciences* 3, no. 5 (2022): 575–84.
Bent, S. "Herbal Medicine in the United States: Review of Efficacy, Safety, and Regulation: Grand Rounds at University of California, San Francisco Medical Center." *Journal of General Internal Medicine* 23, no. 6 (2008): 854–9.
Bhardwaj, S., R. Verma, and J. Gupta. "Challenges and Future Prospects of Herbal Medicine." *International Research in Medical and Health Sciences* 1, no. 1 (2018): 12–15.
Bian, T., P. Corral, Y. Wang, J. Botello, R. Kingston, T. Daniels, R. G. Salloum, E. Johnston, Z. Huo, J. Lu, A. C. Liu, and C. Xing. "Kava as a Clinical Nutrient: Promises and Challenges." *Nutrients* 12, no. 10 (2020): 3044.
Briskin, D. P. "Medicinal Plants and Phytomedicines. Linking Plant Biochemistry and Physiology to Human Health." *Plant Physiology* 124, no. 2 (2000): 507–14.
Byeon, S. E., Y. G. Lee, J. C. Kim, J. G. Han, H. Y. Lee, and J. Y. Cho. "Hinokitiol, a Natural Tropolone Derivative, Inhibits TNF-α Production in LPS-activated Macrophages via Suppression of NF-κB." *Planta Medica* 74, no. 8 (2008): 828–33.

Caesar, L. K., and N. B. Cech. "Synergy and Antagonism in Natural Product Extracts: When 1+ 1 Does Not Equal 2." *Natural Product Reports* 36, no. 6 (2019): 869–88.

Calixto, J. B. "The Role of Natural Products in Modern Drug Discovery." *Anais da Academia Brasileira de Ciencias* 91, no. Suppl 3 (2019): e20190105.

Canenguez Benitez, J. S., T. E. Hernandez, R. Sundararajan, S. Sarwar, A. J. Arriaga, A. T. Khan, A. Matayoshi, H. A. Quintanilla, H. Kochhar, M. Alam, A. Mago, A. Hans, and G. A. Benitez. "Advantages and Disadvantages of Using St. John's Wort as a Treatment for Depression." *Cureus* 14, no. 9 (2022): e29468.

Catalano, A., D. Iacopetta, J. Ceramella, D. Scumaci, F. Giuzio, C. Saturnino, S. Aquaro, C. Rosano, and M. S. Sinicropi. "Multidrug Resistance (MDR): A Widespread Phenomenon in Pharmacological Therapies." *Molecules* 27, no. 3 (2022): 616.

Chakraborty, K., A. Shivakumar, and S. Ramachandran. "Nano-technology in Herbal Medicines: A Review." *International Journal of Herbal Medicine* 4, no. 3 (2016): 21–7.

Chen, S. L., H. Yu, H. M. Luo, Q. Wu, C. F. Li, and A. Steinmetz. "Conservation and Sustainable Use of Medicinal Plants: Problems, Progress, and Prospects." *Journal of the Chinese Medical Association* 11 (2016): 37.

Chiang, L. C., L. T. Ng, P. W. Cheng, W. Chiang, and C. C. Lin. "Antiviral Activities of Extracts and Selected Pure Constituents of *Ocimum basilicum*." *Clinical and Experimental Pharmacology and Physiology* 32, no. 10 (2005): 811–16.

Choi, S., D. S. Oh, and U. M. Jerng. "A Systematic Review of the Pharmacokinetic and Pharmacodynamic Interactions of Herbal Medicine with Warfarin." *PLOS One* 12, no. 8 (2017): e0182794.

Cooper, R., and G. Nicola. *Natural Products Chemistry: Sources, Separations and Structures*. Boca Raton: CRC Press, 2014.

Cushnie, T. T., B. Cushnie, and A. J. Lamb. "Alkaloids: An Overview of Their Antibacterial, Antibiotic-enhancing and Antivirulence Activities." *International Journal of Antimicrobial Agents* 44, no. 5 (2014): 377–86.

Cushnie, T. T., and A. J. Lamb. "Antimicrobial Activity of Flavonoids." *International Journal of Antimicrobial Agents* 26, no. 5 (2005): 343–56.

Dar, R. A., M. Shahnawaz, M. A. Ahanger, and I. Majid "Exploring the Diverse Bioactive Compounds from Medicinal Plants: A Review." *The Journal of Phytopharmacology* 12 (2023): 189–95.

De Gianni, E., and C. Fimognari. "Anticancer Mechanism of Sulfur-containing Compounds." *The Enzymes* 37 (2015): 167–92.

Dhami, N., and A. D. Mishra. "Phytochemical Variation: How to Resolve the Quality Controversies of Herbal Medicinal Products." *Journal of Herbal Medicine* 5, no. 2 (2015): 118–27.

Disegha, G. C., and N. P. Akani. "Antifungal Activity of *Mangifera indica* Leaf Extracts on Selected Fungi." *Current Studies in Comparative Education, Science and Technology* 4, no. 2 (2017): 136–48.

Dores, A. R., M. Peixoto, M. Castro, C. Sá, I. P. Carvalho, A. Martins, E. Maia, I. Praça, and A. Marques. "Knowledge and Beliefs about Herb/Supplement Consumption and Herb/Supplement-Drug Interactions among the General Population, including Healthcare Professionals and Pharmacists: A Systematic Review and Guidelines for a Smart Decision System." *Nutrients* 15, no. 10 (2023): 2298.

Egbuna, C., S. Kumar, J. C. Ifemeje, S. M. Ezzat, and S. Kaliyaperumal. *Phytochemicals as Lead Compounds for New Drug Discovery*. Amsterdam: Elsevier, 2019.

Enioutina, E. Y., E. R. Salis, K. M. Job, M. I. Gubarev, L. V. Krepkova, and C. M. Sherwin. "Herbal Medicines: Challenges in the Modern World. Part 5. Status and Current Directions of Complementary and Alternative Herbal Medicine Worldwide." *Expert Review of Clinical Pharmacology* 10, no. 3 (2017): 327–38.

Fan, X., X. Lin, Q. Ruan, J. Wang, Y. Yang, M. Sheng, W. Zhou, G. Kai, and X. Hao "Research Progress on the Biosynthesis and Metabolic Engineering of the Anti-cancer Drug Camptothecin in *Camptotheca acuminate*." *Industrial Crops and Products* 186 (2022): 115270.

Fang, J., A. Sureda, A. S. Silva, F. Khan, S. Xu, and S. M. Nabavi. "Trends of Tea in Cardiovascular Health and Disease: A Critical Review." *Trends in Food Science and Technology* 88 (2019): 385–96.

Gan, R. Y., H. B. Li, Z. Q. Sui, and H. Corke. "Absorption, Metabolism, Anti-cancer Effect and Molecular Targets of Epigallocatechin Gallate (EGCG): An Updated Review." *Critical Reviews in Food Science and Nutrition* 58, no. 6 (2018): 924–41.

Geller, A. I., N. Shehab, N. J. Weidle, M. C. Lovegrove, B. J. Wolpert, B. B. Timbo, R. P. Mozersky, and D. S. Budnitz. "Emergency Department Visits for Adverse Events Related to Dietary Supplements." *New England Journal of Medicine* 373, no. 16 (2015): 1531–40.

Gouws, C., and J. H. Hamman. "What Are the Dangers of Drug Interactions with Herbal Medicines?" *Expert Opinion on Drug Metabolism and Toxicology* 16, no. 3 (2020): 165–7.

Gu, S., and J. Pei. "Innovating Chinese Herbal Medicine: From Traditional Health Practice to Scientific Drug Discovery." *Frontiers in Pharmacology* 8 (2017): 381.

Gusev, E., and Y. Zhuravleva. "Inflammation: A New Look at an Old Problem." *International Journal of Molecular Sciences* 23, no. 9 (2022): 4596.

Hemaiswarya, S., P. K. Prabhakar, and M. Doble. "Herb-herb and Food-drug Interactions." In *Herb-Drug Combinations: A New Complementary Therapeutic Strategy*, edited by S. Hemaiswarya, P. K. Prabhakar, and M. Doble, 15–26. Springer Nature: Singapore, 2022.

Hilal, M., and S. Hilal. "Knowledge, Attitude, and Utilization of Herbal Medicines by Physicians in the Kingdom of Bahrain: A Cross-sectional Study." *Journal of the Association of Arab Universities for Basic and Applied Sciences* 24 (2017): 325–33.

Ho, K. J. "Cardiovascular Diseases." In *Nutritional Aspects of Aging*, edited by Kang-Jey Ho, 75–100. Boca Raton: CRC Press, 2018.

Hong, S. S., S. A. Lee, X. H. Han, M. H. Lee, J. S. Hwang, J. S. Park, K. W. Oh, K. Han, M. K. Lee, H. Lee, W. Kim, D. Lee, and B. Y. Hwang. "Melampolides from the Leaves of *Smallanthus sonchifolius* and Their Inhibitory Activity of LPS-induced Nitric Oxide Production." *Chemical and Pharmaceutical Bulletin* 56, no. 2 (2008): 199–202.

Hussain, F., S. Pathan, K. Sahu, and B. K. Gupta. "Herbs as Cosmetics for Natural Care: A Review." *GSC Biological and Pharmaceutical Sciences* 19, no. 2 (2022): 316–22.

Jamshidi-Kia, F., Z. Lorigooini, and H. Amini-Khoei. "Medicinal Plants: Past History and Future Perspective." *Journal of Herbmed Pharmacology* 7, no. 1 (2017): 1–7.

Jeong, S. M., J. M. Lee, C. H. Lee, D. S. Hwang, and J. B. Jang. "Innate Immunity Activation and Anti-Inflammation Effects of *Evodia* Rutaecarpine Water Extract." *The Journal of Korean Obstetrics and Gynecology* 34, no. 2 (2021): 115.

Jindal, A., and C. S. Seth. "Medicinal Plants: The Rising Strategy for Synthesis of Modern Medicine." *International Journal of Plant and Environment* 8, no. 1 (2022): 76–80.

Jitareanu, A., A. Trifan, M. Vieriu, I. C. Caba, I. Mârțu, and L. Agoroaei. "Current Trends in Toxicity Assessment of Herbal Medicines: A Narrative Review." *Processes* 11, no. 1 (2022): 83.

Jung, J., N. K. Lee, and H. D. Paik. "Bioconversion, Health Benefits, and Application of Ginseng and Red Ginseng in Dairy Products." *Food Science and Biotechnology* 26 (2017): 1155–68.

Kadam, S. T., and A. D. Pawar. "Conservation of Medicinal Plants: A Review." *International Ayurvedic Medical Journal* 8 (2020): 3890–5.

Karole, S., S. Shrivastava, S. Thomas, B. Soni, S. Khan, J. Dubey, N. Khan, and D. Jain. "Polyherbal Formulation Concept for Synergic Action: A Review." *Journal of Drug Delivery and Therapeutics* 9, no. 1-s (2019): 453–66.

Kassuya, C. A., D. F. Leite, L. V. de Melo, V. L. G. Rehder, and J. B. Calixto. "Anti-inflammatory Properties of Extracts, Fractions and Lignans Isolated from *Phyllanthus amarus*." *Planta Medica* 71, no. 8 (2005): 721–6.

Kesharwani, R. K., K. Misra, and D. B. Singh. "Perspectives and Challenges of Tropical Medicinal Herbs and Modern Drug Discovery in the Current Scenario." *Asian Pacific Journal of Tropical Medicine* 12, no. 1 (2019): 1–7.

Kim, S. H., S. J. Lee, J. H. Lee, W. S. Sun, and J. H. Kim. "Antimicrobial Activity of 9-O-acyl-and 9-O-alkylberberrubine Derivatives." *Planta Medica* 68, no. 03 (2002): 277–81.

Kim, Y., S. Narayanan, and K. O. Chang. "Inhibition of Influenza Virus Replication by Plant-derived Isoquercetin." *Antiviral Research* 88, no. 2 (2010): 227–35.

Koparde, A. A., R. C. Doijad, and C. S. Magdum. "Natural Products in Drug Discovery." In *Pharmacognosy-medicinal Plants*, edited by S. Perveen, and A. Al-Taweel. London: IntechOpen, 2019.

Kulkarni, S. S., and C. Canto "The Molecular Targets of Resveratrol." *Biochimica et Biophysica Acta (BBA)-Molecular Basis of Disease* 1852, no. 6 (2015): 1114–23.

Lanje, C. N., S. R. Patil, and A. M. Wankhade. "Medicinal Natural Drug of Valerian (*Valerina officinalis*): An-over Review." *American Journal of PharmTech Research* 10, no. 1 (2020): 148–73.

Li, F. S., and J. K. Weng. "Demystifying Traditional Herbal Medicine with Modern Approach." *Nature Plants* 31, no. 3 (2017): 17109.

Li, H., A. Sureda, H. P. Devkota, V. Pittalà, D. Barreca, A. S. Silva, D. Tewari, S. Xu, and S. M. Nabavi. "Curcumin, the Golden Spice in Treating Cardiovascular Diseases." *Biotechnology Advances* 38 (2020): 107343.

Liu, W. J. *Traditional Herbal Medicine Research Methods: Identification, Analysis, Bioassay, and Pharmaceutical and Clinical Studies*. Hoboken, NJ: John Wiley & Sons, 2011.

Lu, M., L. Zhang, J. Pan, H. Shi, M. Zhang, and C. Li. "Advances in the Study of the Vascular Protective Effects and Molecular Mechanisms of Hawthorn (*Crataegus anamesa* Sarg.) Extracts in Cardiovascular Diseases." *Food and Function* 14, no. 13 (2023): 5870–90.

Mamedov, N. A., and D. Egamberdieva. "Phytochemical Constituents and Pharmacological Effects of Licorice: A Review." *Plant and Human Health: Pharmacology and Therapeutic Uses* 3 (2019): 1–21.

Manayi, A., M. Vazirian, and S. Saeidnia. "*Echinacea purpurea*: Pharmacology, Phytochemistry and Analysis Methods." *Pharmacognosy Reviews* 9, no. 17 (2015): 63.

Mani, J., J. Johnson, H. Hosking, B. E. Hoyos, K. B. Walsh, P. Neilsen, and M. Naiker. "Bioassay Guided Fractionation Protocol for Determining Novel Active Compounds in Selected Australian Flora." *Plants* 11, no. 21 (2022): 2886.

Marsik, P., L. Kokoska, P. Landa, A. Nepovim, P. Soudek, and T. Vanek. "In vitro Inhibitory Effects of Thymol and Quinones of *Nigella sativa* Seeds on cyclooxygenase-1-and-2-catalyzed Prostaglandin E2 Biosynthesis." *Planta Medica* 71, no. 8 (2005): 739–42.

Martino, E., G. Casamassima, S. Castiglione, E. Cellupica, S. Pantalone, F. Papagni, M. Rui, A. M. Siciliano, and S. Collina. "Vinca Alkaloids and Analogues as Anti-cancer Agents: Looking Back, Peering Ahead." *Bioorganic and Medicinal Chemistry Letters* 28, no. 17 (2018): 2816–26.

Merillon, J. M., and K. G. Ramawat. *Co-evolution of Secondary Metabolites*. Cham: Springer International Publishing, 2020.

Meurer, M. C., M. Mees, L. N. B. Mariano, T. Boeing, L. B. Somensi, M. Mariott, R. C. M. V. A. F. da Silva, A. C. Dos Santos, B. Longo, T. C. Santos-França, L. C. Klein-Júnior, P. de Souza, S. F. de Andrade, and L. M. da Silva. "Hydroalcoholic Extract of *Tagetes erecta* L. Flowers, Rich in the Carotenoid Lutein, Attenuates Inflammatory Cytokine Secretion and Improves the Oxidative Stress in an Animal Model of Ulcerative Colitis." *Nutrition Research* 66 (2019): 95–106.

Mir, R. H., and M. H. Masoodi. "Anti-inflammatory Plant Polyphenolics and Cellular Action Mechanisms." *Current Bioactive Compounds* 16, no. 6 (2020): 809–17.

Mir, T. A., M. Jan, R. K. Khare, and M. H. Bhat. "Medicinal Plant Resources: Threat to Its Biodiversity and Conservation Strategies." In *Medicinal and Aromatic Plants: Healthcare and Industrial Applications*, edited by T. Aftab and K. R. Hakeem, 717–39. Singapore: Springer, 2021.

Mosihuzzaman, M. "Herbal Medicine in Healthcare-an Overview." *Natural Product Communications* 7, no. 6 (2012): 807–12.

Mukherjee, P. K., R. K. Harwansh, and S. Bhattacharyya. "Bioavailability of Herbal Products: Approach toward Improved Pharmacokinetics." In *Evidence-based Validation of* Herbal *Medicine*, 217–45. Amsterdam: Elsevier, 2015.

Mundy, L., B. Pendry, and M. Rahman. "Antimicrobial Resistance and Synergy in Herbal Medicine." *Journal of Herbal Medicine* 6, no. 2 (2016): 53–8.

Munoz, J. E., D. C. P. Rossi, K. Ishida, C. C. Spadari, M. S. C. Melhem, D. M. Garcia, A. C. F. Caires, C. P. Taborda, and E. G. Rodrigues. "Antifungal Activity of the Biphosphinic Cyclopalladate C7a against *Candida albicans* Yeast Forms In Vitro and In Vivo." *Frontiers in Microbiology* 8, no. 771 (2017): 1–10.

Negi, V. S., R. Pathak, K. C. Sekar, R. S. Rawal, I. D. Bhatt, S. K. Nandi, and P. P. Dhyani. "Traditional Knowledge and Biodiversity Conservation: A Case Study from Byans Valley in Kailash Sacred Landscape, India." *Journal of Environmental Planning and Management* 61, no. 10 (2018): 1722–43.

Nguyen-Vo, T. H., L. Nguyen, N. Do, T. N. Nguyen, K. Trinh, H. Cao, and L. Le. "Plant Metabolite Databases: From Herbal Medicines to Modern Drug Discovery." *Journal of Chemical Information and Modeling* 60, 3 (2019): 1101–10.

Niemiec, W., and T. Trzepiecinski. "Machines and Horticultural Implements for the Cultivation of Small-scale Herbs and Spices." *Journal of Ecological Engineering* 19, no. 5 (2018): 225–33.

Nostro, A., M. P. Germanò, V. D'Angelo, A. Marino, and M. A. Cannatelli. "Extraction Methods and Bioautography for Evaluation of Medicinal Plant Antimicrobial Activity." *Letters in Applied Microbiology* 30, no. 5 (2000): 379–84.

Nostro, A., A. S. Roccaro, G. Bisignano, A. Marino, M. A. Cannatelli, F. C. Pizzimenti, P. L. Cioni, F. Procopio, and A. R. Blanco. "Effects of Oregano, Carvacrol and Thymol on *Staphylococcus aureus* and *Staphylococcus epidermidis* Biofilms." *Journal of Medical Microbiology* 56, no. 4 (2007): 519–23.

Pant, P., S. Pandey, and S. Dall'Acqua. "The Influence of Environmental Conditions on Secondary Metabolites in Medicinal Plants: A Literature Review." *Chemistry and Biodiversity* 18, no. 11 (2021): e2100345.

Parasuraman, S., G. S. Thing, and S. A. Dhanaraj. "Polyherbal Formulation: Concept of Ayurveda." *Pharmacognosy Reviews* 8, no. 16 (2014): 73.

Patel, K., N. Panchal, and P. Ingle. "Techniques Adopted for Extraction of Natural Products." *International Journal of Advanced Research in Chemical Science* 6, no. 4 (2019): 1–12.

Patra, J. K., G. Das, S. Lee, S. S. Kang, and H. S. Shin. "Selected Commercial Plants: A Review of Extraction and Isolation of Bioactive Compounds and Their Pharmacological Market Value." *Trends in Food Science and Technology* 82 (2018): 89–109.

Pengelly, A. *The Constituents of Medicinal Plants: An Introduction to the Chemistry and Therapeutics of Herbal Medicine*. London and New York: Routledge, 2020.

Pietrella, D., L. Angiolella, E. Vavala, A. Rachini, F. Mondello, R. Ragno, F. Bistoni, and A. Vecchiarelli. "Beneficial Effect of *Mentha suaveolens* Essential Oil in the Treatment of Vaginal Candidiasis Assessed by Real-time Monitoring of Infection." *BMC Complementary and Alternative Medicine* 11, no. 18 (2011): 1–10.

Poswal, F. S., G. Russell, M. Mackonochie, E. MacLennan, E. C. Adukwu, and V. Rolfe. "Herbal Teas and Their Health Benefits: A Scoping Review." *Plant Foods for Human Nutrition* 74 (2019): 266–76.

Qazi, M. A., and K. Molvi. "Herbal Medicine: A Comprehensive Review." *International Journal of Pharmaceutical Sciences and Research* 8, no. 2 (2016): 1–5.

Ramawat, K. G., and S. Goyal. "Co-evolution of Secondary Metabolites during Biological Competition for Survival and Advantage: An Overview." In *Co-evolution of Secondary Metabolites, Reference Series in Phytochemistry*, edited by J. M. Merillon, and K. Ramawat, 3–17. Cham: Springer, 2020.

Reid, A. M., C. B. Oosthuizen, B. D. Fibrich, D. Twilley, I. A. Lambrechts, M. N. de Canha, S. Rademan, and N. Lall. "Traditional Medicine: The Ancient Roots of Modern Practice." In Medicinal Plants for Holistic Health and Well-Being, edited by N. Lall, 1–11. London: Academic Press, 2018.

Richards, L. A., A. E. Glassmire, K. M. Ochsenrider, A. M. Smilanich, C. D. Dodson, C. S. Jeffrey, and L. A. Dyer. "Phytochemical Diversity and Synergistic Effects on Herbivores." Phytochemistry Reviews 15 (2016): 1153–66.

Roana, J., N. Mandras, D. Scalas, P. Campagna, and V. Tullio. "Antifungal Activity of *Melaleuca alternifolia* Essential Oil (TTO) and Its Synergy with Itraconazole or Ketoconazole against Trichophyton Rubrum." *Molecules* 26, no. 2 (2021): 461.

Rosso, A. M. "Methods and Management in Ancient Egyptian and Greek Medicine." *History and Philosophy of Medicine* 5, no. 3 (2023): 14.

Rungsung, W., K. K. Ratha, S. Dutta, A. K. Dixit, and J. Hazra. "Secondary Metabolites of Plants in Drugs Discovery." *World Journal of Pharmaceutical Research* 4, no. 7 (2015): 604–13.
Sabuj, M. Z. R., and N. Islam. "Nanophytomedicine: An Effective Way for Improving Drug Delivery and Bioavailability of Herbal Medicines." In *Nanophytomedicine: Concept to Clinic*, edited by S. Beg, Md A. Barkat, and F. J. Ahmad, 55–70. Singapore: Springer, 2020.
Sahebkar, A., M. C. Serban, S. Ursoniu, and M. Banach. "Effect of Curcuminoids on Oxidative Stress: A Systematic Review and Meta-analysis of Randomized Controlled Trials." *Journal of Functional Foods* 18 (2015): 898–909.
Sahoo, S., and S. Brijesh. "Pharmacogenomic Assessment of Herbal Drugs in Affective Disorders." *Biomedicine and Pharmacotherapy* 109 (2019): 1148–62.
Salles, T. S., M. D. F. Meneses, L. A. Caldas, T. E. Sá-Guimarães, D. M. de Oliveira, J. A. Ventura, R. C. Azevedo, R. M. Kuster, M. R. Soares, and D. F. Ferreira. "Virucidal and Antiviral Activities of Pomegranate (Punica granatum) Extract against the Mosquito-borne Mayaro Virus. Parasite Vectors." *Journal of Microbiology and Biotechnology* 14, no. 1 (2021): 443.
Schnekenburger, M., M. Dicato, and M. Diederich. "Plant-derived Epigenetic Modulators for Cancer Treatment and Prevention." *Biotechnology Advances* 32, no. 6 (2014): 1123–32.
Seelinger, G., I. Merfort, and C. M. Schempp. "Anti-oxidant, Anti-inflammatory and Anti-allergic Activities of Luteolin." *Planta Medica* 74, no. 14 (2008): 1667–77.
Sen, T., and S. K. Samanta. "Medicinal Plants, Human Health and Biodiversity: A Broad Review." *Advances in Biochemical Engineering/Biotechnology* 147 (2015): 59–110.
Shahrajabian, M. H., W. Sun, and Q. Cheng "*Ginkgo biloba*: A Famous Living Fossil Tree and an Ancient Herbal Traditional Chinese Medicine." *Current Nutrition and Food Science* 18, no. 3 (2022): 259–64.
Shukla, S., P. Gahlot, A. Khandekar, A. Agrawal, and S. Pasricha. "Exploring Coumarin and Chalcone Analogues as Potential Antimycobacterial Agents." *Anti-Infective Agents* 15, no. 2 (2017): 69–86.
Silveira, D., J. M. Prieto, M. M. Freitas, and A. L. Mazzari. "Herbal Medicine and Public Healthcare: Current and Future Challenges." In *Natural Products as Source of Molecules with Therapeutic Potential*, edited by V. Cechinel Filho, 495–515. Cham: Springer, 2018.
Skalli, S., and S. A. Jordan. "Herbal and Traditional Medicines, Now and Future." In *Pharmacovigilance: Critique and* Ways *Forward*, edited by I. Edwards and M. Lindquist, 145–59. Cham: Adis.
Snow, J. E., M. J. Leach, and B. A. Clare. "Attitudes, Skill and Use of Evidence-based Practice among US Western Herbal Medicine Providers: A National Survey." *Journal of Complementary and Integrative Medicine* 14, no. 1 (2017): 20150101.
Soares-Bezerra, R. J., A. S. Calheiros, N. C. da Silva Ferreira, V. da Silva Frutuoso, and L. A. Alves. "Natural Products as a Source for New Anti-inflammatory and Analgesic Compounds through the Inhibition of Purinergic P2X Receptors." *Pharmaceuticals* 6, no. 5 (2013): 650–8.
Solanki, P., Y. Sultana, and S. Singh. "Traditional Medicine: Exploring Their Potential in Overcoming Multi-drug Resistance." In *Strategies to Overcome Superbug Invasions: Emerging Research and Opportunities*, 118–29. Pennsylvania: IGI Global, 2021.

Spinella, M. "The Importance of Pharmacological Synergy in Psychoactive Herbal Medicines." *Alternative Medicine Review* 7, no. 2 (2002): 130–7.

Staub, P. O., M. S. Geck, C. S. Weckerle, L. Casu, and M. Leonti. "Classifying Diseases and Remedies in Ethnomedicine and Ethnopharmacology." *Journal of Ethnopharmacology* 174 (2015): 514–19.

Stéphane, F. F. Y., B. K. J. Jules, G. E. S. Batiha, I. Ali and L. N. Bruno. "Extraction of Bioactive Compounds from Medicinal Plants and Herbs." In *Natural Medicinal Plants*, edited by H. A. El-Shemy, 1–39. London: IntechOpen, 2021.

Suntar, I. "Importance of Ethnopharmacological Studies in Drug Discovery: Role of Medicinal Plants." *Phytochemistry Reviews* 19, no. 5 (2020): 1199–209.

Swamy, M. K., and M. S. Akhtar. *Natural Bio-Active Compounds: Volume 2: Chemistry, Pharmacology and Health Care Practices*. Singapore: Springer Nature, 2019.

Tachjian, A., V. Maria, and A. Jahangir. "Use of Herbal Products and Potential Interactions in Patients with Cardiovascular Diseases." *Journal of the American College of Cardiology* 55, no. 6 (2010): 515–25.

Taher, Z. M., F. Agouillal, A. Q. Marof, D. J. Dailin, M. Nurjayadi, E. N. Razif, S. E. Gomaa, and H. A. El Enshasy. "Anticancer Molecules from *Catharanthus roseus*." *Indonesian Journal of Pharmacy* 30, no. 3 (2019): 147.

Vecchiato, N. L. "Traditional Medicine." In *The Ecology of Health and Disease in Ethiopia*, edited by H. Kloos, and Z. A. Zein, 157–78. New York: Routledge, 2019.

Virgadamo, S., R. Charnigo, Y. Darrat, G. Morales, and C. S. Elayi. "Digoxin: A Systematic Review in Atrial Fibrillation, Congestive Heart Failure and Post Myocardial Infarction." *World Journal of Cardiology* 7, no. 11 (2015): 808.

Vuddanda, P. R., S. Chakraborty, and S. Singh. "Berberine: A Potential Phytochemical with Multispectrum Therapeutic Activities." *Expert Opinion on Investigational Drugs* 19, no. 10 (2010): 1297–307.

Wang, G. F., L. P. Shi, Y. D. Ren, Q. F. Liu, H. F. Liu, R. J. Zhang, Z. Li, F. H. Zhu, P. L. He, W. Tang, P. Z. Tao, C. Li, W. M. Zhao, and J. P. Zuo. "Anti-hepatitis B Virus Activity of Chlorogenic Acid, Quinic Acid and Caffeic Acid In Vivo and In Vitro." *Antiviral Research* 83, no. 2 (2009): 186–90.

Wang, J., Y. K. Wong, and F. Liao. "What Has Traditional Chinese Medicine Delivered for Modern Medicine?" *Expert Reviews in Molecular Medicine* 20 (2018): e4.

Wang, J., R. Zhu, D. Sun, X. Sun, Z. Geng, H. Liu, and S. L. Wang. "Intracellular Uptake of Curcumin-loaded Solid Lipid Nanoparticles Exhibit Anti-inflammatory Activities Superior to Those of Curcumin through the NF-κB Signaling Pathway." *Journal of Biomedical Nanotechnology* 11, no. 3 (2015): 403–15.

Wang, Y., and W. Feng. "Cancer-related Psychosocial Challenges." *General Psychiatry* 35, no. 5 (2022): 1–6.

Wangchuk, P., P. A. Keller, S. G. Pyne, M. Taweechotipatr, A. Tonsomboon, R. Rattanajak, and S. Kamchonwongpaisan. "Evaluation of an Ethnopharmacologically Selected Bhutanese Medicinal Plants for Their Major Classes of Phytochemicals and Biological Activities." *Journal of Etnopharmacology* 137 (2011): 730–42.

Wink, M. "Biochemistry of Plant Secondary Metabolism." *Annual Plant Reviews*, Sheffield Academic Press, 2, no. 374 (1999).

World Health Organization. *WHO Global Report on Traditional and Complementary Medicine*. WHO, 2019.

Yadav, S., A. P. Mishra, S. Kumar, A. Negi, and V. K. Maurya. "Herbal Wound Healing Agents." In *Preparation of Phytopharmaceuticals for the Management of Disorders*, 169–184. London: Academic Press, 2021.
Yucel, Ç., G. Ş.Karatoprak, Ö. B.
Açıkara, E. K. Akkol, T. H. Barak, E. Sobarzo-Sánchez, M. Aschner, and S. Shirooie. "Immunomodulatory and Anti-inflammatory Therapeutic Potential of Gingerols and Their Nanoformulations." *Frontiers in Pharmacology* 13 (2022): 902551.
Zahn, R., N. Perry, E. Perry, and E. B. Mukaetova-Ladinska. "Use of Herbal Medicines: Pilot Survey of UK Users' Views." *Complementary Therapies in Medicine* 44 (2019): 83–90.
Zhang, L., A. S. Ravipati, S. R. Koyyalamudi, S. C. Jeong, N. Reddy, P. T. Smith, J. Barlett, K. Shanmugam, G. Munch, and M. J. Wu. "Antioxidant and Anti-inflammatory Activities of Selected Medicinal Plants Containing Phenolic and Flavonoid Compounds." *Journal of Agricultural and Food Chemistry* 59, no. 23 (2011): 12361–7.
Zhou, T., M. Zhou, C. Tong, and M. Zhuo. "Cauliflower Bioactive Compound Sulforaphane Inhibits Breast Cancer Development by Suppressing NF-κB/MMP-9 Signaling Pathway Expression." *Cellular and Molecular Biology* 68, no. 4 (2022): 134–43.

22

Presence of Trans-α-bergamotene from Young Leaves of *Aegle marmelos* (L.) Correa

An Insight to the Future Therapeutic Potential of a Plant Used in Traditional Healing Practices

Mitu De[1*] and Santi Ranjan Dey[2]

[1*]Department of Botany, Gurudas College, Kolkata, West Bengal, India

[2]Department of Zoology, Rammohan College, Kolkata, West Bengal, India

* Corresponding Author's Email: mitubotany@gmail.com

Introduction

The plant *Aegle marmelos* (L.) Corr. belongs to the Rutaceae family and has been used in various traditional Indian systems from time immemorial, including Ayurveda, Siddha, and Unani practices.[1] This plant is revered for its therapeutic properties and has been extensively used for centuries in treating various ailments. *Aegle marmelos* (L.) Corr. is native to India.[2] This plant is commonly called Bael in the Bengali language. It is also called Bengal quince, Bilva, Indian quince, Golden apple, Holy fruit, Bel, Belwa, Sriphal, Stone apple, and Maredo in India (Vinita Bisht and Johar 2017). *Aegle marmelos* has been used for centuries in traditional medicine for its wide range of therapeutic applications, including anti-inflammatory, antidiabetic, antimicrobial, and antioxidant effects (Hazra et al. 2017; Choudhary, Chaudhary, and Kaurav 2021).

Many workers have done research on the reported medicinal use of this plant and supported the traditional medicinal use claim (Baliga and Bhat 2011; Hazra et al. 2017; Choudhary et al. 2021). Traditionally, the *Aegle marmelos* (L.) Corr. was used to cure digestive disorders using both ripe and unripe fruits, diabetes management, for curing fever and respiratory ailments, and so on. A review by Bhowmick and coworkers in 2013 explained the dual use of ripe and unripe bael fruits in addressing digestive issues. The unripe fruit, rich in tannins, is particularly effective in treating diarrhea and dysentery by reducing intestinal motility and water loss. On the other hand, the ripe fruit acts as a mild laxative, providing relief from constipation while maintaining digestive health (Bhowmick et al. 2013). Antidiabetic activity was reported by Arumugam and coworkers (Arumugam et al. 2008).

Objectives and Present Study

Aegle marmelos (L.) Correa has been mentioned in Ayurvedic texts and Charaka Samhita. Recent researches by different groups are now identifying various bioactive chemicals with potential medicinal properties. Common plant chemicals called bergamotenes are usually present in essential oils that are derived from various plant components, such as flowers, fruits, leaves, bark, and so on. Bergamotenes, a type of bicyclic sesquiterpenes, are found in plants, insects, and fungi with trans-α-bergamotene as the most abundant compound. Bergamotenes and their related structures have been shown to possess diverse biological activities such as antioxidant, anti-inflammatory, immunosuppressive, cytotoxic, antimicrobial, antidiabetic, and insecticidal effects. The group of chemical compounds known as bergamotenes, whose molecular formula is $C_{15}H_{24}$, display isomerism. A number of enzymes are involved in the process that produces bergamotenes from farnesyl pyrophosphate. Notable ones are endo-beta-bergamotene synthase, endo-alpha-bergamotene synthase, and exo-alpha-bergamotene synthase. Additionally, bergamotenes act as intermediaries in numerous biochemical processes. For example, fumagillin, ovalicin, and similar antibiotics are biosynthesized using β-trans-bergamotene as a precursor. This chemical, trans-α-bergamotene, is being described for the first time in this study from young *Aegle marmelos* (L.) Correa leaves using GC-MS analysis.

Medicinal Importance of *Aegle marmelos* (L.)

The plant *Aegle marmelos*, also known as bael, is a medicinal plant that has many uses in traditional Indian medicine. The leaves, bark, roots, fruits, and seeds are used to treat a variety of conditions. *Aegle marmelos* can be used to treat tuberculosis. *Aegle marmelos* is rich in antioxidants, which help in insulin secretion, leading to low blood sugar levels. Various significances of *Aegle marmelos* are given here:

(a) Digestive Disorders: The unripe fruit is known for its astringent properties and is commonly used to treat diarrhea, dysentery, and other gastrointestinal disorders. Ripe fruit acts as a mild laxative, aiding in relieving constipation. Decoctions of the leaves and pulp are used to address peptic ulcers and other digestive issues.

(b) Diabetes Management: *Aegle marmelos* leaves are widely used in traditional medicine for their antidiabetic properties. They help regulate blood sugar levels by improving insulin sensitivity.

(c) Respiratory Ailments: The fruit pulp and leaves are used in the treatment of chronic respiratory conditions like asthma and bronchitis due to their anti-inflammatory and expectorant properties.

(d) Fever and Infections: Bael has antimicrobial properties, making it effective against bacterial, fungal, and viral infections. Decoctions prepared from the leaves and bark are used to manage fevers, especially those related to seasonal changes.
(e) Cardiovascular Health: Traditional texts mention the use of bael in promoting heart health. Its juice and extracts are used to regulate cholesterol levels and support overall cardiovascular function.
(f) Wound Healing: The plant's antimicrobial and anti-inflammatory properties are utilized in treating wounds, burns, and ulcers.
(g) Other Uses: Bael fruit and its extracts are also used to manage conditions like hemorrhoids, skin diseases, and inflammation.

Phytochemicals and Therapeutic Value

Literature review has revealed that many people are more interested in medicine that is of plant origin and in alternative therapies instead of purely synthetic drugs (Mentz and Schenkel 1989). However, only a small portion of the approximated 250,000–500,000 plant genera have been thoroughly explored in terms of their pharmacological qualities, and only a small portion have been investigated phytochemically (Rates 2001). Despite the widespread use of *Aegle marmelos* (L.) Corr., the precise bioactive compounds responsible for these medicinal properties have remained incompletely understood for many years. This gap in knowledge underscores the importance of identifying the phytochemicals present in *Aegle marmelos* (L.) Corr. Modern scientific research has validated many traditional claims about *Aegle marmelos* (L.) Corr. by identifying its bioactive compounds and elucidating their pharmacological effects over several years (Sabu and Kuttan 2004; Baliga and Bhat 2011; Dey, Dutta, and De 2020; Rajeswari et al. 2021). These studies have aided in identifying the phytochemicals found in *Aegle marmelos* (L.) Corr. and can scientifically validate these traditional claims, ensuring that its benefits are evidence-based.

By identifying bioactive compounds like alkaloids, flavonoids, and coumarins in *Aegle marmelos* (L.) Corr., we can aid in isolating potent molecules for the development of novel pharmaceutical drugs targeting chronic conditions such as diabetes, cardiovascular diseases, and microbial infections. The identification of key phytochemicals allows for the standardization of herbal formulations. This ensures consistent efficacy, quality, and safety of *Aegle marmelos*-based products in therapeutic and commercial applications. Phytochemical studies help elucidate the molecular mechanisms underlying the therapeutic effects of *Aegle marmelos* (L.) Corr. This is critical for enhancing its use in integrative medicine and targeted therapies.

By understanding the specific compounds responsible for its medicinal value, sustainable sourcing and conservation strategies can be implemented, ensuring the long-term availability of this valuable medicinal plant. Modern techniques, including Gas Chromatography-Mass Spectrometry (GC-MS), High-Performance Liquid

Chromatography (HPLC), and bioassays, are pivotal in identifying and characterizing the active compounds. These efforts not only bridge traditional knowledge with modern science but also contribute to global healthcare innovation. Thus, the plant Aegle *marmelos* (L.) Corr. is a treasure trove of bioactive phytochemicals, many of which have demonstrated significant therapeutic properties. These compounds are distributed across its leaves, fruit, bark, and roots, contributing to its use in traditional medicine for treating a range of ailments. Thus, *Aegle marmelos* (L.) contains many phytochemicals with a variety of therapeutic effects, which are given below:

(i) Alkaloids. For example, Aegeline has shown antihyperlipidemic and antidiabetic properties. It helps regulate lipid profiles and improves glucose metabolism (Singh et al. 2021).
(ii) Flavonoids like Rutin, Quercetin. These compounds exhibit strong antioxidant, anti-inflammatory, and cardioprotective effects. They neutralize free radicals, reducing oxidative stress and inflammation (Sharma, Sharma, and Agarwal 2023).
(iii) Phenolic compounds like Ferulic acid, Caffeic acid. These phenols are potent antioxidants that protect against neurodegenerative diseases and exhibit antimicrobial activity against various pathogens (Murthy, Bhat, and Dalawai 2019; Ahmad et al. 2021).
(iv) Tannins. For example, Skimmianine. Tannins in *Aegle marmelos* have antidiarrheal and antimicrobial properties, making the fruit pulp effective against gastrointestinal disorders (Monika, Thirumal, and Kumar 2023).
(v) Coumarins like Marmelosin, Umbelliferone. Coumarins exhibit anti-inflammatory, anticoagulant, and hepatoprotective properties. Marmelosin has also shown promising anticancer effects (Tiwari et al. 2023).
(vi) Terpenoids like Limonene, which exhibit antimicrobial, anti-inflammatory, and sedative properties, contribute to the calming effects of bael leaf extracts (Swarnkar et al. 2019; Monika, Thirumal, and Kumar 2023).

Bergamotenes

Bergamotenes are bicyclic sesquiterpenes present in the volatile oils of several plants, mostly bergamot, cannabis, lime, and basil (Hassan et al. 2023). The group of chemical compounds known as bergamotenes, whose molecular formula is $C_{15}H_{24}$, display isomerism. Common plant chemicals called bergamotenes are present in essential oils that are derived from various plant components, such as flowers, fruits, leaves, bark, and so forth. Carrot, bergamot, lime, citron, cottonseed, and kumquat oils contain α-bergamotene. A number of enzymes are involved in the process that produces bergamotenes from farnesyl pyrophosphate. Notable ones are endo-α-bergamotene synthase and exo-α-bergamotene syntheses. Additionally, bergamotenes act as intermediaries in numerous biochemical processes. For example, fumagillin, ovalicin, and similar antibiotics are biosynthesized using trans-β-bergamotene as a precursor (Figure 22.1).

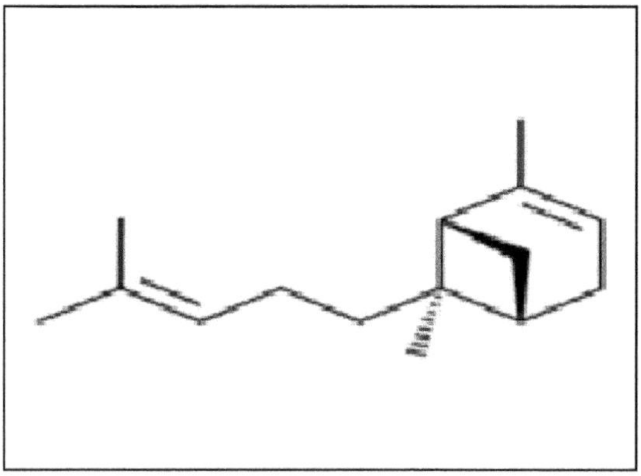

Figure 22.1. Structure of bergamotene. Source: Author.

Table 22.1. Molecular Characters of Trans-α-Bergamotene

Compounds	Molecular Weight	Structure	Retention Time
Trans-α-bergamotene $C_{15}H_{24}$	204.35 g/mol	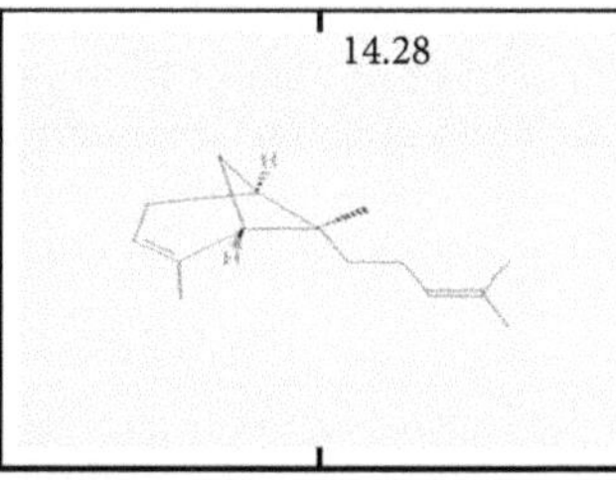	14.28

Source: Authors.

Trans-α-bergamotene, with a molecular formula of $C_{15}H_{24}$, bergamotenes are a class of chemical compounds that display isomerism (Table 22.1). Several studies on plant extractions have been performed that showed the presence of trans-α-bergamotene as an active ingredient of the essential oils derived from them. Trans-α-Bergamotene, with a percentage value of 7.97, has been found as one of the chief chemical constituents of different parts of cinnamon, especially flowers. On the other hand, α-Bergamotene, with a percentage value of 27.38, has been found from the buds of Cinnamon that indicates the likely presence of this compound in the floral parts of certain plants (Ragunath et al. 2020). Plants have a unique defense mechanism that allows them to repel herbivorous insects by releasing pheromones called bergamotenes, which draw in the herbivores' predators. Trans-α-bergamotene, which is released at night by the tobacco plant *Nicotiana attenuata*, attracts pollinators, particularly the tobacco hawk moth, *Manduca sexta*. Conversely, during the day, the leaves release trans-α-bergamotene, which attracts predatory insects and allows them to consume the larvae and eggs produced by the pollinators. In a gas chromatography study on confiscated cannabis seeds, aerial parts of *Cannabis sativa* L. were examined. The results revealed a significant presence of trans-α-bergamotene against the retention time of 0.67, where it is thought to be one of the primary compounds responsible for the biological activities of the plant (Ragunath et al. 2020).

Role of Trans-α-Bergamotene

Trans-α-bergamotene has now been found in many plants that have been used as medicine, namely, in *Azadirachta indica* A. Juss., *Moringa oleifera* Lam., *Rhododendron anthopogon* D. Don, Mem. Wern, and *Cymbidium* oriental orchids and in lavender prized for its essential oils. Numerous investigations into the essential oil content of fruits, seeds, and leaves have shown that α-bergamotene is present in *Zanthoxylum armatum* DC. (Boudieb, AitSlimane-Ait Kaki, and Amellal-Chibane 2019; Shunmugapriya et al. 2017). Trans-α-bergamotene, with a retention time of 34.354, is one of the main volatile chemicals found in the essential oil extracted from *Cinnamon zeylanicum* leaves, according to the results of chromatographic analysis (Rao and Gan 2014). Sesquiterpenes are thought to be involved in defense mechanisms and interactions between plants and their surroundings (Yakubu, Otitoju, and Onwuka 2017). Because of their well-known insecticidal, antibacterial, anticancer, and anti-inflammatory qualities, sesquiterpenes have a large industrial role.

Rationale of the Study and Result

Since it has been used in traditional medicine from time immemorial and has a wide range of therapeutic uses, it was hoped that Gas Chromatography-Mass Spectrometry (GC-MS) analysis could elucidate further on bioactive compounds. The objective of this study was to determine if there was any novel bioactive compound in Bael using the Gas Chromatography-Mass Spectrometry analysis method (Figure 22.2).

IUPAC NAME: 2, 6-dimethyl-6-(4-methylpent-3-enyl) bicycle [3.1.1] hept-2-ene.

Young leaf of *Aegle marmelos* (L.), 1 gm crushed in 10 ml methanol, using mortar and pestle, kept in a sealed tube, at −20 °C for 24 hours, methanolic extract subjected to GC-MS analysis at Bose Institute (Basu Vigyan Mandir), Kolkata, West Bengal, India. The compound has a molecular weight of 204.35 g/mol and an exact molecular mass of 204.187800 Da (Table 22.1). It contains fifteen heavy atoms and is a charge-neutral molecule. The compound features three stereocenters and consists of a single covalent bond unit. The retention time in the chromatographic column is 14.28 minutes, and the compound identification has been confirmed by comparison with the NIST database. The NIST Mass Spectrometry Data Center, part of the Biomolecular Measurement Division (BMD), develops curated mass spectral libraries and related software tools (Figure 22.2). These resources aid in compound identification by offering reference mass spectra for GC/MS (electron ionization) and LC-MS/MS (tandem mass

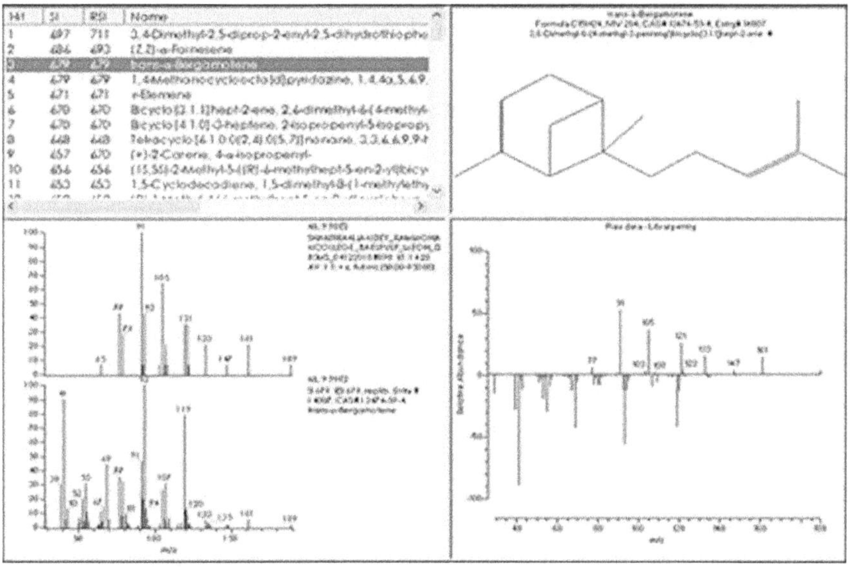

Figure 22.2. GCMS result of analysis of young leaf showing probable presence of Trans-α-Bergamotene. Source: Author.

spectrometry), as well as gas-phase retention indices for GC. The compound has been identified as Trans-α-bergamotene.

Discussion and Conclusion

Aegle marmelos (L.) Corr. is a tree of the Rutaceae family that has medicinal and horticultural value. The item is indigenous to India and known as Bael. This plant is of great importance, so it seems that a diverse range of phytochemicals may be found using modern techniques of chemical resources (Dey, Dutta, and De 2020). In the present study, trans-α-bergamotene is for the first time being reported from young leaves of *Aegle marmelos* (L.) Corr. The beverage, culinary, fragrance, and personal care and skin care industries all use α-bergamotene extensively as a flavor. α-bergamotene was found in pomegranate juices, unifloral honey, and a number of commercial lemon liquors (Limoncello). Furthermore, together with the other three sesquiterpenoids, α-exo-bergamotol, the counterpart of α-bergamotene, makes up almost 90 percent of the oil of *Santalum album* L., which is extensively utilized in the perfume and fragrance industries.

Additionally, α-bergamotene was identified in chardonnay grape berry skin distillates and identified at modest concentrations (0.08 mg/L) in the grape leaves. Some food categories employ α-trans-bergamotene as a flavoring component. Hops, cloves, lemon peel oil, bergamot oil, and lime oil all naturally contain this chemical.

The expected daily intake of α-bergamotene as a flavoring ingredient, according to experts, is 138 μg/person, which is below the toxicological threshold. In fact, when α-trans-bergamotene was examined using the GLP-compliant Ames assay of the in vitro micronucleus assay, no indication of genotoxicity was found. The GRAS (Generally Regarded as Safe) designation was given to α-trans-bergamotene since it was determined to be free of any genotoxicity issues. To investigate the toxicity, mutagenicity, and genotoxicity of all bergamotenes and their associated structures, thorough investigations are required (Annaz et al. 2023).

The rich phytochemical profile of Aegle marmelos underpins its extensive medicinal potential. Modern research continues to unravel the molecular mechanisms of these compounds, fostering the development of standardized herbal formulations and novel drugs. This integrative approach bridges traditional wisdom with evidence-based medicine, enhancing the therapeutic scope of this valuable plant. Modern techniques, including Gas Chromatography-Mass Spectrometry (GC-MS), High-Performance Liquid Chromatography (HPLC), and bioassays, are pivotal in identifying and characterizing the active compounds. These efforts not only bridge traditional knowledge with modern science but also contribute to global healthcare innovation. In conclusion, the systematic identification of *Aegle marmelos* phytochemicals is essential to fully harness its medicinal potential, foster drug development, and ensure its sustainable use for future generations.

Notes

1 Acknowledgments: Authors would like to thank Prof. Sujoy Dasgupta of Bose Institute and Mr. Smriti Kumar Majhi, Central Instrument Facility, Bose Institute, Kolkata, India, for their support and assistance to carry on the GC-MS analysis.

2 Conflict of Interest: Authors declare that there are no conflicts of interest regarding the publication of this work.

References

Ahmad, W., M. Amir, A. Ahmad, A. Ali, A. Ali, S. Wahab, H. A. Barkat, M. A. Ansari, M. Sarafroz, A. Ahmad, M. A. Barkat, and P. Alam. "*Aegle marmelos* Leaf Extract Phytochemical Analysis, Cytotoxicity, In Vitro Antioxidant and Antidiabetic Activities." *Plants (Basel)* 10, no. 12 (2021): 2573.

Annaz, H., K. Fakhouri, W. B. Bakrim, I. Mahdi, M. El Bouhssini, and M. Sobeh. "Bergamotenes: A Comprehensive Compile of Their Natural Occurrence, Biosynthesis, Toxicity, Therapeutic Merits and Agricultural Applications." *Critical Reviews in Food Science and Nutrition* 64, no. 21 (2023): 7343–62.

Arumugam, S., et al. "Antidiabetic Activity of Leaf and Root Extracts of Aegle Marmelos in Diabetic Rats." *Indian Journal of Clinical Biochemistry* 23, no. 4 (2008): 379–85.

Baliga, M. S., and H. P. Bhat. "Phytochemistry and Medicinal Uses of Aegle Marmelos: A Review." *Food Research International* 44, no. 7 (2011): 1768–75.

Bhowmik, D., K. P. S. Kumar, S. Duraivel, and M. Umadevi. "Traditional and Medicinal Uses of *Aegle marmelos*." *Journal of Pharmacognosy and Phytochemistry* 1, no. 6 (2013): 48–53.

Boudieb, K., S. AitSlimane-Ait Kaki, and H. Amellal-Chibane. "Effect of Maturation Degree on the Fixed Oil Chemical Composition, Phenolic Compounds, Mineral Nutrients and Antioxidant Properties of Pistacialentiscus L. Fruits." *Notulae Botanicae Horti Agrobotanici Cluj-Napoca* 47, no. 3 (2019): 836–47.

Choudhary, S., G. Chaudhary, and H. Kaurav. "*Aegle marmelos* (bael patra): An Ayurvedic Plant with Ethnomedicinal Value." *International Journal of Research in Ayurveda and Pharmacy* 12, no. 3 (2021): 147–56.

Dey, S. R., S. Dutta, and M. De. "Neuro-Steroid Compound Found by GC-MS Analysis of the Methanolic Extract of the Leaves of Aegle marmelos (L) Corr." *International Journal of Advancement in Life Sciences Research* 3, no. 4 (2020): 51–6.

Hassan, A., E. F. Karim, W. Benbakrim, I. Mahdi, M. E. Bouhssini, and S. Mansour. "Bergamotenes: A Comprehensive Compile of Their Natural Occurrence, Biosynthesis, Toxicity, Therapeutic Merits and Agricultural Applications." *Critical Reviews in Food Science and Nutrition* 64, no. 6 (2023): 1–20.

Hazra, K., S. Dutta, A. K. Mandal, D. Nath, J. Mondal, and J. Hazra "Comprehensive Dossier on Ayurvedic Medicinal Plant Aegle Marmelos (L.) Corrêa.: A Review." *The Pharmaceutical & Chemical Journal* 4, no. 3 (2017): 55–74.

Mentz, L. A., and E. P. Schenkel. "The Coherence and Reliability of Therapeutic Indications." *Notebook Farmacia* 5 (1989): 3–119.

Monika, S., M. Thirumal, and P. R. Kumar. "Phytochemical and Biological Review of *Aegle marmelos* Linn." *Future Science OA* 23 9, no. 3 (2023): FSO849.

Murthy, H. N., M. A. Bhat, and D. Dalawai. "Bioactive Compounds of Bael (*Aegle marmelos* (L.) Correa)." In *Bioactive Compounds in Underutilized Fruits and Nuts*, edited by H. Murthy, and V. Bapat. Cham: Springer, 2019.

Ragunath, C., Y. A. S. Kumar, I. Kanivalan, and S. Radhakrishnan. "Phytochemical Screening and gc-ms Analysis of Bioactive Constituents in the Methanolic Extract of *Caulerpa racemosa* (Forssk.) J. Agardh and *Padina boergesenii* Allender & Kraft." *Current Applied Science and Technology* 20, no. 3 (2020): 380–93.

Rajeswari, G., J. A. J. Sunilson, N. Nagarajan, A. V. A. G. Kumari, and D. Dhanuprabha. "Antidiabetic Activity of Leaf Extracts of Aegle Marmelos Linn in Streptozotocin – Nicotinamide Induced Diabetic Wistar Albino Rats." *Annals of the Romanian Society for Cell Biology* 5, no. 23 (2021): 2414–21.

Rao, P. V., and S. H. Gan. "Cinnamon: A Multifaceted Medicinal Plant." *Evidence Based Complementary Alternative Medicine*, 2014 (2014): 642942.

Rates, S. M. K. "Plants as Source of Drugs." *Toxicon* 39, no. 5 (2001): 603–13.

Sabu, M. C., and R. Kuttan. "Antidiabetic Activity of Aegle Marmelos and Its Relationship with its Antioxidant Properties." *Indian Journal of Physiology and Pharmacology* 48, no. 1 (2004): 81–8.

Sharma, P., V. Sharma, and N. Agarwal. "Characterization of Phytoconstituents, Total Flavonoids and Anti-Oxidant Activity of Aegle marmelos Correa." *Current Research in Nutrition and Food Science* 11, no. 3 (2023): 713–24.

Shunmugapriya, K., P. Vennila, S. Thirukkumar, and M. Ilamaran "Identification of Bioactive Components in *Moringa oleifera* Fruit by GC-MS." *Journal of Pharmacognosy and Phytochemistry* 6, no. 3 (2017): 748–51.

Singh, A. P., L. Singh, P. Singh, and R. Bhatti. "Biological Evaluation of *Aegle marmelos* Fruit Extract and Isolated Aegeline in Alleviating Pain-Depression Dyad: In Silico Analysis of Aegeline on MAO-A and iNOS." *ACS Omega* 6, no. 3 (2021): 2034–44.

Swarnkar, R., D. Singh, A. Choudhary, S. Anand, A. Rathore, and H. K. Jediya. "Pharmacological Properties of Aegle marmelos: A Review." *International Journal of Current Microbiology and Applied Sciences* 8, no. 05 (2019): 1600–8.

Tiwari, R., S. Mishra, G. Danaboina, G. P. Singh, J. M. Kalaivani, V. Kalaiselvan, M. Dhobi, and R. S. Raghuvanshi. "Comprehensive Chemo-profiling of Coumarins Enriched Extract Derived from Aegle Marmelos (L.) Correa Fruit Pulp, as an Anti-diabetic and Anti-inflammatory Agent." *Saudi Pharmaceutical Journal* 31, no. 9 (2023): 101708.

Vinita Bisht, N., and V. Johar. "Bael (*Aegle marmelos*) Extraordinary Species of India: A Review." *International Journal of Current Microbiology and Applied Sciences* 6, no. 3 (2017): 1870–87.

Yakubu, O. E., O. Otitoju, and J. Onwuka. "Gas Chromatography-Mass Spectrometry (GC-MS) Analysis of Aqueous Extract of Danielliaoliveri Stem Bark." *Pharmaceutica Analytica Acta* 8, no. 11 (2017): 4–8.

Ethnomedicinal Practices and Effect of Socioeconomic Factors on Health among the Rabhas of Garo Basti in Alipurduar of West Bengal, India

Nabanita Goswamy[1], Somenath Bhattacharjee[1], and Arun Makal[2*]

[1] Department of Anthropology, Nagaland University, Nagaland, India

[2]Department of Anthropology, Bangabasi Evening College, Kolkata, India

*Corresponding Author's Email: arunmakal6@gmail.com[2]

Introduction

Ethnomedicine is the study of cultural interpretations of health and healing practices and is deeply influenced by socioeconomic factors affecting the prevalence, accessibility, and use of traditional medicines. In other words, ethnomedicine broadly refers to the traditional medical practices concerned with the cultural interpretation of health, diseases, and illness that address the healthcare process and healing practices. It also encompasses the cultural beliefs, notions, and healing practices of different ethnic or indigenous communities regarding health and illness. It also explores the diverse cultural understandings and practices related to health, illness, and healing within different ethnic or indigenous communities. It examines how people conceptualize their bodies, diagnose illnesses, and seek treatment within their cultural contexts. Besides, it includes practices like acupuncture (China), Ayurveda (India), Unani (Arabic countries), herbal medicines, and traditional birth attendants' medicines. Accordingly, ethnomedicine can study the traditional medical systems of various cultures, such as Ayurveda, Traditional Chinese Medicine, and various African healing traditions. It can also examine how different groups perceive specific diseases, like malaria, or common ailments like colds. Therefore, this ethnomedicine examines how cultural beliefs influence the treatment of mental health conditions, and the role of healing rituals in overcoming trauma.

On the other hand, socioeconomic status plays a significant role in determining people's access to traditional medicine, modern healthcare, and associated costs. In this context, lower-income individuals may rely more heavily on traditional medicines due to their affordability and accessibility, while higher-income individuals have access to modern healthcare. Moreover, levels of education and cultural beliefs can influence people's perceptions of traditional healing methods and their willingness to use them. In reality, rural populations of our country have limited access to formal healthcare facilities and may heavily depend on traditional practices. It is also observed that strong cultural traditions and beliefs can continue the use of ethnomedical practices, even in the face of alternative healthcare options. In addition, the attitudes of healthcare workers toward traditional medicines can influence the willingness of the community to seek care. Furthermore, the physical distance to hospitals and clinics can influence the choice of ethnomedical practices, especially in communities with limited transportation options (Logiel et al. 2021; Biswas 2004).

Keeping all these understandings of ethnomedicinal practices and effect of socioeconomic factors on the indigenous communities in Indian context in mind, the present study has tried to understand the cultural beliefs, notions, and healing practices of forest-dwelling Rabha community of the village Garo Basti in the Rajabhat Khawa region of the district Alipurduar in Indian state of West Bengal. In the Alipurduar district of West Bengal, the Rabha community is mostly confined to the forest areas of Chilapata (Das and Raha 1967; Raha 1989; Mandal and Manadeb 2013; Roy et al. 2018). Similarly, the Rabhas of Garo Basti live beside the forest and consider themselves as a part of Bodo family. They are primarily involved in agriculture and daily labor. Some Rabha families of Garo Basti are better able to perform hunting and gathering due to the deep forest and low population density. They have their own culture and conduct their lives by their own customs and rules. Besides, they possess a rich cultural heritage, including traditional healing practices and beliefs, and utilizes various medicinal plants for treating ailments, with a focus on herbal remedies and traditional healers.

Objectives and Methods

Rabhas of forest fringe village of Garo Basti, Rajabhat Khawa of Alipurduar, West Bengal, consider themselves as a part of Bodo family. Their livelihood is intensely related to the surrounding natural resources and their subsistence pattern includes agriculture followed by daily labor. They use their traditional knowledge to cure their illness and to protect their health. They collect various medicinal plants from the deep forest to cure their disease. Besides, they apply and consume different parts of medicinal plants and local remedies on a regular basis. Furthermore, a number of socioeconomic factors like education, occupation, and marital status affect their health status and health care system as well as traditional medical practices. In this context, the present chapter has tried to explore different ethnomedicinal practices and effect of various socioeconomic factors on health of the Rabha community of the village Garo Basti in Alipurduar. It has also tried to document their perception related to their health and treatment and has tried to examine their perspectives regarding their consideration of natural and supernatural causes of diseases through empirical fieldwork by applying appropriate anthropological methods and techniques like purposive sampling, participant observation, semi-structured interview, focused group discussion, case study, and genealogy.

Study Area and People

The present study was done among the Rabha community of the village Garo Basti of the region Rajabhat Khawa of the district Alipurduar in Indian state of West Bengal. Here, Rabhas are one of the indigenous ethnic tribes who reside in the forest fringe village of Garo Basti of Rajabhat Khawa. It is located between 26.6160° N latitude and 89.5324° E longitude, with an average elevation of 221 meters (725 feet). Rajabhat Khawa, a small town, lies just outside the Buxa Tiger Reserve in the Alipurduar district of West Bengal. Situated approximately 15 kilometers from Jayanti, it is renowned for its pristine natural environment and is enveloped by the Buxa Tiger Reserve Forest (Figure 23.1).

The name of the region Rajabhat Khawa literally means the place where the king had a meal. The folklore is that the kings of the princely state Koch Bihar used to come

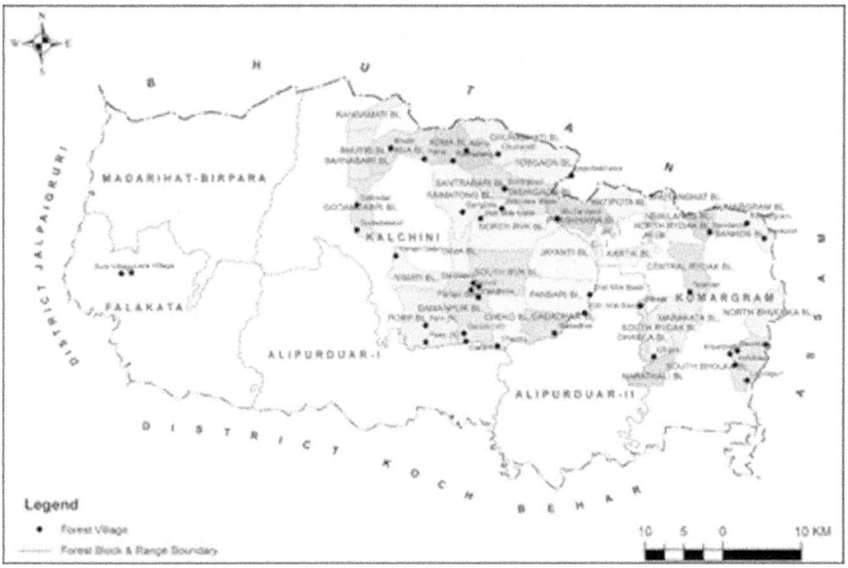

Figure 23.1. Map of the district Alipurduar showing the village Garo Basti in the Rajabhat Khawa region. Source: Author.

here for having picnic in the forests. It is observed that the National Highway 31C passes through Rajabhat Khawa. Rajabhat Khawa also has a railway station, Rajabhat Khawa Railway Station which is situated on the New Jalpaiguri-Alipurduar-Samuktala Road Line. In addition, the Rajabhat Khawa village encompasses approximately 11,968.42 hectares, predominantly covered by forests. Numerous rivers originating from the outer Himalayan ranges in Bhutan flow through this region. Buxa Forest is home to a population of 9,242 individuals, with 4,655 males and 4,587 females. The literacy rate in the Buxa forest village stands at 54.32 percent, with 60.00 percent of males and 48.55 percent of females being literate. The village comprises around 2,072 households, and its postal code is 735227 (Moktan and Nuruzaaman 2020; Goswamy, Kalita, and Banerjee 2024).

Rajabhat Khawa is also a favorite place for wildlife lovers. As part of Buxa Tiger Reserve Forest, Rajabhat Khawa offers the view of a variety of wild animals like elephants, bison, deer, and leopards. A watchtower deep inside the jungle offers a good chance to get glimpses of wild life. This Rajabhat Khawa is also a major attraction for birdwatchers. There are a number of bird species along with migratory species seen here. Forktails, Goosanders, and Ibis Bill are a few among them. There are a number of trekking routes which pass through Buxa forest originating from Rajabhat Khawa. Tourists entering Buxa Tiger Reserve Forest must obtain the necessary permit from the Rajabhat Khawa forest check post. Rajabhat Khawa has a small but beautiful railway station where only passenger trains halt and a local market where tourists can explore. The residents of Rajabhat Khawa encounter various animals from the reserve forest while collecting branches from fallen trees. These include elephants, tigers, leopards, deer, and bison. Rajabhat Khawa predominantly remains a rural area, with 79.38 percent of its population residing in rural settings.

In this region of Rajabhat Khawa, the concentrations of the Rabha community are greater in the Garo Basti village. Garo Basti is a forest fringe village. By definition, forest villages do not mean the villages situated in the forest, but refer to such colonies of colliers or villages or laborers settled by the Forest Department for maintenance of the assured supply of labor required in forest works done departmentally (Sinha 1987; Manoj, Bhattacharyya, and Padhy 2013; Biswas 2014). The Rabhas of North Bengal and also Garo Basti of Rajabhat Khawa have been classified into two types based on socio-cultural-economic status like the forest-dwelling Rabhas and the plain land Rabhas. The forest-dwelling Rabhas are the second largest forest village-dwelling tribal community after Oraon in the Jalpaiguri district of West Bengal. The subsistence strategies of Rabhas have traditionally been linked to the forest. The slash-and-burn agricultural systems are the main practice among the forest-dwelling Rabhas. However, in recent times, they have been obliged to engage themselves with intensive subsistence types of agriculture.

The life of the Rabha community of Garo Basti village is bound to the use of different varieties of flora like Shal tree (*Shorea robusta*), Teak (*Tectona grandis*), Papaya (*Carica papaya*), Date Palm (*Phoenix dactylifera*), Coconut (*Cocos nucifera*), and Bamboo (*Bambusa tulda*). Besides, the Rabha community of Garo Basti village domesticates various types of animals like cows, goats, hens, ducks, and pigs. It is also observed that there are many other hamlets besides Garo Basti like Nepali Basti, Bich Line, Rai Line, and Chitri Line. However, the Rabhas of Garo Basti village are said to be a part of the Bodo family. Their livelihood is intensely related to the surrounding natural resources and their subsistence pattern includes agriculture followed by daily labor. They use their traditional knowledge to cure their illness and to protect their health. They collect various medicinal plants from the deep forest to cure their disease. Besides, they apply and consume different parts of medicinal plants and local remedies on a regular basis.

Notion of Ethnomedicine in Context

Ethnomedicine explores the diverse cultural understandings and practices related to health, illness, and healing within different ethnic or indigenous communities. It examines how people conceptualize their bodies, diagnose illnesses, and seek treatment within their cultural contexts. In other words, ethnomedicine is an interdisciplinary field that examines the cultural interpretation of health, diseases, and illnesses, including the practices and beliefs surrounding healing and healthcare. In such a way, ethnomedicine can study the traditional medical systems of various cultures, such as Ayurveda, Traditional Chinese Medicine, and various African healing traditions. It can also examine how different groups perceive specific diseases, like malaria, or common ailments like colds. It studies how cultural beliefs influence the treatment of mental health conditions, and the role of healing rituals in overcoming trauma. It encompasses a wide range of topics like (a) Cultural beliefs about health and illness—different societies have unique ideas about what causes sickness, how the body functions, and what constitutes health; (b) Traditional healing practices—this includes the use of herbs, rituals, spiritual practices, and other methods to treat illness and promote well-being; (c) Health-seeking behaviors—how people identify illnesses, choose a healer, and participate in the healing process.

In addition, ethnomedicine draws upon various disciplines like medical anthropology (understanding culture's role in shaping health and illness), ethnobotany (studying the use of plants for medicinal purposes), and ethnopharmacology (examining the use of traditional medicines and their bioactive compounds). On the other hand, understanding ethnomedicine is important for improving healthcare (by understanding cultural beliefs and practices, healthcare providers can better communicate with and serve diverse communities), respecting cultural diversity (it helps to promote cultural sensitivity and avoid imposing one's own cultural ideas of health and illness on others), and identifying potential new medicines (ethnomedicine can uncover traditional knowledge about plants and other substances with medicinal properties, which may lead to new drug discoveries).

Therefore, ethnomedicine refers to the specific traditional medical practices and beliefs of a particular culture. It recognizes that health and illness are not just biological phenomena but are also shaped by cultural beliefs, social structures, and historical experiences. Accordingly, ethnomedical systems view health as a holistic state of being, considering physical, mental, and spiritual aspects of well-being. It also studies the interrelations of man and plants, as well as being concerned with the cultural interpretations of health and disease, and also addresses the traditional health care–seeking process and healing practices. Therefore, ethnomedicine is used as a starting point in drug discovery, specifically those using reverse pharmacological techniques.

Understanding Socioeconomic Influences on Ethnomedicinal Practices

Socioeconomic factors significantly influence ethnomedicinal practices. Accordingly, various factors like income, education, and access to healthcare shape the use of traditional medicines. For example, individuals with lower incomes and less access to modern healthcare may depend more on ethnomedicinal practices. More detailed points regarding how socioeconomic factors impact ethnomedicinal practices are given here:

(a) **Income and Affordability:** A number of socioeconomic factors in the context of income and affordability like lower income, access to resources, and dependency on medicinal plants impact the ethnomedicinal practices. People with lower incomes may rely more on ethnomedicinal practices because they are often cheaper and more accessible than modern healthcare. Conversely, socioeconomic status can influence access to resources, including medicinal plants and traditional healers. Various studies have shown that households with lower incomes and fewer material goods are more likely to have higher knowledge of medicinal plants and their uses.

(b) **Education and Knowledge:** Various factors in the context of education and knowledge, such as traditional understanding, access to information, and cultural values, influence ethnomedicinal practices. Ethnomedicinal knowledge is often passed down through generations and is more prevalent among older individuals and those with lower levels of education. On the other hand, higher education levels might lead to greater access to information about modern medicine, potentially reducing the reliance on traditional practices. Moreover, education can also influence cultural values and attitudes toward traditional practices, potentially leading to a shift away from ethnomedicinal practices.

(c) **Healthcare Access and Infrastructure:** Several factors in the context of healthcare access and infrastructure, like distance to healthcare facilities, quality of healthcare, and trust in healthcare systems, affect the ethnomedicinal practices. People living in remote areas with limited access to healthcare facilities may rely more on ethnomedicinal practices. Conversely, the quality and affordability of healthcare services can also influence the use of ethnomedicinal practices. In addition, if people have negative experiences with modern healthcare, they may be more likely to turn to traditional practices.

In relation to these said factors, many other socioeconomic factors affect the ethnomedicinal practices like gender, family size, migration, and rural-urban continuum. Therefore, in some cultures, women are more likely to be involved in the collection and preparation of medicinal plants. Besides, larger families may have greater reliance on ethnomedicinal practices due to the need for cost-effective healthcare solutions. Moreover, migrants may maintain their traditional practices, especially if they are from areas where ethnomedicinal practices are deeply ingrained. Finally, ethnomedicinal practices are often more prevalent in rural areas where access to modern healthcare is limited.

Yet again, ethnomedicinal practices also have various socioeconomic importances like health benefits, revenue generation, cultural development, and insights for novel medication development. Ethnomedicine or herbal medicines can address health issues and contribute to the well-being of rural and suburban populations. On the other hand, the commercialization of medicinal plants can provide economic opportunities for local communities. Additionally, ethnomedicinal practices are an important part of cultural heritage and can contribute to the preservation of traditional knowledge. Lastly, ethnomedicinal knowledge can provide valuable insights for the development of new drugs and treatments.

Ethnomedicinal Practices among the Rabhas

The Rabha community of the village Garo Basti of Rajabhat Khawa of the district Alipurduar is well-known for their close association with nature and forest resources. They have a rich tradition of using plants for medicinal purposes. They depend on locally available vegetation for various needs, including food, fuel, and medicine. Many family members of the Rabha community of the village Garo Basti gather wood from forest areas as a means of subsistence, primarily for use as fuel in cooking, eliminating the need for gas ovens. This practice is widespread among households in the village, with the gathered wood also utilized for special occasions. Additionally, community members collect various plants from the forest for medicinal purposes, particularly for treating allergies, coughs, pneumonia, and other ailments. Fuel procurement involves venturing into the forest to collect wood throughout the year, excluding the monsoon season when gathering becomes impractical. Some individuals also work as daily wage earners (*hazira*) under contractors, earning approximately 200 to 300 rupees per day. Seasonal patterns in gathering indicate that the largest quantities of wood are collected during the winter months when demand for fuel is higher. Despite the challenges posed by the monsoon season, efforts are made to gather wood consistently throughout the year. The division of labor in wood gathering is inclusive, with individuals over the age of fifteen permitted to participate regardless of gender or caste.

Besides, the Rabha community of the village Garo Basti possesses a rich cultural heritage, including traditional healing practices and beliefs, and utilizes various medicinal plants for treating ailments, with a focus on herbal remedies and traditional healers. The faith of the Rabha community of the village Garo Basti is largely animistic, believing in a supernatural power that animates the material universe and that all natural phenomena, including plants, rocks, and so on, share one vital force. They have traditional healers who diagnose and treat illnesses using their own methods and specific medicines. The traditional healer among the Rabha community is locally called *kabiraj*, who is often associated with practices involving herbal remedies and rituals. The community members also perform traditional rituals by wearing traditional dresses and practice traditional dances and theaters to preserve their culture. They have unique dance forms, music, and festivals, including the main festival of Baikho, which involves rituals in both Rabha and Aryan languages. Rabha society is matrilineal, with women holding a special position in the family and participating in economic and political activities. Their cultural practices of resource utilization and beliefs have elements of sustainability, which act as natural deterrents against overexploitation.

Concept of Health and Disease among the Rabhas

Health is a state of complete physical, mental, and social well-being and not merely the absence of disease or infirmity. The enjoyment of the highest attainable standard of health is one of the fundamental rights of every human being without distinction of race, religion, political, economic, or social condition (WHO 1948). In this regard, Bircher (2005) suggests health as a dynamic state of well-being characterized by a physical, mental, and social potential, which satisfies the demands of a life commensurate with age, culture, and personal responsibility. If the potential is insufficient to satisfy these demands, the state is disease. Within this context, health is viewed among the Rabhas of Garo Basti as a balance between natural, physical, and supernatural realms, while disease is seen as an imbalance or disruption of this harmony, often linked to transgressions of social or religious norms or the anger of deities and spirits.

Thus, the traditional faith of Rabhas of Garo Basti is primarily animistic, meaning they believe in spirits and attribute a soul or vital force to natural phenomena and objects. The Rabhas traditionally believe in a supernatural power that organizes the material universe and that all natural phenomena, including plants and rocks, share a vital quality—the soul or spirit that energizes them. They believe in both malevolent and benevolent spirits and used to worship spirits presumed to stay on stones, trees, and other natural objects. While animism is central, the Rabha community also has a blend of Hindu and some animistic rituals (Sarkar and Mistri 2018; Sarkar 2020; Medhi 1980; Medhi 1984; Baruah 2019; Bora 2020, 2023). The Rabhas of Garo Basti are known for their festivals, including Baikho, which is a major festival with rituals. Among the indigenous Rabha, pig and fowl are traditionally used as sacrificial animals, while among the Rabha who maintain Hindu ways of rites, only duck and goat are used. On the other hand, the Rabhas of Garo Basti village possess a sacred grove. They worship their sacred groves, which are locally called *thaan*. Such groves have five *shal* trees (*Shorea robusta*) and are located around a water body. These Rabha community members are very animistic in faith and hold the fauna found in the forest in great reverence. Nesting of vultures atop *shal* trees is considered sacred by the Rabha community members as interaction of the flora and fauna is an indicator of its health.

Accordingly, Rabha community members of Garo Basti believe in the presence of deities, ghosts, and spirits, both benevolent and malevolent, who can influence health and well-being. They also believe that health is a state of equilibrium between the individual, their environment, and the supernatural world. Consequently, the Rabhas of Garo Basti recognize the importance of nature and its elements in maintaining well-being and health. They also think that faithfulness to social and religious customs is considered crucial for maintaining well-being and health. A number of important deities found in the traditional religion among the Rabhas of Garo Basti are *Bay-Ma-Bay* (benevolent deity), *Darmang-Bay* (god of good health), *Bero-Hachu-Bay* (protector of domestic animals), *Khaisam-Bay* (sacrifice to cure height blindness), *Achka-Bay* (goddess of water), *Budha-Bay* (household deity), *Biswali-Bay* (to cure pain), *Singra-Bay* (to cure fever), and *Khclaram Bay* (to save crops). Besides, the Rabha community of Garo Basti, at present, is not careful to observe the long-established religion and rituals as they are facing their identity crises before the other advanced communities such as the well-developed local Bengalis, Rajbanshis, and Christians. The Rabha groups of Garo Basti have lost some of their original worship patterns side by side with their originality in social structure. In the process of assimilation, the Rabha community succeeded in retaining some of the distinct identity markers in spite of the push and pull of development perspectives. Still, the Rabhas of Garo Basti are trying to take the help of herbal medicine instead of using Western oral medicine due to their physical ailments or some major diseases.

The case studies show that various diseases like fever, jaundice, and itching are more common among the Rabhas of Garo Basti. They collect different kinds of herbal medicines from the forest that they learned from their previous generation. They use local homemade herbal medicine for broken limbs and jaundice. It is also seen that almost all the Rabha people of the village go to the *kabiraj* or *ojha* (local medicine man) for medicine. Villagers frequently experience severe jaundice, which is cured by herbal medicines. In addition, if someone's arm or leg is broken, the *kabiraj* immediately gives medicine. The disease jaundice is called *kangar* in the Rava language. The Rabha people said that there are three types of jaundice in Garo Basti: one is yellow jaundice, black jaundice, and white jaundice. The most dangerous form of this is black jaundice. Different types of jaundice have different symptoms. In the case of yellow jaundice, the eyes turn yellow, the hands, feet, and nails turn yellow, and the urine turns yellow. In the case of white jaundice, the whole body starts turning pale, the urine becomes completely white, and the body starts getting weak. Furthermore, in black jaundice, which is the most serious form, the body becomes completely black, leading to apathy toward food. Additionally, the urine also turns black, and the hands and feet turn black.

In case of jaundice, there are some herbal remedies that *kabiraj* or *ojha* use to benefit the Rabha people. The medicine that *kabiraj* gives for jaundice is the cold roots of the *kangar* plant boiled with the crabs found in the river, and the water cures the jaundice. According to him, the best way is to boil the roots of an orange-colored flower called *agalkal* in water and pour it on the head, and then jaundice never occurs again. For white jaundice, there is *talmichari* along with the leaves of *nal-singha*, which are brought from the jungle, leaves of the garlic plant, and roots of the *koja* plant. Leaves or roots of the *kangaroo* plant and roots of the *lajyavati* plant are boiled together and fed to the bet. In this same way, and with some other herbs, black jaundice medicine is prepared. The medicine man or *kabiraj* also told that if the limbs are broken, the limbs need to be covered with the help of the roots and leaves of various plants. A kind of creeping leaf *googly* and *lajjabati* plants should be well mixed and applied to the fractured area for three days. The area should be covered with a clean cloth every day. Once the coating is dry, the area should be cleaned thoroughly with hot water, and the herbal mixture should be applied again. And there is no need to take any medicine with it.

Like these examples, the *kabiraj* or *ojha* (local medicine man) among the Rabhas provide herbal medicine to the villagers for the treatment of various other common diseases like black fever, cough, typhoid, diarrhea, joint pain, skin infection, snake bites, hydrocele, and diabetes. Case studies show that *kabiraj* gives the leaf of a local plant *nakdana* to the people who have black fever and the flower extract of a local plant *kauri* for the treatment of snake bite. Accordingly, the life cycle, well-being, and potential health issues of Rabhas of Garo Basti are interconnected with the plants, forest, and forest products. However, with the seeping in of modernization, in the form of trained doctors or forest officials or medicinal plant contractors, and increased inflow of money replacing the erstwhile barter, the symbiosis of the Rabhas with their ecosystem has eroded. The fragile balance which man maintained with nature has become tense. Today, the resistance of the Rabhas is broken by intermittent use of allopathic medicine, often substantiated by indigenous herbs. The community has not fully been able to accept either of the systems, yet it intermittently uses both, thereby making them vulnerable.

Medicinal Plant Use among the Rabhas

Ethnobotanical studies are crucial for documenting and preserving the traditional knowledge of tribal communities about medicinal plants. These ethnobotanical studies also highlight the importance of conserving medicinal plants, as many are facing threats due to habitat loss and overexploitation (Moktan 2018; Datta, Prakash, and Singharoy 2022). This is the reason the present study has tried to document the rich tradition of using medicinal plants for various ailments by the Rabhas of Garo Basti. The Rabha community members of the village Garo Basti have extensive knowledge of medicinal plants, which they use to treat various diseases, including fever, fungal infections, skin problems, diabetes, anemia, and respiratory disorders. Different parts of plants, such as leaves, flowers, shoots, seeds, fruits, stems, buds, tubers, and bark, are used for medicinal purposes by them. Some medicinal plants commonly used by the Rabha community of the village Garo Basti include *Centella asiatica*, *Cissus quadrangularis* L., *Houttuynia cordata*, *Phyllanthus emblica*, *Terminalia arjuna*, and many others. Among the Rabhas, *titepati* (*Artemisia vulgaris* or *mugwort*) is known for its medicinal properties, used to treat abdominal pain, dyspepsia, diarrhea, and dysentery, as well as its insect repellent and protective qualities. The Rabhas are known to utilize various other plants for medicinal purposes, including Tulsi, Rongdani, Maitori, Koch, Hana, Pati, Dahuri, Totla, and Bitalia.

The Rabha community members generally use locally available herbs, cultivated drugs, and even cultivate depleting medicinal plants. They also have traditional bone-setting practices, with *Cissus quadrangularis* L. being a commonly used plant for treating bone fractures. In other words, among the Rabhas, *Cissus quadrangularis* L., known as *hadjod* or *asthisamhara* (bone setter), is a plant species traditionally used for bone fracture healing and other medicinal purposes, reflecting their close relationship with nature and utilization of local resources. In addition, the case studies show that many diseases like malaria and jaundice are prominent diseases among the Rabha community of the village Garo Basti. In that case, the traditional healers use various herbs for treating malaria and jaundice. Therefore, the Rabha community's indigenous knowledge of medicinal plants contributes to their health and well-being, aligning with sustainable development goals. Table 23.1 shows the list of medicinal plants used by the Rabhas of the village Garo Basti, Rajabhat Khawa, Alipurduar.

Thus, the Rabha community of the village Garo Basti relies heavily on herbal medicine. Many community members prefer traditional treatments over modern medicine, especially for women's health issues. The family members of the Rabha community are largely dependent on plant-based indigenous medicines. Some especially experienced people in the village know the use and benefits of various plants. They can prepare medicines for various diseases. Such experienced people are called *Kabiraj*. They treat almost everything with medicinal plants, like fever, cold, cough, headache, blood sugar, blood pressure, kidney stones, and even conditions like Covid-19. If any part of the body is broken, they treat it without an X-ray and make the patient completely cured. Not only humans but also any other animals or their cattle are treated by such experienced people or "Kabiraj." They are physicians as well as veterinarians. On the other hand, some experienced people also treat plants. They make various medicines at home and apply them to the roots and leaves to make any plant healthy. They use cow urine, cow dung, and *neem* juice as fertilizers and pesticides (Figure 23.2).

Although the present study shows that there is a primary health care center near Garo Basti, the Rabha community members rarely visit it. They prefer to visit a medicine man in the village, as these medicines have no side effects on their bodies. Moreover, from Table 23.1, we can see that the medicine man mostly makes medicine from plants that are available in the village as well as in the forest, on which they rely more than allopathic medicines. Even medicine men also have the responsibility for the villagers. They try their level best to cure any disease, and if they fail, they refer them to the nearby health center. Some community members go to modern primary health centers for the treatment of their common fever, cold, and cough. Sometimes, a few community members go to modern primary health centers near Rabha Basti for

Table 23.1. List of Medicinal Plants Used by the Rabhas of the Village Garo Basti, Rajabhat Khawa, Alipurduar

Local Name	Scientific Name	Family Name	Parts Used	Medicinal Uses
Loshun	*Allium sativum* L.	Alliaceae	Leaves	The leaves are eaten raw in the early morning to cure cough problem
Matikanduri	*Altemanthera sessilis* L.	Amaranthaceae	Shoot	Leaf Paste is applied on wound
Titepati	*Artemisia vulgaris*	Asteraceae	Whole Plant	Used to treat abdominal pain, dyspepsia, diarrhea, and dysentery, as well as it has insect repellent and protective qualities.
Puroi sak	*Basella alba L. var. alba*	Basellaceae	Leaf, Stem	Leaves, stem, and fruits useful in anemia
Thinsengi	*Borreria latifolia K.Schum*	Rubiaceae	Shoot	Leaf juice mixed with seed powder of *Piper nigrum* L. and salt used in treatment of tonsillitis.
Manimuni	*Centella asiatia*	Apiaceae	Leaves	Fresh raw leaves are eaten in the early morning to cure gastric problem.
Asthisamhara	*Cissus quadrangularis* L.	Vitaceae	Whole Plant	Cissus quadrangularis, known as "Hadjod" or "Asthisamharaka" ("bone setter"), is traditionally used for bone fracture healing, pain relief, and inflammation, with potential benefits for diabetes, and obesity.
Kath Alu	*Dioscorea alata* L.	Discoreaceae	Tuber	Tubers useful in anemia
Siju	*Euphorbia nerifolia* L.	Euphorbiaceae	Latex	The latex is applied at night during bed time for early suppuration of boils.
Katamasala	*Eryngium foetidum* L.	Apiaceae	Leaves	Leaves are useful in cold and fever
Dimoru	*Ficus racemosa* L.	Moraceae	Fruits	Decoction of bark is used in fever
Mosandri	*Houttuynia cordata*	Saurauaceae	Leaves	Leaves juice are useful in gastroenteritis
Mesta tenga	*Hibiscus subdarifa* L.	Malvaceae	Leaves, Flower	Leaves and flower juice are used as in gastroenteritis and dysentery.
Parchinkou	*Justicia adhatoda* L.	Acanthaceae	Leaves	Luke warm juice of the raw leaves is taken orally 2–3 times daily before meal to cure jaundice.
Pategoja	Kalanchoe pinnata	Crassulaceae	Leaves	Decoction of leaves is used in cough and gastroenteritis

Kanshisa	Leucus plukentii	Lamiaceae	Leaves	Juice of the leaves mixed with the leaf juice of *Andrographis paniculata* and given to children once daily in the early morning for deworming.
Jetuka	Lawsonia inermis L.	Lythraceae	Leaves	Leaf paste useful in fever, high blood pressure and effective in fungal infection of skin.
Lejumalati	*Mimosa pudica* L.	Mimosaceae	Root	Juice of the root is taken twice daily during dysentery.
Narasingha	*Murraya koenegii* L.	Rutaceae	Leaves	Leaf juice used as tonic, curing many stomach problems.
Chipriteeta	*Nyctanthus arbour-tristis* L.	Oleaceae	Leaves, Seed	The juice of the tender leaves is taken once daily in the early morning to get relief from worms. Leaves are used in malaria.
Tulsi	*Ocimum sanctum* L.	Lamiaceae	Leaves	Juice of the raw leaves is applied on the eye to cure eye allergy. The juice of the fresh leaves mixed with honey is taken orally twice daily to get relief from cough.
Zamlok	*Oroxylum indicum* (L.) Vent	Bigoniaceae	Bark	Juice of the bark is taken orally 2–3 times daily against jaundice.
Emblica	*Phyllanthus emblica*	Phyllanthaceae	Leaves Fruits	Leaves are used medicinally to treat coughs and fever. Fruits are used as a liver tonic and laxative.
Tita phool	*Phlobacanthus thyrsiformis T.Andr.*	Acantthaceae	Flower	Extract of flower useful in asthma and small pox.
Arjun gaas	*Terminalia arjuna*	Combretaceae	Bark	Decoction of bark mixed with milk and water is effective in heart problem. Crushed stem bark juice is taken orally 3 times a day before meal against stomach pain.
Paroli	*Stereospermum chelonoides*	Bignoniaceae	Leaves	Used in tuberculosis
Tupurilota	*Stephania hernandifolia*	Menispermaceae	Leaves	Leaves are effective in diabetes.
Postia	*Vitex negundo* L.	Verbaneceae	Leaves	A drink prepared by mixture of the plant juice and water effective in body pain, headache, and earache.

Source: Authors.

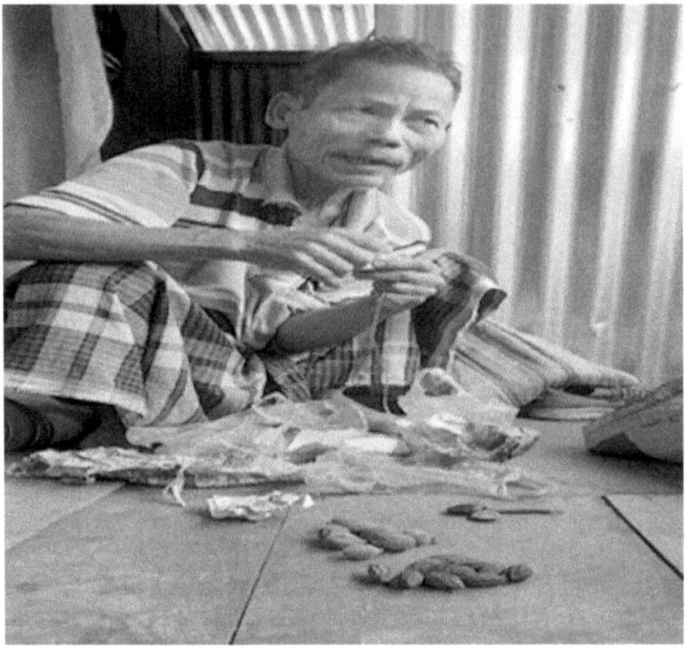

Figure 23.2. Ojha, a Rabha medicine man, providing knowledge about the medicinal plant use. Source: Author.

the treatment of their common fever, cold, and cough, as well as to get women checked during pregnancy.

Effect of Socioeconomic Factors on Health among the Rabhas

By and large, the socioeconomic factors encompassing income, education, employment, and housing significantly impact health outcomes, with individuals in disadvantaged positions often experiencing poorer health and shorter lifespans. In the same way, a number of socioeconomic factors significantly impact the health of the Rabha community of the village Garo Basti. These socioeconomic factors are low education, limited access to healthcare, and poverty hindering their overall well-being and leading to a lower standard of living. The detailed look at the issue is discussed here:

(i) **Poverty and Limited Resources:** The Rabha community of the village Garo Basti often faces poverty and limited access to basic resources like clean water, sanitation, and nutritious food, which directly impact their health.

(ii) **Lack of Education:** Low levels of education among Rabha people of the village Garo Basti can lead to poor health literacy, hindering their ability to make informed decisions about their health and access appropriate healthcare services.
(iii) **Limited Access to Healthcare:** The Rabha community members of the studied area may face geographical barriers, lack of transportation, and financial constraints that limit their access to quality healthcare facilities and services.
(iv) **Traditional Beliefs and Practices:** Some traditional beliefs and practices may hinder the adoption of modern healthcare practices and preventive measures, impacting the health of the community.
(v) **Impact on Specific Health Issues:** Studies have shown that socioeconomic factors are linked to higher rates of malaria, malnutrition, and other health problems within the Rabha community.
(vi) **Need for Targeted Interventions:** Addressing the socioeconomic factors that impact the health of the Rabha community requires targeted interventions focused on improving education, access to healthcare, economic opportunities, and addressing traditional beliefs that may hinder health outcomes.
(vii) **SHGs and Empowerment:** Self-help groups (SHGs) can play a crucial role in improving the socioeconomic status of Rabha women of the village Garo Basti leading to better nutrition and healthcare for their families.

Thus, the present study observes that the Rabha community of the village Garo Basti is socioeconomically backward. The educational and occupational status, annual family income, and health conditions of these Rabha people are not up to the mark. They still believe in traditional practices and beliefs. Nowadays, the youth of the Rabha people of Garo Basti are shifting from traditional agricultural practices to government jobs and business. For this, the sources of their livelihood are now diversified. In modern times, there is a great need to overcome the backwardness to achieve self-sufficiency for the people of Rabha. They also feel immensely that they have capacities and efficiency like other social groups to achieve something different.

Conclusion and Recommendation

The forest-dwelling Rabha community of the village Garo Basti of the region Rajabhat Khawa in the district Alipurduar has been performing their health practice very well by utilizing their indigenous knowledge. Most of the common diseases like cough, cold, fever, stomach problems, jaundice, diarrhea, skin infection, and diabetes are cured by the local medicine men *kabiraj* or *ojha* and the elder people of the village who have good knowledge of ethnomedicine. But presently, the lack of proper practice and modernization among the new generation will lead to the loss of such valuable indigenous knowledge. Therefore, proper documentation of such practices through a comprehensive picture of the medicinal plants to identify, a proper list of those plants along with their ways of practice, by doing semi-structured interviews of the local healers or folk medicinal practitioners of the village Garo Basti of the region Rajabhat Khawa, should be done. Conversely, nowadays the Rava community has been actively involved in the promotion of sustainable development through the utilization of their traditional and culturally rooted knowledge.

But, somehow the indigenous knowledge of the Rabha community persists in its harmful impact on the environment. Moreover, one of the leading factors of deforestation is the Rabha people's dependency on forests. Nonetheless, the contribution of indigenous knowledge of the Rabha community is crucial for sustainable development. Besides, the sustainable development of the forest-dwelling Rabha community of the village Garo Basti can be achieved by implementing specific policies that address difficulties such as boosting women's economic opportunities, aiding landless families, ensuring wage parity, preserving cultural practices, and avoiding human-animal conflict. These endeavors will not only enhance the community's ability to sustain themselves and survive but also guarantee the peaceful cohabitation of the Rabha people with their natural surroundings.

Moreover, some important plants with high medicinal value from the nearby forest of Garo Basti have reached a threatened condition due to some man-made activities like overexploitation, habitat destruction, and rapid urbanization. Hence, there is an urgent need to record all information related to the indigenous knowledge as well as information related to ethnomedicine of the Rabhas of Garo Basti. In addition, there is a need for further documentation of the traditional knowledge of the Rabha community people of the village Garo Basti of the region Rajabhat Khawa in the district Alipurduar, especially regarding their ethnomedicinal practices to prevent the loss of this valuable knowledge.

In addition, the government should prioritize the provision of educational facilities for the Rabha community of the Garo Basti. This includes establishing schools within their communities, ensuring the presence of qualified teachers, and facilitating access to quality education for all members. Furthermore, the development of pucca houses and pucca road infrastructure is essential for enhancing connectivity and facilitating overall progress in the region of Rajabhat Khawa. Improved road networks not only ease transportation challenges but also stimulate economic activities, encourage investment, and promote social integration. Moreover, there is a pressing need to raise awareness about the importance of education, particularly among the female members of the Rabha community of the Garo Basti.

References

Baruah, G. "A Study on Socio-Economic Conditions of Rabha People of Kamrup District of Assam." *IOSR Journal of Humanities and Social Science* 24, no. 11 (2019): 21–4.

Bircher, J. "Towards a Dynamic Definition of Health and Disease." *Medicine, Healthcare & Philosophy* 8 (2005): 335–41.

Biswas, S. K. "Samataler Rabha: Samaj O Sanskriti Paribartaner Prekshapat (in Bengali)." In *Uttar Banger Janajati O Luptopray Lokosanskriti,* edited by G. Roy, 120–36. Siliguri: Baitanik, 2004.

Biswas, S. K. "A Tribe in Transition: Study on Plain Land Rabhas." *Bulletin of the Cultural Research Institute* XXV, no. 1 & 2 (2014): 30–42.

Bora, B. "Development Model in Rural Assam: An Analysis of the Rabha Community in Baksa District, Assam." *International Journal for Innovative Research in Multidisciplinary Field* 6, no. 3 (2020): 11–15.

Bora, D. "Determinants of Livelihood Diversification among Rabha Tribes of Assam: A Case Study." *Palarch's Journal of Archaeology of Egypt/Egyptology* 17, no. 7 (2023): 4058–69.

Das, A. K., and M. K. Raha. *The Rabhas of West Bengal.* Calcutta: SC & ST Welfare Department. Government of West Bengal, 1967.

Datta, C., N. Prakash, and D. K. Singharoy. "An Outline of the Trend of Change: A Case of an Indigenous Rabha Tribe of India." *Journal of Pharmaceutical Negative Results* 13, no. 4 (2022): 721–4.

Goswamy, N., J. Kalita, and S. Banerjee. "Forest-Dwelling Rabha Community in Alipurduar, West Bengal: An Ethnographic Study." *International Journal of Recent Advances in Multidisciplinary Topics* 5, no. 8 (2024): 60–5.

Logiel, A., E. Jørs, P. Akugizibwe, and P. Ahnfeldt-Mollerup. "Prevalence and Socio-economic Factors Affecting the Use of Traditional Medicine among Adults of Katikekile Subcounty, Moroto District, Uganda." *African Health Sciences* 21, no. 3 (2021): 1410–17.

Mandal, B., and R. Manadeb. "The Rabha and Their Social Movement (1925–1950): A Case Study of North Bengal." *IOSR Journal of Humanities and Social Science* 10, no. 3 (2013): 5–8.

Manoj, K., R. Bhattacharyya, and P. K. Padhy. "Forest and Wildlife Scenarios of Northern West Bengal, India: A Review." *International Research Journal of Biological Sciences* 2, no. 7 (2013): 70–9.

Medhi, B. K. "Beliefs, Rituals and Ceremonies Connected With the Principle Events of the Life of the Pati Rabhas of Assam." *Bulletin of the Department of Anthropology* 9 (1980): 41–53.

Medhi, B. K. "Snake Godess Marai of the Pati Rabha of Assam." *The Eastern Anthropologist* 37, no. 2 (1984): 159–64.

Moktan, R. "Rabha Ethnic Community of North Bengal: Analysis on the Socio-Economic Status." *Journal of Emerging Technologies and Innovative Research* 5, no. 8 (2018): 1–4.

Moktan, R., and N. Kasemi. "Socio-Cultural Development among the Tribal Community: A Study on Rabha Ethnic Community in North Bengal." *International Journal of Humanities and Social Science Invention* 9, no. 6 (2020): 4–9.

Raha, M. K. *Matriliny to Patriliny A Study of the Rabha Society.* New Delhi: Gian Publishing House, 1989.

Roy, A., A. Sinha, R. K. Manna, B. K. Das, and S. Majumder. "Socio-cultural Tradition of the Rabha Tribes of North Bengal, India: In Relation to Fisheries." *Journal of the Inland Fisheries Society of India* 50, no. 2 (2018): 79–83.

Sarkar, A., and T. Mistri. "A Discourse on the Religious Practices of the Rabha Community of West Bengal." *International Journal of Research in Social Science* 8, no. 7 (2018): 1–15.

Sarkar, K. "A Probe into the Socio-Economic and Cultural Transformation of the Forest Dwellers Rabha Community of Jalpaiguri District, West Bengal, in the 21st Century." *IOSR Journal of Humanities and Social Science* 25, no. 7 (2020): 19–25.

Sinha, S. P. "Forest Village in Bihar: An Analysis of Their Present Status." In *Tribals and Forests*, edited by S. P. Sinha, 297–8. Govt. of Bihar, Welfare Department, BTWRI, Ranchi, 1987.

World Health Organization. *Summary Reports on Proceedings Minutes and Final Acts of the International Health Conference held in New York from 19 June to 22 July 1946.* World Health Organization, 1948.

24

Indigenous Knowledge and Healthcare Practices among the Limbu Community of Darjeeling Hills

Insights from the Covid-19 Pandemic

Niten Chhetri* and Somenath Bhattacharjee

Department of Anthropology, Nagaland University, Nagaland, India

*Corresponding Author's Email: niten_rs2023@nagalanduniversity.ac.in

Introduction

Over generations, indigenous knowledge system (IKS) formed by distinct cultures has contributed to their folktales, customs, traditions, rituals, and beliefs. The knowledge transmitted orally over the years has guaranteed its longevity.[1] Stevenson (1996) states that the term indigenous knowledge encompasses traditional and nontraditional, ecological and non-ecological knowledge. The practical involvement of daily life gave rise to indigenous knowledge, strengthened by trial and error methods, hands-on experience, and considerate reflection. This pragmatic wisdom is typically shaped by generations of sharp reasoning. The prosperity of this knowledge that directly impacts the health of those who follow it is a great measure of Darwinian fitness (Ellen et al. 2000).

The landscape of tribal communities in terms of sociocultural setting has sustained continuous transition resulting in instability of culture and tradition. Modernization, education, cultural interactions, and the impact of technology, government, and nongovernmental organization development initiatives are the reasons for these changes. Understanding the health of the tribe would require consideration and interpretation of health within tribal concepts and beliefs. There has been documentation of diseases

[1] Acknowledgments: Authors are thankful to all the participants from the Limbu communities of Darjeeling Sadar subdivision for their cooperation and also the Department of Anthropology, Nagaland University, for working facilities.
Conflict of interest: Authors declare that there is no conflict of interest.

such as influenza, cholera, dengue, and smallpox throughout history, and with time there has been progress in eradicating these diseases, but many still pose a significant threat to the communities. The origin of Covid-19 goes back to China's Wuhan city, and then it reached India and other parts of the country. In India, the first case was reported in Kerala's Thrissur district on January 30, 2020, and it rapidly spread across all states and Union Territories (WHO 2020). The implementation of the nationwide lockdown enforced social and physical distancing to curb the disease's spread. While this measure had profound effects on the daily lives of the entire 1.3 billion population and the country's economy, the people of India are grappling with a global health crisis within the context of a national lockdown and state health emergency. It is crucial to examine how local communities respond to this pandemic by drawing upon their long-standing indigenous knowledge systems to safeguard them. Therefore, amid the outbreak, a pressing public health objective is to halt the virus's transmission from an epidemic source region to other areas within the country or globally. Additionally, there is a need to explore alternative solutions, including tapping into the indigenous community's medicinal knowledge.

Thapa (2017) in her famous dissertation entitled "Phedangma among Limboos of Sikkim: Change and Continuity" looks at the Phedangma tradition and the concept of reinvented religion among Limbus in three different geographical regions. The study explores the traditional religious practices in the context of reimagined religion, which certain Limbus have opted to embrace. The study examines the social and religious disparity within the Limbu community, emphasizing the central roles played by various segments in the ongoing religious transformations in contemporary Sikkim. On the other hand, R. K. Limbu (2013) in his article titled "Exploring Indigenous Knowledge System and Limbu Cultural Identity in Nepal" investigated the connection between the Limbu indigenous knowledge system and the preservation of cultural identities. The study highlights a thoughtful reflection to determine and uphold the cultural heritages to ensure diverse unity. Further, Chatterjee (2017) in his article named "Indigenous Knowledge and Practices among the Limbus of Sikkim Himalayas" explored the remarkable ecological, biological, and ethnomedicinal knowledge that the Limbu community in Sikkim possesses. This article recognizes the community's traditional folk wisdom and aims to document this wealth of knowledge and practices. Moreover, Sundas (2023) in his research entitled "Language and Traditional Healing Practice: A Study of Limbu Community" explored the intrinsic relationship between language and traditional healing practices among the Limbus of Sikkim.

Yet again, Debnath (2020) in his study called "The Limbus of North Bengal: An Anthropological Study in Two Districts of West Bengal" focused on the origin, ethnohistory, and various aspects of social, economic, religious, and political life among the Limbus in North Bengal. This research employs social anthropological tools and techniques to gather empirical data. Once more, R. K. Limbu (2010) in his famous research named "Performance in Limbu Mundhum: A Study of Cultural Representation" emphasized the major Mundhum performances and their reflection on the sociocultural and religio-historical aspects of the Limbu people. This study also highlights how the Kirant Limbu community's cultural, historical, and mythical characteristics are shaped by ritual performers, participants, and audience members. Therefore, it is acknowledged that not much is known about how these Limbu communities were affected by the pandemic and how they responded in the lockdown period. Accordingly, the present study reflects a modest attempt to document and preserve the wealth of insights about livelihoods, with a primary focus on significant healthcare practices adopted by the Limbu communities of Darjeeling Sadar subdivision amid the challenges posed by the Covid-19 pandemic.

Objectives and Methods

This study tries to examine the indigenous healthcare beliefs and practices of the Limbu community amid the Covid-19 pandemic. It also gained an understanding of ethnomedicinal practices within the Limbu community, looked into their perspectives on Covid-19 vaccination, found out what influences their choices between traditional medicine and modern medicine, and investigated any potential long-term implications of these practices during the pandemic. Furthermore, this study examines the Limbu community's customary approaches to healthcare practices, including their perceptions of illness and healthcare, rituals associated with quarantine, and the historical use of medicinal plants both during and before the Covid-19 period.

Many Limbu communities live in the Darjeeling Sadar subdivision, where we performed this study. They are mostly concentrated in Kalimpong, Darjeeling Sadar, and some tribal regions in the Jalpaiguri district of the Indian state of West Bengal. This study concentrated on the Darjeeling district, positioned in the northernmost part of West Bengal, which presents itself as an irregular triangle. The district is divided geographically into two main divisions: the hills and the plains. The hilly region is part of the Gorkhaland Territorial Administration—a semiautonomous body under the governance of the West Bengal state. This administrative division includes the three subdivisions of Darjeeling, Kurseong, Mirik, and as well as the Kalimpong district. The Terai is the Siliguri subdivision's name for the Darjeeling Himalayan foothills. East of Darjeeling, that is, Bijanbari is a quaint town within the Darjeeling district with a pleasant environment. Positioned at an elevation of 5,200 feet, Lamagaon is located approximately 33 kilometer from the main town of Darjeeling and 10 kilometers from Bijanbari. Limbus (Subba) comprises the majority of Lamagaon's population. For primary data collection, the researcher undertook a cab journey from Bijanbari to Kaijalay, followed by a 2.2-kilometer trek on foot to reach Lamagoan.

The primary methods of gathering data were interviews, case histories, focused group discussions, and participant observation. The interview adheres to a semi-structured framework, utilizing strategies of openness and probing. This research diligently documented and transcribed the interviews verbatim. It collected data mostly from the elderly inhabitants of the residents, herbalists, and practitioners who are knowledgeable in magico-religious traditions as well as mainly those participants who are well-versed in local herbal practices and experiences. The collaboration with herbalists and healers facilitated the initial identification of the local herbs and plants. Besides, the traditional healers and older community members provided much data and information regarding plants' local names and their respective uses, consumption, and procedures of application, which were also systematically recorded and documented in written forms and by audiovisual systems.

Brief Outline of the Limbus

The Limbus retains a plethora of indigenous knowledge, encompassing their unique mother tongue, folk culture incorporating folk literature, beliefs, customs, traditional dance, music, art, artifacts, tools, games, cuisine, clothing, and dwellings. Their cultural fabric is woven with various festivals, rituals, and traditional healing practices. They identify as Yakthumba, indicating that their resilience is similar to that of Yaks (Singh 1993). They were believed to have originated from the Tsong province in Tibet, migrating to Eastern Nepal and the neighboring regions of present-day Western Sikkim (Singh 1993). Risley (1894) proposed that the Limbus had their origins from Kashi Thongba clans (common people call Kasigotra). From the Limbu standpoint, their ancestral homeland is Limbuwan, located east of Khambuan and thought to have been conquered using bows and arrows. This geographical area extends from the Arun River west to the Singalila range, along the Sikkim and Darjeeling borders (Pradhan 2009). The Limbus adhere to the oral scripture of Kirat Mundhum, akin to the Bon shamanic tradition. However, their religious practices also bear the influences of later Tibetan Buddhism and Hinduism. Within their religious framework, there are various classes of ritual specialists such as "Phedangma," "Yema/Yeba," and "Samba." Although "Tagera Ningwaphuma" is their supreme deity, the Limbus revere the deity "Yuma" on all occasions due to its paramount significance and popularity. The Limbu revere "Yuma" as the mother of all, instilling a reverence for one's mother as a deity.

The Limbus, recognized as nature worshippers and initially categorized as animists, reveal upon closer examination of their traditional religion, a trajectory that aligns with Tylor's (1871) evolution of religion. This progression spans from animism to polytheism and eventually reaches the contemporary stage of monotheism. Over time, the Limbus experienced significant influences from Hinduism and Buddhism, dividing them into distinct religious groups. They cultivate various seasonal vegetables and aromatic herbs, including spinach, ginger, potato, turmeric, tomato, onion, radish, squash, pumpkin, and chili. Moreover, the Limbu communities in these regions often preserve these vegetables through drying methods, ensuring consumption during the off-season. The *Gundruk*, a traditional dish, is prepared from spinach leaves and radishes, contributing to the creation of *Sinki*. Conversely, Lamagoan is also renowned for producing *Ishkus* (squash), ginger, and black cardamoms (Limbu 2013). Additionally, the cultural opulence of the Limbus has gradually unfurled across centuries, molded by their continual observations, actions, and responses to the natural environment. Medicinal plants take on the role of primary health care providers for the majority, whereas traditional healers or shamans become the initial recourse for any ailment. The Limbu worldview attributes illnesses to the influence of ghosts and spirits. The treatment process typically entails a fusion of rituals, incantations, and the utilization of herbal remedies and preparations. Within Limbu communities, recognition exists for four distinct categories of shamans: Yeba and Yema, Samba, Phedangma, and Mangba.

The present study categorizes the Limbu medical frameworks into two primary divisions: (i) the disease theory system and (ii) the healthcare system (Bhasin and Bhasin 1995). The disease theory system encompasses beliefs regarding health's essence, illness's origins, and the corresponding remedies and curative procedures. On the other hand, the healthcare system focuses on the methods employed by society to address sickness and uphold well-being. In addition, among the Limbus, there are usually two types of healthcare systems: traditional and Western. But traditional medicine encompasses all forms of folk medicine and unconventional healing practices passed down through generations.

Findings and Discussion

Tribal societies intricately tie the perception of health to the magico-religious fabric of their existence, not viewing it in isolation. Furthermore, many tribal communities define health, medical care, and the causes of diseases within their social context (Sonowal and Praharaj 2007). In this regard, Singh (2008) opined that tribal health is significantly shaped by the interaction of social, economic, political factors, and their cultural practices influence their health behavior. Therefore, gaining insight into the culture of tribal groups becomes crucial for comprehending the concept of tribal health. Considering the same, R. K. Limbu (2013) revealed that Limbu people possess extensive knowledge of nature, local flora, fauna, herbal practices, traditional medicines, and the utilization of herbal remedies for treating various diseases. Their understanding extends to identifying the locations of medicinal and ritual plants, the appropriate times for collection, and the techniques involved in preparing and storing medicines. Additionally, they possess insights into human health, nutrition, and the classification of animal and human diseases. However, the Lamagoan study reveals a comparatively limited level of knowledge or practice in certain aspects, including familiarity with the locations of medicinal and ritual plants, the optimal timing for collection, and the methods for preparing and storing medicines. The residents, particularly the elderly leaders in Lamagaon, believed that even a slight fever was immediately associated with the possibility of coronavirus because of the Covid-19 pandemic. Despite the lockdown, people remained in their village and stayed indoors. Agricultural activities, including cultivating and marketing crops, especially squash (*Ishkus*), continued during the lockdown. While there was a need to travel approximately 10 kilometer to Bijanbari for hospital facilities, Lamagaon had its primary health center and residents preferred seeking medical assistance there. High sugar levels and hypertension were prevalent health issues in the village and the villagers deemed the medications provided by the primary health center satisfactory. This region extensively employs the indigenous healing approach, now recognized as homeopathy, to address various health issues such as elevated sugar levels, hypertension, jaundice, injuries, toothaches, headaches, and similar illnesses (Figure 24.1 and Figure 24.2).

During the lockdown, home remedies and traditional medicines from their surroundings became significant. For instance, in the case of mild fever (though no Covid cases were recorded), they utilized plants like *Titepati* (Mugwort) and *Tulsi* (Holy basil), which were boiled and consumed. Adhering to government protocols, they followed social distancing, wore facemasks, and used hand sanitizer during marriage or death rituals. Only a few could attend such events due to Covid-19 restrictions. They referred to fever and cold as *Kumrek/Haija*, and for cough, they relied on plants like *Banmara* (Crofton weed), *Swertia chirayita*, *Tulsi*, and Ginger. The belief that going to the hospital might lead to harm persisted, as there was a widespread sense of panic and fear around Covid. They refrained from using locally available fauna for medicine, acknowledging the changing times and a shift toward reduced animal sacrifice and violence, influenced by the adoption of Hinduism and Buddhism.

Concerns were raised about the diminishing traditional knowledge among the younger generation. According to the village elder, who served as the president of the Limbu community, the transfer of traditional knowledge to the youth depends solely on parental guidance. If parents fail to impart this knowledge, the younger generation will remain unaware of these practices. Besides, there are a few locally available plants that are used for medicinal purposes. During the lockdown, herbalists and residents employed plants such as *Gol-Patta*, *Titepati*, *Tulsi*, and Chiraito to treat fever.

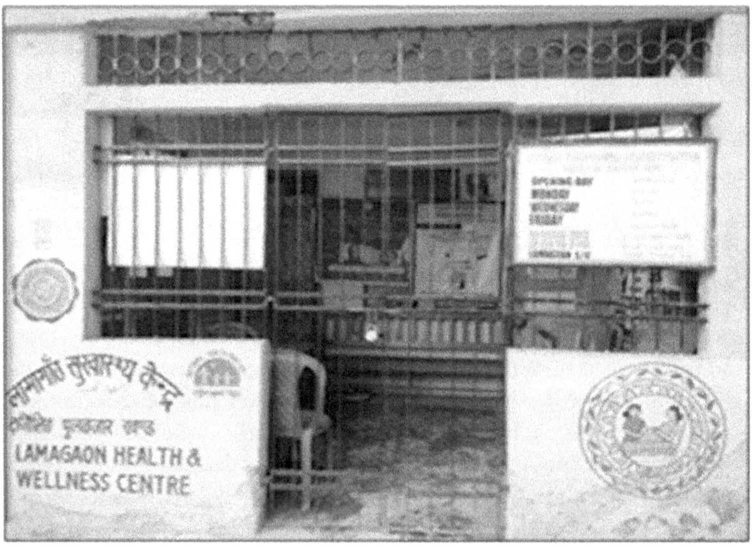

Figure 24.1 Primary Health Center (PHC), Lamagaon. Source: Author.

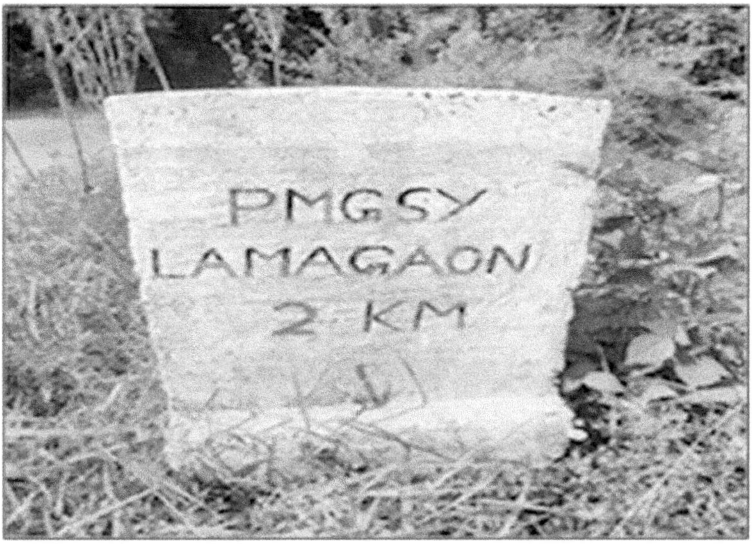

Figure 24.2. Pillar of Pradhan Mantri Gram Sadak Yojana (PMGSY). Source: Author.

Interestingly, herbalists leaned more toward traditional medicines than modern medical solutions during the Covid-19 pandemic. Other noteworthy plants include *Avijalo* for sinusitis, *Akhley* for managing fever and tonsil issues, *Pashanbheda* for toothache and vomiting, Aloe vera for cuts and burns, Makiba leaves for addressing sugar-related concerns, and *Chuwa-Ko-Phool* (*Phlogacanthus thyrsiformis*) for hypertension. Despite the prevalence of sugar and hypertension in Lamagaon, the community showed a reliance on modern medicines both before and during the pandemic. Various methods were applied for using plants and herbs including creating pastes, extracting juices, and chewing. The process typically involves crushing or mincing plant parts with a stone pestle and mortar to produce a paste. The juice is extracted by squeezing or crushing plant components and filtering the liquid through a cloth. In cases where infusion is the objective, plant parts are immersed in water for a specific duration. In addition, certain plant parts are boiled in water to create a medicinal solution called decoction (Figure 24.3 and Figure 24.4).

In this study, it is also revealed that the selected Phedangba received training from Ban-Jhakri, a shamanic deity associated with the wilderness. In the past, he engaged in Mundhums (a compilation of cultural and ritual references) as well as other traditional practices, religious festivals, and rituals. However, contemporary times witness a decline in these traditional rituals, with little to no ceremonies performed. Phedangba predominantly relied on herbal medicines over modern alternatives. He emphasized the belief that worshiping deities is integral to maintaining optimal health. Throughout the Covid-19 pandemic, he adhered to staying indoors and leaned on traditional medicines for support (Figure 24.5, Figure 24.6, and Figure 24.7).

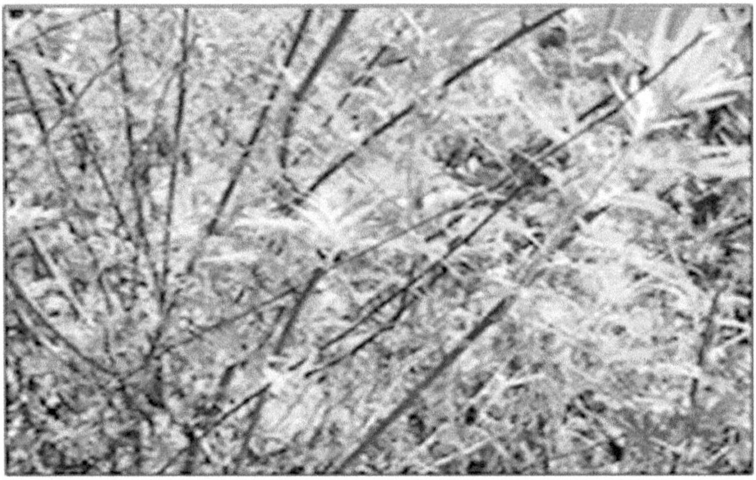

Figure 24.3. A local medicinal plant named Titepati. Source: Author.

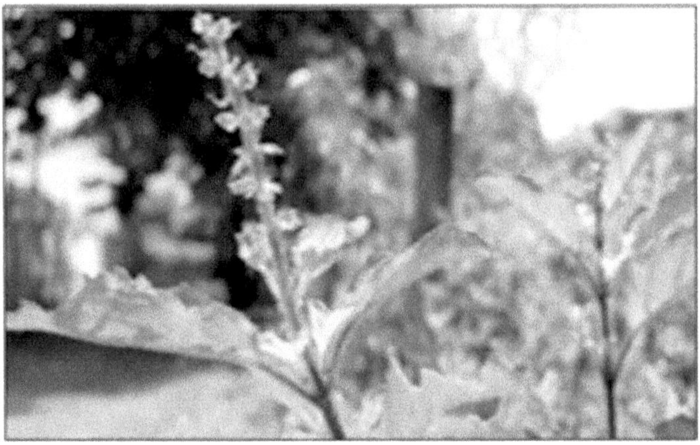

Figure 24.4. Mostly used medicinal plant locally called as Tulsi. Source: Author.

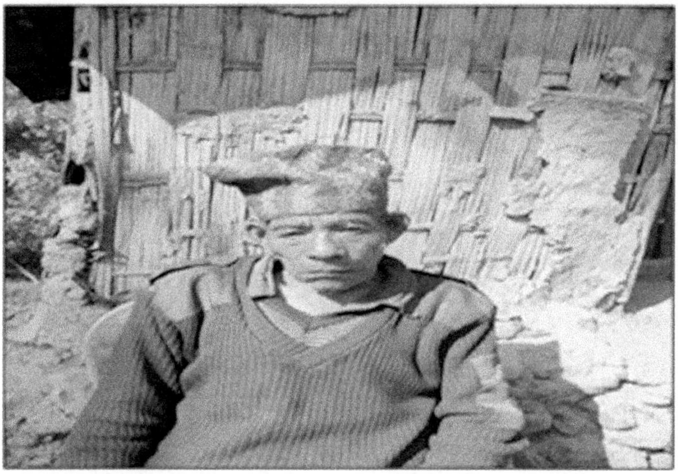

Figure 24.5. Phedangba, a Limbu priest, mostly relies on herbal medicines rather than modern alternatives. Source: Author.

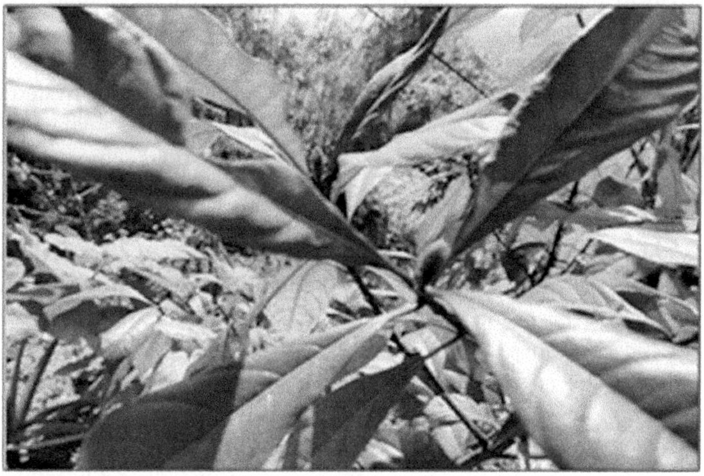

Figure 24.6. A local medicinal flower used by the Limbu community called Chuwa-Ko-Phool. Source: Author.

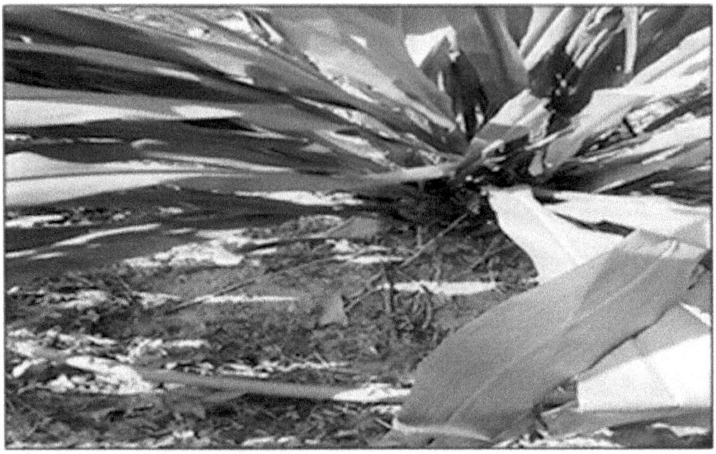

Figure 24.7. A well-known medicinal plant used by the Limbu community, locally called Makiba. Source: Author.

Conclusion

Limbu, a Tibeto-Burmese language, is spoken by the Limbu community residing in Nepal, Sikkim, Kashmir, and also in the Darjeeling and Kalimpong Districts of the Indian state of West Bengal. The majority of Limbus are bilingual and proficient in Nepali as well. Engaged in traditional subsistence farming, they cultivate principal crops such as squash, ginger, and black cardamom. Plants are vital among the Limbus of Lamagoan in Darjeeling Sadar subdivision for treating various ailments, showcasing their profound ethnobotanical knowledge. The Limbu community relies significantly on ethnomedicine, considering it a crucial system for primary healthcare. The Limbus possess a rich tapestry of indigenous knowledge and cultural treasures, including their distinct mother tongue folk culture encompassing literature, beliefs, customs, dance, music, art, artifacts, tools, games, cuisine, clothing, and dwellings. This cultural richness extends to various festivals and rituals.

Amid the lockdown, reliance on home remedies and traditional medicines from the local surroundings became prevalent. In instances of mild fever (although no recorded Covid cases), they turned to plants like *Titepati* (Mugwort) and *Tulsi* (Holy basil), boiling and consuming them. Government guidelines were diligently followed during marriage or death rituals, encompassing social distancing, facemasks, and hand sanitizers. Owing to Covid restrictions, attendance at such events was limited to a select few. Fever and cold were colloquially referred to as *Kumrek/Haija*, with remedies for cough involving plants like *Banmara* (Crofton weed), *Swertia Chirayita*, *Tulsi*, and Ginger. A prevailing fear of harm associated with hospitals persisted, reflecting the widespread panic surrounding Covid. The community refrained from using locally available fauna for medicine, recognizing societal shifts toward reduced animal sacrifice and violence, influenced by the adoption of Hinduism and Buddhism. Phedangba, an octogenarian, faced communication challenges due to impaired hearing and speech. His recollections highlighted training under a *Ban-jhakri* (a shamanic deity associated with the wilderness) and his previous engagements in *Mundhums*, traditional practices, religious festivals, and rituals. However, contemporary times witness a decline in such rituals. He predominantly relied on herbal medicines over modern alternatives, emphasizing the belief that worshiping deities contributes to holistic well-being. Throughout the Covid-19 pandemic, he stayed indoors and leaned on traditional medicines for support.

Thus the indigenous knowledge system of Lamagoan in Darjeeling Sadar subdivision is an invaluable heritage passed down through generations and is pivotal in shaping their identity. In the past, they served as the sole healthcare providers in the villages, initiating treatments through the traditional process. However, the shift toward allopathic treatment gained momentum as hospitals, specifically Primary Health Care Centers (PHSCs), were established, changing people's beliefs and preferences. This tradition is at risk of fading due to neglect from the newer generations and the overshadowing influence of modernity and globalization. To ensure sustainable development and the proper utilization of Limbu indigenous knowledge, it is imperative for the Limbu community to understand its significance. Additionally, the state and other stakeholders should contribute to preserving and enhancing Limbu's native skills and knowledge. Homeopathy, a traditional treatment system, is extensively utilized in these areas. In short, during the lockdown, the Limbu people of Lamagoan in Darjeeling Sadar subdivision relied on local remedies and traditional medicines for mild fever, using plants like *Titepati* and *Tulsi*. Government guidelines were followed for rituals, including social distancing and masks. Fever and cold were casually called *Kumrek/Haija*. Also, herbal remedies like *Banmara*, *Swertia Chirayita*, *Tulsi*, and ginger were used for cough. These herbal practices could prove beneficial during future pandemics and also complement modern medicine.

References

Bhasin M. K., and V. Bhasin. *Sikkim Himalayas Ecology and Resource Development.* New Delhi: Kamla Raj Enterprise, 1995.

Chatterjee, R. "Indigenous Knowledge and Practices among the Limbus of Sikkim Himalayas." *Genus Homo* 1 (2017): 57–64.

Debnath, D. "The Limbus of North Bengal: An Anthropological Study in Two Districts of West Bengal." *Man, Environment and Society* 1, no. 2 (2020): 127–152.

Ellen, R., P. Parkes, and A. Bicker. *Indigenous Enviromental Knowledge and its Transformations: Critical Anthropological Perspectives.* London: Routledge Taylor & Francis Group, 2000.

Limbu, R. K. "Exploring Indigenous Knowledge System and Limbu Cultural Identity in Nepal." *Journal of the University of Human Development* 2 (2013): 22–137.

Limbu, R. K. "Performance in Limbu Mundhum: A Study of Cultural Representation." M. Phil diss., Central Department of English Kirtipur, Kathmandu, 2010.

Pradhan, K. *The Gorkha Conquests: The Process and Consequences of the Unification of Nepal, with Particular Reference to Eastern Nepal.* Kathmandu: Himali Books, 2009.

Risley, H. H. *Gazetteer of Sikkim.* Calcutta: Bengal Secretariat Press, 1894.

Singh, U. P. *Tribal Health in North East India: A Study of Socio-Cultural Dimension of Health Care Practices.* New Delhi: Serials Publications, 2008.

Singh, S. K. 1993. *People of India-Sikkim.* Calcutta: Anthropological Survey of India, 1993.

Sonowal, C. J., and P. Praharaj. "Traditional vs. Transition: Acceptance of Health Care Systems among the Santhals of Orissa." *Study on Ethno-Medicine* 1, no. 2 (2007): 135–46.

Stevenson, M. G. "Indigenous Knowledge in Environmental Assessment." *Arctic* 49, no. 3 (1996): 278–91.

Sundas, B. "Language and Traditional Healing Practice: A Study of Limbu Community." In *Ethnomedicine and Tribal Healing Practices in India: Challenges and Possibilities of Recognition and Integration*, edited by S. Reddy, N. Guite, and B. Subedi. Singapore: Springer, 2023.

Thapa, N. "Phedangma among Limboos of Sikkim: Change and Continuity." Unpublished M.Phil diss., Department of Anthropology, Sikkim University, 2017.

Tylor, E. B. *Primitive Culture.* New York: J. Murray, 1871.

World Health Organization (WHO). *Coronavirus Disease (COVID-19) Situation Report-178*, 2020.

Index

Accredited Social Health Activists (ASHA) 361
Acharya
  Charaka 242
  Sushruta 242
adaptogenic qualities 253
afforestation 97
African medicine 43
  African traditional medicine (TAM) 321
agriculture 16
  agroforestry 97
  labour 349
ailments 86
  stomach problems 86
alkaloid 433
  Camptothecin 433
Allicin 188
  ajoene 188
  diallyl polysulfides 188
allopathic medicine 215, 329, 362
alternative healthcare 464
anaerobic conditions 102
analgesic 35, 112–13
ancient
  civilization 85
  doctors 418
  healers 418
  heritage 101
  literature 24
  sages 418
  scientists 418
Andaman
  archipelago 14, 333
  Great 333
  Great Andamanese 367
  Little 333
Andaman Adim Janjati Vikas Samiti (AAJVS) 376
Andaman and Nicobar Administration 376
Andaman and Nicobar Tribal Research Institute (ANTRI) 342
angiogenesis 433
angiosperm 102
animism 393
antagonism 231
Anthraquinone compounds 110
anthropogenic 97, 102
Anthropological pressure 97
  anthroposophic medicine 43
Anthropological Survey of India 334
anthropology 1
  anthropologist 6
  cultural 11
  medical 11
antibacterial 34, 91
  antibiotics 5, 189
  anticancer 34, 90–1, 94
antifungal 91, 189
  antioxidant activity 89, 91
  antiseptic 79
anti-inflammatory 33, 90–1, 94, 112
  antimicrobial 4, 91, 97, 113, 183, 248
antinociceptive 112
antitumor agent 33
  antihepatotoxic 35
  antihypertensive 33
antiviral 91
aphrodisiac 250
apoptosis 113
aquatic 127
  semiaquatic 117
arboriculture 16
archipelagos 16
aromatherapy 329
  alternative therapy 330
Arthritis 81
  rheumatism 81
  sprains 81

aromatic
  plant/s 25, 352
  organic compound 94
Ashwagandha 417
Assam 345
  Pragjyotish or *Kamrupa* 345
Astringent, laxative and bronchodilator 129
Awareness programs 97
Ayurveda 1, 192, 415
  doshas 192
  rasayana 192
  tridoshas 324
Ayurvedic medicine 404, 416
AYUSH 9, 69, 399
Azadirachtin 196
  nimbin 196

Bacterial pathogens 251
Bangladesh 101
Bay of Bengal 85, 89, 101
bergamotene 17, 454
bicyclic sesquiterpenes 456
bio
  diversity 11, 85
  energy 5
  fuel 137
bioactive
  chemicals 111
  components 97, 102
  compound 4, 90–1, 94, 109
  elements 91
biochemical constituents 112
bioclimatic zone 101
biocultural conservation 23, 42
Biological Diversity Act 69
bioprospecting 150
biosocial correlates 347
biosynthetic pathways 151
block
  Keshpur 128
  Salboni 128
blood glucose levels 254
botanical garden 361
Botanical Survey of India (BSI) 213
Broad spectrum 55, 251
Buyi community 46

cancer 141
  cell lines 95
carbon sinks 102
carboxylic group 91
cardiovascular diseases (CVDs) 431
carminative 137
carrageenan 302
chemical
  compounds 90, 104
  constituents 111
  diversity 440
Chinese medicine 5
Christianity 393
civilization 14, 39
climate change 97
clinical
  advice 229
  application 229
coastal
  lands 90
  region 101
commercial purposes 128
communities
  Aadi Nippani 58
complementary and alternative medicine (CAM) 438
conservation
  efforts 257
  measures 103
  nature 26
  strategies 97
contemporary
  consumers 86
  society 152
contraception 397
cosmetic applications 77
cottage industries 97
COVID-19, 17, 255, 429, 481
  lockdown 482, 485;
  pandemic 255, 429
  SARS-CoV-2, 429, 481
crop cultivation 90
cryptogams 150
  phanerogams 150
cultural
  belief 5, 13

development 17
ethnocide 375
heritage 1
interpretation 467
revitalization 342
curcumin 191
turmerones 191
cyanobacterial taxa 102
cyclonic storms 102
cytotoxic
activity 113
property 113

daily labor 464
Darjeeling 491
Darwinian fitness 481
defense and adaptation 171
deforestation 27
deltaic confluence 85
Dhanvantari 242
diabetes 141
diagnosis 382, 384
Malam 384
Naa 384
Naadi 384
Neer 384
Niram 384
digitization 48
Dipyranocoumarins 111
diuretic properties 96
divination 77
documentation 32, 43
dosha 8
drug
discovery 2, 91, 214
efficacy 97
new 26
dyeing processes 77

early humans 423
eco-friendly approaches 97
ecological
benefits 102
integrity 442
knowledge 67
legacy 32
niche 372
process 85
progress 39
economic
advantages 102
benefits 102
importance 144
regression 215
ecosystem 97, 102
ecosystem management 85
ecotourism 39, 97, 102
education 17, 86, 97
elephantiasis 137
elicitor 171
endogenous hormones 426
neurotransmitters 426
signaling molecules 426
environment 7
constraint 13
degradation 53
environmental
importance 102
management 7
stewardship 64
well-being 103
epigallocatechin gallate (EGCG) 428
essential oil 185
ethnic community 1, 8
ethnobiology 11
ethnobotanical
knowledge 39
use 103
wealth 97
ethnobotany 1
ethnobotanist 6
ethnomedical practices 464
Ethnomedicinal
plants 397
practices 468
properties 103
Ethnomedicine 1–7, 10–13, 18, 29, 40, 43, 149, 463
ethnopharmacology 26
ethno-veterinary usage 269
eugenol 186
caryophyllene 186
linalool 186
rosmarinic acid 186

extraction techniques 226
  pressurized liquid extraction 227
  soxhlet extraction 227
  supercritical fluid extraction 227

fever 86
  asthma 86
  bronchitis 86
  colds 86
  malaria 86
field observation 77
financial importance 102
fish processing 97
  fishing industries 103
flora 101, 117
  fauna 101
folk knowledge 8
  folklore 130, 241, 391
  folktales 40
folklore medicine 102–3
food security 39
forest
  ecosystem 39
  products 103
Fourier Transform Infrared (FTIR) 91
free radicals 138, 142

Gas Chromatography-Mass Spectrometry (GC-MC) 160, 455, 457
gene pool 371
Geographical locales 345
Georgian folk medicine 43
German physician 323
Gestation 351
gingerol 193
  shogaol 193
  zingerone 194
global
  demand 257
  issues 97
  medical cabinet 97
globalization 27, 262, 399
glycoproteins 436
gold standard 229
Gorkhaland Territorial Administration 483
Government 97
Green planet 23
  greener society 32

Habitat destruction 97
Healing rituals 463
Health
  benefits 95
  concerns 95
  issues 86, 131, 252, 383, 404
  treatment 41
Healthcare practices 85–6
Hepatoprotective activity 114, 304
herbal
  medicine 220, 441
  ointments 40
  supplements 86
herbs and plants 416
High-density Lipoprotein (HDL) 255
  Low-density Lipoprotein 255
High-Performance Liquid Chromatography (HPLC) 455
High Pressure Liquid Chromatography (HPLC) 160
high tide 373
high-throughput screening (HTS) 439
Hinduism
  Buddhism 486, 491
HIV 248, 428
  gene expression 248
  treatments 248
holistic
  approach 72, 220
  healing 416
  knowledge 13
Holocene era 346
homeopathy 321
  naturopathy 321
household healthcare 57
HPLC method 303
human
  cytomegalovirus 301
  health 39, 97
  knowledge 401
hydrophytes 130
  macrophytes 130
hydroxyl groups 91

hydroxylation 171
  oxidation 171
hygiene 393
hypertension 142, 485

illnesses 463
immune-modulating properties 90
Indian *materia medica* 150
Indian
  populations 418
  subcontinent 415
indigenous
  healing 337–8
  knowledge 85, 478, 491
  medicine 3
  people 7
Indus Valley Civilization 401–3, 405
  Harapan civilization 401
  Harappa and Mohenjodaro 405
  people 405
Infectious diseases 86
Inflammation 81, 112, 141, 302
In-situ and ex-situ methods 259
intellectual property right 12
interrelationship 23
intrinsic knowledge 26
Islamic medicine 43
Island communities 86
International Union for Conservation of Nature (IUCN) 27

jaundice
  black 471
  yellow 471
Joint Forest Management (JFM) 70

Kabiraj 472–3
  ojha 472
kaempferol and quercetin 427

lactucarium 269
Lamagaon's population 483
language
  Austro-Asiatic 391
  Mon-Khmer 391
  Munda 391
  Nicobarese 391
laxative 453
lifestyle 39
  livelihood 10, 67
Limbus of North Bengal 482
  Limbus (Subba) 483
livestock 131
local
  community 9, 97, 103
  healer (Rukmini Amma) 63
  inhabitants 39
  people 97
  remedies 491

macro and micro molecules 110
magico-religious traditions 483
Maharshi Patanjali 323
malaria 398
malnutrition 44
mangrove
  Dhundal 89
  ecosystem 89, 97, 101–2
  family 94
  forest 12, 85
  forest resources 97
  Garan 89
  Garjan 89
  genera 91, 103
  Genwa 89
  Golpata 89
  Kankra 89
  Keora 89
  Mat-goran 89
  plants 86, 89, 102
  region 103
  saplings 97
  species 89
  Sundari 89
  trees 89
marine life 102
marriage rituals 337
maternal health 349
medical
  botany 403
  practices 85
  systems 415
medicinal
  applications 86

benefits 86, 96
implications 91
knowledge 394, 418
mangroves 103
plants 4, 85, 97, 102–3, 395
properties 103
uses 102
melanoma cells 114
membrane stability 89
menstruation 81
menstrual problems 397
mental health 463
mesohaline zones 89
polyhaline zones 89
Mesopotamian civilization 323
metabolic pool 177
metastasis 433
methanolic extracts 114, 305
methyl jasmonate (MJ) 174
micronutrients 301
minerals 301
vitamins 301
microorganisms 90
minimum inhibitory concentration (MIC) 231
modern healthcare 3, 58
modernization 27, 254, 399
molecular markets 268
Mongoloid Population 347
morbidity 44
morphological data 268
mortality 44
Muslim communities 385
mutagenicity 460
genotoxicity 460
mythological and historical events 101

nanoparticles 143
National Biodiversity Authority (NBA) 68
natural
elicitors 270
remedy 5
resources 86, 101, 213
stress factors 102
nature
drought 172
radiation 172
salinity 172
temperature 172
Nicobar 14
Nicobarese people 16, 389
North East India 347
Nutraceutical 127, 144
nutritional quality 268

occupation 17
oral knowledge 253
oriental medicine 434
ornamental 144
osteoporosis 115
overexploitation 25, 55
oxidative
damage 302
stress 142

parasites/epiphytes/mistletoes 102
Particularly Vulnerable Tribal Groups (PVTGs) 366, 391
pathogens 230
pathogenic organisms 168
patriarchal society 349
pharmaceutical
compounds 97
industry 27, 40, 86
pharmacodynamic 232
synergy 435
pharmacokinetic
profiles 232
synergy 435
pharmacological
activities 103
use 13
pharmacopoeia 261
phenolic compounds 91, 94, 173
polyphenolic 104
phenylpropanoid pathways 170
shikimic acid pathways 170, 175
photosynthesis 143
phytochemical
compounds 64
constituents 103, 110–11
content 102
screenings 103, 111
studies 4

phytoremediation 130
policy suggestion 68
plant-based remedies 86, 382
  products 405
plant metabolism 230
  Giloy 61
  kalmegh 63
  Sarpagandha 79
  Triphala 63
  turmeric 57
plant/s
  ecology 64
  Neem 56, 61
  pharmacophore 97
  Tulsi, Aswagandha, Indian Catmint 79
pollution levels 97
polyherbal formulations 423
practitioner 6
  prehistoric time 16, 23, 401
preservation strategies 97
Primary Health Care Centres (PHSCs)
primary substances 305
proanthocyanidins 109

qualitative 18
quality council 9

Rabha families of Garo Basti 464, 470
radioprotective qualities 254
Ramayana 389, 403, 412
  Mahabharata 403, 412
Rasayana 255
rationalization 42
rejuvenation 192
relationship
  humans and plants 401
religious rituals 413
research and development 187
respiratory diseases 157
rhizomatous plant 190
Rigveda 16, 247, 323, 401, 412
  Atharvaveda 260, 323, 401–2
  Samveda 323
  Yajurveda 323
ringworm 83
Rio Earth Summit 39
Rishis (Sages) 404
ritual 8, 17
River systems 85
  Brahmaputra 85, 89, 101
  Ganga 85, 89, 101, 129
  Kangsabati 129
  Meghna 85, 89, 101
  Shilabati 129
  Subarnarekha 129
rotational harvesting 59

Salinity stress 270
Salt-tolerant plants 89
Sanskrit
  authors 412
  literature 412
science of life 320, 381
scientific
  field 241
  research 86, 97
sea level rise 102
seawards 101
secondary metabolites 26, 86, 110, 151, 153, 425
  alkaloids 86, 153
  flavonoids 86, 113, 153
  glycosides 86, 153
  phenols 153
  saponins 86, 153
  steroids 86, 153
  tannins 86, 153
  terpenoids 153
  triterpenes 86
sedative 35
Self-help groups (SHGs) 477
Siddha 3, 404
skin
  condition 86
  disorders 86
  infection 79
  issues 86
  irritation 168
skin care solutions 260
social behavior 5, 6
  socioeconomic status 11
sociocultural practice 16
socio-biological practices 361
socio-economic conditions 103
socio-environmental 11

socio-religious practices 336
socio-techno-economic background 342
societal benefit 167
soluble proteins 270
  carbohydrates 270
  carotenoids 270
  glutathione 271
sonneratiosides 110
spiritual
  aspects 415
  identity 242
strong zone of inhibition (ZOI) 249
suburban populations 469
Sundarban 12, 85–6, 89, 97, 101, 103, 109, 111, 117
surgical procedures 382
  lithotomy 382
  rhinoplasty 382
Sushruta Samhita 252, 403
  Arthasastra and Brihat Samhita 403
  Charaka Samhita 252, 403
  Krishi Parasara 403
  Medinikosa and Amarakosa 403
  Vibhagavidya 416
suspension cultures 174
sustainable
  development 2, 7, 478
  harvesting 97
  nature 345
  utilization 86
sustainable development goals (SDGs) 55
synthetic drugs 183, 424, 439
synergistic effects 423

Tai-speaking groups 347
  Tai people 348
tannin production 102
therapeutic
  agents 90
  benefits 439
  effects 437
  interventions 97
  potentials 91, 94, 96
  properties 90
  purposes 86, 89
Tibetan medicine 47
toxicity 381
  toxicological research 442
traditional
  culture 39
  healer 8, 45, 415
  knowledge 7, 86, 97, 346, 390
  lifestyle 367
  medicine 1, 86, 149, 394
  remedies 405
Traditional Chinese Medicine 47
Traditional Knowledge Digital Library (TKDL) 71
tranquilizer 269
trauma 463
tree care 402
  arboreal medicine 402
tribal
  communities 103
  health 45
  populace 366
  studies 11
tribe
  Bhil 67
  Bhilalas 67
  Gond 66
tuberculosis 398
tyrosinase activity 116

Unani 1, 404
underprivileged sections 150
UNESCO 13, 89
United Nations (UN) 27
United Nations Children's Fund (UNICEF) 43
urbanization 24
UV treatments 270

Vedas 412
  Upanisads 412
Vedic
  age 411
  Indians 402, 411
  literatures 404
  medicine 261
  period 411
  post-Vedic 413
  texts 414

virus
  hepatitis C 428
  herpes simplex 428
  influenza 428
  respiratory syncytial 428
Vrikshayurveda 402–4
  Salihotra 403
vulnerable zones 97

water
  pollution 138
  purification 138
  quality 137
waterborne infection 44
wellness products 86
Western
  medicine 10
  oral medicine 471
wetland 132
World Health Organization (WHO) 8, 381
WWF 27

Yunani medicine 385

About the Editors

Arun Makal is presently working as an assistant professor of anthropology at Bangabasi Evening College, affiliated with the University of Calcutta, West Bengal, India. He received his MSc and PhD from the Department of Anthropology, University of Calcutta, with a specialization in social-cultural anthropology. His PhD research covers knowledge, experience, and practices of agricultural communities of different regions of the Indian state of West Bengal. He has participated in and presented papers in many national and international seminars and workshops. He has published one international edited book volume, one national edited book volume, four national level textbooks, six book chapters, and sixteen research articles in peer-reviewed indexed journals. His current research interests focus on Indian civilization, Indian knowledge systems, farmer's knowledge, ethnomedicinal knowledge, food security, sustainable development and environment as well as culture and health of various Indian communities. Email: arunmakal6@gmail.com

Gour Gopal Satpati is an assistant professor of botany, Bangabasi Evening College, affiliated with the University of Calcutta, West Bengal, India. He is also associated as guest faculty with the PG department of Botany, University of Calcutta, since 2022. Dr. Satpati received his MSc and PhD from the Department of Botany, University of Calcutta. He has participated in and presented papers in many national and international seminars and workshops. He is a fellow of the Scholars Academic and Scientific Society (FSASS) and the World Researchers Association (FWRA). He is the recipient of "The Endowment of Foreign Travel Scholarship" from the University of Calcutta for presenting a paper in Adelaide, South Australia. He has been awarded the "Thomas Edison Award in Biochemistry" as a young researcher. He is a renowned editor and reviewer of highly reputed journals belonging to Nature Group, PeerJ, and Elsevier. He has been awarded three best paper awards at national and international conferences. He has published fifty-one research papers in peer-reviewed indexed journals and seven book chapters. His research areas of interest are algal taxonomy, ecology, biofuel production, and waste management. In addition, he is interested in ethnobotany, traditional knowledge, and sustainable Development. Email: gour _satpati@yahoo.co.in

About the Contributors

Krishnendu Acharya is a professor of the Department of Botany, University of Calcutta, Kolkata, India. His research interests are in macrofungal diversity and medicinal prospects, innate immunity in plants, and myco-nanotechnology. He has 333 research publications, 4 books, and 2 patents to his credit. Thirteen PhD scholars have been awarded PhD degrees under his supervision. Now he has eight PhD scholars, of which two have submitted their PhD theses and six are registered. Email: krish_paper@yahoo.com

Tanzila Alvi has done her master's in microbiology from Sister Nivedita University, Kolkata, West Bengal, India. She specializes in microbiology, medical technology, and bioactive compounds of medicinal plants. She has a number of journal articles to her credit. Email: tanzilaalvi8@gmail.com

Sreemanti Banerjee is a faculty member in the Department of Botany, Diamond Harbour Women's University, West Bengal, India. Before this, she had served as a guest faculty member in the Department of Botany at Vivekananda College (Thakurpukur), Lady Brabourne College, Serampore College, and Scottish Church College. Dr. Banerjee did her MSc and PhD from the Department of Botany, University of Calcutta. She has more than five years of teaching experience. She has also participated in several national and international conferences within and outside the country. She has published one book chapter, one review, and eight research articles in peer-reviewed journals. Her research interest is related to the taxonomy of cyanobacteria and phyco-nanotechnology. Email: sreemantibanerjee@gmail.com

Somenath Bhattacharjee works as a professor in the Department of Anthropology at Nagaland University. He has done his PhD in the Department of Anthropology, University of North Bengal, West Bengal, India. His research interests include tribal ethnography, medical anthropology, and folk and material culture. A number of his research articles have been published in different reputable national and international journals and conference proceedings. He has authored four books from national and international publishers. Four PhD scholars and two MPhil scholars have been awarded under his supervision. Email: somenath@nagalanduniversity.ac.in

Dola Boral works as an associate professor in the Department of Botany, Murshidabad University (Erstwhile Krishnath College), Berhampore, Murshidabad, West Bengal, India. She has done her PhD in botany from the Department of Botany, Visva-Bharati

University. She specializes in aerobiology. She has a number of books and journal articles to her credit. Email: dbbot@msduniv.ac.in

Shruti Chattaraj is a state aided college teacher (SACT) of the Department of Botany, Ananda Mohan College, Kolkata, West Bengal, India. She did her MSc from the Department of Botany, University of Calcutta. She has done her PhD in botany from the Department of Life Science and Biotechnology, Jadavpur University, in collaboration with Bose Institute, Kolkata. Her research interests include cell biology and molecular genetics, fungal biotechnology, and mycology. She has published a number of research articles in journals of national and international repute. Email: shruti.chattaraj@gmail.com

Sabatini Chatterjee is a junior research fellow in the Andaman and Nicobar Regional Centre, Anthropological Survey of India (Ministry of Culture, Govt. of India), Port Blair, Andaman and Nicobar Islands. She has done MSc in anthropology from the Department of Anthropology, University of Calcutta. She is pursuing her PhD from the Department of Anthropology, University of Calcutta. Email: sabatinichatterjee11@gmail.com

Niten Chhetri is a junior research fellow in the Department of Anthropology, Nagaland University, Nagaland, India. He has done MSc in anthropology from the Department of Anthropology, Nagaland University. He specializes in social-cultural anthropology. He is pursuing his PhD from the Department of Anthropology, Nagaland University. Email: niten_rs2023@nagalanduniversity.ac.in

Debapriya Das is a senior research fellow and PhD scholar in the Post Graduate Department of Botany, Lady Brabourne College, Kolkata, West Bengal, India. She is marked by an impressive academic journey and completed her MSc and BSc with distinction and multiple awards. She specializes in the field of plant biology with a strong foundation in botany. She has a number of journal articles to her credit. Email: debapriyadas0209@gmail.com

Kankana De is a researcher at the Department of Anthropology, Vidyasagar University, West Bengal, India. She has done her MSc and PhD from the same Department of Anthropology, Vidyasagar University. Her major research areas are anthropometric measurements, nutritional status, adolescents, adults, body index, malnutrition, and ethnomedicine. She has a number of publications to her credit. Email: dekankana@gmail.com

Mitu De is an associate professor in the Department of Botany at Gurudas College, Kolkata, West Bengal, India. She specializes in the taxonomy of angiosperms. Her research interests include the documentation and characterization of rice landraces, ethnobotany and traditional knowledge, and autism. She was a junior research fellow at Bose Institute for three years before joining Gurudas College. Her PhD thesis title is

"Rice Landraces of West Bengal: Genetic Diversity and DNA Fingerprinting." She has a number of books and journal articles to her credit. Email: mitubotany@gmail.com

Santi Ranjan Dey is an assistant professor, Department of Zoology, Rammohan College, Kolkata, West Bengal, India. Recently he has been working on numerical taxonomy of Neuroptera (Insecta) and Fish. His research interests include molecular biology, ecology, and systematics (taxonomy). He has a number of books and journal articles to his credit. Email: santiranjandey@rammohancollege.ac.in

Shinjini Dey is a researcher at the Postgraduate Department of Botany, Scottish Church College, Kolkata, West Bengal, India. She has done an MSc in botany from the Department of Botany, Scottish Church College, Kolkata, West Bengal, India. Email: deyshinjini26@gmail.com

Atreyi Ghosh is an assistant professor of the Department of Microbiology and Biotechnology, Sister Nivedita University, Kolkata, West Bengal, India. She did her MSc in molecular biology and biotechnology from Kalyani University, Kalyani, West Bengal, India, and PhD in environmental biotechnology from IIT Guwahati, India. She has a number of publications in international journals and has presented papers at several international and national conferences. Email: atreyi.g@suuniv.ac.in

Mimosa Ghosh is an independent researcher in plant taxonomy. She has done her MSc from the Department of Botany, Vidyasagar University. Her major research areas are indigenous knowledge and medicinal plants. She is a regular basis writer for Bengali newspapers. She has a number of publications to her credit. Email: ghoshmimosa@gmail.com

Piyasa Ghosh is a researcher at the Department of Botany, Scottish Church College, Kolkata, West Bengal, India. She has done her MSc from the same Department of Botany, Scottish Church College, Kolkata. She has done her BSc from the Department of Botany of Vidyasagar College for Women, Kolkata, West Bengal, India. She has a number of publications to her credit. Email: ghoshpiyasa092@gmail.com

Srijita Ghosh is a state aided college teacher (SACT) of the Department of Botany of Scottish Church College, Kolkata, West Bengal, India. She has done her MSc and PhD from the Department of Botany, University of Calcutta. Her major research areas include plant physiology and plant biochemistry. She has a number of books and journal articles to her credit. Email: srijita.ghosh@scottishchurch.ac.in

Yikham Gogoi works as an assistant anthropologist in the Andaman and Nicobar Regional Centre, Anthropological Survey of India (Ministry of Culture, Govt. of India), Port Blair, Andaman and Nicobar Islands, India. She has done MSc in anthropology from the Department of Anthropology, Gauhati University, with a specialization in biological anthropology. She did her PhD from the Department of Anthropology,

Dibrugarh University. She has a number of books and journal articles to her credit. Email: yikhamansi@gmail.com

Nabanita Goswamy is a state aided college teacher in the Department of Anthropology, New Alipore College, Kolkata, West Bengal. She has done MSc in anthropology from the Department of Anthropology, University of Calcutta. She specializes in social-cultural anthropology. Currently, she is pursuing her PhD from the Department of Anthropology, Nagaland University, Nagaland, India. Email: nabanita_rs2023@nagalanduniversity.ac.in

Sunanda Halder is a researcher at the Department of Botany, Bethune College, University of Calcutta, Kolkata, West Bengal, India. She has done her MSc from the same Department of Botany, Bethune College, University of Calcutta, Kolkata. She has done her BSc from the Department of Botany, Scottish Church College, Kolkata, West Bengal, India. Her research interests include plants and microbiomes as well as phytochemical and pharmaceutical properties of medicinal plants. She has a number of publications to her credit. Email: halders0812@gmail.com

Jurol is a junior research student in Port Blair, Andaman and Nicobar Islands, India. Email: jurolzach@gmail.com

Anstice Justin is a former deputy director in Andaman and Nicobar Regional Centre, Anthropological Survey of India (Ministry of Culture, Govt. of India), Port Blair, Andaman and Nicobar Islands, India. He has a number of books and national and international journal articles to his credit. Email: ansticejustin@rediffmail.com

Raspinder Kaur is a research fellow at the Post Graduate Department of Botany, Dev Samaj College for Women, Ferozepur, Punjab, India. She has done her MSc from the same Department of Botany, Dev Samaj College for Women, Ferozepur, Punjab, India. She has a number of publications to her credit. Email: creater606@gmail.com

Barsha Majumder is a state aided college teacher (SACT) in the Department of Botany of Netaji Nagar College for Women, Kolkata, West Bengal, India. She has done her MSc and PhD in botany from the Department of Botany, University of Calcutta. Her research interests include arsenic toxicity on plants; heavy metal pollution; genotoxicology, molecular-physicochemical antioxidative defense network of plants, oxidative stress biomarkers, and genomic profiling. She has published a number of research articles in journals of national and international repute. Email: barshamjmdr@gmail.com

Pooja Mawal is a faculty member in the Department of Botany of Central University of Jammu, J & K, India. She has done her MSc and PhD in botany from the Department of Botany, Punjabi University, Patiala, Punjab, India. Her research interests include phytochemical and pharmacological analysis of plants. She has published a number of research articles in journals of national and international repute. Email: poojabc.786@gmail.com

Sutibra Narayan Mondal is a researcher at Department of Botany, Murshidabad University (Erstwhile Krishnath College), Murshidabad, West Bengal, India. He is the MSc gold medalist in botany from Murshidabad University, Murshidabad, West Bengal, India. His area of specialization is molecular genetics and genomics. He has published a number of papers and articles in different reputed national and international journals. Email: sutibrolifescience@gmail.com

Sandip More works as an assistant professor in the Department of Botany, Murshidabad University (Erstwhile Krishnath College), Murshidabad, West Bengal, India. He has done MSc in botany from the Department of Botany, University of Kalyani. He has done his PhD in botany from the Department of Botany, University of Calcutta. His research interests include forensic palynology, palaeobotany, palynology, and climate change. He has a number of national and international journal articles to his credit. Email: smbot@msduniv.ac.in

Abhishek Mukherjee is a researcher at the Department of School of Materials Science and Nanotechnology, Jadavpur University, Kolkata, West Bengal, India. Email: abhi.mukh@yahoo.com

Sudipta Mukherjee is a senior project scientist at West Bengal Biodiversity Board, Department of Environment, Government of West Bengal, Salt Lake City, Kolkata, West Bengal, India. He is doing research at Molecular and Applied Mycology and Plant Pathology Laboratory, Department of Botany, University of Calcutta, Kolkata, West Bengal, India. His research areas include agricultural economics, agricultural philosophy, and agricultural plant science. He has a number of national and international journal articles to his credit. Email: mr.mukherjee.88@gmail.com

Renia Mullick is a researcher at the Post Graduate Department of Botany, Lady Brabourne College, Kolkata, West Bengal, India. She has done her MSc from the same Post Graduate Department of Botany, Lady Brabourne College, Kolkata, West Bengal, India. Her research interests include plant biotechnology, molecular biology, plant tissue culture, and phytoplankton study. She has a number of journal articles to her credit. Email: reniarens@gmail.com

Camellia Nandi works as a state aided college teacher (SACT) in the Department of Botany, Scottish Church College, Kolkata, West Bengal, India. She has done her MSc and is pursuing her PhD in botany from the Department of Botany, University of Calcutta. Her research interests include phycology and algal biotechnology. She has a number of journal articles to her credit. Email: camellia.nandi@scottishchurch.ac.in

Aishwarya B Patil is a visiting faculty, MIT Art Design and Technology University, Pune, India. She is a dedicated anthropologist with a passion for academia, research, and knowledge dissemination. As a seasoned professional in the field, she brings a wealth of experience in content writing, evaluation, and teaching. She has done her MSc in anthropology from the Department of Anthropology of Savitribai Phule Pune University, Pune, India. She has published a number of research articles in journals of national and international repute. Email: pruthasmi@gmail.com

Satyaki Paul works as an assistant professor and functionary chair of Dr. Ambedkar Research Chair of Kalinga Institute of Social Sciences (KISS), Deemed to be University, Bhubaneswar, Odisha, India. He has done MSc in anthropology from the Department of Anthropology, University of Calcutta. He is pursuing his PhD from the Department of Anthropology, University of Calcutta. He specializes in social-cultural anthropology and has a number of journal articles to his credit. Email: satyakipaul54@gmail.com

Saroj Kumar Pradhan works as an assistant professor in the Department of Botany and Environmental Sciences at Sri Guru Granth Sahib World University (SGGSWU), Fatehgarh Sahib, Punjab, India. Previously, he was engaged as a research associate in the Department of Botany of the same University. Email: pradhan_sarojkumar@yahoo.com

Shreeya Purkait is a researcher at the Agricultural and Ecological Research Unit, Indian Statistical Institute, Giridih, Jharkhand, India. She is also engaged in research at the School of Materials Science and Nanotechnology, Jadavpur University, Kolkata, West Bengal, India. She has a number of publications to her credit. Email: shreeyapurkait98@gmail.com

Jyoti Rani is a researcher at the Department of Botany, Chaudhary Devi Lal University, Sirsa, Haryana, India. She has a number of publications to her credit. Email: jyotipanghal91286@gmail.com

Souhardya Ray is a researcher at the Department of Botany, Murshidabad University (Erstwhile Krishnath College), Berhampore, Murshidabad, West Bengal, India. Email: souhardyaraymsd@gmail.com

Debleena Roy is an assistant professor (WBES) in the Post Graduate Department of Botany, Lady Brabourne College, Kolkata, West Bengal, India. She has done her MSc from the University College of Science, Technology, and Agriculture, University of Calcutta. She has done her PhD in botany from the Department of Botany, University of Calcutta. She has been teaching for nearly thirteen years in different fields of botany such as plant tissue culture—biotechnology and paleobotany—palynology. Her research areas of interest are the study of plant function using both in vivo and in vitro approaches with a system level understanding of plant metabolism by application of biotechnology. She is deciphering the intricate metabolism of important crop and medicinal plants using transcriptome analysis, metabolic profiling, and tissue culture-based methods for producing sustainable species across climatic barriers. She has to her credit ten research papers published in international journals and two papers published in national refereed journals. She has three research projects under her supervision. She has also been felicitated by several awards throughout these years. Email: debleena.roy@ladybrabourne.com

Dipu Samanta is a faculty member in the Department of Botany of Dr. Kanailal Bhattacharyya College, Ramrajatala, Howrah, West Bengal, India. She has done her MSc and PhD in botany from the Department of Botany, University of Calcutta. She specializes in plant cell and tissue culture. She has a number of books and journal articles to her credit. Email: dipusamanta2010@gmail.com

Suparna Sardar is a researcher at the Department of Botany, Diamond Harbour Women's University, Sarisha, South 24 Parganas, West Bengal, India. She has done her MSc in botany from the Department of Botany, Diamond Harbour Women's University. She specializes in plant biology and has a number of publications to her credit. Email: sardarsuparna3210@gmail.com

Chirabrata Sarkar is a guest faculty member in the Department of Botany of the Post Graduate section of Serampore College under the University of Calcutta, West Bengal, India. He is also teaching in the Department of Botany as well as in the Department of Biochemistry of West Bengal State University. Dr. Sarkar did his MSc from the Department of Botany, West Bengal State University, and PhD from the Department of Botany, University of Calcutta. He has almost 1.5 years of teaching experience and has also participated in national and international conferences. He has published five research articles in peer-reviewed journals. His research interest is related to molecular genetics and plant biotechnology. Email: sarkarchirabrata@gmail.com

Jit Sarkar is a research fellow at the Department of Botany, University of Calcutta, Kolkata, West Bengal, India. He has done his MSc in botany from the Department of Botany, University of Calcutta, and M.Tech from IIT Kharagpur. He specializes in bioprocess engineering and has research interest in Green technology and environmental science. He has a number of books and national and international journal articles to his credit. Email: sarkar09jit@gmail.com

Sunipa Sen works as a state aided college teacher (SACT) in the Department of Botany, Bangabasi Evening College, University of Calcutta, Kolkata, India. She has done her MSc in botany from the Barasat Govt. College under West Bengal State University, West Bengal, India. Her research interests include molecular biology, plant genetics, and genomics. She has published a number of book chapters and research articles in journals of national and international repute. Email: mailsunipasen@gmail.com

Rohita Singla is a researcher at the Department of Botany, Eternal University, Baru Sahib, Himachal Pradesh, India. Email: singlarohita7@gmail.com

Suchita Sinha works as an associate professor in the Postgraduate Department of Botany, Lady Brabourne College, Suhrawardy Avenue, Kolkata, West Bengal, India. She has done her PhD in metal toxicity on mungbean plants from the Department of Botany, University of Calcutta. She has published a number of book chapters and research articles in journals of national and international repute. Email: suchita1sinha@gmail.com

Laiba Usmani is a researcher at the Department of Biotechnology, Sister Nivedita University, DG Block, Newtown, West Bengal, India. Email: laibausmani2003@gmail.com

www.ingramcontent.com/pod-product-compliance
Ingram Content Group UK Ltd.
Pitfield, Milton Keynes, MK11 3LW, UK
UKHW020222290926
15470UKWH00001B/336

9 781666 98207